Clinical Aspects of Brain Function Augmentation

Clinical Aspects of Brain Function Augmentation

Edited by Benjamin Green

STATES
ACADEMIC PRESS
www.statesacademicpress.com

States Academic Press,
109 South 5th Street,
Brooklyn, NY 11249, USA

Visit us on the World Wide Web at:
www.statesacademicpress.com

ISBN: 978-1-63989-109-2

Cataloging-in-Publication Data

Clinical aspects of brain function augmentation / edited by Benjamin Green.
p. cm.
Includes bibliographical references and index.
ISBN 978-1-63989-109-2
1. Nervous system--Diseases--Treatment. 2. Neuroergonomics. 3. Brain--Physiology.
4. Brain--Localization of functions. I. Green, Benjamin.

RC346 .C55 2022
616.8--dc23

Table of Contents

Preface

Every book is a source of knowledge and this one is no exception. The idea that led to the conceptualization of this book was the fact that the world is advancing rapidly; which makes it crucial to document the progress in every field. I am aware that a lot of data is already available, yet, there is a lot more to learn. Hence, I accepted the responsibility of editing this book and contributing my knowledge to the community.

The brain is an organ which consists of a mass of nerve tissue which is surrounded by the skull. Its major divisions are cerebrum, cerebellum and brain stem. The cerebrum is divided into two hemispheres, which are further divided into lobes. It is responsible for problem solving, coordinating motor skills, attention, interpreting sensory information, interpreting emotions, etc. The cerebellum helps in the management of fine motor skills as well as helping the body maintain its balance and posture. The functions of the brain can be broadly categorized into sensory information processing, maintaining breathing and blood pressure, and regulating the release of hormones. The book aims to shed light on some of the unexplored aspects of brain functions and the recent researches in this field. Its extensive content provides the readers with a thorough understanding of the subject. This book will prove to be immensely beneficial to students and researchers in this field.

While editing this book, I had multiple visions for it. Then I finally narrowed down to make every chapter a sole standing text explaining a particular topic, so that they can be used independently. However, the umbrella subject sinews them into a common theme. This makes the book a unique platform of knowledge.

I would like to give the major credit of this book to the experts from every corner of the world, who took the time to share their expertise with us. Also, I owe the completion of this book to the never-ending support of my family, who supported me throughout the project.

Editor

1

A practical application of text mining to literature on cognitive rehabilitation and enhancement through neurostimulation

Puiu F. Balan[1]*, Annelies Gerits[1] and Wim Vanduffel[1,2,3]

[1] Laboratory for Neuro-and Psychophysiology, Katholieke Universiteit Leuven Medical School, Leuven, Belgium
[2] Athinoula A. Martinos Center for Biomedical Imaging, Massachusetts General Hospital, Charlestown, MA, USA
[3] Department of Radiology, Harvard Medical School, Charlestown, MA, USA

Edited by:
Ioan Opris, Wake Forest University, USA

Reviewed by:
Estate M. Sokhadze, University of Louisville, USA
Mikhail Lebedev, Duke University, USA

***Correspondence:**
Puiu F. Balan, Laboratory for Neuro-and Psychophysiology, KU Leuven Medical School, Herestraat 49, Bus 1021, Leuven 3000, Belgium
e-mail: puiu.balan@med.kuleuven.be

The exponential growth in publications represents a major challenge for researchers. Many scientific domains, including neuroscience, are not yet fully engaged in exploiting large bodies of publications. In this paper, we promote the idea to partially automate the processing of scientific documents, specifically using text mining (TM), to efficiently review big corpora of publications. The "cognitive advantage" given by TM is mainly related to the automatic extraction of relevant trends from corpora of literature, otherwise impossible to analyze in short periods of time. Specifically, the benefits of TM are increased speed, quality and reproducibility of text processing, boosted by rapid updates of the results. First, we selected a set of TM-tools that allow user-friendly approaches of the scientific literature, and which could serve as a guide for researchers willing to incorporate TM in their work. Second, we used these TM-tools to obtain basic insights into the relevant literature on cognitive rehabilitation (CR) and cognitive enhancement (CE) using transcranial magnetic stimulation (TMS). TM readily extracted the diversity of TMS applications in CR and CE from vast corpora of publications, automatically retrieving trends already described in published reviews. TMS emerged as one of the important non-invasive tools that can both improve cognitive and motor functions in numerous neurological diseases and induce modulations/enhancements of many fundamental brain functions. TM also revealed trends in big corpora of publications by extracting occurrence frequency and relationships of particular subtopics. Moreover, we showed that CR and CE share research topics, both aiming to increase the brain's capacity to process information, thus supporting their integration in a larger perspective. Methodologically, despite limitations of a simple user-friendly approach, TM served well the reviewing process.

Keywords: text mining, transcranial magnetic stimulation, cognitive, rehabilitation, enhancement

INTRODUCTION

Gathering accurate and reliable information from web repositories became increasingly complex because of the exponential growth in the number of publications. For example, a PubMed search retrieved 9407 papers including 1172 reviews for TMS in "All Fields," and the ratio became 8186/988 when the filter "[Title/Abstract]" was applied. Reading without some selection criteria becomes challenging. Even when selectively focusing on specific topics in a review, this increases the chances to miss trends shown only by huge bodies of literature. Thus, when processing vast corpora of publications, we are facing challenges that require automated solutions. One of the most promising approaches to alleviate these problems is to assist the human operator with computers running artificial intelligence applications. Here, we selected one of these applications, text mining (TM), and showed that TM will enable us to efficiently deal with huge amounts of information from the TMS-related literature.

Our approach was also motivated by the fact that, neuroscience has to make efforts to integrate data mining and TM when dealing with huge and diverse experimental datasets (Akil et al., 2011) and text documents. TM is able to catch the complexity of all relevant studies in an efficient manner. Statistical and natural language processing (NLP) procedures to "mine" the literature have been developed to address big data general problems (Dias et al., 2011). Here, we used a practical approach to promote TM as a tool for the reviewing process. Specifically, we selected a set of TM-tools that allowed user-friendly approaches to reveal relevant outcomes in large corpora of publications. Our intention was to use TM-tools that are not too demanding on programming skills, required knowledge and training period. Therefore, the example set of TM-tools could serve as an attractive guide map for researchers willing to incorporate TM in their work.

Next, we demonstrate the use of TM-tools in gaining basic insights into the relevant literature on cognitive rehabilitation

(CR) and cognitive enhancement (CE) using transcranial magnetic stimulation (TMS). TMS is a valuable non-invasive perturbation method used to address fundamental and clinical neuroscience questions, both in human and animal models. Cognitive rehabilitation (CR-TMS) and cognitive enhancement (CE-TMS) are two important TMS applications. Indeed, TMS is establishing itself as major tool used in rehabilitation improving a wide variety of impaired mental functions (Miniussi and Rossini, 2011; Kammer and Spitzer, 2012; Vicario and Nitsche, 2013). Moreover, recent studies reported TMS-induced enhancements of normal brain functions (Brem et al., 2014; Luber and Lisanby, 2014).

The TM application to CR- and CE-TMS literature was focused on two main aspects. First, we aimed to show that TM could reveal the diversity of TMS applications in CR and CE, automatically retrieving trends already described in published reviews. Second, we specifically aimed to find trends only noticeable in big corpora of publications. The main feature of our findings is given by the statistical power of such analyses. Detailed analyses of the CR- and CE-TMS literature revealed relevant terms in the form of lists, topics and classes of terms associated with specific subtopics. It also showed relations between the relevant terms in the form of co-occurrences maps, groups of relevant terms with high probability co-occurrences and lists of relevant relational verbs. Moreover, the TM approach revealed conclusive sentences that appeared with a high probability. Finally, a large-scale corpora perspective showed that CR-TMS and CE-TMS share research topics allowing us to make inferences about their similarities. Although they start from specific states of the brain (impaired for CR and normal for CE), both aim to increase the brain's capacity to process information and to optimize adaptation. This unitary perspective is supported by fields that use TMS in diagnostic (TMS-DIAG) or in clinical and fundamental research (TMS-RES), which show that TMS is effective for changing and studying normal and abnormal brain processes. Accordingly, CR-TMS and CE-TMS also share research topics with these fields, showing their appurtenance to a larger context, which integrates diagnostic, fundamental research and fMRI studies.

TEXT MINING AS A METHOD TO PARTIALLY AUTOMATE THE REVIEWING OF BIG CORPORA OF PUBLICATIONS

Scholarly journals and data sources are increasingly available in electronic and Open Access form. Nonetheless, availability is not enough to extract specific information, mainly due to the abundance of information. TM comes with solutions for this problem offering automated methods to extract condensed information hidden within huge volumes of publications. TM can be achieved using several complementary approaches (Cohen and Hunter, 2008). Co-occurrence-based methods look for concepts that occur in the same unit of text (sentence/abstract) and posit a relationship between them. The statistical or machine learning systems rely on statistic properties of the text and work by building classifiers that operate on any level, from labeling part of speech to classifying full sentences or documents. The rule-based systems use knowledge about how language is structured and about how domain relevant things, facts and their relationships are stated in publications. The main areas/stages of TM are (Lourenco et al., 2009): Information Analysis that includes Information Retrieval and Information Extraction (e.g., Name Entity Recognition, Relationship Extraction, document classification and summarization); Information Synthesis that uses the databases generated by Information Extraction for answering simple questions, discovering new information and generating hypotheses.

A wide variety of publications and software tools approach TM at different levels of complexity, hampering the selection of relevant TM-tools. We chose a specific set of TM-tools, aiming to evaluate how they can help the TM-non-specialist accelerate the review of big corpora of literature, using the following criteria:

a. Allow a user-friendly approach by selecting TM-tools requiring medium investments in training, programming and specific knowledge.
b. Use free open-source software, selected based on features like: easiness of installation; quality of the documentation and support; accessible formats for input and output.
c. Use TM-tools with general functionalities like: allowance of document corpora; pre-processing the text; built-in biomedical Name Entity Recognition; queries to a document or corpora; support for ontologies and terminologies.

We used three groups of TM-tools that served different purposes:

I Basic resources that gave foundation to TM: the MeSH browser; the PubMed repository of publications; repositories of NLP resources (e.g., Neuroscience Information Framework, National Institute of Neurological Disorders and Stroke).

II TM-tools II (**Table 1**) that are web-based ready-to-use tools requiring no programming efforts and performing simple TM tasks (Lu, 2011).

III TM-tools III that were used in the final stage of the study optimized for the reviewed topics:

1. Statistical or machine-learning-based approaches: Mallet (McCallum, 2002), Text to Matrix Generator (TMG) (Zeimpekis and Gallopoulos, 2006) and Matlab applications for NLP.
2. TM-tools with predefined NLP processing stream: KH Coder (Higuchi, 2012).
3. Integrated environments for visual programming of NLP: VisualText (Meyers, 2003; Alfred et al., 2014).
4. Biomedical TM rule-based approaches using fully automated stages in text processing: Anote2 (Lourenco et al., 2009) and Biological Research Assistant for TM (BioRAT) (Corney et al., 2004).

A PRACTICAL APPLICATION OF THE TEXT MINING TO LITERATURE ON COGNITIVE REHABILITATION AND ENHANCEMENT THROUGH NEUROSTIMULATION

To show that TM enables us to efficiently deal with big corpora of publications and for publishing practical reasons, the TM application to CR- and CE-TMS literature was limited

Table 1 | TM-tools II presented in the order (indicated by numbers) of their use.

TM tool	INPUT								Targeted processing	Topics						
	Query- T	Query – S	Predefined	Filters	Statistic	Corpus (C)	Terms (T)	Sentences (S)		CR-TMS	CE-TMS	TMS	CR	CE	TMS -	DIAG/RS TMS-fMRI
Mesh	1			1			1		Terms (T)							
PubMed	1			1					Search optimization; Corpus (C)							
MEDSUM	1			1			1		Statistic							
PubReMiner	1			1					Statistic							
LingerCat	1			1					T cloud; papers -T relationships							
Carrot	1			1					Clustering papers; Plot clusters							
Anne O'Tate	1			1	1		1		Clustering papers; statistic; Topics							
BioTextQuest	1			1		1	1		Clustering papers; Biomedical T							
askMEDLINE	1	1		1		1		1	Bottom Line summary of abstracts							
Ultimate Res. Assistant	1			1			1	1	Text summarization; Taxonomies; Mind maps							
Quertle	2	2		2				2	Ranking papers; Subject verb - object relationships							
GoPubMed	2			2	2	2		2	Clustering papers; Statistic							
PubMatrix	3		T				3		Matrix of terms co-occurrence							
Medline Ranker	3		C	3		3	3	3	Ranking papers; Evaluate ranking performance							
XplorMed			C			3	3	3	Clustering papers; T relationships							
Textpresso Neuroscience									Information Extraction; Transition to TM-tools III							

Gray scale qualitatively codes their weights in TM (the darker, the higher the importance). Each subgroup (1–4) includes kernels of TM-tools (circled red) and "targeted processing" (red text) that have the highest importance for our study. INPUT: query terms (T) = query using combinations of terms; query sentences (S) – query using free text or questions; predefined = fixed user-predefined input consisting of lists of terms or publications; filters = tuning the search using supplementary terms, constrains regarding the type/part of the publication to be processed etc. OUTPUT: Statistic about authors, journals, papers per year, topics; corpus (C) = retrieving sets of relevant papers; terms (T) = extracting lists of frequent and relevant terms and their relationships; sentences (S) = extracting relevant sentences and paper summaries. Targeted processing = processing from the TM-tool repertoire used for this review. The last 7 columns show topics whose corpora of publications were studied with TM (gray scale codes the weight of the approach). References: MEDSUM (Bridges-Webb, 1986), PubReMiner (Koster, 2008), LingerCat (Sarkar et al., 2009), Carrot2 (Carpineto et al., 2009), Anne O'Tate (Smalheiser et al., 2008), BioTextQuest (Iliopoulos et al., 2001), askMEDLINE (Fontelo et al., 2005), Ultimate Research Assistant (Hoskinson, 2005), Quertle (Giglia, 2011), GoPubMed (Doms and Schroeder, 2005), PubMatrix (Becker et al., 2003), Medline Ranker (Fontaine et al., 2009), XplorMed (Perez-Iratxeta et al., 2001), Textpresso for Neuroscience (Muller et al., 2008).

to few aspects. First, we aimed to show that TM could retrieve the diversity of TMS applications in vast corpora of publications about CR and CE (see Cognitive Rehabilitation and Enhancement Accomplished with TMS), automatically retrieving trends already described in published reviews (see Discussions and Conclusions). Second, we looked for trends noticeable only in big corpora of publications, relying on the statistical power of the analyses and including results like topics' occurrence frequency and relationships, relevant relational verbs, and high probability conclusive sentences (see Cognitive Rehabilitation and Enhancement Accomplished with TMS). Furthermore, we analyzed large context relationships between topics showing how CR- and CE-TMS integrate with diagnostic, fundamental research and fMRI studies (see A General Context).

Using TM to efficiently review corpora of publications requires roughly three stages: pre-TM-processing, TM-processing, and post-TM-processing. In this paper, we focused on the TM-processing by showing mainly the "raw" TM results. Accordingly, the seemingly redundant diversity of results is determined by our intention to illustrate few similar results given by different TM-tools.

We used a multi-stage and multi-tool approach ordered by the complexity in TM, which was gradually increased, starting with TM-tools II and continuing with TM-tools III. The same analysis was performed with few TM-tools (**Table 2**), which can be regarded as alternative solutions for the same problem. This helped us to cope with the limited perspective offered by different TM-tools, to perform comparisons and cross-validations, and to build synthetic results.

The main classes of TM processing on the selected corpora were:

- Statistics about the number of publications, authors, journals; thematic/MeSH headings division of the field; clustering

Table 2 | Number of publications retrieved from PubMed using search queries defined previously.

Search query	Publications per search filter:		
	TIAB	PBRK	TIABREV
CR-TMS	**4074**	**0.913**	**641**
CE-TMS	**181**	**0.956**	**41**
TMS	8386	0.909	1018
CR	4220	0.896	914
CE	1235	0.895	312
TMS-DIAG	212	0.994	68
TMS-RES	360	0.994	93
TMS-fMRI	875	0.906	211

PBRK, the probability of correct ranking of a random positive-negative pair of publications determined with Medline Ranker.

of publications; selection and ranking of relevant corpora of papers necessary for TM-tools III (all performed with TM-tools II).
- Extract relevant terms and their relationships, involving: categorization of key concepts; building correlation matrices for relevant terms and showing the most informative correlations; showing the topological maps of the main terms, using their relationships inferred from co-occurrence in the same text units.
- Retrieve automatically relevant sentences, study their probability of occurrence, and identify parts-of-sentence (e.g., predicates) relevant for deriving conclusions.
- Build a "map of science," which characterize large-scale relationships between multiple topics. Each topic-topic relationship was evaluated based on common relevant terms retrieved from each corpus, similar thematic clustering of the publications, common authors, journals and publications approaching both topics.

To create a larger context allowing a better understanding of CR- and CE-TMS, we selected topics like TMS, CR, CE, TMS-RES, TMS-DIAG, and TMS-fMRI. **Figure 1** presents a "qualitative hypothesis" about the topology of this context and we used TM to test it. Corpora of publications for each topic were retrieved using the following PubMed queries:

- For CR-TMS: ("transcranial magnetic stimulation") AND ("cognitive rehabilitation" OR "rehabilitation" OR "cognitive therapy" OR "therapy" OR "cognitive recovery" OR "recovery" OR "cognitive treatment" OR "treatment" OR "cognitive repair" OR "neurorehabilitation" OR "improvement" OR "decrease").
- For CE-TMS: ("transcranial magnetic stimulation") AND [("cognitive enhancement") OR ("cognitive augmentation") OR ("cognitive improvement") OR ("cognitive enrichment") OR ("cognitive amelioration") OR ("neuroenhancement")].
- For TMS: "transcranial magnetic stimulation."
- Queries for CR/CE include the second operand of the AND operator in the CR-TMS/CE-TMS queries.

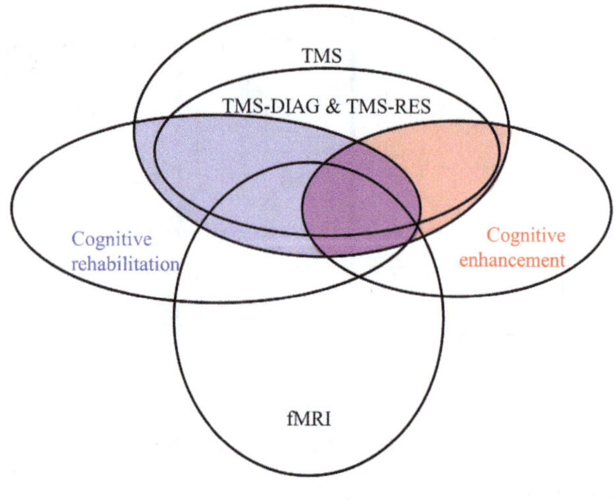

FIGURE 1 | Qualitative approximation of a larger context for CR- and CE-TMS. Topics are represented by ellipses with CR-TMS (filled blue) and CE-TMS (red) representing intersections of topics.

All queries were used separately with two filters ("[Title/Abstract]" (TIAB-filter) and "[Title/Abstract] AND Review" TIABREV-filter) creating two separate corpora of abstracts: TIAB-corpora (the main target for TM) and TIABREV-corpora (used for comparisons). Empty or less relevant abstracts were removed from the corpora. Corpora were also compared with local databases and missing publications were added manually.

Finally, the TM results were evaluated in few ways. First of all, we used TM-tools that are already tested and evaluated, building our results on this general basis. Second, we used the *post-hoc* judgment of the system outputs (Cohen and Hunter, 2008) in few stages, and compared: results of similar processing (e.g., term extraction) performed with different TM-tools using TIAB-corpora (see A Practical Application of the Text Mining to Literature on Cognitive Rehabilitation and Enhancement Through Neurostimulation); results of similar processing using TIAB-corpora vs. TIABREV-corpora (see A Practical Application of the Text Mining to Literature on Cognitive Rehabilitation and Enhancement Through Neurostimulation); TM-results vs. manual-curated results (see Discussions and Conclusions).

A GENERAL CONTEXT

We used TM-tools II to determine relationships that put CR- and CE-TMS topics in the same neighborhood on a "map of science." An outline of the main results includes:

1. MeSH headings mention TMS as a preferred term, defined by its use in brain mapping, neurophysiology and treatment of depression (replacing electroconvulsive therapy), while paired-pulse TMS, rTMS and single-pulse TMS are narrower concepts. The MeSH tree considers that TMS belongs to the fields of neurological diagnostic and therapeutic techniques. CR is related with MeSH headings like Cognitive Therapy, Rehabilitation and Treatment/Rehabilitation Outcome, and CE is related with Cognitive Therapy, Nootropic Agents and Cognitive Enhancers.

2. The number of the publications retrieved from PubMed (**Table 2**) for each topic.

It is noteworthy that a large number of reviews were written for each topic.

3. The number of publications per year evaluating the interest for each topic (**Figure 2**), which showed the following trends:
   - The interest for all topics increased in the last decades;
   - TMS generated numerous publications per year;
   - CR-TMS has a stronger representation than CE-TMS;
   - Across-topics perspectives (CR & CE; CR & CE-TMS; TMS-DIAG & RES) are less represented.

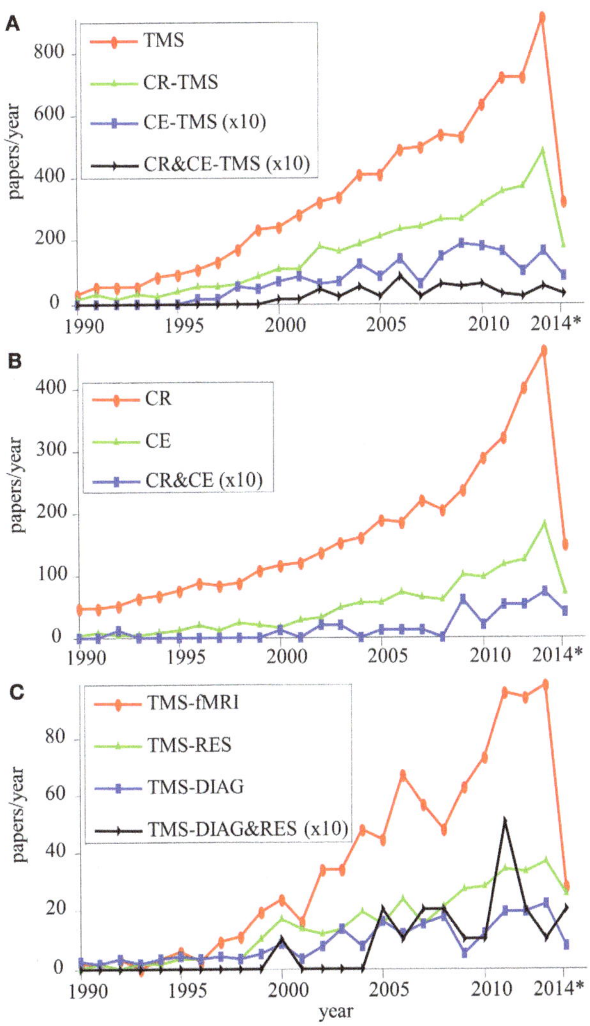

FIGURE 2 | Number of publication per year (2014*, only the first 3 months) for different topics: TMS, CR-TMS, and CE-TMS (A); CE and CR (B); applications of TMS in research (TMS-RES), diagnostic (TMS-DIAG) and concurrent TMS-fMRI (C). Results for topics represented by small numbers of publications are multiplied by 10 (×10). We show also results for conjunctions of topics: (CR&CE-TMS) **(A)**; (CR&CE) **(B)**; (TMS-DIAG&RES) **(C)**.

   - Fundamental research (e.g., TMS-RES, TMS-DIAG) is less represented than practical applications (e.g., CR-TMS).

4. Co-occurrence matrix for terms used to build the search queries, retrieved with PubMatrix (**Figures 3A,B**). We made the following observations:
   - TMS co-occurred very frequently (publications $\sim 10^3$) with terms like therapy, treatment, brain function, brain physiology, and diagnostic (mainly CR-TMS);
   - TMS co-occurred frequently (publications $\sim 10^2$) with rehabilitation, recovery, cognitive treatment, improvement, decrease, brain anatomy, brain performance, brain networks, psychology, brain mapping, MRI, mental disorder, mental disease and psychiatric disorder (mainly CR-TMS and CE-TMS);

5. Frequent terms co-occurring in different corpora (included between brackets):
   a. Among the first 10 MeSH headings, we mention:
      - [CR-TMS]: Motor Cortex/physiology, TMS/methods, Evoked Potentials, Treatment Outcome, Evoked Potentials, Electromyography, Functional Laterality, Stroke, Brain, Motor, (Major) Depressive Disorder;
      - [CE-TMS]: TMS/methods, Brain Mapping, Brain, Functional Laterality, Cognition, Psychomotor Performance, Reaction Time/physiology, Motor Cortex/physiology, Cognition Disorders, Prefrontal Cortex/physiology.
   b. Among the first 100 common MeSH headings (average frequency range [51, 2010]) for groups of topics (included between brackets), we mention:
      - [CR-TMS; CE-TMS; TMS; TMS-fMRI]: Brain, Cognition, Brain Mapping, Electromyography, Evoked Potentials, Motor Skills, MRI, Motor Cortex/physiology, Neural Inhibition, Neuronal Plasticity, Neuropsychological Tests, Parietal Lobe, Prefrontal Cortex, Psychomotor Performance, Reaction Time, TMS/methods, Treatment Outcome;
      - [CR-TMS; CR]: Brain, Chronic Disease, Cognition, (Major) Depressive Disorder, MRI, Motor Cortex, Neuropsychological Tests, Psychomotor Performance, Recovery Of Function, Schizophrenia, Severity Of Illness Index, Treatment Outcome, Neuronal Plasticity/physiology, Recovery of Function/physiology, Stroke;
      - [CE-TMS; CE]: Attention, Brain, Cognition, Learning, MRI, Memory, Neurons, Neuropsychological Tests, Psychomotor Performance, Reaction Time, Prefrontal Cortex, Treatment Outcome, Cognition Disorders/diagnosis and etiology.
   c. Other trends noticed using the TM-tools II:
      - Different groups of topics (e.g., [CR-TMS; CE-TMS]; [TMS; TMS-fMRI; TMS-RES; TMS-DIAG]) are connected as shown by common headings/terms;
      - CR-TMS related terms: motor cortex, treatment, excitability, facilitation, antidepressant, plasticity, MEP, stroke, Parkinson, severity of illness index, treatment outcome, (major) depressive disorder, schizophrenia,

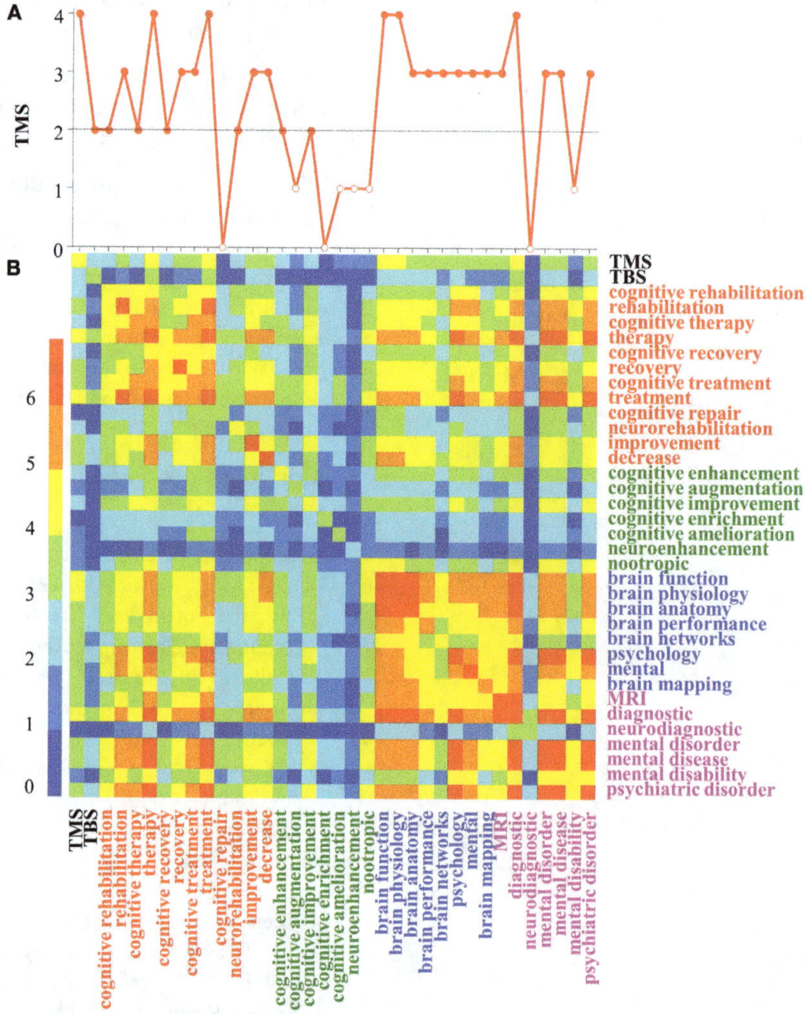

FIGURE 3 | Co-occurrence matrix built with PubMatrix. The matrix **(B)** represents the decimal logarithm of the number of publications retrieved from PubMed using queries combining all possible conjunctions of pairs of terms (e.g., TMS and neurorehabilitation), which label the lines and the rows of the matrix. Panel **(A)** represents the first line in the matrix, showing co-occurrences involving the term TMS. Different colors (see the left color-coding bar) represent different powers of 10. The color of the text marks terms associated dominantly with: TMS (black); CR-TMS (red); CE-TMS (green); TMS-RES (blue); TMS-DIAG (purple).

stroke/complications, neuronal plasticity, rehabilitation, cognition, recovery, parietal lobe, prefrontal cortex, psychomotor performance;

- CE-TMS related terms: prefrontal cortex, DLPFC, cognition, psychomotor performance, attention, learning, memory, performance, placebo, cognition disorders, severity of illness index, treatment outcome, neuroenhancement, Hebbian, neurofeedback, enhancement, improvement;
- [CR-TMS; CE-TMS] and [CR; CE] groups of topics have “mental diseases” and “treatments” as common subtopics, thus supporting the hypothesis that the relative improvement of the mental performance is a common aspect of their definitions.

6. The first 5 authors for different topics (all including Pascual-Leone A on the first place):
   - [CR-TMS]: Fregni F, Daskalakis ZJ, Fitzgerald PB, Rothwell JC;
   - [CE-TMS]: Walsh V, Fregni F, Cowey A, Miniussi C;
   - [TMS]: Rothwell JC, Hallett M, Cohen LG, Fitzgerald PB;

Some authors covered several of the selected topics (e.g., common authors for [CR-TMS; CE-TMS; TMS; TMS-fMRI]: Pascual-Leone A, Cohen LG, Fregni F, Lisanby SH, Miniussi C, Rothwell JC), and this is an indirect argument for potential connections between topics.

7. Finally, comparisons between corpora for different topics showed relevant numbers of common publications (**Figure 4**), thus emphasizing a unitary context. Consistently, clustering the publications for each topic using Carrot2 showed also different clusters sharing publications.

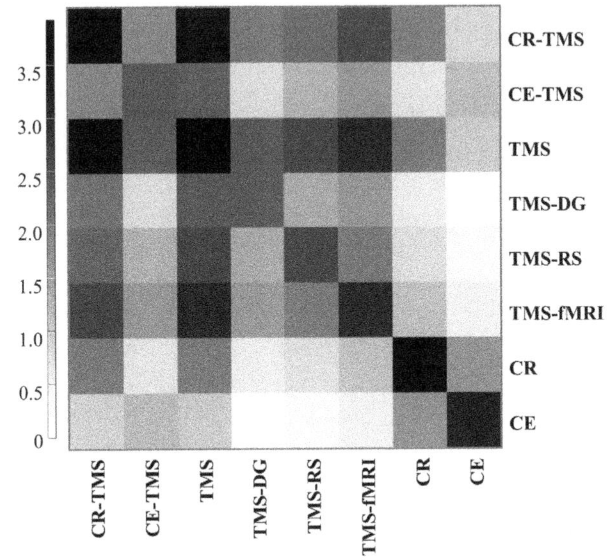

FIGURE 4 | Number of common publications (in decimal logarithmic scale) for pairs of corpora representing topics labeling the rows and the columns of the matrix. Different shades of gray (see the color-coding bar) represent different powers of 10.

COGNITIVE REHABILITATION AND ENHANCEMENT ACCOMPLISHED WITH TMS

First, we need to reiterate that the relevance of all the retrieved terms is based on the idea that words co-occurring frequently in the abstracts are related in ways intrinsically constrained by the topic of the abstracts. Moreover, our specific selection of publications guarantees that term like TMS (all protocols) are present in all abstracts included in corpora. Thus, TMS is strongly related with all frequent terms retrieved with different TM-tools. Specifically, if, for example, the frequent terms are treatment and depression, this means that TMS is used frequently in depression treatment.

We used TM-tools III to increase our insights in CR-TMS and CE-TMS literature, and selected the following groups of results:

1. Statistical or machine-learning-based NLP:

   a. Topic modeling with Mallet (500 iterations, 7 topics, topics proportion threshold 0.05, and removed the standard Mallet stop-words). Each topic is a set of terms used with high probability by the authors, thus reflecting a specific thinking pattern involving TMS. Without knowing anything about the meaning of the words in a text, topic modeling assumes that any piece of text is written by selecting words from possible topics. Thus, it becomes possible to mathematically decompose a text into probable topics from which the words originated.

Example topics separated in CR/CE related terms (brackets) and TMS related terms (double brackets):

a1. CR-TMS:

- [treatment, depression, clinical, therapy, disorder, major, antidepressant, electroconvulsive therapy], [transcranial, magnetic, stimulation, effective];
- [motor, stroke, patients, recovery, function, hemisphere, affected, rehabilitation, limb], [magnetic, transcranial, stimulation].

The [CR] kernel of 2 topics includes CE-related terms (e.g., [cortex, learn, activity, visual, memory, performance, area]).

a2. CE-TMS:

- [cortex, DLPFC, prefrontal, dorsolateral, memory, processing], [stimulation, applied, TMS, effect, frequency], significant;
- [cognitive, brain, healthy, functions, enhance, neuroenhancement, parietal, cognition], [stimulation, magnetic, TMS], studies.

The [CE] kernel of 3 topics includes CR-related terms (e.g., [improvement, depression, treatment, deprivation, sleep, occipital, functional, disease, fluoxetine]).

   b. Term-related queries with TMG toolbox. Document retrieval relies often on matching terms from documents with those from queries. However, natural languages present some challenges (e.g., polysemy, synonymy) that render term-matching inaccurate. TMG is using latent semantic analysis to overcome these problems (Landauer et al., 1998), based on the application of singular value decomposition of a term-by-document matrix (TDM).

We performed the indexing for each corpus creating new TDMs using "common-words" stop-list, logarithmic local weights, "GfIdf" global term weighs, normalization of terms, removing of alpha-numerics and numbers. For dimensionality reduction and TDM best rank approximation, we selected the dimensionality via the use of profile likelihood (Zhu and Ghodsi, 2006). Example results:

b1. For CR-TMS, the TDM included 607 documents, 6387 terms with average 111 indexing terms/document for the query matrix, and the best rank approximation 360. Among the best retrieved terms (apparition frequency > 86; range [870, 896] terms), we mention: [stimulation, rTMS, treatment, TMS, brain, motor, depression, patients, stroke, cortical, therapy, clinical, effects, disorders, pain, cortex] in the first 20; [recovery, disorder, schizophrenia, tinnitus, excitability, cognitive, plasticity, antidepressant, rehabilitation, mechanisms, psychiatric, symptoms, aphasia, language, noninvasive, sham, EEG, Parkinson, resistant, human, induced, movement, neglect] in the next 80; [cerebral, epilepsy, deep, migraine, neural, bipolar, visual, OCD, seizures, acute, neurological, diagnosis, auditory, neuroimaging, reorganization, prefrontal, inhibition, improvement, mood, neuropsychiatric, neuromodulation] in the next 50 terms.

b2. For CE-TMS, the TDM included 174 documents, 3235 terms with average 117 indexing terms/document for the query matrix, and the best rank approximation 174. Among the best retrieved terms (apparition frequency > 37; range [776, 1010] terms), we mention: [TMS, rTMS, motor, cortex, brain, visual, memory, cognitive, performance, parietal, healthy, patients, learning, improvement, enhancement] in the first 20; [excitability, neural, DLPFC, facilitation, plasticity, attention, control, prefrontal, network, evoked, neuroscience, perception, EEG, mechanisms, modulation, semantic, training, frontal, FEF, treatment, fluoxetine, neuroenhancement, sleep, emotional, skill, inhibition, Parkinson] in the next 80; [fMRI, MEP, Wernicke, search, discrimination, pain, cognition, increased, encoding, oscillatory, language, psychiatric, decrease, experimental, stroke, illness, major, effective, resistant, improve] in the next 50 terms.

2. Processing performed with KH Coder:

   a. Determine the co-occurrence network for CR-TMS and CE-TMS corpora using 7 sets of coding rules. A coding rule is a list of terms connected with OR (|), AND (&) or NOT used to "focus" the TM of the corpora toward specific topics. We used coding rules (marked by brackets) that were common for CR-TMS and CE-TMS: [TMS] (transcranial & magnetic & stimulation | rTMS | TBS etc.); [mental disabilities] (depression | stroke | schizophrenia etc.); [brain functions] (memory | learning | attention etc.); [research methods] (fMRI | EEG etc.); [verbs-] describing negative effects of the stimulation (fail | worsen | damage | debilitate | miss etc.). To these we added a set of rules specific to CR-TMS/CE-TMS: [verbs+] describing positive effects for CR-TMS (rehabilitate | treat | recover | restore etc.) or CE-TMS (enhance | improve | augment | strengthen etc.); [CR-TMS-effects] (rehabilitation | cognitive & rehabilitation | cognitive & therapy | neurorehabilitation etc.); [CE-TMS-effects] (performance | enhancement | neuroenhancement | neuromodulation etc.). The co-occurrence networks revealed that the terms from the coding rules [TMS], [CR-TMS-effects], [mental disabilities] and [Verbs+] have the highest co-occurrence frequency in the CR-TMS corpus. The CE-TMS corpus is characterized by high co-occurrence frequency of the terms from the coding rules [TMS], [CE-TMS-effects] and [Verbs+].
   b. Determine the keyword-in-context (KWIC) collection for terms in both CR-TMS (**Table 3**) and CE-TMS (**Table 4**). The KWIC statistic revealed information about both the relevant terms co-occurring with specific query terms (e.g., TMS) and statistical regularities (e.g., probable word positions) about the way the scientists build their statements.

3. Summary of results obtained with VisualText, ANote2, BioRAT and our Matlab applications (MAPP). All TM-tools used similar resources, including: dictionaries (mental disabilities, brain anatomy, cognitive processes, built using Neuroscience Information Framework (NIF) resources; CR-TMS-effects, CE-TMS-effects and TMS, built using our term statistic, similar with KH Coder coding rules); ontologies (NIF gross-anatomy and NIF dysfunction; human disease and neuro-behavior ontology from The Open Biological and Biomedical Ontologies Foundry); lexical words (Mallet stop-words; verbs+ and verbs- for CR-TMS and CE-TMS, similar with KH Coder rules). Each dictionary/ontology could be considered a class of terms (indicated by brackets; e.g., [mental disabilities]).

The text processing relied on predefined streams of processing or on existing libraries of examples (e.g., TAIParse general text analyzer for VisualText). Our Matlab applications (MAPP) were used to handle the results, to perform relation extraction and to extract sentences with high probability of occurrence (low perplexity coefficients, PP).

We summarized here few results from the following processing: Evaluate term frequency and co-occurrences and perform Name Entity Recognition using lexical resources (ANote2,

Table 3 | KWIC examples for CR-TMS.

Word	Total	LT	RT	L5	L4	L3	L2	L1	KW	R1	R2	R3	R4	R5
Treatment	160	63	97	25	11	11	16	0	TMS	5	17	53	12	10
Depression	113	37	76	8	11	18	0	0	TMS	0	22	13	14	27
Alzheimer	100	55	45	20	13	19	3	0	TMS	2	12	10	5	16
Therapy	98	58	40	25	4	3	26	0	TMS	5	3	6	22	4
fMRI	79	57	22	14	6	19	18	0	TMS	0	3	8	0	11
Stroke	50	35	15	9	5	11	10	0	TMS	0	4	3	4	4
Disorder	38	27	11	9	3	2	13	0	TMS	0	0	6	4	1
Recovery	34	28	6	15	6	4	3	0	TMS	0	2	0	0	4
Schizophrenia	15	12	3	5	1	2	4	0	TMS	0	1	0	0	2
Parkinson	14	6	8	2	4	0	0	0	TMS	0	5	1	1	1
Improvement	13	5	8	3	0	1	1	0	TMS	0	0	2	1	5
Neurorehabilitation	20	14	6	7	0	1	6	0	TMS	0	2	1	1	2

Columns show the number of co-occurrences of the context word (left) at different positions left/right (L5-L1/R1-R5) in the sentence relative to the query keyword (KW) and their total (LT/RT).

Table 4 | KWIC examples for CE-TMS.

Word	Total	LT	RT	L5	L4	L3	L2	L1	KW	R1	R2	R3	R4	R5
Induce	29	6	23	2	1	3	0	0	TMS	3	15	1	2	2
Performance	24	12	12	5	4	3	0	0	TMS	0	1	7	2	2
EEG	18	5	13	2	0	1	2	0	TMS	0	11	1	1	0
Paired-pulse	17	16	1	0	1	2	0	13	TMS	0	0	0	0	1
Cognitive	16	4	12	2	0	2	0	0	TMS	1	2	6	2	1
Memory	13	9	4	2	3	3	1	0	TMS	0	1	1	2	0
Stimulation	13	5	8	1	2	0	2	0	TMS	2	0	3	2	1
fMRI	9	7	2	1	1	3	2	0	TMS	0	2	0	0	0
Enhance	8	3	5	1	1	1	0	0	TMS	1	2	0	2	0
Facilitate	7	1	6	1	0	0	0	0	TMS	1	1	0	3	1
Improve	6	1	5	0	0	1	0	0	TMS	1	3	0	0	1
Perception	5	3	2	0	2	1	0	0	TMS	0	0	0	0	2

MAPP); Relations Extraction (ANote2, MAPP); Extract relevant sentences (VisualText, BioRAT, MAPP). The selected results are:

a. Terms statistic from Name Entity Recognition applied to CR-TMS (ANote2; 27506 annotations):

   - Top terms (number of occurrences): treatment (1177), rTMS (1000), brain (982), TMS (1410), therapy (503), depression (456), stroke (420);
   - Classes of terms (class per document, number of occurrences for all terms of the class): [neuro-behavior ontology] (22.8, 14903), [CR-TMS-effects] (4.8, 3163), [TMS] (4.3, 2811), [mental disabilities] (3.2, 2073), [cognitive processes] (1.6, 1028), [CE-TMS-effects] (0.2, 137);
   - Examples from the detailed class statistic (ANote2, MAPP; parentheses indicate number of occurrences):
     - [TMS]: rTMS (1301), TMS (1466), TBS (32);
     - [CR-TMS-effects]: treatment (1177), decrease (27), inhibition (96), antidepressant (175), antipsychotic (23), neurorehabilitation (45), recovery (286), rehabilitation (171), therapy (503);
     - [mental disabilities]: ADHD (25), Alzheimer's (14), OCD (92), Parkinson (104), Tourette (9), anxiety (49), auditory hallucinations (24), bipolar depression (27), bipolar disorder (25), depression (462), epilepsy (77), major depressive disorder (111), neglect (68), psychiatric disorders (80), schizophrenia (158), seizures (69), stress (25), stroke (422), tinnitus (153);

b. Terms statistic from Name Entity Recognition applied to CE-TMS (ANote2; 7404 annotations):

   - Top terms (number of occurrences): TMS (727), rTMS (360), brain (207), cognitive (131), performance (130), facilitation (67);
   - Classes of terms (class per document, number of occurrences for all terms of the class): [neuro-behavior ontology] (22.97, 4111), [TMS] (6.23, 1116), [CE-TMS-effects] (3.70, 663), [cognitive processes] (3.49, 624), [mental disabilities] (0.35, 63), [CR-TMS-effects] (0.32, 57);
   - Examples from the detailed class statistic (ANote2, MAPP):
     - [TMS]: TMS (739), rTMS (365);
     - [CE-TMS-effects]: activation (28), cognitive (131), cognitive enhancement (19), enhancement (34), facilitation (67), improvement (29), neuroenhancement (27), performance (130), performance enhancement (8), rehabilitation (27), therapy (37);
     - [cognitive processes]: attention (53), cognition (25), learning (70), memory (85), working memory (46), perception (37), visual search (19), skill acquisition (12), consolidation (9), decision (14), emotion (8), encoding (23), language (21), movement (17), recognition (13), semantic processing (2), speech (7);

c. Relationship Extraction for CR-TMS (ANote2; 27506 annotations). From 6754 relations, 2163 were verb associated relations, and we found among the top 30 the following verbs: induced, related, controlled, based, treating, underlying, compared, modulate, affected, applied, provide, discuss, to study, has been used, combined, to treat, improving. The statistics showed positive (89.1%), negative (1.7%), conditional (9.2%) for the polarity of the relations, and one-one (11.8%), one-many (16.7%), many-one (13.4%), many-many (12.1%) for their cardinality.

d. Examples of terms from classes [TMS] (omitted, next) & [CR-TMS-effects] & [mental disabilities] co-occurring in the same sentence (MAPP; 1290 sentences; | = OR):

   - [treat] & [depression (24%)| disorder (12%)| tinnitus (4.3%)| schizophrenia (3%)| stress (1%)| pain (1%)| stroke (1%)| epilepsy (1%)| anxiety (1%)| seizures (0.2%)| neglect (0.1%)];
   - [therapy] & [depression (5%)| stroke (3%)| pain (1%)| epilepsy (0.4%)| seizures (0.5%)| schizophrenia (0.2%)| mood (0.2%)];
   - [improve] & [stroke (3%)| depression (0.6%)| tinnitus (0.3%)| reading (0.1%)| attention (0.1%)| schizophrenia (0.1%)];

e. Relationship Extraction for CE-TMS (ANote2; 7404 annotations). From 2025 relations, 903 were verbs associated relations, and we found among the top 30 the following verbs:

is, induced, applied, guided, learning, improved, increasing, enhancing, was applied, paired, stimulated, delivered, reduced, impaired, performed, encoding. The statistics showed positive (92.0%), negative (1.2%), conditional (6.8%) for the polarity of the relations, and one-one (14.0%), one-many (17.6%), many-one (14.5%), many-many (12.4%) for their cardinality.

f. Example of terms from classes [TMS] (omitted, next) & [CE-TMS-effects] & [cognitive processes] occurring in the same sentence (MAPP; 1591 sentences):

   - [performance] & [memory (3.7%)| attention (1%)| language (1%)| motor (1%)| visual (1%)];
   - [facilitation] & [motor (6%)| memory (2%)| linguistic (2%)| concept (1%)| control (1%)| knowledge (1%)| logical (1%)| awareness (1%)| visual (1%)];
   - [improve] & [memory (1%)| visual (1%)| language (1%)];

g. Example of high probability sentences (PP, range [4, 99]) from the CR-TMS corpus including terms from classes [TMS] & [CR-TMS-effects] & [mental disabilities] (see d):

   - "Daily rTMS improves mood in depression" (PP 13.0).
   - "Excitatory rTMS induces improvements in chronic post-stroke aphasia" (PP 13.5).
   - "Slow TMS can rapidly reduce resistant auditory hallucinations in schizophrenia" (PP 16.8).

Using VisualText we showed also that from 4085 sentences, 1417 include terms from [TMS] hierarchy, and 847 include terms from [TMS] & [CR-TMS-effects OR mental disabilities]. Examples from the last group:

- "TMS has been shown to be an effective treatment for mental illnesses including major depressive disorder."
- "...rTMS has been developed for the treatment of major depression and schizophrenia."

h. Example of high probability sentences (PP; range [3, 50]) from the CE-TMS corpus including terms from classes [TMS] & [CE-TMS-effects] & [cognitive processes] (see f):

   - "...rTMS to left dorsal premotor cortex enhances motor consolidation of new skills" (PP 9).
   - "rTMS over Wernicke's area leads to a brief facilitation of picture naming by shortening linguistic processing time" (PP 11).
   - "...rTMS at alpha frequency can modulate short-term memory capacity by influencing the ability to suppress distracting information" (PP 15).

Using VisualText we showed that from 1008 sentences, 445 included terms from [TMS], and 238 include terms from [TMS] & [CE-TMS-effects OR cognitive processes]. Examples from the last group:

- "...rTMS of the DLPFC can affect the performance in an affective go-no-go task."
- "...here we report the ipsilateral enhancement of visual attention after rTMS of parietal cortex at parameters known to reduce cortical excitability."

k. Example of sentences extracted with BioRAT from the CR-TMS corpus using a specific rule, which indicate classes of terms that have to be found at specific locations (block) in the sentence (**Table 5**).

DISCUSSIONS AND CONCLUSIONS

We here used a set of selected TM-tools to obtain basic insights into the relevant literature on the CR- and CE-TMS. For obvious reasons, we limited this application to few simple aspects. First, we showed that TM could retrieve from vast corpora of publications the diversity of TMS applications in CR and CE, automatically extracting trends already described in published reviews. Second, we searched for trends noticeable only in big corpora of publications.

Along this exercise, we attempted to validate our results in different ways. For example, we compared similar results obtained using different TM-tools applied to different corpora (TIAB-corpora or TIABREV-corpora). Relevant and common aspects, synthesized in unique results per type of analysis and topics were shown in the paper. Finally, we compared TM to human curation efforts. Accordingly, we selected for human curation 30 of the top ranked (with Medline Ranker) publications from

Table 5 | Example sentences retrieved with BioRAT using a specific rule.

Blocks of the rule						Context
<LOOKUP: TMS>	**<MACRO: WORD>**	**<MACRO: WORD?>**	**<LOOKUP: CR-TMS-effects>**	**<MACRO: WORD>**	**<LOOKUP: mental disabilities>**	
rTMS	for	–	treatment	of	depression	"...the first cases report of using rTMS for the treatment of depression ..."
TMS	for	–	treatment	of	obsessive compulsive disorder	"...TMS for the treatment of obsessive compulsive disorder ..."

"< >" delimitate a block of the rule; LOOKUP, looking for a term included in a class ([TMS], [CR-TMS-effects] or [mental disabilities]); MACRO WORD, any word; "?," the block is optional.

the TIABREV-corpora, separately for CR-TMS and CR-TMS. We performed a selective manual curation aimed to retrieve relevant terms co-occurring with TMS (all types of protocol) in the abstracts, which belong to the following classes: mental functions, healthy or impaired, modulated by TMS; mental disabilities treated with TMS; rehabilitation or enhancement effects of TMS. We also searched for relationships between classes of relevant terms and conclusive sentences summarizing research results.

Very briefly, the manual curation gave the following perspective over the main topics:

a. CR-TMS. TMS is continuously establishing itself as one of the "tools of the trade" in psychiatric therapeutic practice (Kammer and Spitzer, 2012) improving mental functions in: Parkinson's disease (Pascual-Leone et al., 1994), aphasia (Medina et al., 2012), motor control after stroke (Takeuchi et al., 2005), epilepsy (Nitsche and Paulus, 2009), depression (Lisanby et al., 2009; Conforto et al., 2014), schizophrenia (Levkovitz et al., 2011; Kammer and Spitzer, 2012), autism (Krause et al., 2012), chronic migraine (Conforto et al., 2014), dyslexia (Costanzo et al., 2013), neglect (Fasotti and Van Kessel, 2013), obsessive-compulsive disorder (OCD) (Mantovani et al., 2013), chronic pain (Moreno-Duarte et al., 2014), and social anxiety disorder (Paes et al., 2013). The TMS therapy applied to younger patients (children and adolescents) improves cognitive functions (Vicario and Nitsche, 2013) in: stroke affecting the motor cortex (Kirton et al., 2008), epilepsy (Fregni et al., 2005), ADHD (Weaver et al., 2012), Tourette syndrome (Le et al., 2013), autism (Baruth et al., 2010), treatment-resistant depression (Bloch et al., 2008), and medication-resistant schizophrenia (Jardri et al., 2012).
b. CE-TMS. CE is defined as any augmentation of core information processing systems in the brain underlying perception, attention, conceptualization, memory, reasoning and motor performance (Sandberg and Bostrom, 2006; Luber and Lisanby, 2014). Studies reported TMS-induced modulations and enhancements of brain functioning and neural processing involved in: language comprehension (Floel et al., 2008), learning and memory (Vicario et al., 2013), cortical plasticity improving learning (Vallence and Ridding, 2014), motor memory (Butefisch et al., 2004), working memory (Gaudeau-Bosma et al., 2013), memory (Gagnon et al., 2011; Blumenfeld et al., 2014), phonological memory (Kirschen et al., 2006), perception (Hamilton et al., 2013), perceptual discrimination (Luber and Lisanby, 2014), eye movements and visual search, (Gerits et al., 2011; Luber and Lisanby, 2014), attention (Cooper et al., 2004; Lee et al., 2013), reward behavior (Stanford et al., 2013), analogic reasoning (Boroojerdi et al., 2001), motor learning (Luber and Lisanby, 2014), consolidation of new skills (Boyd and Linsdell, 2009), visual awareness (Grosbras and Paus, 2003), activity of specific frequencies supporting functions of the brain (Rahnev, 2013), and Pavlovian conditioning (Luber et al., 2007).

CR-TMS and CE-TMS used various TMS paradigms, including single-pulse, theta-burst, paired-pulse, and trains of rTMS at both low and high frequencies (Luber and Lisanby, 2014).

Comparisons with the manual curation showed that the TM-tools were also able to extract:

- All the relevant terms for CR-TMS and CE-TMS in the form of: lists; topics; classes of terms associated with specific subtopics (e.g., mental disabilities, cognitive processes).
- Relations between relevant terms in the form of: co-occurrences maps (**Figure 3**); groups of relevant terms with high probabilities co-occurrences; KWIC (**Tables 3**, **4**); lists of relevant relational verbs.
- High probability and relevance conclusive sentences (see examples and **Table 5**). We studied also structural statistical regularities in both conclusive sentences and abstracts shown by: the relative position in the sentence for groups of relevant terms (**Tables 3–5**); combinations of relevant terms with high probability occurrence; the occurrence frequency for conclusive sentences.

In addition, the TM approach has clear advantages emerging from the statistical properties of big corpora. Accordingly, the tirade (terms, terms-relationships, sentences) gained statistical strength, enabling us to quantify the frequency of a term or occurrence probabilities for specific relationships between terms or for conclusive sentences. For example, the hierarchy of the top terms for the CR-TMS-corpus includes TMS, treatment, rTMS, brain, therapy, depression, and stroke. We also found hierarchies for classes of terms like [CR-TMS-effects] (e.g., treatment, therapy, recovery, antidepressant, rehabilitation, neurorehabilitation) and [mental disabilities] (e.g., depression, stroke, schizophrenia, tinnitus, major depressive disorder, Parkinson, OCD, epilepsy, seizures, neglect, anxiety, ADHD, stress, Alzheimer's). For the CE-TMS-corpus the top terms are TMS, rTMS, brain, cognitive, performance, and facilitation. We also added hierarchies for classes of terms like [CE-TMS-effects] (e.g., performance enhancement, improvement, facilitation, neuromodulation, neurostimulation, therapy, neuroenhancement, rehabilitation, CE) and [cognitive processes] (e.g., memory, learning, attention, working memory, perception, language skill acquisition, decision, emotion, speech, semantic processing).

The relevance of all the retrieved terms and of their relationships is based on the idea that words co-occurring frequently in the abstracts are related in specific ways intrinsically constrained by the (TMS-related) topic of the abstracts. Thus, TMS is strongly related with all frequent terms retrieved with different TM-tools. Although in a relatively crude form, determined by our intention to show "raw" TM results, our study is showing that TMS emerged as one of the important non-invasive tools that can both improve cognitive and motor functions in numerous neurological diseases and induce enhancements of many fundamental brain functions.

We were able to characterize topics considering their dynamic relationships, trends in research and the interest shown by the scientific community. For example, CR-TMS and CE-TMS share studies (**Figure 4**), being an argument for their similarity. The reviewed topics share also publications with other fields suggesting their appurtenance to a larger context, which integrates diagnostic, fundamental research and fMRI studies. TMS can be used both to investigate and to modify brain physiology and performance in healthy and diseased subjects (Vicario and Nitsche, 2013).

Methodologically speaking, we conclude that TM was helpful in getting an overall perspective on a huge corpus of literature with some level of detail, intentionally limited to handle complexity. Richer information can be extracted using more complex TM methods focused on narrower topics, but this requires extensive training and knowledge.

A decision factor to use TM relates to how profitable and how difficult the tools may be. The study aimed to address these simple issues in a pragmatic way. First and foremost, we argue that TM-tools may become a basic component in the methodological library. Unfortunately, it is equally clear that TM is a difficult task. With this in mind, we aimed to evaluate relatively immediate advantages of a user-friendly TM approach, based on easy-to-use TM-tools applied to CR- and CE-TMS corpora of abstracts. The hierarchical structure of our example set of TM-tools could serve as a guide for researchers aiming to use TM. Accordingly, for a rapid enrichment of the PubMed search, TM-tools II could be used, with special considerations for Carrot2, PubReMiner, Quertle, Medline Ranker, and Textpresso for Neuroscience. All TM-tools III could help a more elaborate TM without a considerable increase in demands to the user. For complex studies combining multiple aspects of the "mining," we recommend systems like Knime, RapidMiner, and Taverna.

ACKNOWLEDGMENT

This work was supported by IUAP 7-11, PF10/008, FWO-K714811, and G.083111.

REFERENCES

Akil, H., Martone, M. E., and Van Essen, D. C. (2011). Challenges and opportunities in mining neuroscience data. *Science* 331, 708–712. doi: 10.1126/science.1199305

Alfred, R., Razali, M., Alias, S., and On, C. (2014). "A visualization approach to automatic text documents categorization based on HAC," in *The 8th International Conference on Knowledge Management in Organizations, Social and Big Data Computing for Knowledge Management, KMO 2013*, eds L. Uden, L. S. L. Wang, J. M. Corchado Rodríguez, H.-C. Yang, and I. H. Ting (Kaohsiung: Springer), 273–284. doi: 10.1007/978-94-007-7287-8_22

Baruth, J. M., Casanova, M. F., El-Baz, A., Horrell, T., Mathai, G., Sears, L., et al. (2010). Low-frequency repetitive transcranial magnetic stimulation (rTMS) modulates evoked-gamma frequency oscillations in autism spectrum disorder (ASD). *J. Neurother.* 14, 179–194. doi: 10.1080/10874208.2010.501500

Becker, K. G., Hosack, D. A., Dennis, G. Jr., Lempicki, R. A., Bright, T. J., Cheadle, C., et al. (2003). PubMatrix: a tool for multiplex literature mining. *BMC Bioinform.* 4:61. doi: 10.1186/1471-2105-4-61

Bloch, Y., Grisaru, N., Harel, E. V., Beitler, G., Faivel, N., Ratzoni, G., et al. (2008). Repetitive transcranial magnetic stimulation in the treatment of depression in adolescents: an open-label study. *J. ECT* 24, 156–159. doi: 10.1097/YCT.0b013e318156aa49

Blumenfeld, R. S., Lee, T. G., and D'Esposito, M. (2014). The effects of lateral prefrontal transcranial magnetic stimulation on item memory encoding. *Neuropsychologia* 53, 197–202. doi: 10.1016/j.neuropsychologia.2013.11.021

Boroojerdi, B., Phipps, M., Kopylev, L., Wharton, C. M., Cohen, L. G., and Grafman, J. (2001). Enhancing analogic reasoning with rTMS over the left prefrontal cortex. *Neurology* 56, 526–528 doi: 10.1212/WNL.56.4.526

Boyd, L. A., and Linsdell, M. A. (2009). Excitatory repetitive transcranial magnetic stimulation to left dorsal premotor cortex enhances motor consolidation of new skills. *BMC Neurosci.* 10:72. doi: 10.1186/1471-2202-10-72

Brem, A. K., Fried, P. J., Horvath, J. C., Robertson, E. M., and Pascual-Leone, A. (2014). Is neuroenhancement by noninvasive brain stimulation a net zero-sum proposition? *Neuroimage* 85 Pt 3, 1058–1068. doi: 10.1016/j.neuroimage.2013.07.038

Bridges-Webb, C. (1986). A computer summary for general practice medical records: MEDSUM. *J. Fam. Pract.* 23, 389–392

Butefisch, C. M., Khurana, V., Kopylev, L., and Cohen, L. G. (2004). Enhancing encoding of a motor memory in the primary motor cortex by cortical stimulation. *J. Neurophysiol.* 91, 2110–2116. doi: 10.1152/jn.01038.2003

Carpineto, C., Osinski, S., Romano, G., and Weiss, D. (2009). A survey of Web clustering engines. *ACM Comput. Surv.* 41, 1–38. doi: 10.1145/1541880.1541884

Cohen, K. B., and Hunter, L. (2008). Getting started in text mining. *PLoS Comput. Biol.* 4:e20. doi: 10.1371/journal.pcbi.0040020

Conforto, A. B., Amaro, E. Jr., Goncalves, A. L., Mercante, J. P., Guendler, V. Z., Ferreira, J. R., et al. (2014). Randomized, proof-of-principle clinical trial of active transcranial magnetic stimulation in chronic migraine. *Cephalalgia* 34, 464–472. doi: 10.1177/0333102413515340

Cooper, A. C., Humphreys, G. W., Hulleman, J., Praamstra, P., and Georgeson, M. (2004). Transcranial magnetic stimulation to right parietal cortex modifies the attentional blink. *Exp. Brain Res.* 155, 24–29. doi: 10.1007/s00221-003-1697-9

Corney, D. P., Buxton, B. F., Langdon, W. B., and Jones, D. T. (2004). BioRAT: extracting biological information from full-length papers. *Bioinformatics* 20, 3206–3213. doi: 10.1093/bioinformatics/bth386

Costanzo, F., Menghini, D., Caltagirone, C., Oliveri, M., and Vicari, S. (2013). How to improve reading skills in dyslexics: the effect of high frequency rTMS. *Neuropsychologia* 51, 2953–2959. doi: 10.1016/j.neuropsychologia.2013.10.018

Dias, A. M., Mansur, C. G., Myczkowski, M., and Marcolin, M. (2011). Whole field tendencies in transcranial magnetic stimulation: a systematic review with data and text mining. *Asian J. Psychiatr.* 4, 107–112. doi: 10.1016/j.ajp.2011.03.003

Doms, A., and Schroeder, M. (2005). GoPubMed: exploring PubMed with the Gene Ontology. *Nucleic Acids Res.* 33, W783–W786. doi: 10.1093/nar/gki470

Fasotti, L., and Van Kessel, M. (2013). Novel insights in the rehabilitation of neglect. *Front. Hum. Neurosci.* 7:780. doi: 10.3389/fnhum.2013.00780

Floel, A., Rosser, N., Michka, O., Knecht, S., and Breitenstein, C. (2008). Noninvasive brain stimulation improves language learning. *J. Cogn. Neurosci.* 20, 1415–1422. doi: 10.1162/jocn.2008.20098

Fontaine, J.-F., Barbosa-Silva, A., Schaefer, M., Huska, M. R., Muro, E. M., and Andrade-Navarro, M. A. (2009). MedlineRanker: flexible ranking of biomedical literature. *Nucleic Acids Res.* 37, W141–W146. doi: 10.1093/nar/gkp353

Fontelo, P., Liu, F., and Ackerman, M. (2005). askMEDLINE: a free-text, natural language query tool for MEDLINE/PubMed. *BMC Med. Inform. Decis. Mak.* 5:5. doi: 10.1186/1472-6947-5-5

Fregni, F., Thome-Souza, S., Bermpohl, F., Marcolin, M. A., Herzog, A., Pascual-Leone, A., et al. (2005). Antiepileptic effects of repetitive transcranial magnetic stimulation in patients with cortical malformations: an EEG and clinical study. *Stereotact. Funct. Neurosurg.* 83, 57–62. doi: 10.1159/000086674

Gagnon, G., Schneider, C., Grondin, S., and Blanchet, S. (2011). Enhancement of episodic memory in young and healthy adults: a paired-pulse TMS study on encoding and retrieval performance. *Neurosci. Lett.* 488, 138–142. doi: 10.1016/j.neulet.2010.11.016

Gaudeau-Bosma, C., Moulier, V., Allard, A. C., Sidhoumi, D., Bouaziz, N., Braha, S., et al. (2013). Effect of two weeks of rTMS on brain activity in healthy subjects during an n-back task: a randomized double blind study. *Brain Stimul.* 6, 569–575. doi: 10.1016/j.brs.2012.10.009

Gerits, A., Ruff, C., Guipponi, O., Wenderoth, N., Driver, J., and Vanduffel, W. (2011). Transcranial magnetic stimulation of macaque frontal eye fields decreases saccadic reaction time. *Exp. Brain Res.* 212, 143–152. doi: 10.1007/s00221-011-2710-3

Giglia, E. (2011). Quertle and KNALIJ: searching PubMed has never been so easy and effective. *Eur. J. Phys. Rehabil. Med.* 47, 687–690

Grosbras, M. H., and Paus, T. (2003). Transcranial magnetic stimulation of the human frontal eye field facilitates visual awareness. *Eur. J. Neurosci.* 18, 3121–3126. doi: 10.1111/j.1460-9568.2003.03055.x

Hamilton, R. H., Wiener, M., Drebing, D. E., and Coslett, H. B. (2013). Gone in a flash: manipulation of audiovisual temporal integration using transcranial magnetic stimulation. *Front. Psychol.* 4:571. doi: 10.3389/fpsyg.2013.00571

Higuchi, K. (2012). "The internet in newspaper articles and people's minds: a corpus-based exploratory approach to social consciousness in japan," in *The 4th International Conference on Corpus* (Linguistics), 115–116.

Hoskinson, A. (2005). Creating the ultimate research assistant. *Computer* 38, 97–99. doi: 10.1109/MC.2005.375

Iliopoulos, I., Enright, A. J., and Ouzounis, C. A. (2001). Textquest: document clustering of Medline abstracts for concept discovery in molecular biology. *Biocomputing* 2001, 384–395. doi: 10.1142/9789814447362_0038

Jardri, R., Bubrovszky, M., Demeulemeester, M., Poulet, E., Januel, D., Cohen, D., et al. (2012). Repetitive transcranial magnetic stimulation to treat early-onset auditory hallucinations. *J. Am. Acad. Child Adolesc. Psychiatry* 51, 947–949. doi: 10.1016/j.jaac.2012.06.010

Kammer, T., and Spitzer, M. (2012). Brain stimulation in psychiatry: methods and magnets, patients and parameters. *Curr. Opin. Psychiatry* 25, 535–541. doi: 10.1097/YCO.0b013e328358df8c

Kirschen, M. P., Davis-Ratner, M. S., Jerde, T. E., Schraedley-Desmond, P., and Desmond, J. E. (2006). Enhancement of phonological memory following transcranial magnetic stimulation (TMS). *Behav. Neurol.* 17, 187–194 doi: 10.1155/2006/469132

Kirton, A., Chen, R., Friefeld, S., Gunraj, C., Pontigon, A. M., and Deveber, G. (2008). Contralesional repetitive transcranial magnetic stimulation for chronic hemiparesis in subcortical paediatric stroke: a randomised trial. *Lancet Neurol.* 7, 507–513. doi: 10.1016/S1474-4422(08)70096-6

Koster, J. (2008). *PubMed. PubReMiner.* Available online at: http://hgserver2.amc.nl/cgi-bin/miner/miner2.cgi

Krause, L., Enticott, P. G., Zangen, A., and Fitzgerald, P. B. (2012). The role of medial prefrontal cortex in theory of mind: a deep rTMS study. *Behav. Brain Res.* 228, 87–90. doi: 10.1016/j.bbr.2011.11.037

Landauer, T. K., Foltz, P. W., and Laham, D. (1998). An introduction to latent semantic analysis. *Discourse Process.* 25, 259–284. doi: 10.1080/0163853980 9545028

Le, K., Liu, L., Sun, M., Hu, L., and Xiao, N. (2013). Transcranial magnetic stimulation at 1 Hertz improves clinical symptoms in children with Tourette syndrome for at least 6 months. *J. Clin. Neurosci.* 20, 257–262. doi: 10.1016/j.jocn.2012.01.049

Lee, J., Ku, J., Han, K., Park, J., Lee, H., Kim, K. R., et al. (2013). rTMS over bilateral inferior parietal cortex induces decrement of spatial sustained attention. *Front. Hum. Neurosci.* 7:26. doi: 10.3389/fnhum.2013.00026

Levkovitz, Y., Rabany, L., Harel, E. V., and Zangen, A. (2011). Deep transcranial magnetic stimulation add-on for treatment of negative symptoms and cognitive deficits of schizophrenia: a feasibility study. *Int. J. Neuropsychopharmacol.* 14, 991–996. doi: 10.1017/S1461145711000642

Lisanby, S., Husain, M., Rosenquist, P., Maixner, D., Gutierrez, R., Krystal, A., et al. (2009). Daily left prefrontal repetitive transcranial magnetic stimulation in the acute treatment of major depression: clinical predictors of outcome in a multisite, randomized controlled clinical trial. *Neuropsychopharmacology* 34, 522–534 doi: 10.1038/npp.2008.118

Lourenco, A., Carreira, R., Carneiro, S., Maia, P., Glez-Pena, D., Fdez-Riverola, F., et al. (2009). @Note: a workbench for biomedical text mining. *J. Biomed. Inform.* 42, 710–720. doi: 10.1016/j.jbi.2009.04.002

Lu, Z. (2011). PubMed and beyond: a survey of web tools for searching biomedical literature. *Database (Oxford)* 2011:baq036. doi: 10.1093/database/baq036

Luber, B., Balsam, P., Nguyen, T., Gross, M., and Lisanby, S. H. (2007). Classical conditioned learning using transcranial magnetic stimulation. *Exp. Brain Res.* 183, 361–369. doi: 10.1007/s00221-007-1052-7

Luber, B., and Lisanby, S. H. (2014). Enhancement of human cognitive performance using transcranial magnetic stimulation (TMS). *Neuroimage* 85(Pt 3), 961–970. doi: 10.1016/j.neuroimage.2013.06.007

Mantovani, A., Rossi, S., Bassi, B. D., Simpson, H. B., Fallon, B. A., and Lisanby, S. H. (2013). Modulation of motor cortex excitability in obsessive-compulsive disorder: an exploratory study on the relations of neurophysiology measures with clinical outcome. *Psychiatry Res.* 210, 1026–1032. doi: 10.1016/j.psychres.2013.08.054

McCallum, A. K. (2002). *MALLET: A Machine Learning for Language Toolkit.* Available online at: http://mallet.cs.umass.edu

Medina, J., Norise, C., Faseyitan, O., Coslett, H. B., Turkeltaub, P. E., and Hamilton, R. H. (2012). Finding the right words: transcranial magnetic stimulation improves discourse productivity in non-fluent aphasia after stroke. *Aphasiology* 26, 1153–1168. doi: 10.1080/02687038.2012.710316

Meyers, A. (2003). *Multi-Pass Multi-Strategy Nlp.* Available online at: http://www.textanalysis.com/tai-multi2003.pdf

Miniussi, C., and Rossini, P. M. (2011). Transcranial magnetic stimulation in cognitive rehabilitation. *Neuropsychol. Rehabil.* 21, 579–601. doi: 10.1080/09602011.2011.562689

Moreno-Duarte, I., Morse, L. R., Alam, M., Bikson, M., Zafonte, R., and Fregni, F. (2014). Targeted therapies using electrical and magnetic neural stimulation for the treatment of chronic pain in spinal cord injury. *Neuroimage* 85 Pt 3, 1003–1013. doi: 10.1016/j.neuroimage.2013.05.097

Muller, H. M., Rangarajan, A., Teal, T. K., and Sternberg, P. W. (2008). Textpresso for neuroscience: searching the full text of thousands of neuroscience research papers. *Neuroinformatics* 6, 195–204. doi: 10.1007/s12021-008-9031-0

Nitsche, M. A., and Paulus, W. (2009). Noninvasive brain stimulation protocols in the treatment of epilepsy: current state and perspectives. *Neurotherapeutics* 6, 244–250. doi: 10.1016/j.nurt.2009.01.003

Paes, F., Baczynski, T., Novaes, F., Marinho, T., Arias-Carrion, O., Budde, H., et al. (2013). Repetitive transcranial magnetic stimulation (rTMS) to treat social anxiety disorder: case reports and a review of the literature. *Clin. Pract. Epidemiol. Ment. Health* 9, 180–188. doi: 10.2174/174501790130 9010180

Pascual-Leone, A., Valls-Sole, J., Brasil-Neto, J. P., Cammarota, A., Grafman, J., and Hallett, M. (1994). Akinesia in Parkinson's disease. II. Effects of subthreshold repetitive transcranial motor cortex stimulation. *Neurology* 44, 892–898 doi: 10.1212/WNL.44.5.892

Perez-Iratxeta, C., Bork, P., and Andrade, M. A. (2001). XplorMed: a tool for exploring MEDLINE abstracts. *Trends Biochem. Sci.* 26, 573–575 doi: 10.1016/S0968-0004(01)01926-0

Rahnev, D. (2013). Entrainment of neural activity using transcranial magnetic stimulation. *J. Neurosci.* 33, 11325–11326. doi: 10.1523/JNEUROSCI.2012-13.2013

Sandberg, A., and Bostrom, N. (2006). Converging cognitive enhancements. *Ann. N.Y. Acad. Sci.* 1093, 201–227. doi: 10.1196/annals.1382.015

Sarkar, I. N., Schenk, R., Miller, H., and Norton, C. N. (2009). LigerCat: using "MeSH Clouds" from journal, article, or gene citations to facilitate the identification of relevant biomedical literature. *AMIA Annu. Symp. Proc.* 2009, 563–567.

Smalheiser, N. R., Zhou, W., and Torvik, V. I. (2008). Anne O'Tate: a tool to support user-driven summarization, drill-down and browsing of PubMed search results. *J. Biomed. Discov. Collab.* 3:2. doi: 10.1186/1747-5333-3-2

Stanford, A. D., Luber, B., Unger, L., Cycowicz, Y. M., Malaspina, D., and Lisanby, S. H. (2013). Single pulse TMS differentially modulates reward behavior. *Neuropsychologia* 51, 3041–3047. doi: 10.1016/j.neuropsychologia.2013.09.016

Takeuchi, N., Chuma, T., Matsuo, Y., Watanabe, I., and Ikoma, K. (2005). Repetitive transcranial magnetic stimulation of contralesional primary motor cortex improves hand function after stroke. *Stroke* 36, 2681–2686. doi: 10.1161/01.STR.0000189658.51972.34

Vallence, A. M., and Ridding, M. C. (2014). Non-invasive induction of plasticity in the human cortex: uses and limitations. *Cortex* 58C, 261–271. doi: 10.1016/j.cortex.2013.12.006

Vicario, C. M., Candidi, M., and Aglioti, S. M. (2013). Cortico-spinal embodiment of newly acquired, action-related semantic associations. *Brain Stimul.* 6, 952–958. doi: 10.1016/j.brs.2013.05.010

Vicario, C. M., and Nitsche, M. A. (2013). Non-invasive brain stimulation for the treatment of brain diseases in childhood and adolescence: state of the art, current limits and future challenges. *Front. Syst. Neurosci.* 7:94. doi: 10.3389/fnsys.2013.00094

Weaver, L., Rostain, A. L., Mace, W., Akhtar, U., Moss, E., and O'Reardon, J. P. (2012). Transcranial magnetic stimulation (TMS) in the treatment of attention-deficit/hyperactivity disorder in adolescents and young adults: a pilot study. *J. ECT* 28, 98–103. doi: 10.1097/YCT.0b013e31824532c8

Zeimpekis, D., and Gallopoulos, E. (2006). "TMG: a MATLAB toolbox for generating term-document matrices from text collections," in *Grouping Multidimensional Data: Recent Advances in Clustering*, eds J. Kogan, C. Nicholas, and M. Teboulle (Berlin, Heidelberg: Springer), 187–210.

Zhu, M., and Ghodsi, A. (2006). Automatic dimensionality selection from the scree plot via the use of profile likelihood. *Comput. Stat. Data Anal.* 51, 918–930 doi: 10.1016/j.csda.2005.09.010

2

Neural rhythmic symphony of human walking observation: *Upside-down* and *Uncoordinated* condition on cortical theta, alpha, beta and gamma oscillations

David Zarka[1], Carlos Cevallos[1], Mathieu Petieau[1], Thomas Hoellinger[1], Bernard Dan[1,2] and Guy Cheron[1,3]*

[1] *Laboratory of Neurophysiology and Movement Biomechanics, Université Libre de Bruxelles, Brussels, Belgium*
[2] *Department of Neurology, Hopital Universitaire des Enfants reine Fabiola, Université Libre de Bruxelles, Bruxelles, Belgium*
[3] *Laboratory of Electrophysiology, Université de Mons-Hainaut, Bruxelles, Belgium*

Edited by:
Mikhail Lebedev, Duke University, USA

Reviewed by:
Daniel P. Ferris, University of Michigan, USA
Lewis A. Wheaton, Georgia Tech, USA
Miguel Escudero, University of Seville, Spain

Correspondence:
Guy Cheron, Laboratory of Neurophysiology and Movement Biomechanics, Université Libre de Bruxelles, CP 640, 50 Av. F. Roosevelt, 1050 Brussels, Belgium
e-mail: gcheron@ulb.ac.be

Biological motion observation has been recognized to produce dynamic change in sensorimotor activation according to the observed kinematics. Physical plausibility of the spatial-kinematic relationship of human movement may play a major role in the top-down processing of human motion recognition. Here, we investigated the time course of scalp activation during observation of human gait in order to extract and use it on future integrated brain-computer interface using virtual reality (VR). We analyzed event related potentials (ERP), the event related spectral perturbation (ERSP) and the inter-trial coherence (ITC) from high-density EEG recording during video display onset (−200–600 ms) and the steady state visual evoked potentials (SSVEP) inside the video of human walking 3D-animation in three conditions: *Normal*; *Upside-down* (inverted images); and *Uncoordinated* (pseudo-randomly mixed images). We found that early visual evoked response P120 was decreased in *Upside-down* condition. The N170 and P300b amplitudes were decreased in *Uncoordinated* condition. In *Upside-down* and *Uncoordinated* conditions, we found decreased alpha power and theta phase-locking. As regards gamma oscillation, power was increased during the *Upside-down* animation and decreased during the *Uncoordinated* animation. An SSVEP-like response oscillating at about 10 Hz was also described showing that the oscillating pattern is enhanced 300 ms after the heel strike event only in the *Normal* but not in the *Upside-down* condition. Our results are consistent with most of previous point-light display studies, further supporting possible use of virtual reality for neurofeedback applications.

Keywords: ERP, ERSP, ITC, SSVEP, walking, observation, virtual reality

INTRODUCTION

Neuronal processing of the visual system allows us to perceive objects, movements, colors, contrasts, and to represent the space around us with a very high resolution. In addition to the classical dichotomy between the ventral stream (the "What" pathway) supporting object vision and a dorsal stream (the "Where" pathway), a more recent conception based on clinical evidence (Kravitz et al., 2011) divides the dorsal stream into three sub-pathways projecting on to the premotor (supporting visually-guided actions), the prefrontal and the medial temporal lobes (supporting spatial working memory) both directly and through the posterior cingulate and retrosplenial areas (supporting navigation). This emphasizes the contribution of numerous functionally specialized, hierarchically organized visual areas giving rise to a conscious perception of the different attributes of the visual scene (Zeki et al., 1991; Singer, 1999). The discovery of the phase-locking mechanism at the level of the cortical neurons producing gamma oscillation (Gray et al., 1989) constitutes a strong scientific foundation for the binding by synchrony hypothesis (Singer, 1999) and has also paved the way for non-invasive investigation of the implicated mechanisms by electroencephalography (EEG) and event-related potentials (ERP) (Makeig et al., 2002; Cheron et al., 2007, 2014; Cebolla et al., 2009, 2014). New approaches of signal analysis (Delorme and Makeig, 2004) have permitted to better understand the genesis of the sensory evoked responses including visual motion in VR environment (Gramann et al., 2009; Cheron et al., 2014) and the origin of the movement gating of sensory evoked responses (Cebolla et al., 2009).

The discovery of mirror neurons responding similarly when the monkey performs an action and when it observes the experimenter performing the same action (Rizzolatti et al., 1996) has led to human studies of visual processes involved in recognition (Blake and Shiffrar, 2007; Avanzini et al., 2013; Di Dio et al., 2013), prediction of others' movements (Csibra, 2007; Kilner et al., 2007), and their implication in social cognition (Jacob and Jeannerod, 2005; Schütz-Bosbach and Prinz, 2007; Heyes, 2010; Press et al., 2011). Behavioral, neuroimaging and neurophysiological data have demonstrated a high sensitivity to reference frame (Pavlova and Sokolov, 2000; Pavlova et al., 2004; McGlothlin et al., 2012), human body form (Downing et al., 2001), kinematics of human movement (Avanzini et al., 2012; McAleer et al., 2014), gender and personal traits (Pollick et al., 2005; Troje et al., 2005; McGlothlin et al., 2012). Several studies demonstrated that shape and motion information are treated separately by ventral and dorsal visual streams, and converge to the posterior portion of superior temporal sulcus (Vaina et al., 2001; Giese and Poggio, 2003; Blake and Shiffrar, 2007). Moreover, the motor theory of perception, based on the fact that movement perception is influenced by the implicit knowledge about the working principles of the motor control system (Viviani and Stucchi, 1992; Rizzolatti and Craighero, 2004), give a critical place to ventral premotor cortex in biological motion perception processes (Saygin et al., 2004).

By extending Darwin's evolutionary perspective about face emotion (Darwin, 1872) to human locomotion, we may advance that the recognition of the human primate by its bipedal locomotion already present in early hominid before stone tools and large brains (Leakey and Walker, 1997) is probably one of the most vital activities of human in a selection retrospective view. Moreover, such human gestures may represent a constitutive element of the emotional body language (De Gelder, 2006, for a review). This whole body movement of *homo sapiens* is characterized by distinctive patterns of smooth, regular, alternated lower and upper limbs movements performed around a relatively fixed and erected posture of the head and trunk segment (Pozzo et al., 1990). Another remarkable element is the heel-strike considered as an acquired character of African and Asian apes linked closely to knuckle walking quadrupedalism (Thorpe et al., 2007; Crompton et al., 2010). These highly recognizable elements would implicate that human mirror neuron systems should be active when watching somebody else walk (Cheng et al., 2005).

Thanks to dynamics analysis of high-density EEG associating event-related potential (ERP), event-related spectral perturbation (ERSP) and inter-trial coherency (ITC), it has become possible to identify electrophysiological mechanisms related to recognition processes (Engel et al., 1997; Singer, 2009). In this context, coherent stimulus representation, including biological motion (Pavlova et al., 2004), are thought to result from binding of widely distributed cell ensembles by synchronizing their high-frequency oscillation activity (Tallon-Baudry and Bertrand, 1999; Singer, 2009). In parallel, other oscillatory processes may be activated following a motor template as suggested for mu rhythm (Ulloa and Pineda, 2007; Arnstein et al., 2011; Braadbaart et al., 2013; Urgen et al., 2013; Frenkel-Toledo et al., 2014). Point-light display of human locomotion has been used to characterized the cortical activity involved in recognition of locomotion either through MEG (Pavlova et al., 2004, 2006) or ERP studies (Hirai et al., 2003, 2005, 2013; Jokisch et al., 2005; Hirai and Hiraki, 2006; Krakowski et al., 2011; Buzzell et al., 2013).

Here, we studied the ERP and dynamics of theta, alpha, beta and gamma oscillations induced by the observation of an animated avatar in a virtual reality (VR). We hypothesized that physical plausibility of the spatial-kinematic of human locomotion plays a major role in different modes of neural processing (bottom-up and top-down) implicated in locomotion recognition: we expect that these processes will be reflected in different contributions of rhythmic power and phase-locked perturbation in different frequency bands and cortical areas. To address this question, we used an animation representing a human mannequin during walking action performed in normal, *Uncoordinated* kinematics and in *Upside-down* views. This will offer the possibility to extract the dynamic signature of human walking observation with respect to the neural activity evoked by the same image content but in an unusual frame of reference (*Upside-down* view) or without respect to normal kinematics (*Uncoordinated* walk) from the EEG signals.

MATERIALS AND METHODS

ARTICIPANTS

Sixteen healthy volunteers took part in this study (ten males, mean age 25.9 years, range 18–35 years). All subjects were right-handed, had *Normal* or corrected-to-*Normal* vision, were naive with respect to the purpose of the experiment, and gave informed consent. The experiment was performed with the approval of the ethics committee of Université Libre de Bruxelles and realized in accordance with the ethical standards of the 1964 Declaration of Helsinki.

STIMULI

Visual stimuli consisted of an animation in the center of the screen representing human walking mannequin (from Cal3D Library) that was presented in three different ways: *Normal* walking (N), *Upside-down* (U), and *Uncoordinated* (J) (**Figure 1**). Each animation was organized in 22 blocks of 10 s duration interspersed by 7–12 s of random periods of gray screen. This allowed us to obtain a repetitive control of the baseline state throughout the whole recording session and facilitated the recording of the averaged responses (see below). For the *Normal* walking condition, each block was initiated by an image representing the heel strike event of the right leg and was ended by the last image preceding the next heels strike of the right leg picture (**Figure 1A**). The animation had a 10 Hz frequency. In the *Upside-down* condition the same successive pictures were merely inverted, keeping the same kinematics sequences. In the *Uncoordinated* condition the first image remained the same as the *Normal* condition while all the others were randomly mixed giving rise to an incoherent *Uncoordinated* movement. The random sequence was conserved for each trial and each subject (**Figure 1B**).

We have calculated the luminosity of each image in the three colors (RGB) by using "imread" MATLab function. This function stores in a matrix the composition in red, green and blue of each pixel of an image. For each frame of the animation, we subtracted this matrix to that of the previous frame. We have then computed the mean of the resulting matrix and called this composition "dynamic contrast." This represents overall change between two successive frames of the composition in luminosity of the same located pixels.

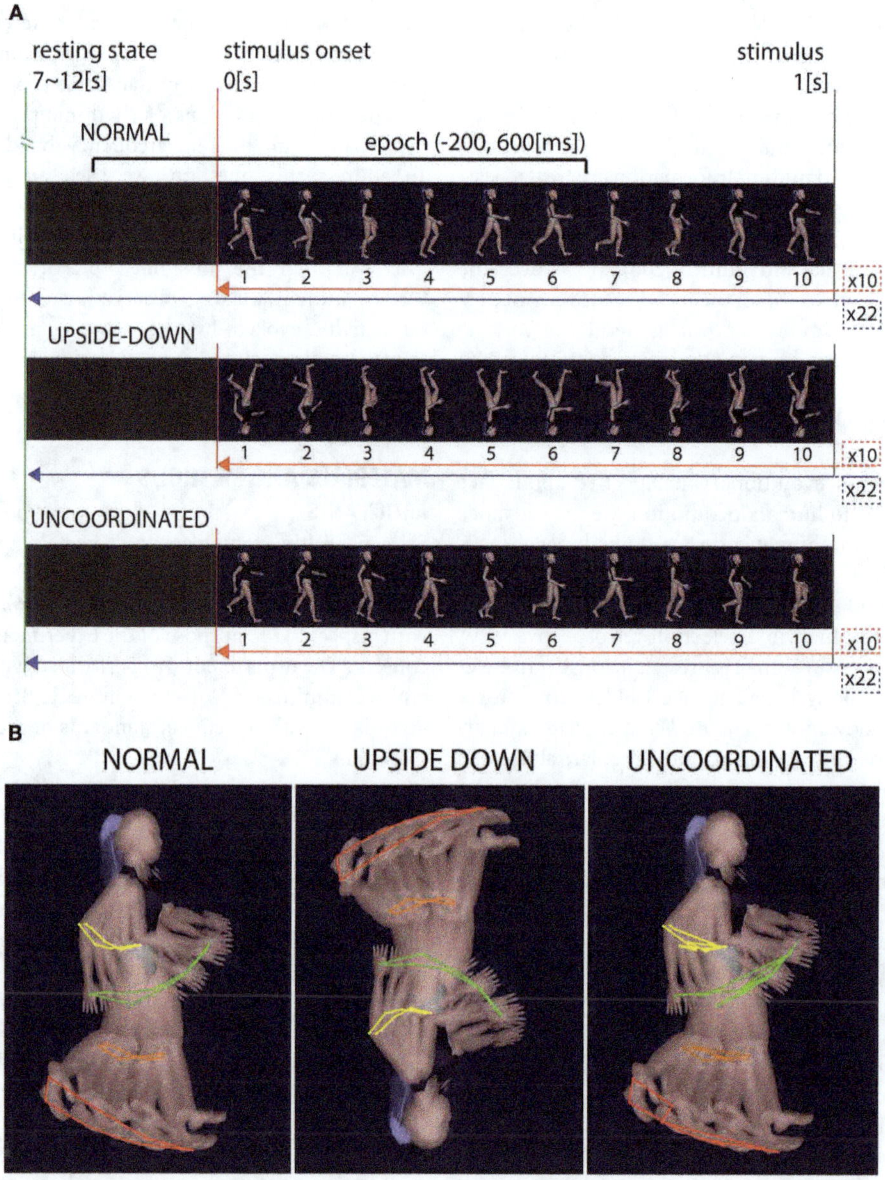

FIGURE 1 | Condition's stimuli. (A) Time representation of the stimuli in each three conditions. *Normal* condition shows ten successive gait cycles of 1 s each. Trials were separated by 7–12 s of gray screen and repeated 22 times. *Upside-down* condition show the same images sequence, rotated to 180° in the image plane. *Uncoordinated* condition show the same first image as the *Normal* condition while all the others images were mixed. **(B)** Kinematics representation of the gait in the three conditions. While *Normal* and *Upside-down* conditions have the same coherent kinematic sequence, *Uncoordinated* condition show an incoherent kinematic sequence.

EXPERIMENTAL SETUP

The recording was realized in a single session. EEG was recorded in 128 channels (ANT system, *The Netherlands*) at a sampling frequency of 2048 Hz and with a resolution of 22 bits (71.5 nV per bit). An active-shield cap using 128 Ag/AgCl sintered ring electrodes and shielded co-axial cables (5–10 electrode system placements) was comfortably adjusted to subject head. All electrodes were referred to left earlobe. Impedance was lowered below 10 kΩ for each electrode and checked before each recording. Displays were presented on a 17″ Dell computer screen. Participants looked straight ahead at the computer screen through a form-fitting facemask and a circular barrel (cylinder). The screen was centered on the line of gaze at a distance of ~30 cm from the eyes. Viewing through the barrel removed any external visual references. In addition, subjects had earplugs to isolate from external hearing disturbance. For eight subjects, we presented in three successive sessions the *Normal* walking condition, then *Upside-down* walking and then *Uncoordinated* one *(No-Random group)*. For eight other subjects, conditions were presented randomly in three successive sessions (*Random* group). We made a pause between each session in order to limit the effect of fatigue. As the aim of this study was to evaluate the effect of purposeless perception on the brain rhythms, no particular attentional task was required. However, the state of awareness was continuously checked by online EEG (absence of slow rhythm linked to drowsiness) and EOG, for which we placed electrodes above, below, right and left of the right eye. In particular, we checked that the blink number and configuration remained unchanged throughout the experimental session. We used an in-house script that counts the number of blinks by incrementing an index for each potential higher than 250 μV, and calculates the interval between blinks to provide a view of their configuration over time. We then calculated the number of saccades by EOG derived function. The results show there is no difference between conditions for blink (means by subject for *Normal*: 81 ± 33.3; *Upside-down*: 99.8 ± 27.2; *Uncoordinated*: 120.4 ± 34.6) and saccades (means by subject for *Normal*: 316 ± 137.8; *Upside-down*: 455.4 ± 98.3; *Uncoordinated*: 385.2 ± 136.6).

DATA TREATMENT

Off-line data treatment and analysis was performed by means of EEGLAB software (Delorme and Makeig, 2004; Brunner et al., 2013) and in-house MATLAB-based tools (Cheron et al., 2014). DC offset was removed, then band pass filter 0.1–80 Hz and notch filter around 50 Hz (47.5–52.5 Hz) were applied to attenuate electrical artifacts. Portions of data and defective electrodes (max. 6%) were removed by careful visual inspection. Ocular (blink and saccade) and any other remaining artifacts (muscular, cardiac) were isolated by ICA algorithm decomposition. We used the scalp topography, temporal activity localization and spectra magnitude criterion to identify ICA related to artifact. In case of doubt the rejection occurred only if all experimenters involved in data treatment reached agreement. After ICA rejection, defective electrodes were spherically interpolated.

Two analyses were performed: animation onset analysis and SSVEP analysis. In the animation onset analysis, data were organized in epochs corresponding to intervals [−1000; 3000] ms, centered on animation onset. We rejected epochs according to ±100 μV threshold criterion, and we made a visual review to confirm epoch rejection. In total, we obtained 17 ± 5 epochs per subject ($n = 16$) and per condition ($n = 3$). A study design was used to average data from subjects for each condition. A time window of 1000 ms before stimulus onset was used as baseline.

In SSVEP analysis, data were organized in epochs corresponding to intervals [−200; 600] ms, centered on each heel strike except for the first and the last one. As in preceding analysis, we applied ±100 μV threshold criterion confirmed by a visual review. In total, we obtained 159 ± 16) epochs per subject ($n = 16$) and per condition ($n = 3$). We performed a grand average study including 2065 ± 26 trials for each condition. The interval [−200; 0] ms was used as baseline, and the first and last heel strikes were excluded from the analysis In this case, the SSVEP analysis was independent of the neutral black screen periods allowing to join mixed *Random* and *Non-Random* groups.

A subset of 32 electrodes was explored for each measure analysis: O2, Oz, O1, POz, P8, P4, Pz, P3, P7, CP6, CP2, CP1, CP5, T8, C4, Cz, C3, T7, FC6, FC2, FC1, FC5, F8, F4, Fz, F3, F7, Fp2, Fpz, Fp1. We first checked ERP and ERSP of [−1000; 3000] ms epoch, and then we focused on events related to animation onset, and SSVEP centered on heel strike between −200 and 600 ms. ERP, ERSP, and ITC analysis was performed. Difference between *Random* and *No-Random* groups and between *Normal* and both *Upside-down* and *Uncoordinated* condition were performed by EEGLab non-parametric permutation test ($n = 2000$) at each trial latency of the average ERPs and every time-frequency point for ERSP and ITC.

RESULTS

EVENT-RELATED POTENTIAL

The first noticeable ERP component referenced to the earlobe elicited after the onset of the VR-animation was the P120 component recorded in occipito-parietal electrodes. Analysis revealed a peak reduction in *Upside-down* condition with respect to *Normal* condition over occipito-parietal regions. The next component was the N170 mainly recorded over the occipito-parietal regions (**Figure 2**). We observed a significant decrease in *Uncoordinated* condition over occipital and parieto-lateral regions. This was followed by a large P300 component ending at about 500 ms in occipital regions and 400 ms in frontal regions. In order to simplify the description of condition effect, we subdivided P300 in the two classical P300a and P300b components (**Figure 2**). The P300a component was significantly smaller in the *Upside-down* condition over parietal regions with respect to the *Normal* situation, whereas the P300b component remained the same. On the contrary in the *Uncoordinated* condition, the P300a component was not modified whereas the P300b showed a significant decrease in occipital and parietal regions (**Table 1**). Comparison between *Random* and *No-Random* group revealed no significant difference between their respective conditions except in the P300 amplitude in parietal region which was greater for the *No-Random* group for the 3 conditions.

EVENT-RELATED SPECTRAL PERTURBATION AND INTER-TRIAL COHERENCE

Whatever the observed condition (**Figures 3–5**), the video onset triggered throughout the scalp a theta ERS in the [0; 500] ms interval followed by an alpha ERD initiated at about 200 ms and maintained during all the duration of the video. This alpha ERD was accompanied by a beta ERD which was more pronounced in the *Uncoordinated* condition (**Figure 5**). The *Normal* presentation induced a gamma ERD at about 700 ms and maintained for all the duration of the video in the left sensori-motor region (**Figure 3**, CP5 electrode). This gamma ERD was not present in the two others conditions (**Figures 4, 5**).

In the [−200;600] ms time-window, the *Normal* condition was characterized by the following observations (**Figures 6–9**): (1) at the latency of the P120, ERSP plots showed an earlier alpha ERS reaching maximal value in the parietal region and extending to the beta band in the parieto-central region. (2) This was sustained by theta activation and phase-locking presenting its maximal value at about 200 ms. (3) ERD in the upper alpha band at about 200 ms in the occipito-parietal regions. (4) ERS clusters in the gamma range (30–70 Hz) in the parieto-occipital and centro-frontal regions.

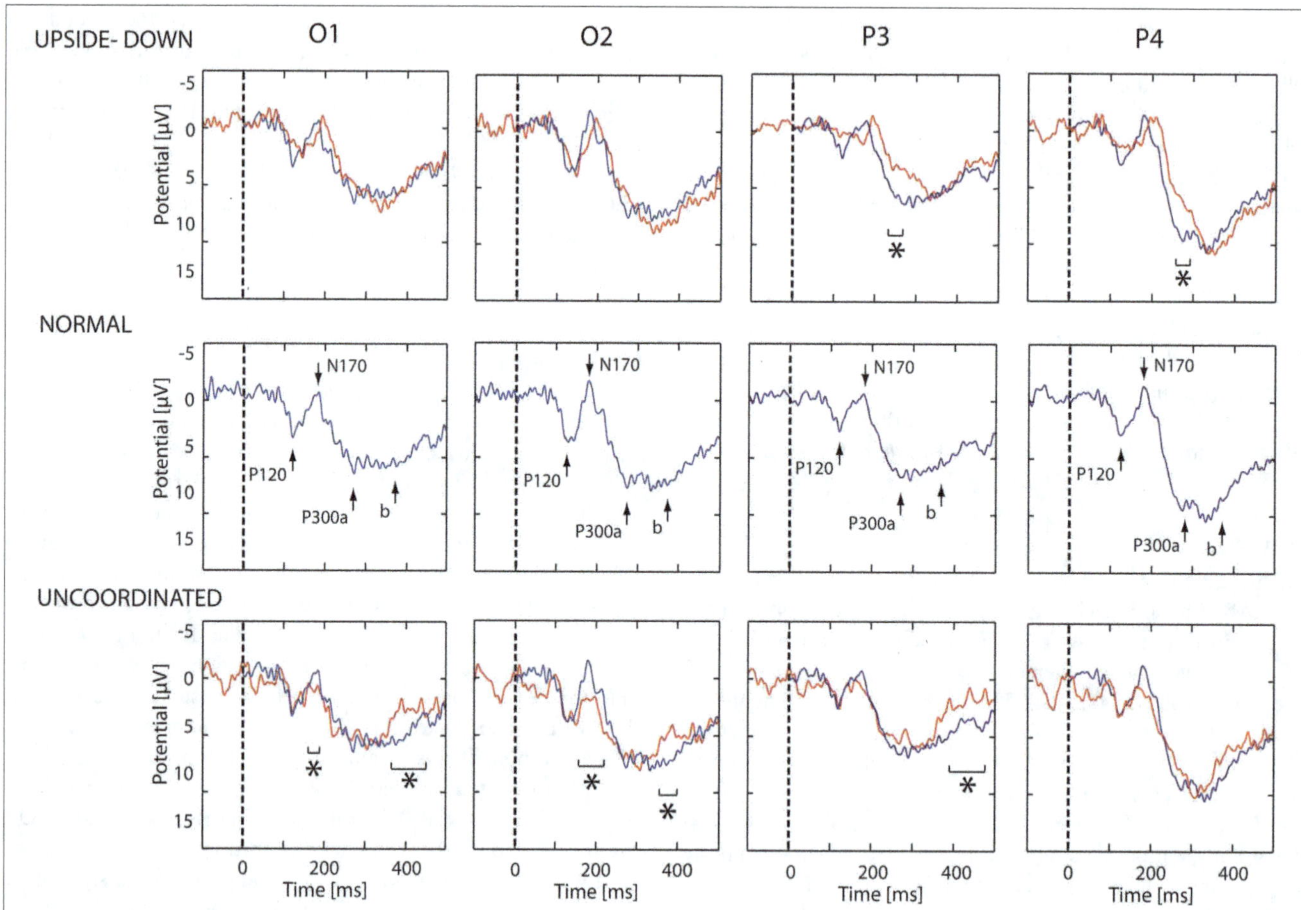

FIGURE 2 | ERP evoked by animation onset in each condition. ERP recorded in O1, O2, P3, and P4 electrodes. In middle part, the ERP evoked by the normal animation onset show three successive potentials: P120, N170, and P300a,b. In upper part, the blue and red lines show respectively the ERP response in the *Normal* and *Upside-down* condition. In lower part, the blue and red lines show respectively the ERP response in the *Normal* and *Uncoordinated* conditions. Significant differences are mark by asterisks ($p < 0.05$).

With respect to the *Normal* condition, in the *Upside-down* condition, three significant changes were noted (**Figures 6–9**): (1) a decrease in alpha-beta power between 100 and 500 ms over occipital to frontal regions, resulting in a lack of ERS in alpha bands at the latency of the P120, and an increased alpha-beta ERD at about 200–500 ms; (2) a decrease of the theta phase-locking in the parieto-central regions; (3) an increase in (gamma) 40 and 60 Hz ERS over occipito-central regions, respectively at about 150 and 350 ms latency (**Table 1**).

With respect to the *Normal* condition, in the *Uncoordinated* condition the following was observed (**Figures 6–9**): (1) a decrease of alpha-beta band at the latency of the P120, followed by an earlier and greater alpha-beta ERD over the occipito-parietal region; (2) a reduction of theta phase-locking. However, in contrast to the *Upside-down* and *Normal* condition, (3) the *Uncoordinated* animation produced a gamma 40–60 Hz ERD at about 200–500 ms over occipito-central regions (**Table 1**). The analysis of the dynamic contrast of the image showed that the *Uncoordinated* condition presented an increased contrast between the third and the fourth image (400 ms after the onset) with respect to the two other conditions.

STEADY STATE VISUAL EVOKED POTENTIALS

When the heel strike of the right leg was used as trigger, the average trace corresponded to an oscillatory pattern peaking at about 9 Hz. (8.86 Hz). This was observed for all subjects and conditions and may be considered as a SSVEP induced by the frequency of the video. **Figure 10** illustrates the SSVEP traces resulting from a grand average of all the 16 subjects which conserve the 9 Hz oscillating pattern presented in each single subject. However, the amplitude of the grand average oscillation was not constant throughout the time period. The first negative peak occurred close to 100 ms after the heel strike in any of the 3 different conditions (**Figure 10A**). For *Normal* and *Upside-Down* condition the SSVEP amplitude increased after the heel strike and culminated at a latency of 300 ms (negative peak) only in the *Normal* condition. Thereafter, the oscillating pattern decreased in *Normal* and *Upside-down* condition but was maintained in the *Uncoordinated* condition.

The *Upside-down* condition showed a significant decrease of the third negative SSVEP component at 300 ms with respect to the *Normal* condition over parieto-occipital regions (**Figure 10A,**

Table 1 | Summary of statistical analysis about the 32 selected electrodes for both conditions *Upside-down* (U) and *Uncoordinated* (J) vs. Normal (N).

A

Conditions	**U–N**		**J–N**	
ERP	**P120**	**P300a**	**N170**	**P300b**
Frontal				
Central				
Temporal			***T8	
Parietal	**P3, *P7, ***Pz, *P4	*P3, *Pz, **P4, ***P8, ***CP6	**P7, **P8	*P3, *Pz
Occipital	**O1		**O1, **Oz, ***O2	**O1, **Oz, **POz, *O2

B

ERSP/U-N	**Alpha-Beta ERS/ERD**	**Gamma (40 Hz) ERS**	**Gamma (60 Hz) ERS**
Frontal	***Fz		
Central	***C3, ***Cz, ***FC1, ***FC2		
Temporal			
Parietal	***P3, ***CP1, ***CP5, ***Pz	***P3, ***P7, ***CP5, ***P4	***P3, ***P7, ***CP1, ***CP5, ***P4, ***CP2, ***CP6
Occipital	***O1, ***O2	***O1, ***POz, ***O2	***O1, ***Oz, ***O2, ***POz

C

ERSP/J–N	**Alpha-Beta ERS/ERD**	**Gamma (40–60 Hz) ERD**
Frontal		
Central	***C3, ***Cz	***C3, ***C4
Temporal		
Parietal	***P3, ***P7, ***CP1, ***CP5, ***Pz, **P4, ***P8, ***CP2	***P3, ***P7, **Pz, ***CP1, ***CP5, ***CP2, ***CP6
Occipital	***O1, ***Oz, ***POz, ***O2	***O1, ***Oz, ***POz, ***O2

D

SSVEP	**U–N 300 ms**	**J–N 400 ms**
Frontal		
Central	***C3, **Cz	
Temporal		
Parietal	***CP1, **P3, ***Pz, **P4, **CP2	***CP5, **CP1, ***P3, ***Pz, **P4, **CP2
Occipital	***O1, ***Oz, ***POz, ***O2	***O1, ***Oz, ***POz, ***O2

*(A) ERP for P120, N170, P300a, and P300b amplitudes. (B) ERSP and ITC for U vs. N. (C) ERSP and ITC for J vs. N. Only the electrodes showing significant results are represented (***0.001, **0.01). The reduction in theta phase locking (ITC) is indexed by gray shading (dark $p < 0.001$, light $p < 0.01$). (D) SSVEP behavior differences.*

left part; **Table 1**). The reduction of the ascending phase slope of this negativity in the *Upside-Down* condition was accompanied over parieto-occipital regions by a power increase in beta-gamma band at about 250 ms and later by a power increase in gamma band (60 Hz) at about 400 ms (**Figure 10B**, *left part*). These effects were preceded by a decrease of theta-alpha bands ITC at about 120 ms with respect to the *Normal* condition (**Figure 10B**, *left part*).

The *Uncoordinated* condition showed a significant increase of the SSVEP negativity at about 400 ms with respect to the *Normal* condition (**Figure 10A**, *right part*; **Table 1**). This was preceded by an ERD in the theta–alpha band (**Figure 10B**) over parieto-occipital regions. While the higher amplitude of the first negative peak recorded in this condition remained under the significance level (**Figure 10A**, *right part*) it was accompanied by a significant increase of theta-alpha bands power at about 100 ms with respect to the *Normal* condition. These effects were followed by successive decrease and then increase of theta-alpha ITC respectively at about 350 and 450 ms (**Figure 10B**, *right part*).

DISCUSSION

To our knowledge, this work represents the first study on the dynamic neural response elicited by VR-animation of human walking. The presentation of the VR-animation elicits ERP components classically described in response to a visual stimulation (Jeffreys, 1996). We demonstrate significant changes in the amplitude of the P120 and P300a when the avatar

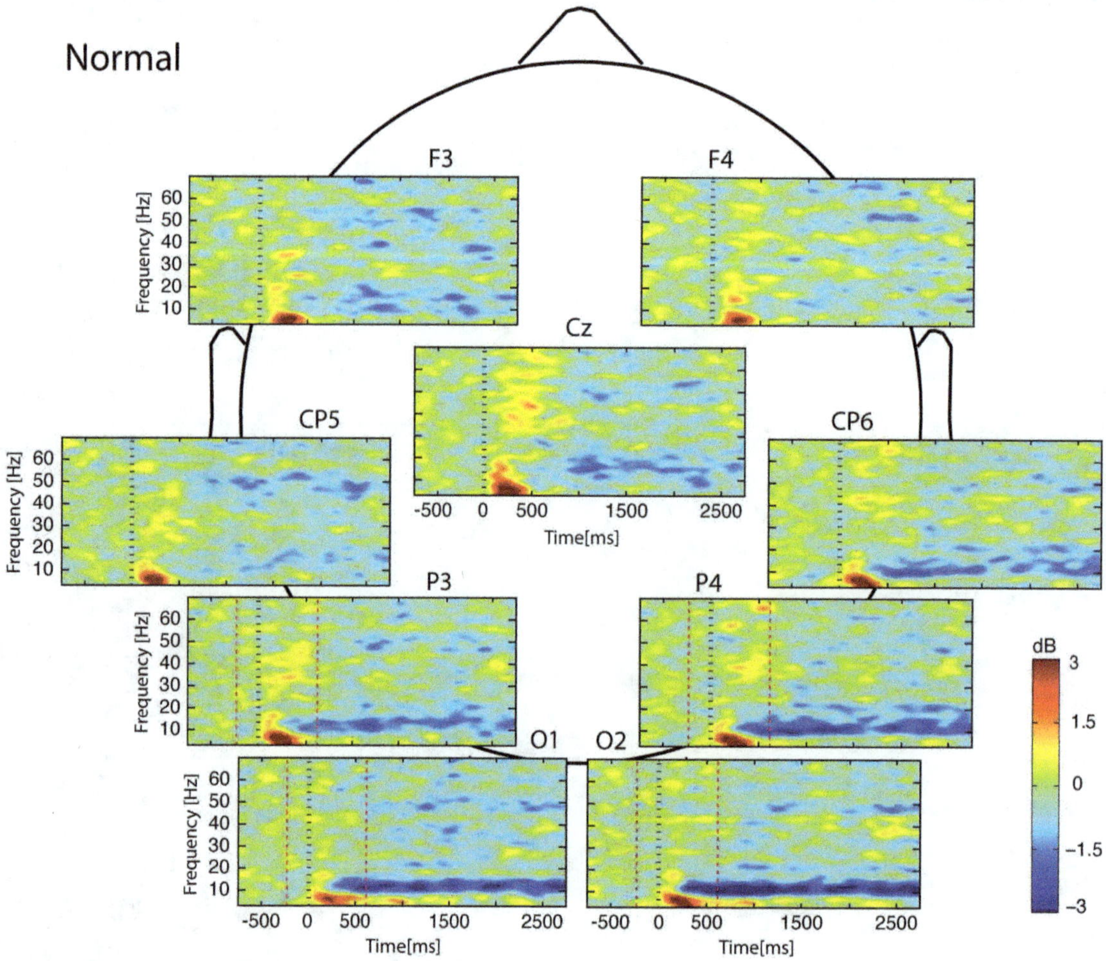

FIGURE 3 | Scalp ERSP on [−1000; 3000] ms in *Normal* condition. Rhythmic activity can be splits in two parts: [0; 500] ms which contains responses evoked by animation onset; and [500; 3000] ms of maintaining task. Note that bilateral alpha-beta ERD was continue from 200 to 3000 ms, and gamma ERD at about 700 ms, maintained for the 3000 ms in the left sensori-motor region. Red lines delimit epochs analyzed: [−200; 600] ms.

was upside-down, and the N170 and P300b when the walking sequence was perturbed (*Uncoordinated*) with respect to the *Normal* condition.

The presence of the early alpha ERS characterize the *Normal* condition. The alpha-beta ERD was reinforced and the theta phase-locking was disturbed in *Upside-down* and *Uncoordinated* condition. As regards gamma oscillation, a contrasting situation was seen as its power was increased in association with the *Upside-down* animation and decreased with the *Uncoordinated* animation.

An SSVEP-like response oscillating at about 9 Hz was also described when the heel strike event was used as trigger, showing that the oscillating pattern is enhanced 300 ms after the heel strike event only in the *Normal* but not in the *Upside-Down* condition.

ERP

The present ERP components evoked by avatar observation are in accordance with those recorded in previous studies using point-light paradigm (Johansson, 1973). The timing of P120, N170, and P300 are commonly regarded as corresponding to the main three components P1 around 130 ms, N1 at 200 ms and N2 (P3 depending of the type and the placement of reference electrode) at 300–400 ms described in point-light walking studies (Hirai et al., 2003, 2005, 2009, 2013; Jokisch et al., 2005; Krakowski et al., 2011; Buzzell et al., 2013).

Although point-light and VR displays concern the same biological motion, VR display induced a stronger visual representation, including form and color than point-light walking. VR display conserved body structure in the *Normal*, *Upside-down*, and *Uncoordinated* conditions. This was not the case in point-light studies, where inverted condition associate form recognition to motion, and scramble condition deconstruct body form. In this context, the present VR-paradigm offers the possibility to dissociate recognition of body form occurring at the first video frame, and motion coherence (smoothness, coordination, speed, etc.) produced by the successive frames. This allows to focus specifically on the effect induced by changing the frame of reference in *Upside-down* and the global coherency of the walking motion in *Uncoordinated*.

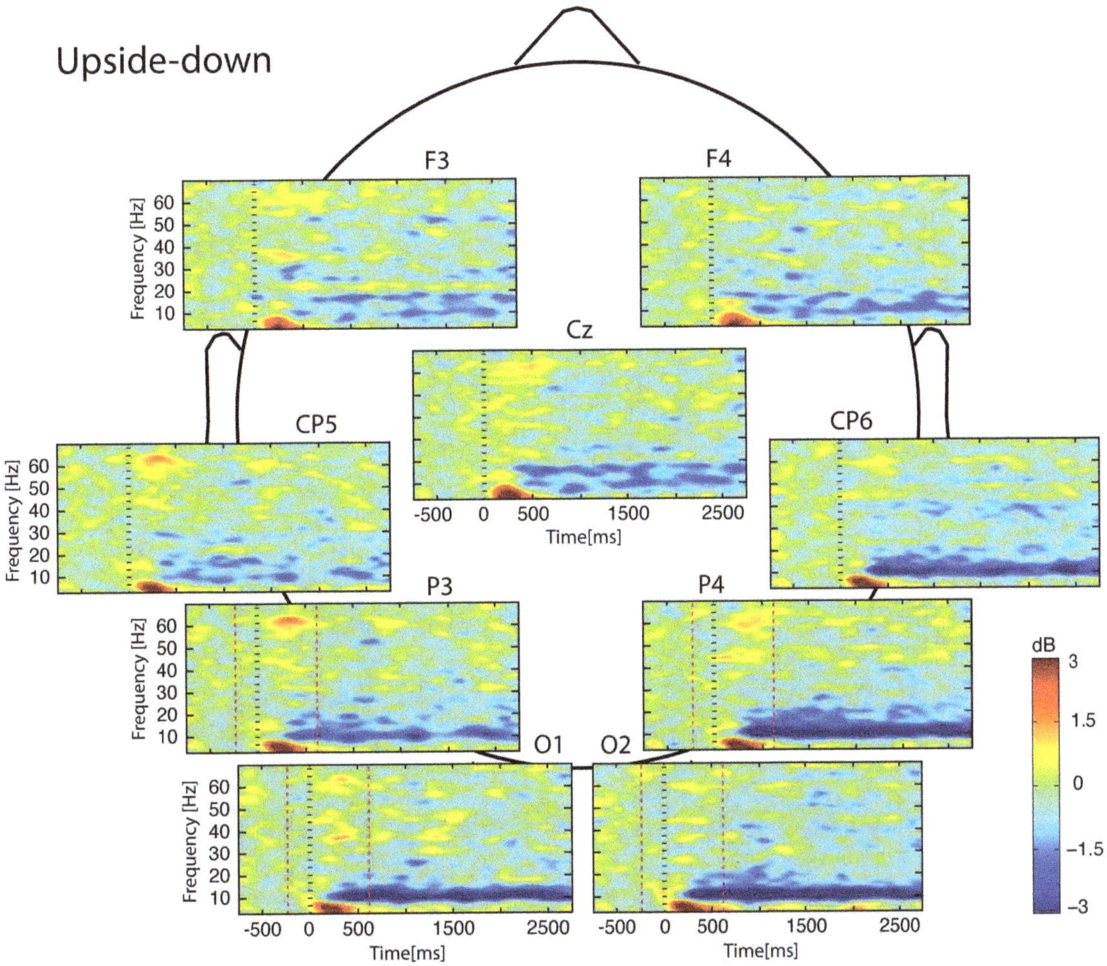

FIGURE 4 | Scalp ERSP on [−1000; 3000] ms in *Upside-down* condition. Rhythmic activity can be splits in two parts: [0; 500] ms which contains responses evoked by animation onset; and [500; 3000] ms of maintaining task. Note that bilateral alpha-beta ERD was continue from 200 to 3000 ms. Red lines delimit epochs analyzed: [−200; 600] ms.

The similarity of P120 evoked by the *Normal* and the *Uncoordinated* conditions is consistent with the fact that the first image is the same in these conditions. In contrast, point-light studies showed a delay and a decrease in P1 response elicited by scramble condition with respect to upright condition (Hirai et al., 2009, 2013; Krakowski et al., 2011). These results support common interpretation that first component reflects a global representation coding of form (Baccus et al., 2009; Buzzell et al., 2013; White et al., 2014). However, the finding of decrease P120 in the *Upside-down* condition with respect to the *Normal* condition was not reported by previous point-light studies. The origin of this early alteration can be explained by both bottom-up and/or top-down process. Distinctions between these influences are not easy. The *Normal* presentation of the avatar may unconsciously induce an easy visual representation than the *Upside-down* mannequin which implies a mental transformation of the reference frame. In parallel, the repeated presentation of normal or inverted locomotion can predictively influence this early response by a top-down effect exerted by the frontal cortex to the primary visual cortex (Peyrin et al., 2010; Cardin et al., 2011; Zanto et al., 2011; Ramalingam et al., 2013). However, previous studies suggest that explicitly attended tasks process does not appear to influence the earlier activity at about 100 ms (Krakowski et al., 2011; Buzzell et al., 2013).

Concerning later activation, N1 and N2 were generally related to integration of form and motion (Baccus et al., 2009; Buzzell et al., 2013; White et al., 2014). It is interesting to note that the effects of *Uncoordinated* condition on N170 (analogous to N1 in point-light studies) and of point-light scramble on N1 are comparable, as N170 was reduced in *Uncoordinated* condition as N1 in scramble condition (Hirai et al., 2003, 2013; Jokisch et al., 2005). This result suggests that N170 was mainly related to motion. In contrast, P300a (analogous to N2 in point-light studies) amplitude was the same in *Normal* and *Uncoordinated* conditions, whereas N2 was larger in upright point-light walker than point-light scramble (Jokisch et al., 2005; Hirai et al., 2013). Moreover, P300a amplitude was smaller in *Upside-down* than in *Normal*. This could also be related to the alteration of the SSVEP pattern occurring at this latency in the

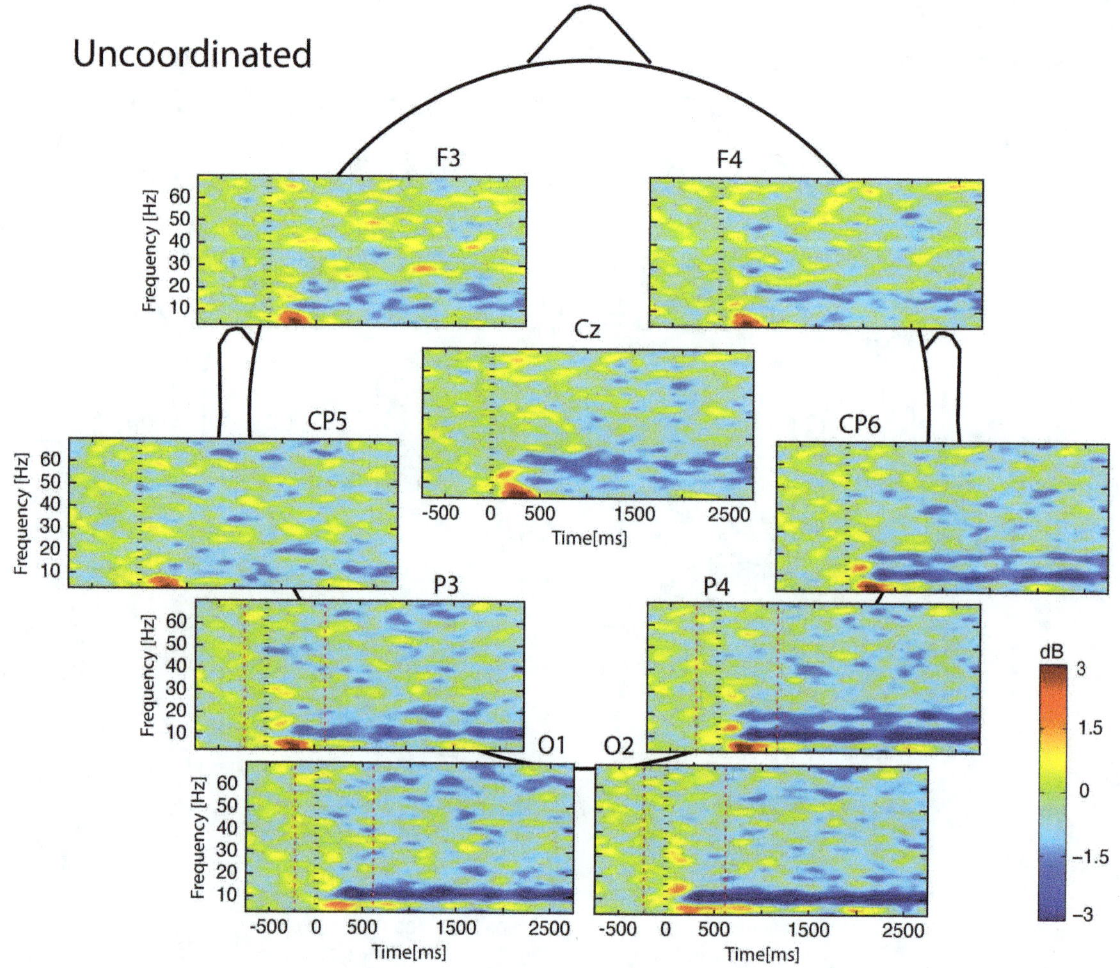

FIGURE 5 | Scalp ERSP on [−1000; 3000] ms in *Uncoordinated* condition. Rhythmic activity can be splits in two parts: [0; 500] ms which contains responses evoked by animation onset; and [500; 3000] ms of maintaining task. Note bilateral that alpha-beta ERD was continue from 200 to 3000 ms. Red lines delimit epochs analyzed: [−200; 600] ms.

Upside-down vs. *Normal* condition. Taken together these results suggest that P300a was mainly related to the global form of walking.

Finally, the effect we recorded on P300b and in the SSVEP at about the same latency in the *Uncoordinated* condition is comparable to the late phase describe by Krakowski et al. (2011), which was characterized by a greater positivity in response to upright and inverted point-light walker than point-light scramble. This last phase after 400 ms is generally considered as indexing a high-order representation coding (Krakowski et al., 2011). This effect observed in *Uncoordinated* suggests that P300b component is sensitive to coherence of motion rather to mere recognition of walking.

ERSP AND ITC

Alpha ERS/ERD

The significant alpha ERS occurring at about 120 ms in the occipito-parietal regions characterized the *Normal* walking observation. It was followed by an alpha-beta ERD at 200 ms, which extends throughout the video. This was significantly more pronounced in *Upside-down* and *Uncoordinated* conditions than in *Normal*.

The first alpha ERS is in accordance with recent studies showing similar transient alpha increase in response to upright facial motion (Girges et al., 2014). The suppression of the early alpha ERS in *Upside-down* suggest that the inversion of the body presentation rapidly affect the early visual process. However, similar alteration found for the *Uncoordinated* condition while the first image was exactly the same suggests a top-down influence. Alpha oscillation has been interpreted as reflecting global inhibition of the cortex, improving behavioral performance by facilitation of the cognitive control (Klimesch et al., 1996, 2003, 2007; Klimesch, 1999, 2012; Cheron et al., 2006; Haegens et al., 2010). Thus, increase in alpha power (ERS) may participate to a general clearance of noise or distracting event in order to selectively update relevant incoming information (Sadaghiani et al., 2012), and access to memory (Klimesch, 2012). In this context, suppression of alpha ERS in *Upside-down* and *Uncoordinated* conditions would be correlated with increase of attention to motion cue and involvement of cognitive resources.

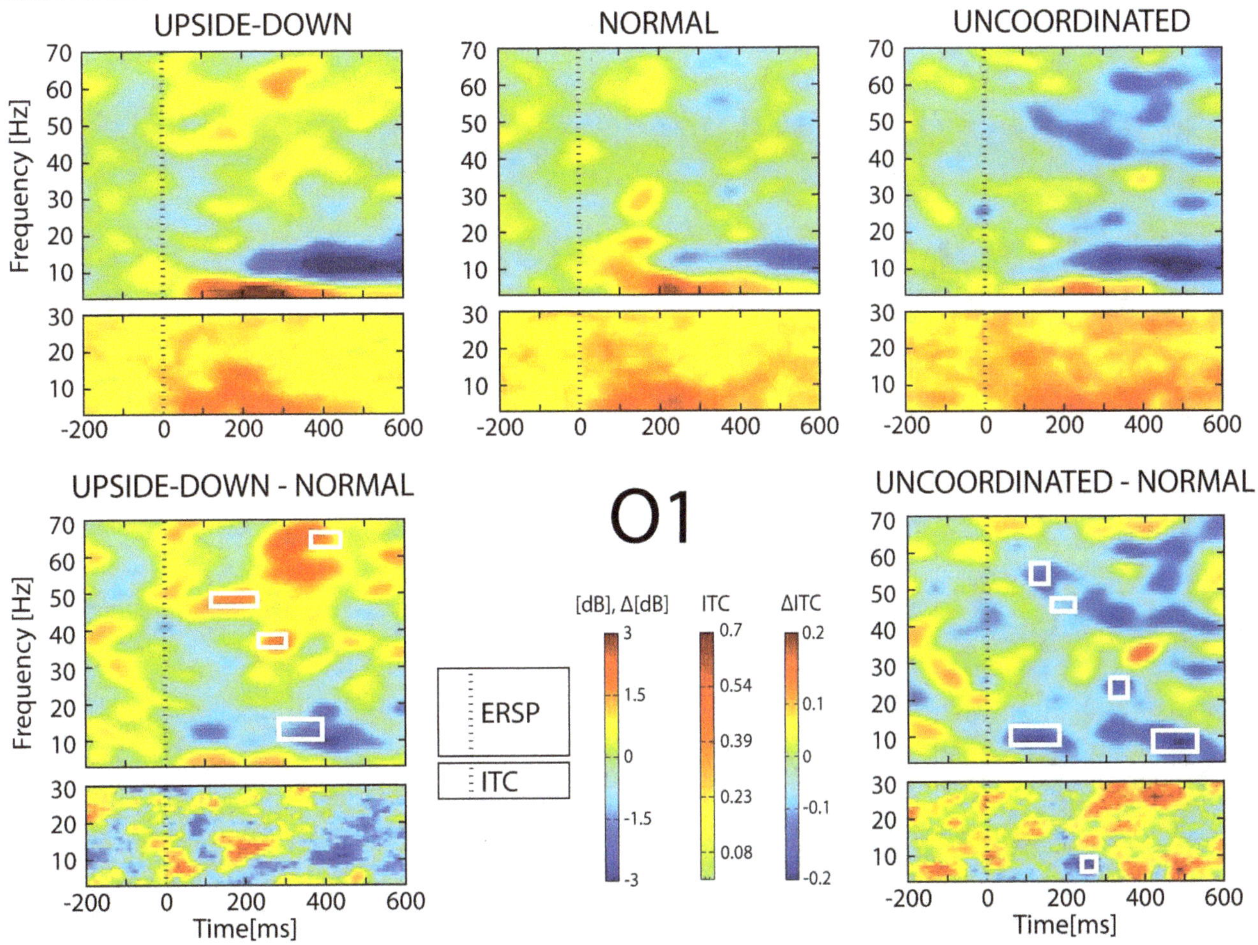

FIGURE 6 | ERSP and ITC from O1 electrode. The upper panel shows the ERSP and ITC in each three conditions. The lower panel shows difference *Upside-down-Normal* (left), and *Uncoordinated-Normal* (right) for ERSP and ITC. Areas of statistical significances ($p < 0.001$) are marked by white squares.

The next alpha ERD are in line with previous research showing decrease in alpha band power during perception of human motion (Cochin et al., 1998; Ulloa and Pineda, 2007). This was generally related to the desynchronization of mirror neurons activity as studied with EEG and fMRI combination (Arnstein et al., 2011), and would reflect a release from inhibition. However, it is interesting to note that our results are in contrast to studies of face perception (Girges et al., 2014), which report a greater alpha ERD in response to upright facial motion than in inverted condition. This difference between face and body motion recognition may be explain by high specialization of the brain to face recognition, and in particular to treatment of semantic content of facial gesture (Rojas et al., 2011). According to Klimesch et al. (1997, 1999, 2012), the alpha ERD increased as a function of the semantic content of retrieved information from the storage system. In our study, each stimulus has the same semantic content as a walking avatar. In this context, amplification of alpha ERD would indicate a recruitment of the mirror neurons system in order to recognize or predicted observed motion, by transformation of reference frame (in *Upside-down*) and reconstruction of motion (in *Uncoordinated*). The enhancement of the alpha ERD in *Upside-down* and *Uncoordinated* condition might then facilitate a dynamical process throughout the neural network involved in alpha rhythm generation evoked by the *Normal* walking avatar.

Theta ERS

The present ITC analysis shows that phase locking occur mainly in the theta range (peaked at ~5 Hz). However, as it is classically the case, this is not a pure phase locking because it was accompanied by theta ERS throughout all electrodes. Indeed, the visual evoked potentials (P100-N200) elicited by the classical checkerboard pattern or by more complex visual stimuli were accompanied by a clear theta ERS and related ITC (Klimesch et al., 2004; Cheron et al., 2014). Although present in each of the three present conditions in the 100–400 ms time period, the theta ITC was significantly perturbed in both *Upside-down* and *Uncoordinated* condition, while theta ERS were not significantly different. This indicates that the recognition of *Normal* walking is accompanied by a stronger theta phase locking peaking between 200 and 300 ms.

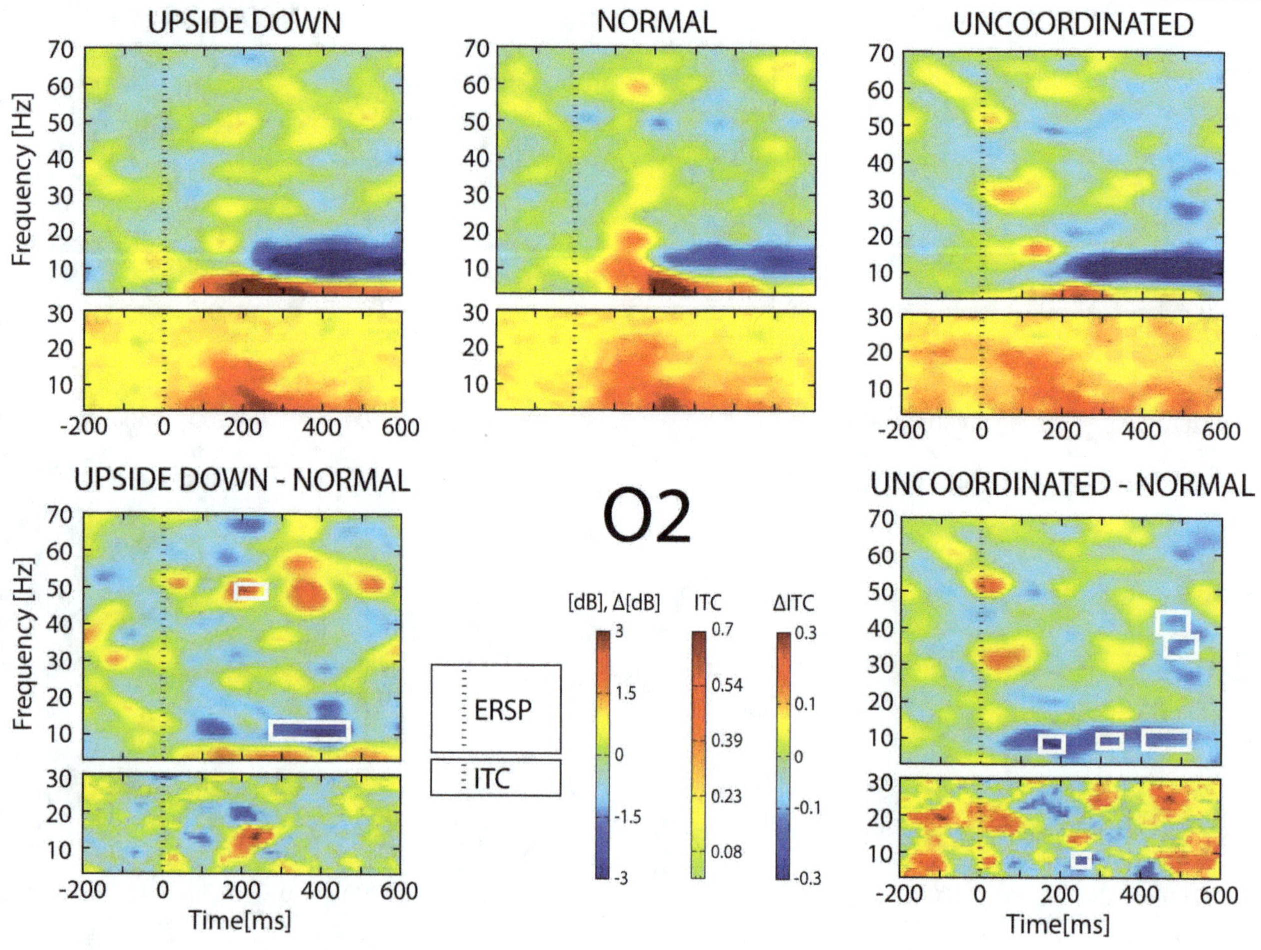

FIGURE 7 | ERSP and ITC from O2 electrode. The upper panel shows the ERSP and ITC in each three conditions. The lower panel shows difference *Upside-down-Normal* (left), and *Uncoordinated-Normal* (right) for ERSP and ITC. Areas of statistical significances ($p < 0.001$) are marked by white squares.

In humans the theta EEG rhythm (4–7 Hz) was initially defined as an intermediate rhythm between delta and alpha (Walter and Dovey, 1944; Mitchell et al., 2008). Later, the term FM-theta (FM for fronto-midline) was introduced by Ishihara and Yoshi (1972) when EEG was recorded during arithmetic task (Ishihara and Yoshi, 1972). Later, the presence of FM-theta during arithmetic and musical activities was demonstrated with MEG (Sasaki et al., 1996a,b,c). The midline frontal areas, such as the anterior cingulate cortex encompassing the lateral part of the prefrontal cortex are commonly cited as potential generators of the FM-theta (Gevins et al., 1997; Mizuhara et al., 2004; Sauseng et al., 2007).

In rat hippocampal regions, theta oscillation (3–9 Hz) is recognized to play an important role in the phase precession of the place cells firing assuming cued recall of the coming positions along the locomotion path of the rat (O'Keefe and Recce, 1993). The intrinsic theta generator of the hippocampal cortex is reinforced by the extrinsic theta pacemaker situated in the medial septal nucleus and allows a large-scale synchronization of theta oscillations in the hippocampus (Kocsis et al., 1999; Buzsáki, 2002). Theta oscillation is not restricted to the hippocampus but also emerges in different cortical areas in the rat (Leung and Borst, 1987; Silva et al., 1991). The ability of different cortical regions to produce theta is supported by slice recording demonstrating that theta oscillation may be produced by the activation of the NMDA receptors of the layer 5 (Silva et al., 1991; Flint and Connors, 1996) as well as by cholinergic activation of interneurons (Blatow et al., 2003).

Although human theta rhythm is not as robust as in the rat hippocampus, the ability of the human cortex to produce theta oscillation is now well recognized. It has been related to sensorimotor integration (Caplan et al., 2001), navigation (Kahana et al., 1999), memory load (Howard et al., 2003) and working memory (Raghavachari et al., 2001, 2006; Liebe et al., 2012). Interestingly, all the different phases of virtual movement during a navigation game induced an increase of 4–8 Hz oscillation in both the hippocampus and neocortex in human (Ekstrom et al., 2005). Although the present experiment involves the observation of human locomotion it cannot be assumed that the recorded theta oscillations are specifically related to locomotion *per se*. Indeed, theta oscillations are now considered as a basic physiological element involved in global oscillatory synchronization processes

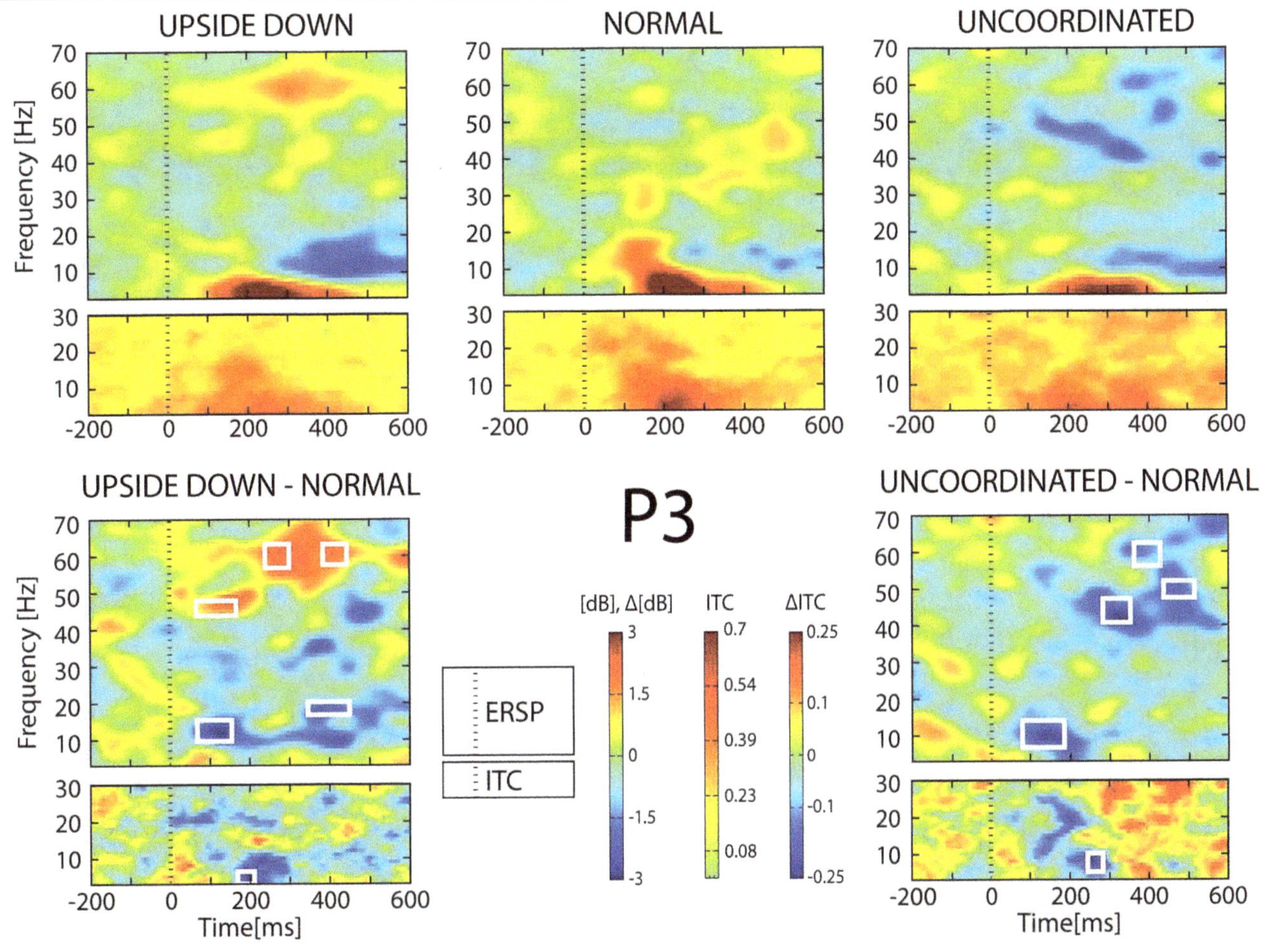

FIGURE 8 | ERSP and ITC from P3 electrode. The upper panel shows the ERSP and ITC in each three conditions. The lower panel shows difference *Upside-down-Normal* (left), and *Uncoordinated-Normal* (right) for ERSP and ITC. Areas of statistical significances ($p < 0.001$) are marked by white squares.

linking together multiple brain regions (Buzsáki and Draguhn, 2004; Fries, 2005). For example, the multiplicity of functional roles for this oscillation was demonstrated by the fact that the amplitude of theta power recorded over the temporal and frontal cortex predicted the behavioral performance of the subject (Sederberg et al., 2003). A recent MEG study demonstrated that hippocampal-prefrontal theta synchronization plays a mnemonic guidance in human decision-making (Guitart-Masip et al., 2013). Single neurons and local field potential recordings in the human medial temporal lobe show that theta phase locking reflects a global activation providing a temporal window for the conscious recognition (Rey et al., 2014). At a lower hierarchical level closer to the present observational task, theta oscillation is related to the perception of color shape of object and visual attention (Fries et al., 2001b). It is also involved in different sensory modalities to provide meaningful chunks of neuronal signals allowing subsequent decoding for an enhanced perception. In our case, such theta oscillation may thus be viewed as taking part of time-division multiplexing mechanism representing sequential information upon which a neuronal code may emerge by cross-frequency interaction with faster (gamma) oscillation (Akam and Kullmann, 2014).

Gamma modulation

Gamma oscillation (30–100 Hz) occupies a privileged position in cognitive neuroscience. The current understanding of gamma oscillation points to its emergence from the synchronous activity of a large ensemble of firing neurons (Eckhorn et al., 1988; Gray et al., 1989; Jensen and Colgin, 2007). It is central to the binding theory, in which gamma oscillations combine different features in a visual scene to form a coherent percept (Singer, 1999). Unexpectedly, our results show that *Upside-down* condition elicited gamma power increase at about 150 and 400 ms and a gamma ERD at the same latency in the *Uncoordinated* condition. This contrasting behavior of gamma oscillation is interesting because these oscillations are considered to underlie perception of coherent stimuli. These data are in accordance to previous MEG study showing enhancements in gamma rhythm at 100 ms after display onset in upright and inverted point-light walker (Pavlova et al., 2004). However, in the latter study additional gamma peak appeared only for upright point-light walker at 130 and 170 ms. Another study of the same group reported increased gamma activity in the left parieto-occipital region at 80 ms, with additional peaks in attended point-light walker on the right parietal and temporal cortex at 120 and

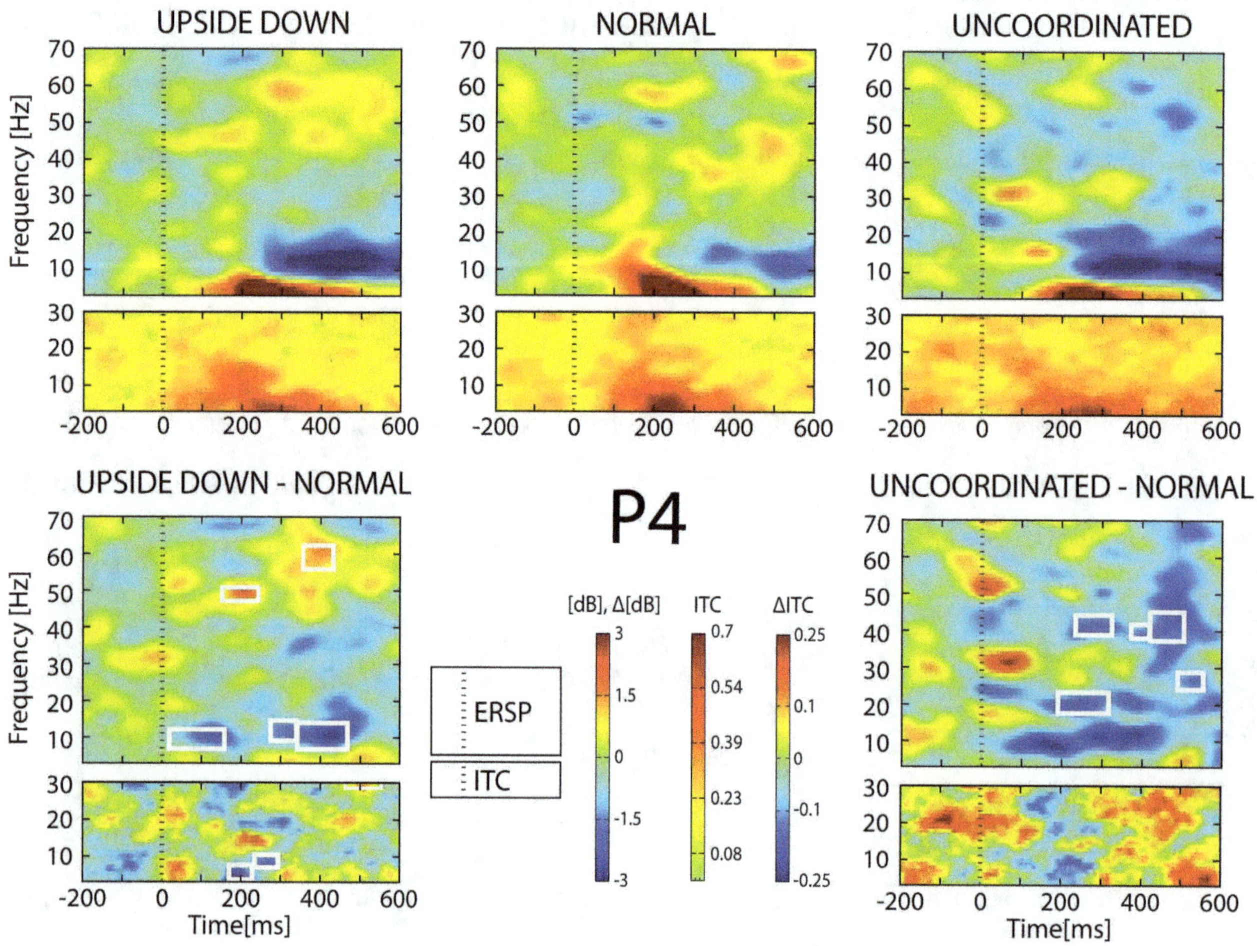

FIGURE 9 | ERSP and ITC from P4 electrode. The upper panel shows the ERSP and ITC in each three conditions. The lower panel shows difference *Upside-down-Normal* (left), and *Uncoordinated-Normal* (right) for ERSP and ITC. Areas of statistical significances ($p < 0.001$) are marked by white squares.

155 ms, respectively (Pavlova et al., 2006). The present results are in agreement with the data of Tallon-Baudry et al. (1996), where they demonstrated the presence of non-phase-locked gamma activation (60 Hz) at about 300–400 ms after the presentation of an illusory Kanizsa triangle figure (Tallon-Baudry et al., 1996). In this experiment, the gamma activity was stronger when the recognition task required additional mental reconstruction (stronger gamma oscillation for illusory triangle than normal triangle). In our present study, a non-phase-locked 60 Hz power increase occurred at the same latency only when the walking avatar was presented in *Upside-down* configuration. The subject was not instructed to perform any mental task but implicit recognition can recruit gamma activity for unconscious and conscious neuronal process (Aru et al., 2012; Vidal et al., 2014). The complex interplay between these neuronal qualia occupies a central position in cognitive neuroscience (Kandel, 2013). In the context of the Global Workspace Theory, serial and parallel processing take part from the widespread treatment of unconscious information to the emergence of consciousness (Baars, 1997; Dehaene and Naccache, 2001; Baars et al., 2013; Dehaene et al., 2014).

From a physiological perspective, experiments and modeling have demonstrated that gamma rhythms emerge from the interaction between local excitation and inhibition (Traub et al., 1997; Brunel and Wang, 2003; Kang et al., 2010), in which the gap junctions between interneurons play a pivotal role in ensuring gamma oscillation coherence (Traub et al., 2003; Whittington and Traub, 2003). In macaque, high density electrocorticography recording (Brunet et al., 2013) demonstrated that natural viewing induced a strong gamma oscillation (50–80 Hz) over most of the recorded visual cortex including V1 and V4 but not over most of the remaining cortex extending from superior temporal sulcus to the anterior part of the arcuate sulcus. The functional link between neuronal spikes and local field potential oscillation has been well documented in different preparations, demonstrating that spike-field coherence in the gamma-band frequency is accompanied by power enhancement of the gamma rhythm (Fries et al., 2001a,b, 2002, 2008). It was also demonstrated that when visual stimuli are moving smoothly, the visual cortex produces neuronal synchronization in the gamma-frequency band (Friedman-Hill et al., 2000). This gamma synchronization is considered as a key element for signal transmission to

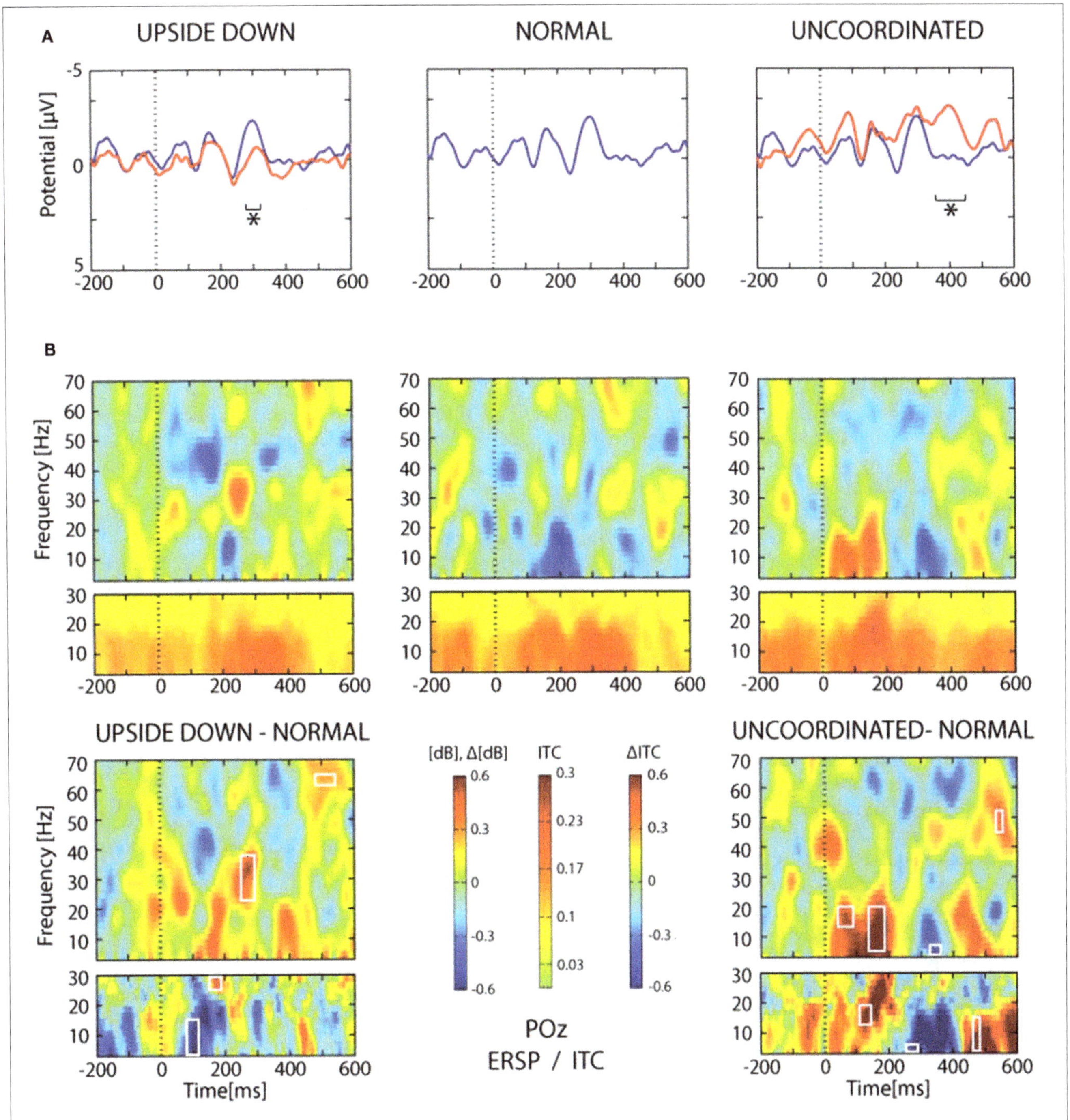

FIGURE 10 | SSVEP analysis from POz electrode. **(A)** Grand average trace corresponding to 16 subjects and about 2065 ± 26 trials for each condition. The heel strike of the right leg was used as trigger. Note the oscillating pattern at about 9 Hz and the superimposition of the *Normal* condition (blue trace) over the *Upside-down* (red trace, left part) and the *Uncoordinated* condition (red trace, right part). Areas of statistical significance ($p < 0.001$) are indicated by an asterisk. **(B)** The upper panel shows ERSP and ITC analysis of the same SSVEP data for the three respective conditions presented in **(A)**. The lower panel shows, ERSP and ITC differences *Upside-down-Normal* (left), and *Uncoordinated-Normal* (right). Areas of statistical significance ($p < 0.001$) are marked by white squares.

postsynaptic targets and to assume the continuity of the visual message (Fries, 2009).

In this context, the gamma ERD recorded during the *Uncoordinated* condition could be explained by a previous experience of Kruse and Eckhorn (1996) realized in the primary visual cortex of the cat. When a smooth movement of the visual field was presented it induced gamma oscillation, but when the smooth movement was intermingled with sudden random acceleration in and against the original direction of the smooth movement the gamma oscillations disappeared (Kruse and Eckhorn, 1996). This latter situation corresponds to the present *Uncoordinated* condition where gamma ERD replace gamma ERS present in *Normal* and *Upside-down* condition. The smoothness aspect of the walking video for both *Normal* and *Upside-down* presentations induces gamma oscillation while the sudden "*Uncoordinated*" image desynchronizes the neuronal population responsible for the gamma oscillation. In addition, Kruse and Eckhorn (1996) have demonstrated an inverse relationship between the decrease in gamma power and an increase in the stimulus-locked responses in lower frequency band (Kruse and Eckhorn, 1996).

Following the canonical microcircuit model (Bastos et al., 2012) based on intracellular recordings in cat visual cortex incorporating the neuronal sources of forward and backward connections in cortical hierarchies, it was proposed that the superficial pyramidal neurons generate gamma responses whereas deep pyramidal neurons generate alpha and beta dynamics. The visual cortex has been suggested to act as a dynamic filter of the visual input where stimulus properties like movement, contrast, localization and size of visual cues may modify the configuration of gamma oscillation (Gray et al., 1989; Ray and Maunsell, 2010; Brunet et al., 2013; Roberts et al., 2013). Among these stimulus properties, contrast is able to enhanced the signal-to-noise ratio of the sensory input inducing an increase in the postsynaptic gain of superficial pyramidal cells implicate in gamma oscillation (Feldman and Friston, 2010). Although, the same avatar was used here in the three different conditions the kinematic change of the *Uncoordinated* condition induced a significant increase in the dynamic contrast at the latency of 400 ms and may thus explain the late gamma ERD present in this condition. The spatial summation and the receptive field organization in V1 depend on contrast stimulus (Sceniak et al., 2002). The effects of contrast on the induced rhythms are complex and specifically influence the postsynaptic gain of neuronal populations, the strength of intrinsic and horizontal connectivity which can be differentially engaged depending on stimulus properties (Pinotsis et al., 2014). These authors have reported that the increase in visual contrast induces an increase of gamma peak frequency (from 46 to 58 Hz) accompanied by a decrease in gamma power. This contrast effect on the gamma power must be taken in account in the present gamma ERD and is complementary to the previous Kruse and Eckhorn's (1996) reported effect on the gamma power when the visual movement is *Uncoordinated.*

SSVEP

In order to strengthen the ERP, ERSP, and ITC studies of the transient presentation of the walking video, a SSVEP approach was made by using the heel strike events as the synchronized item of the video images occurring at every 100 ms. SSVEP offer many advantages in comparison to ERP, including better signal-to-noise ratio with a clear peak in the FFT occurring at the frequency of interest and some of its harmonics, and greater number of averaged items in a shorter period of time. SSVEP are classically obtained by using neutral LED or LCD image flashing between 1 and 100 Hz inducing resonance phenomena. In the present study, the SSVEP was not obtained by directly triggering all of the images occurring at 10 Hz but by using a specific event of the avatar locomotion corresponding to the initiation of the step cycle.

SSVEP is classically considered as an oscillatory response of the visual cortex evoked by contrast or luminance-modulated stimuli that drive the neural response at the imposed frequency of the constant peripheral stimulation (Regan, 1966; Müller et al., 1998). SSVEP are not only imposed by the physical properties of the stimulus but also depends on the brain state, task related-process, bottom-up and top-down influences (Müller et al., 1998; Keil et al., 2003; Andersen and Müller, 2010). This oscillatory pattern is a strong steady state potential that mainly arises from the occipital area, with strong contribution from the early visual cortex but also from more extended parts of the visual system including higher visual areas (Müller et al., 1997; Di Russo et al., 2007). This partly explains why SSVEP approach is increasingly used in cognitive and affective neurosciences to study face processing including face identification and decoding of facial emotional expressions (McTeague et al., 2011; Ales et al., 2012; Gruss et al., 2012; Rossion et al., 2012). To our knowledge, the present study is the first to use a walking avatar video for inducing SSVEP-like response. It showed specific amplitude enhancement of the oscillatory pattern and the related spectral perturbation at a precise time in relation to a kinematic event. Although no direct comparison can be made between SSVEP and ERP results, it is interesting to highlight the convergence of both types of results with regard to significant changes in the EEG brain rhythms at about the latency of 300 ms when the same avatar video was presented in *Upside-down* vs. *Normal* condition. The reported differences in the SSVEP configuration and rhythmic alteration (early theta-alpha ERS and late gamma ERS) in the *Uncoordinated* condition can be due to the higher dynamic contrast of this condition with respect to the other two conditions.

ACKNOWLEDGMENTS

We wish to thank Cal3D team for providing us with the original stimuli. We thank all volunteers for their participation. This work was funded by the Belgian Federal Science Policy Office, the European Space Agency (AO-2004,118), the Belgian National Fund for Scientific Research (FNRS), the research funds of the Université Libre de Bruxelles and of the Université de Mons (Belgium), the FEDER support (BIOFACT), the MINDWALKER project (FP7–2007–2013) supported by the European Commission, and the NeuroAtt BIOWIN project supported Walloon Country. The scientific responsibility rests with its author(s).

REFERENCES

Akam, T., and Kullmann, D. M. (2014). Oscillatory multiplexing of population codes for selective communication in the mammalian brain. *Nat. Rev. Neurosci.* 15, 111–122. doi: 10.1038/nrn3668

Ales, J. M., Farzin, F., Rossion, B., and Norcia, A. M. (2012). An objective method for measuring face detection thresholds using the sweep steady-state visual evoked response. *J. Vis.* 12:18. doi: 10.1167/12.10.18

Andersen, S. K., and Müller, M. M. (2010). Behavioral performance follows the time course of neural facilitation and suppression during cued shifts of feature-selective attention. *Proc. Natl. Acad. Sci. U.S.A.* 107, 13878–13882. doi: 10.1073/pnas.1002436107

Arnstein, D., Cui, F., Keysers, C., Maurits, N. M., and Gazzola, V. (2011). μ-suppression during action observation and execution correlates with BOLD in dorsal premotor, inferior parietal, and SI cortices. *J. Neurosci.* 31, 14243–14249. doi: 10.1523/JNEUROSCI.0963-11.2011

Aru, J., Axmacher, N., Do Lam, A. T. A., Fell, J., Elger, C. E., Singer, W., et al. (2012). Local category-specific gamma band responses in the visual cortex do not reflect conscious perception. *J. Neurosci.* 32, 14909–14914. doi: 10.1523/JNEUROSCI.2051-12.2012

Avanzini, P., Fabbri-Destro, M., Campi, C., Pascarella, A., Barchiesi, G., Cattaneo, L., et al. (2013). Spatiotemporal dynamics in understanding hand-object interactions. *Proc. Natl. Acad. Sci. U.S.A.* 110, 15878–15885. doi: 10.1073/pnas.1314420110

Avanzini, P., Fabbri-Destro, M., Dalla Volta, R., Daprati, E., Rizzolatti, G., and Cantalupo, G. (2012). The dynamics of sensorimotor cortical oscillations during the observation of hand movements: an EEG study. *PLoS ONE* 7:e37534. doi: 10.1371/journal.pone.0037534

Baars, B. J. (1997). Spatial brain coherence during the establishment of a conscious event. *Conscious. Cogn.* 6, 1–2. doi: 10.1006/ccog.1996.0289

Baars, B. J., Franklin, S., and Ramsoy, T. Z. (2013). Global workspace dynamics: cortical "binding and propagation" enables conscious contents. *Front. Psychol.* 4:200. doi: 10.3389/fpsyg.2013.00200

Baccus, W., Mozgova, O., and Thompson, J. C. (2009). Early integration of form and motion in the neural response to biological motion. *Neuroreport* 20, 1334–1338. doi: 10.1097/WNR.0b013e328330a867

Bastos, A. M., Usrey, W. M., Adams, R. A., Mangun, G. R., Fries, P., and Friston, K. J. (2012). Canonical microcircuits for predictive coding. *Neuron* 76, 695–711. doi: 10.1016/j.neuron.2012.10.038

Blake, R., and Shiffrar, M. (2007). Perception of human motion. *Annu. Rev. Psychol.* 58, 47–73. doi: 10.1146/annurev.psych.57.102904.190152

Blatow, M., Rozov, A., Katona, I., Hormuzdi, S. G., Meyer, A. H., Whittington, M. A., et al. (2003). A novel network of multipolar bursting interneurons generates theta frequency oscillations in neocortex. *Neuron* 38, 805–817. doi: 10.1016/S0896-6273(03)00300-3

Braadbaart, L., Williams, J. H. G., and Waiter, G. D. (2013). Do mirror neuron areas mediate mu rhythm suppression during imitation and action observation? *Int. J. Psychophysiol.* 89, 99–105. doi: 10.1016/j.ijpsycho.2013.05.019

Brunel, N., and Wang, X.-J. (2003). What determines the frequency of fast network oscillations with irregular neural discharges? I. Synaptic dynamics and excitation-inhibition balance. *J. Neurophysiol.* 90, 415–430. doi: 10.1152/jn.01095.2002

Brunet, N., Bosman, C. A., Roberts, M., Oostenveld, R., Womelsdorf, T., De Weerd, P., et al. (2013). Visual cortical gamma-band activity during free viewing of natural images. *Cereb. Cortex.* doi: 10.1093/cercor/bht280. [Epub ahead of print].

Brunner, C., Delorme, A., and Makeig, S. (2013). Eeglab—an open source matlab toolbox for electrophysiological research. *Biomed. Tech. (Berl).* doi: 10.1515/bmt-2013-4182. [Epub ahead of print].

Buzsáki, G. (2002). Theta oscillations in the hippocampus. *Neuron* 33, 325–340. doi: 10.1016/S0896-6273(02)00586-X

Buzsáki, G., and Draguhn, A. (2004). Neuronal oscillations in cortical networks. *Science* 304, 1926–1929. doi: 10.1126/science.1099745

Buzzell, G., Chubb, L., Safford, A. S., Thompson, J. C., and McDonald, C. G. (2013). Speed of human biological form and motion processing. *PLoS ONE* 8:e69396. doi: 10.1371/journal.pone.0069396

Caplan, J. B., Madsen, J. R., Raghavachari, S., and Kahana, M. J. (2001). Distinct patterns of brain oscillations underlie two basic parameters of human maze learning. *J. Neurophysiol.* 86, 368–380.

Cardin, V., Friston, K. J., and Zeki, S. (2011). Top-down modulations in the visual form pathway revealed with dynamic causal modeling. *Cereb. Cortex* 21, 550–562. doi: 10.1093/cercor/bhq122

Cebolla, A. M., De Saedeleer, C., Bengoetxea, A., Leurs, F., Balestra, C., d' Alcantara, P., et al. (2009). Movement gating of beta/gamma oscillations involved in the N30 somatosensory evoked potential. *Hum. Brain Mapp.* 30, 1568–1579. doi: 10.1002/hbm.20624

Cebolla, A. M., Palmero-Soler, E., Dan, B., and Cheron, G. (2014). Modulation of the N30 generators of the somatosensory evoked potentials by the mirror neuron system. *Neuroimage* 95C, 48–60. doi: 10.1016/j.neuroimage.2014.03.039

Cheng, Y.-W., Tzeng, O. J. L., Hung, D., Decety, J., and Hsieh, J.-C. (2005). Modulation of spinal excitability during observation of bipedal locomotion. *Neuroreport* 16, 1711–1714. doi: 10.1097/01.wnr.0000183325.13618.5f

Cheron, G., Cebolla, A. M., De Saedeleer, C., Bengoetxea, A., Leurs, F., Leroy, A., et al. (2007). Pure phase-locking of beta/gamma oscillation contributes to the N30 frontal component of somatosensory evoked potentials. *BMC Neurosci.* 8:75. doi: 10.1186/1471-2202-8-75

Cheron, G., Leroy, A., De Saedeleer, C., Bengoetxea, A., Lipshits, M., Cebolla, A., et al. (2006). Effect of gravity on human spontaneous 10-Hz electroencephalographic oscillations during the arrest reaction. *Brain Res.* 1121, 104–116. doi: 10.1016/j.brainres.2006.08.098

Cheron, G., Leroy, A., Palmero-Soler, E., De Saedeleer, C., Bengoetxea, A., Cebolla, A.-M., et al. (2014). Gravity influences top-down signals in visual processing. *PLoS ONE* 9:e82371. doi: 10.1371/journal.pone.0082371

Cochin, S., Barthelemy, C., Lejeune, B., Roux, S., and Martineau, J. (1998). Perception of motion and qEEG activity in human adults. *Electroencephalogr. Clin. Neurophysiol.* 107, 287–295. doi: 10.1016/S0013-4694(98)00071-6

Crompton, R. H., Sellers, W. I., and Thorpe, S. K. S. (2010). Arboreality, terrestriality and bipedalism. *Philos. Trans. R. Soc. Lond. B Biol. Sci.* 365, 3301–3314. doi: 10.1098/rstb.2010.0035

Csibra, G. (2007). "Action mirroring and action interpretation: an alternative account," in *Sensorimotor Foundations of Higher Cognition. Attention and Performance XXII*, eds P. Haggard, Y. Rosetti, and M. Kawato (Oxford; New York, NY: Oxford University Press), 435–459.

Darwin, C. (1872). *The Expression of the Emotions in Man and Animals.* 1st Edn. London: John Murray.

De Gelder, B. (2006). Towards the neurobiology of emotional body language. *Nat. Rev. Neurosci.* 7, 242–249. doi: 10.1038/nrn1872

Dehaene, S., Charles, L., King, J.-R., and Marti, S. (2014). Toward a computational theory of conscious processing. *Curr. Opin. Neurobiol.* 25C, 76–84. doi: 10.1016/j.conb.2013.12.005

Dehaene, S., and Naccache, L. (2001). Towards a cognitive neuroscience of consciousness: basic evidence and a workspace framework. *Cognition* 79, 1–37. doi: 10.1016/S0010-0277(00)00123-2

Delorme, A., and Makeig, S. (2004). EEGLAB: an open source toolbox for analysis of single-trial EEG dynamics including independent component analysis. *J. Neurosci. Methods* 134, 9–21. doi: 10.1016/j.jneumeth.2003.10.009

Di Dio, C., Di Cesare, G., Higuchi, S., Roberts, N., Vogt, S., and Rizzolatti, G. (2013). The neural correlates of velocity processing during the observation of a biological effector in the parietal and premotor cortex. *Neuroimage* 64, 425–436. doi: 10.1016/j.neuroimage.2012.09.026

Di Russo, F., Pitzalis, S., Aprile, T., Spitoni, G., Patria, F., Stella, A., et al. (2007). Spatiotemporal analysis of the cortical sources of the steady-state visual evoked potential. *Hum. Brain Mapp.* 28, 323–334. doi: 10.1002/hbm.20276

Downing, P. E., Jiang, Y., Shuman, M., and Kanwisher, N. (2001). A cortical area selective for visual processing of the human body. *Science* 293, 2470–2473. doi: 10.1126/science.1063414

Eckhorn, R., Bauer, R., Jordan, W., Brosch, M., Kruse, W., Munk, M., et al. (1988). Coherent oscillations: a mechanism of feature linking in the visual cortex? Multiple electrode and correlation analyses in the cat. *Biol. Cybern.* 60, 121–130. doi: 10.1007/BF00202899

Ekstrom, A. D., Caplan, J. B., Ho, E., Shattuck, K., Fried, I., and Kahana, M. J. (2005). Human hippocampal theta activity during virtual navigation. *Hippocampus* 15, 881–889. doi: 10.1002/hipo.20109

Engel, A. K., Roelfsema, P. R., Fries, P., Brecht, M., and Singer, W. (1997). Role of the temporal domain for response selection and perceptual binding. *Cereb. Cortex* 7, 571–582. doi: 10.1093/cercor/7.6.571

Feldman, H., and Friston, K. J. (2010). Attention, uncertainty, and free-energy. *Front. Hum. Neurosci.* 4:215. doi: 10.3389/fnhum.2010.00215

Flint, A. C., and Connors, B. W. (1996). Two types of network oscillations in neocortex mediated by distinct glutamate receptor subtypes and neuronal populations. *J. Neurophysiol.* 75, 951–957.

Frenkel-Toledo, S., Bentin, S., Perry, A., Liebermann, D. G., and Soroker, N. (2014). Mirror-neuron system recruitment by action observation: effects of focal brain damage on mu suppression. *Neuroimage* 87, 127–137. doi: 10.1016/j.neuroimage.2013.10.019

Friedman-Hill, S., Maldonado, P. E., and Gray, C. M. (2000). Dynamics of striate cortical activity in the alert macaque: I. Incidence and stimulus-dependence of gamma-band neuronal oscillations. *Cereb. Cortex* 10, 1105–1116. doi: 10.1093/cercor/10.11.1105

Fries, P. (2005). A mechanism for cognitive dynamics: neuronal communication through neuronal coherence. *Trends Cogn. Sci.* 9, 474–480. doi: 10.1016/j.tics.2005.08.011

Fries, P. (2009). Neuronal gamma-band synchronization as a fundamental process in cortical computation. *Annu. Rev. Neurosci.* 32, 209–224. doi: 10.1146/annurev.neuro.051508.135603

Fries, P., Neuenschwander, S., Engel, A. K., Goebel, R., and Singer, W. (2001a). Rapid feature selective neuronal synchronization through correlated latency shifting. *Nat. Neurosci.* 4, 194–200. doi: 10.1038/84032

Fries, P., Reynolds, J. H., Rorie, A. E., and Desimone, R. (2001b). Modulation of oscillatory neuronal synchronization by selective visual attention. *Science* 291, 1560–1563. doi: 10.1126/science.1055465

Fries, P., Schröder, J.-H., Roelfsema, P. R., Singer, W., and Engel, A. K. (2002). Oscillatory neuronal synchronization in primary visual cortex as a correlate of stimulus selection. *J. Neurosci.* 22, 3739–3754.

Fries, P., Womelsdorf, T., Oostenveld, R., and Desimone, R. (2008). The effects of visual stimulation and selective visual attention on rhythmic neuronal synchronization in macaque area V4. *J. Neurosci.* 28, 4823–4835. doi: 10.1523/JNEUROSCI.4499-07.2008

Gevins, A., Smith, M. E., McEvoy, L., and Yu, D. (1997). High-resolution EEG mapping of cortical activation related to working memory: effects of task difficulty, type of processing, and practice. *Cereb. Cortex* 7, 374–385. doi: 10.1093/cercor/7.4.374

Giese, M. A., and Poggio, T. (2003). Neural mechanisms for the recognition of biological movements. *Nat. Rev. Neurosci.* 4, 179–192. doi: 10.1038/nrn1057

Girges, C., Wright, M. J., Spencer, J. V., and O'Brien, J. M. D. (2014). Event-related alpha suppression in response to facial motion. *PLoS ONE* 9:e89382. doi: 10.1371/journal.pone.0089382

Gramann, K., El Sharkawy, J., and Deubel, H. (2009). Eye-movements during navigation in a virtual tunnel. *Int. J. Neurosci.* 119, 1755–1778. doi: 10.1080/00207450903170361

Gray, C. M., König, P., Engel, A. K., and Singer, W. (1989). Oscillatory responses in cat visual cortex exhibit inter-columnar synchronization which reflects global stimulus properties. *Nature* 338, 334–337. doi: 10.1038/338334a0

Gruss, L. F., Wieser, M. J., Schweinberger, S., and Keil, A. (2012). Face-evoked steady-state visual potentials: effects of presentation rate and face inversion. *Front. Hum. Neurosci.* 6:316. doi: 10.3389/fnhum.2012.00316

Guitart-Masip, M., Barnes, G. R., Horner, A., Bauer, M., Dolan, R. J., and Duzel, E. (2013). Synchronization of medial temporal lobe and prefrontal rhythms in human decision making. *J. Neurosci.* 33, 442–451. doi: 10.1523/JNEUROSCI.2573-12.2013

Haegens, S., Osipova, D., Oostenveld, R., and Jensen, O. (2010). Somatosensory working memory performance in humans depends on both engagement and disengagement of regions in a distributed network. *Hum. Brain Mapp.* 31, 26–35. doi: 10.1002/hbm.20842

Heyes, C. (2010). Where do mirror neurons come from? *Neurosci. Biobehav. Rev.* 34, 575–583. doi: 10.1016/j.neubiorev.2009.11.007

Hirai, M., Fukushima, H., and Hiraki, K. (2003). An event-related potentials study of biological motion perception in humans. *Neurosci. Lett.* 344, 41–44. doi: 10.1016/S0304-3940(03)00413-0

Hirai, M., and Hiraki, K. (2006). The relative importance of spatial versus temporal structure in the perception of biological motion: an event-related potential study. *Cognition* 99, B15–B29. doi: 10.1016/j.cognition.2005.05.003

Hirai, M., Senju, A., Fukushima, H., and Hiraki, K. (2005). Active processing of biological motion perception: an ERP study. *Brain Res. Cogn. Brain Res.* 23, 387–396. doi: 10.1016/j.cogbrainres.2004.11.005

Hirai, M., Watanabe, S., Honda, Y., and Kakigi, R. (2009). Developmental changes in point-light walker processing during childhood and adolescence: an event-related potential study. *Neuroscience* 161, 311–325. doi: 10.1016/j.neuroscience.2009.03.026

Hirai, M., Watanabe, S., Honda, Y., and Kakigi, R. (2013). Developmental changes in point-light walker processing during childhood: a two-year follow-up ERP study. *Dev. Cogn. Neurosci.* 5, 51–62. doi: 10.1016/j.dcn.2013.01.002

Howard, M. W., Rizzuto, D. S., Caplan, J. B., Madsen, J. R., Lisman, J., Aschenbrenner-Scheibe, R., et al. (2003). Gamma oscillations correlate with working memory load in humans. *Cereb. Cortex* 13, 1369–1374. doi: 10.1093/cercor/bhg084

Ishihara, T., and Yoshi, N. (1972). Multivariate analytic study of EEG and mental activity in juvenile delinquents. *Electroencephalogr. Clin. Neurophysiol.* 33, 71–80. doi: 10.1016/0013-4694(72)90026-0

Jacob, P., and Jeannerod, M. (2005). The motor theory of social cognition: a critique. *Trends Cogn. Sci.* 9, 21–25. doi: 10.1016/j.tics.2004.11.003

Jeffreys, D. A. (1996). Simple methods of identifying the independently generated components of scalp-recorded responses evoked by stationary patterns. *Exp. Brain Res.* 111, 100–112. doi: 10.1007/BF00229559

Jensen, O., and Colgin, L. L. (2007). Cross-frequency coupling between neuronal oscillations. *Trends Cogn. Sci.* 11, 267–269. doi: 10.1016/j.tics.2007.05.003

Johansson, G. (1973). Visual perception of biological motion and a model for its analysis. *Percept. Psychophys.* 14, 201–211. doi: 10.3758/BF03212378

Jokisch, D., Daum, I., Suchan, B., and Troje, N. F. (2005). Structural encoding and recognition of biological motion: evidence from event-related potentials and source analysis. *Behav. Brain Res.* 157, 195–204. doi: 10.1016/j.bbr.2004.06.025

Kahana, M. J., Sekuler, R., Caplan, J. B., Kirschen, M., and Madsen, J. R. (1999). Human theta oscillations exhibit task dependence during virtual maze navigation. *Nature* 399, 781–784. doi: 10.1038/21645

Kandel, E. (2013). The new science of mind and the future of knowledge. *Neuron* 80, 546–560. doi: 10.1016/j.neuron.2013.10.039

Kang, J., Robinson, H. P. C., and Feng, J. (2010). Diversity of intrinsic frequency encoding patterns in rat cortical neurons—mechanisms and possible functions. *PLoS ONE* 5:e9608. doi: 10.1371/journal.pone.0009608

Keil, A., Gruber, T., Müller, M. M., Moratti, S., Stolarova, M., Bradley, M. M., et al. (2003). Early modulation of visual perception by emotional arousal: evidence from steady state visual evoked brain potentials. *Cogn. Affect. Behav. Neurosci.* 3, 195–206. doi: 10.3758/CABN.3.3.195

Kilner, J. M., Friston, K. J., and Frith, C. D. (2007). Predictive coding: an account of the mirror neuron system. *Cogn. Process.* 8, 159–166. doi: 10.1007/s10339-007-0170-2

Klimesch, W. (1999). EEG alpha and theta oscillations reflect cognitive and memory performance: a review and analysis. *Brain Res. Brain Res. Rev.* 29, 169–195. doi: 10.1016/S0165-0173(98)00056-3

Klimesch, W. (2012). Alpha-band oscillations, attention, and controlled access to stored information. *Trends Cogn. Sci.* 16, 606–617. doi: 10.1016/j.tics.2012.10.007

Klimesch, W., Doppelmayr, M., Pachinger, T., and Russegger, H. (1997). Event-related desynchronization in the alpha band and the processing of semantic information. *Brain Res. Cogn. Brain Res.* 6, 83–94. doi: 10.1016/S0926-6410(97)00018-9

Klimesch, W., Doppelmayr, M., Schimke, H., and Pachinger, T. (1996). Alpha frequency, reaction time, and the speed of processing information. *J. Clin. Neurophysiol.* 13, 511–518.

Klimesch, W., Sauseng, P., and Gerloff, C. (2003). Enhancing cognitive performance with repetitive transcranial magnetic stimulation at human individual alpha frequency. *Eur. J. Neurosci.* 17, 1129–1133. doi: 10.1046/j.1460-9568.2003.02517.x

Klimesch, W., Sauseng, P., and Hanslmayr, S. (2007). EEG alpha oscillations: the inhibition-timing hypothesis. *Brain Res. Rev.* 53, 63–88. doi: 10.1016/j.brainresrev.2006.06.003

Klimesch, W., Schack, B., Schabus, M., Doppelmayr, M., Gruber, W., and Sauseng, P. (2004). Phase-locked alpha and theta oscillations generate the P1-N1 complex and are related to memory performance. *Brain Res. Cogn. Brain Res.* 19, 302–316. doi: 10.1016/j.cogbrainres.2003.11.016

Kocsis, B., Bragin, A., and Buzsáki, G. (1999). Interdependence of multiple theta generators in the hippocampus: a partial coherence analysis. *J. Neurosci.* 19, 6200–6212.

Krakowski, A. I., Ross, L. A., Snyder, A. C., Sehatpour, P., Kelly, S. P., and Foxe, J. J. (2011). The neurophysiology of human biological motion processing: a high-density electrical mapping study. *Neuroimage* 56, 373–383. doi: 10.1016/j.neuroimage.2011.01.058

Kravitz, D. J., Saleem, K. S., Baker, C. I., and Mishkin, M. (2011). A new neural framework for visuospatial processing. *Nat. Rev. Neurosci.* 12, 217–230. doi: 10.1038/nrn3008

Kruse, W., and Eckhorn, R. (1996). Inhibition of sustained gamma oscillations (35-80 Hz) by fast transient responses in cat visual cortex. *Proc. Natl. Acad. Sci. U.S.A.* 93, 6112–6117. doi: 10.1073/pnas.93.12.6112

Leakey, M., and Walker, A. (1997). Early hominid fossils from Africa. *Sci. Am.* 276, 74–79. doi: 10.1038/scientificamerican0697-74

Leung, L. W., and Borst, J. G. (1987). Electrical activity of the cingulate cortex. I. Generating mechanisms and relations to behavior. *Brain Res.* 407, 68–80. doi: 10.1016/0006-8993(87)91220-0

Liebe, S., Hoerzer, G. M., Logothetis, N. K., and Rainer, G. (2012). Theta coupling between V4 and prefrontal cortex predicts visual short-term memory performance. *Nat. Neurosci.* 15, 456–462, S1–S2. doi: 10.1038/nn.3038

Makeig, S., Westerfield, M., Jung, T. P., Enghoff, S., Townsend, J., Courchesne, E., et al. (2002). Dynamic brain sources of visual evoked responses. *Science* 295, 690–694. doi: 10.1126/science.1066168

McAleer, P., Pollick, F. E., Love, S. A., Crabbe, F., and Zacks, J. M. (2014). The role of kinematics in cortical regions for continuous human motion perception. *Cogn. Affect. Behav. Neurosci.* 14, 307–318. doi: 10.3758/s13415-013-0192-4

McGlothlin, B., Jiacoletti, D., and Yandell, L. (2012). The inversion effect: biological motion and gender recognition. *Psi Chi J. Psychol. Res.* 17, 68–72.

McTeague, L. M., Shumen, J. R.,Wieser, M. J., Lang, P. J., and Keil, A. (2011). Social vision: sustained perceptual enhancement of affective facial cues in social anxiety. *Neuroimage* 54, 1615–1624. doi: 10.1016/j.neuroimage.2010.08.080

Mitchell, D. J., McNaughton, N., Flanagan, D., and Kirk, I. J. (2008). Frontal-midline theta from the perspective of hippocampal "theta." *Prog. Neurobiol.* 86, 156–185. doi: 10.1016/j.pneurobio.2008.09.005

Mizuhara, H., Wang, L.-Q., Kobayashi, K., and Yamaguchi, Y. (2004). A long-range cortical network emerging with theta oscillation in a mental task. *Neuroreport* 15, 1233–1238. doi: 10.1097/01.wnr.0000126755.09715.b3

Müller, M. M., Teder-Salejarvi, W., and Hillyard, S. A. (1998). The time course of cortical facilitation during cued shifts of spatial attention. *Nat. Neurosci.* 1, 631–634. doi: 10.1038/2865

Müller, M. M., Teder, W., and Hillyard, S. A. (1997). Magnetoencephalographic recording of steady-state visual evoked cortical activity. *Brain Topogr.* 9, 163–168. doi: 10.1007/BF01190385

O'Keefe, J., and Recce, M. L. (1993). Phase relationship between hippocampal place units and the EEG theta rhythm. *Hippocampus* 3, 317–330.

Pavlova, M., Birbaumer, N., and Sokolov, A. (2006). Attentional modulation of cortical neuromagnetic gamma response to biological movement. *Cereb. Cortex* 16, 321–327. doi: 10.1093/cercor/bhi108

Pavlova, M., Lutzenberger, W., Sokolov, A., and Birbaumer, N. (2004). Dissociable cortical processing of recognizable and non-recognizable biological movement: analysing gamma MEG activity. *Cereb. Cortex* 14, 181–188. doi: 10.1093/cercor/bhg117

Pavlova, M., and Sokolov, A. (2000). Orientation specificity in biological motion perception. *Percept. Psychophys.* 62, 889–899. doi: 10.3758/BF03212075

Peyrin, C., Michel, C. M., Schwartz, S., Thut, G., Seghier, M., Landis, T., et al. (2010). The neural substrates and timing of top-down processes during coarse-to-fine categorization of visual scenes: a combined fMRI and ERP study. *J. Cogn. Neurosci.* 22, 2768–2780. doi: 10.1162/jocn.2010.21424

Pinotsis, D. A., Brunet, N., Bastos, A., Bosman, C. A., Litvak, V., Fries, P., et al. (2014). Contrast gain control and horizontal interactions in V1: a DCM study. *Neuroimage* 92C, 143–155. doi: 10.1016/j.neuroimage.2014.01.047

Pollick, F. E., Kay, J. W., Heim, K., and Stringer, R. (2005). Gender recognition from point-light walkers. *J. Exp. Psychol. Hum. Percept. Perform.* 31, 1247–1265. doi: 10.1037/0096-1523.31.6.1247

Pozzo, T., Berthoz, A., and Lefort, L. (1990). Head stabilization during various locomotor tasks in humans. I. Normal subjects. *Exp. Brain Res.* 82, 97–106. doi: 10.1007/BF00230842

Press, C., Heyes, C., and Kilner, J. M. (2011). Learning to understand others' actions. *Biol. Lett.* 7, 457–460. doi: 10.1098/rsbl.2010.0850

Raghavachari, S., Kahana, M. J., Rizzuto, D. S., Caplan, J. B., Kirschen, M. P., Bourgeois, B., et al. (2001). Gating of human theta oscillations by a working memory task. *J. Neurosci.* 21, 3175–3183.

Raghavachari, S., Lisman, J. E., Tully, M., Madsen, J. R., Bromfield, E. B., and Kahana, M. J. (2006). Theta oscillations in human cortex during a working-memory task: evidence for local generators. *J. Neurophysiol.* 95, 1630–1638. doi: 10.1152/jn.00409.2005

Ramalingam, N., McManus, J. N. J., Li, W., and Gilbert, C. D. (2013). Top-down modulation of lateral interactions in visual cortex. *J. Neurosci.* 33, 1773–1789. doi: 10.1523/JNEUROSCI.3825-12.2013

Ray, S., and Maunsell, J. H. R. (2010). Differences in gamma frequencies across visual cortex restrict their possible use in computation. *Neuron* 67, 885–896. doi: 10.1016/j.neuron.2010.08.004

Regan, D. (1966). Some characteristics of average steady-state and transient responses evoked by modulated light. *Electroencephalogr. Clin. Neurophysiol.* 20, 238–248. doi: 10.1016/0013-4694(66)90088-5

Rey, H. G., Fried, I., and Quian Quiroga, R. (2014). Timing of single-neuron and local field potential responses in the human medial temporal lobe. *Curr. Biol.* 24, 299–304. doi: 10.1016/j.cub.2013.12.004

Rizzolatti, G., and Craighero, L. (2004). The mirror-neuron system. *Annu. Rev. Neurosci.* 27, 169–192. doi: 10.1146/annurev.neuro.27.070203.144230

Rizzolatti, G., Fadiga, L., Gallese, V., and Fogassi, L. (1996). Premotor cortex and the recognition of motor actions. *Brain Res. Cogn. Brain Res.* 3, 131–141. doi: 10.1016/0926-6410(95)00038-0

Roberts, M. J., Lowet, E., Brunet, N. M., Ter Wal, M., Tiesinga, P., Fries, P., et al. (2013). Robust gamma coherence between macaque V1 and V2 by dynamic frequency matching. *Neuron* 78, 523–536. doi: 10.1016/j.neuron.2013.03.003

Rojas, M., Masip, D., Todorov, A., and Vitria, J. (2011). Automatic prediction of facial trait judgments: appearance vs. structural models. *PLoS ONE* 6:e23323. doi: 10.1371/journal.pone.0023323

Rossion, B., Prieto, E. A., Boremanse, A., Kuefner, D., and Van Belle, G. (2012). A steady-state visual evoked potential approach to individual face perception: effect of inversion, contrast-reversal and temporal dynamics. *Neuroimage* 63, 1585–1600. doi: 10.1016/j.neuroimage.2012.08.033

Sadaghiani, S., Scheeringa, R., Lehongre, K., Morillon, B., Giraud, A.-L., D'Esposito, M., et al. (2012). α-band phase synchrony is related to activity in the fronto-parietal adaptive control network. *J. Neurosci.* 32, 14305–14310. doi: 10.1523/JNEUROSCI.1358-12.2012

Sasaki, K., Gemba, H., Nambu, A., Kyuhou, S., Matsuzaki, R., and Tsujimoto, T. (1996a). Studies on integrative functions of the human frontal association cortex by use of MEG. *Electroencephalogr. Clin. Neurophysiol. Suppl.* 47, 181–190.

Sasaki, K., Nambu, A., Tsujimoto, T., Matsuzaki, R., Kyuhou, S., and Gemba, H. (1996b). Studies on integrative functions of the human frontal association cortex with MEG. *Brain Res. Cogn. Brain Res.* 5, 165–174. doi: 10.1016/S0926-6410(96)00053-5

Sasaki, K., Tsujimoto, T., Nishikawa, S., Nishitani, N., and Ishihara, T. (1996c). Frontal mental theta wave recorded simultaneously with magnetoencephalography and electroencephalography. *Neurosci. Res.* 26, 79–81. doi: 10.1016/0168-0102(96)01082-6

Sauseng, P., Hoppe, J., Klimesch, W., Gerloff, C., and Hummel, F. C. (2007). Dissociation of sustained attention from central executive functions: local activity and interregional connectivity in the theta range. *Eur. J. Neurosci.* 25, 587–593. doi: 10.1111/j.1460-9568.2006.05286.x

Saygin, A. P., Wilson, S. M., Hagler, D. J. Jr., Bates, E., and Sereno, M. I. (2004). Point-light biological motion perception activates human premotor cortex. *J. Neurosci.* 24, 6181–6188. doi: 10.1523/JNEUROSCI.0504-04.2004

Sceniak, M. P., Hawken, M. J., and Shapley, R. (2002). Contrast-dependent changes in spatial frequency tuning of macaque V1 neurons: effects of a changing receptive field size. *J. Neurophysiol.* 88, 1363–1373.

Schütz-Bosbach, S., and Prinz, W. (2007). Perceptual resonance: action-induced modulation of perception. *Trends Cogn. Sci.* 11, 349–355. doi: 10.1016/j.tics.2007.06.005

Sederberg, P. B., Kahana, M. J., Howard, M. W., Donner, E. J., and Madsen, J. R. (2003). Theta and gamma oscillations during encoding predict subsequent recall. *J. Neurosci.* 23, 10809–10814.

Silva, L. R., Amitai, Y., and Connors, B. W. (1991). Intrinsic oscillations of neocortex generated by layer 5 pyramidal neurons. *Science* 251, 432–435. doi: 10.1126/science.1824881

Singer, W. (1999). Neuronal synchrony: a versatile code for the definition of relations? *Neuron* 24, 49–65, 111–125. doi: 10.1016/S0896-6273(00)80821-1

Singer, W. (2009). Distributed processing and temporal codes in neuronal networks. *Cogn. Neurodyn.* 3, 189–196. doi: 10.1007/s11571-009-9087-z

Tallon-Baudry, C., and Bertrand, O. (1999). Oscillatory gamma activity in humans and its role in object representation. *Trends Cogn. Sci.* 3, 151–162. doi: 10.1016/S1364-6613(99)01299-1

Tallon-Baudry, C., Bertrand, O., Delpuech, C., and Pernier, J. (1996). Stimulus specificity of phase-locked and non-phase-locked 40 Hz visual responses in human. *J. Neurosci.* 16, 4240–4249.

Thorpe, S. K. S., Holder, R. L., and Crompton, R. H. (2007). Origin of human bipedalism as an adaptation for locomotion on flexible branches. *Science* 316, 1328–1331. doi: 10.1126/science.1140799

Traub, R. D., Cunningham, M. O., Gloveli, T., LeBeau, F. E. N., Bibbig, A., Buhl, E. H., et al. (2003). GABA-enhanced collective behavior in neuronal axons underlies persistent gamma-frequency oscillations. *Proc. Natl. Acad. Sci. U.S.A.* 100, 11047–11052. doi: 10.1073/pnas.1934854100

Traub, R. D., Jefferys, J. G., and Whittington, M. A. (1997). Simulation of gamma rhythms in networks of interneurons and pyramidal cells. *J. Comput. Neurosci.* 4, 141–150. doi: 10.1023/A:1008839312043

Troje, N. F., Westhoff, C., and Lavrov, M. (2005). Person identification from biological motion: effects of structural and kinematic cues. *Percept. Psychophys.* 67, 667–675. doi: 10.3758/BF03193523

Ulloa, E. R., and Pineda, J. A. (2007). Recognition of point-light biological motion: mu rhythms and mirror neuron activity. *Behav. Brain Res.* 183, 188–194. doi: 10.1016/j.bbr.2007.06.007

Urgen, B. A., Plank, M., Ishiguro, H., Poizner, H., and Saygin, A. P. (2013). EEG theta and Mu oscillations during perception of human and robot actions. *Front. Neurorobotics* 7:19. doi: 10.3389/fnbot.2013.00019

Vaina, L. M., Solomon, J., Chowdhury, S., Sinha, P., and Belliveau, J. W. (2001). Functional neuroanatomy of biological motion perception in humans. *Proc. Natl. Acad. Sci. U.S.A.* 98, 11656–11661. doi: 10.1073/pnas.191374198

Vidal, J. R., Perrone-Bertolotti, M., Levy, J., De Palma, L., Minotti, L., Kahane, P., et al. (2014). Neural repetition suppression in ventral occipito-temporal cortex occurs during conscious and unconscious processing of frequent stimuli. *Neuroimage* 95C, 129–135. doi: 10.1016/j.neuroimage.2014.03.049

Viviani, P., and Stucchi, N. (1992). Biological movements look uniform: evidence of motor-perceptual interactions. *J. Exp. Psychol. Hum. Percept. Perform.* 18, 603–623. doi: 10.1037/0096-1523.18.3.603

Walter, W. G., and Dovey, V. J. (1944). Electro-encephalography in cases of sub-cortical tumour. *J. Neurol. Neurosurg. Psychiatry* 7, 57–65. doi: 10.1136/jnnp.7.3-4.57

White, N. C., Fawcett, J. M., and Newman, A. J. (2014). Electrophysiological markers of biological motion and human form recognition. *Neuroimage* 84, 854–867. doi: 10.1016/j.neuroimage.2013.09.026

Whittington, M. A., and Traub, R. D. (2003). Interneuron diversity series: inhibitory interneurons and network oscillations *in vitro*. *Trends Neurosci.* 26, 676–682. doi: 10.1016/j.tins.2003.09.016

Zanto, T. P., Rubens, M. T., Thangavel, A., and Gazzaley, A. (2011). Causal role of the prefrontal cortex in top-down modulation of visual processing and working memory. *Nat. Neurosci.* 14, 656–661. doi: 10.1038/nn.2773

Zeki, S., Watson, J. D., Lueck, C. J., Friston, K. J., Kennard, C., and Frackowiak, R. S. (1991). A direct demonstration of functional specialization in human visual cortex. *J. Neurosci.* 11, 641–649.

3

Best of both worlds: promise of combining brain stimulation and brain connectome

Caroline Di Bernardi Luft[1], Ernesto Pereda[2], Michael J. Banissy[1] and Joydeep Bhattacharya[1]*

[1] *Department of Psychology, Goldsmiths, University of London, London, UK*
[2] *Lab. of Electrical Engineering and Bioengineering, Department of Industrial Engineering, Institute of Biomedical Technology, University of La Laguna, Tenerife, Spain*

Edited by:
Mikhail Lebedev, Duke University, USA

Reviewed by:
Kohitij Kar, Rutgers University, USA
Diego Kaski, Imperial College London, UK

****Correspondence:***
Joydeep Bhattacharya, Department of Psychology, Goldsmiths, University of London, New Cross, London SE14 6NW, UK
e-mail: j.bhattacharya@gold.ac.uk

Transcranial current brain stimulation (tCS) is becoming increasingly popular as a non-pharmacological non-invasive *neuromodulatory* method that alters cortical excitability by applying weak electrical currents to the scalp via a pair of electrodes. Most applications of this technique have focused on enhancing motor and learning skills, as well as a therapeutic agent in neurological and psychiatric disorders. In these applications, similarly to lesion studies, tCS was used to provide a causal link between a function or behavior and a specific brain region (e.g., primary motor cortex). Nonetheless, complex cognitive functions are known to rely on functionally connected multitude of brain regions with dynamically changing patterns of information flow rather than on isolated areas, which are most commonly targeted in typical tCS experiments. In this review article, we argue in favor of combining tCS method with other neuroimaging techniques (e.g., fMRI, EEG) and by employing state-of-the-art connectivity data analysis techniques (e.g., graph theory) to obtain a deeper understanding of the underlying spatiotemporal dynamics of functional connectivity patterns and cognitive performance. Finally, we discuss the possibilities of using these combined techniques to investigate the neural correlates of human creativity and to enhance creativity.

Keywords: tCS, connectome, graph theory, functional connectivity, structural connectivity, tDCS, tACS, tRNS

INTRODUCTION

The possibility of non-invasively modulating the activity of the brain using transcranial current brain stimulation (tCS) has been intriguing the researchers in a variety of fields as it allows to improve cognition in various domains (Fregni et al., 2005; Santiesteban et al., 2012; Schaal et al., 2013; Snowball et al., 2013) or treat many human psychiatric conditions (Boggio et al., 2007, 2008; Rigonatti et al., 2008; Nitsche et al., 2009; Terhune and Cohen Kadosh, 2013). There are a number of tCS techniques available, including, but not limited to, transcranial direct current stimulation (tDCS), transcranial alternating current stimulation (tACS), and transcranial random noise stimulation (tRNS) (for a review on the tCS methods, see: Nitsche et al., 2008; Ruffini et al., 2013). In tDCS, a small direct current (DC) is passed from anodal (positive) to cathodal (negative) electrodes positioned in the head surface in order to target specific brain areas underneath the electrodes (Nitsche and Paulus, 2000; Faria et al., 2011). Early studies with animals demonstrated an increase in excitation through membrane depolarization in the neurons underneath anodal electrode but an inhibition under the cathodal one (Bindman et al., 1962, 1964; Purpura and McMurtry, 1965). In humans, there is evidence for an increase in excitability in areas underneath the anodal electrode and a decrease underneath the cathodal following tDCS on the motor (Nitsche and Paulus, 2000) and visual cortex (Antal et al., 2004). Although this rationale of higher excitability under anodal and inhibition under cathodal has been used for determining the stimulation protocol in many studies, it remains unclear if this is so in all cases, as other variables such as the position of the cathodal in relation to anodal (Nitsche and Paulus, 2000; Antal et al., 2004; Moliadze et al., 2010) and the intensity of the stimulation (Batsikadze et al., 2013) seem to interfere with the excitability effects observed under anodal and cathodal stimulation sites. In tRNS the areas underneath both electrodes are stimulated with a current whose amplitude varies randomly in time within the frequency range of 100–640 Hz (Terney et al., 2008; Ruffini et al., 2013). In tACS, an alternating current (AC) with a pre-determined frequency passes from anodal to cathodal and the frequency is usually set within the EEG frequency spectrum (1–100 Hz) (Antal et al., 2008; Kanai et al., 2010).

The protocol for tCS stimulation, especially the anodal and cathodal electrodes location, is usually determined based on neuroimaging findings (e.g., EEG, fMRI) evidencing that a certain region is involved in the target brain function which the researcher wants to modulate. Therefore, most tCS studies hitherto are grounded on the modular paradigm, in which complex cognitive functions are thought to be mediated by independent brain areas (e.g., Kanwisher et al., 1997). Despite the great advance in the knowledge made through the modular paradigm in the last decades, the understanding that each cognitive function is mediated by independent brain areas is challenged by an increasing number of studies supporting that most cognitive functions are mediated by widely distributed areas functioning in parallel (Fuster, 2000; Sporns, 2014). For example, dyslexia was for a long time thought to be caused by a problem in the phonetic representations located in the primary and secondary auditory cortices (Goswami, 2000). However, recent work (Boets et al., 2013) has shown that dyslexic individuals have intact phonetic representations, but presented a problem in connectivity, both structural and functional, between inferior frontal gyrus (IFG) and the bilateral auditory cortex, which is associated with retrieving these representations. Other disorders such as schizophrenia (van den Heuvel et al., 2013), epilepsy (Bettus et al., 2008), and autism (Barttfeld et al., 2011) are also associated with abnormal (increased or decreased) brain connectivity rather than abnormal activity of isolated brain regions. In such cases, in seems logical that brain stimulation should not target one or the other isolated area, but the connection between them, which is certainly a challenging aim because most of the brain stimulation effects are assumed to be caused by the excitation/inhibition of the specific areas underneath anodal/cathodal electrodes.

Thus, in order to target specific connections rather than specific areas, it is necessary to understand how (or even whether) brain networks respond under or after tCS. In fact, the notion that tCS effects are brought about by increases/decreases in activation of the stimulated area has been challenged by studies showing that the effects of tDCS are not restricted to the stimulated sites (Lang et al., 2005; Kwon et al., 2008; Keeser et al., 2011). Moreover, there are some recent studies showing that tDCS affects brain connectivity patterns during both task and rest (Keeser et al., 2011; Polania et al., 2011a,b, 2012a; Meinzer et al., 2012, 2013), suggesting that the tCS has an impact not only on the target areas, but also on the brain networks. In this review paper, we discuss the possibility of tracking tCS-induced changes in the brain network by combining neuroimaging with advanced connectivity analysis techniques (e.g., graph theory). We briefly review the mechanisms of tCS and the basics of brain network analysis through graph theory as a framework to develop new brain stimulation protocols able to produce relevant changes in brain connectivity and, ultimately, in the features of a given brain network. In particular, we discuss the rationale for determining the stimulation protocol for improving creativity as an example of a complex cognitive construct which requires complex associations between multiple brain areas.

POSSIBLE MECHANISMS OF tCS

Before discussing the macro effects of tCS on connectivity, a brief discussion of its potential mechanisms is needed. Dissertating in detail on how the distinct tCS techniques can affect brain and behavior is out of the scope of this paper, but some of the key issues are elucidated here as they may be important for understanding how tCS can shape brain functional connectivity. Previous research with animals (Bindman et al., 1962, 1964; Purpura and McMurtry, 1965) showed that a small electrical DC passing through the anodal electrode can depolarize the cell membrane at subthreshold intensity, making the neurons more susceptible to excitatory activity as they become less negative, whereas the current passing the cathodal electrode polarizes the cell membrane making it more negative, inhibiting neural firing. Gartside (1968) found that a weak electrical current induced an increase in cortical firing under the stimulated area (anodal) in rats. Importantly, the same study observed that turning off the electrical current after 5 min of stimulation did not cease this increased neural discharge, termed the "aftereffect." Although in humans the currents reaching the brain through tCS are much weaker than the ones in animal studies (even if the external stimulating current is the same as humans have thicker skull), there is evidence that the brain areas underneath the anodal electrode are more prone to excitatory activity (Nitsche and Paulus, 2000, 2001; Antal et al., 2004). Repeated firing, or high-frequency stimulation, may result in long-term potentiation (LTP) and long-term depression (LTD) (Bliss and Lomo, 1973), which are thought to be the main mechanisms by which tCS modulates brain activity, as it does during learning (Rioult-Pedotti et al., 2000). In the LTP process, sustained activation of the cell through the binding of glutamate to α-Amino-3-hydroxy-5-methyl-4-isoxazolepropionic acid (AMPA) receptors in the post-synaptic membrane causes the magnesium (Mg^{2+}) to leave the N-methyl-D-aspartate receptor (NMDA) ion channel, allowing large quantities of calcium (Ca^{2+}) to enter the cell through this channel (Mg^{2+} blocks the NMDA channel). These large quantities of Ca^{2+} in the post-synaptic dendrites can improve the synaptic efficiency for an extended time period by activating second messengers (calcium-dependent kinases such as the Ca^{2+}/calmodulin-dependent ones: CaMKs), which create more AMPA receptors and protein expressions (growth factor), thereby facilitating neural plasticity (Malenka and Bear, 2004). The role of LTP on tCS effects is supported by pharmacological studies showing that the administration of an antagonist of the NMDA receptor blocks the effects of anodal and cathodal stimulation on the motor evoked potential (MEP), as triggered by a transcranial magnetic stimulation (TMS) pulse, an indirect measure of motor cortex excitability (Liebetanz et al., 2002; Nitsche et al., 2003; Monte-Silva et al., 2013). Saturation of the LTP can induce LTD (Rioult-Pedotti et al., 2000), which might be one of the reasons why the tCS effects were found to be dosage dependant (Batsikadze et al., 2013). It is important to notice that the electrical currents delivered by tDCS/tACS and tRNS are not strong enough to fire an action potential (Radman et al., 2009), but they can cause a bimodal polarization effect, namely soma depolarization and apical dendrite hyperpolarization (Bikson et al., 2004). Therefore tCS, as opposed to TMS (Terao and Ugawa, 2002), affects the post-synaptic potential by promoting a change in the cell gain (Rahman et al., 2013), and not by increasing the firing itself. Furthermore, single neuron response to weak current stimulation seems to be rather dependant on the network dynamics. It was found that low frequency AC currents can induce changes in gamma oscillations (25–35 Hz) in a zero-sum fashion as increases in excitability were balanced by complimentary inhibitory activity according to the network dynamics (Reato et al., 2010). Other studies (Parra and Bikson, 2004; Deans et al., 2007) also revealed that the network plays a role even at the cellular level (*in vitro* studies), as the neuronal firing behavior was largely determined by the network it belongs to.

The ongoing neuronal oscillatory activity during stimulation seems to shape the effects of tDCS and tACS on the resulting network activity (Frohlich and McCormick, 2010; Ali et al., 2013; Frohlich and Schmidt, 2013). This appears to happen through a feedback loop between the neural activity and the endogenous electric field (Frohlich and McCormick, 2010). Thus, tACS at the endogenous oscillation frequency (*in vitro*) produced a higher enhancement of this oscillation as compared to tDCS (Ali et al., 2013). In addition, these authors found that the network oscillatory effects were more pronounced if the stimulated frequency matches the endogenous oscillation frequency, suggesting a resonance-like effect. The importance of network activity was not only evidenced at the cellular level, but also at the cortical level in awake human beings. In relation to tDCS, it was found that stimulating over the premotor cortex (PMC) resulted in increased excitability (as measured by the MEP) over the primary motor cortex (M1) (Boros et al., 2008), which suggests that stimulating one area can affect others structurally connected to it. This might explain why many studies found that the stimulation with weak currents affects a number of areas other than the region underneath the anodal electrode (Lang et al., 2005; Kwon et al., 2008; Keeser et al., 2011). The possibility that network dynamics also plays a role in the effects of tCS at the macro level is supported by studies showing that tDCS brings about changes in functional connectivity, especially when those changes are assessed during task performance (Polania et al., 2012a; Weber et al., 2014). The default mode network (DMN) (Keeser et al., 2011; Amadi et al., 2014) and the attention network (AN) (Pena-Gomez et al., 2012) also seem to be affected by brain stimulation, even when the stimulated area is not within the same network. However, studies investigating the effects of tCS on brain connectivity during different tasks are still scarce (Polania et al., 2011b, 2012a,b; Meinzer et al., 2012, 2013; Weber et al., 2014), but they may shed new light into how tCS affects the brain dynamics and behavior. One of the challenges on this enterprise is to develop a suitable framework that can guide not only the analysis and interpretation of complex connectivity results derived from various neuroimaging techniques, but also to develop more efficient protocols to tackle connectivity.

NETWORK ANALYSIS AND BRAIN STIMULATION

There are many ways of measuring how different brain areas interact or communicate with each other. Connectivity is usually investigated from three perspectives: structural, functional and effective (Friston, 2011). Structural connectivity refers to the anatomical connections within the brain, such as axons and synapses, that can be measured non-invasively through diffusion tensor imaging (DTI) (van den Heuvel and Sporns, 2013). The brain structure is thought to shape or determine the paths for the communication between brain areas while the brain is engaged in various tasks or even at rest (Friston, 2011). While structural connectivity traces the paths between regions based on the physical connections between them, functional and effective connectivity estimate these connections based on the relationship between the time series from each of these brain regions (voxels) or the corresponding electrode / sensor (van den Heuvel and Sporns, 2013). Functional connectivity refers to how interdependent the activity between two areas (or more) is, with no information on the direction of their communication, whereas effective connectivity refers to the directed (source and sink) connection between two areas (Horwitz, 2003; Friston, 2011). Both functional and effective connectivity are dynamic and can be measured from data collected using various neuroimaging techniques, such as EEG, MEG, and fMRI. A variety of algorithms has been developed to estimate functional (e.g., coherence, phase synchronization, correlation, synchronization likelihood), and effective (e.g., dynamic causal modeling, Granger causality, phase slope index) connectivity, and they are available in many neuroimaging analysis toolboxes (e.g., Delorme and Makeig, 2004; Oostenveld et al., 2011; Niso et al., 2013). These measures allow us to estimate the strength of the communication between regions/sensors and they all have different advantages and limitations (Pereda et al., 2005; Friston, 2011).

In order to understand the organizing principles of the brain networks (estimated using the techniques mentioned in the previous paragraph), we can use graph theory, which has emerged as an important model for understanding and quantifying the global properties of brain networks (Bassett and Bullmore, 2006; Bressler and Menon, 2010; Sporns, 2011). In graph theory, networks are mathematically represented as a set of *nodes*, which in this framework are the brain regions or the electrodes/sensors for EEG/MEG, connected through *edges*, which are the paths or lines representing the direct relation between the nodes (**Figure 1A**).

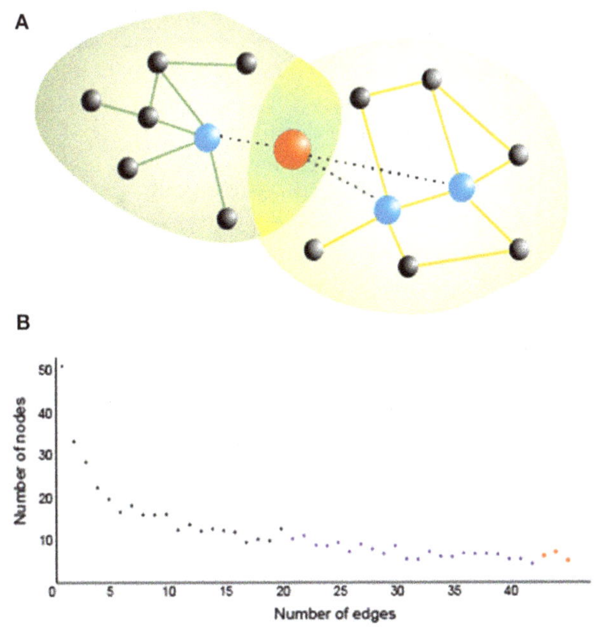

FIGURE 1 | (A) A hub naturally serves as a bridge between two or more networks, as it is connected to many nodes in all of them, thereby playing an important role in brain functioning. Stimulating a hub is likely to affect many nodes even at a long distance, which could maximize the effect of stimulation. Yet networks are also vulnerable against a directed attack on the hubs, so that their inhibition, however partial and/or transient, may crucially affect the corresponding cognitive functions if it is not properly controlled (e.g., by multisite stimulation of nearby nodes). *Green and orange lines*: intra-network edges. *Dotted lines*: edges connecting the hub with nodes in both networks; **(B)** A typical degree distribution for brain nodes as assessed by a functional connectivity index. Most of the nodes (black) have low degree (i.e., are connected only to a few nodes); some of them (blue) have moderate degree, and a few of them (in red) are hubs, which are connected to many nodes.

Out of the many measures that can be used to characterize these networks (Rubinov and Sporns, 2010; Sporns, 2014), two of them are allegedly the most commonly used in neuroscience: (1) the average clustering coefficient, and (2) the average shortest path length. The clustering coefficient is the probability that neighboring nodes will be connected. The average shortest path length is the average minimum number of edges or connections that need to be traversed between two nodes. The arrangement of the edges in the network can take three main forms, which in turn determines the character of the network itself: regular, random, and small-world (Watts and Strogatz, 1998). In a regular network, each node is connected to its neighbors, resulting in high clustering and large average path length. If we randomly rewire most of the edges in a regular network, we would reduce the path length and the clustering coefficient, which characterizes a random network. However, if only a small number of edges are rewired to connect distant nodes, we have a "small-world" network, characterized by a small shortest path length and a high clustering coefficient (Watts and Strogatz, 1998). In small-world networks, the nodes containing the long-range connections have a similar number of connections in comparison to the other nodes, which makes the network resistant to random attack to the nodes. In the brain, however, there are some regions (termed network hubs) that are more heavily connected than others, and also more connected among themselves (van den Heuvel and Sporns, 2013). This type of network organization, with only a few nodes more connected than others and also more connected among themselves, is known as "scale-free," because such networks have a power law degree distribution (Barabasi and Albert, 1999; Sporns et al., 2004), which means that most nodes have only few connections or edges, whereas a few hubs have a large number of connections, as represented in **Figure 1B**. The presence of hubs (blue and red nodes in **Figure 1**), which are heavily connected and usually also centrally located nodes, and associated with locally connected specialized nodes, allows the network to have both local and global information processing (van den Heuvel and Sporns, 2011, 2013). The hubs are essential for brain communication, albeit energetically expensive as they are highly connected, and occupy a privileged position in the network, connecting distant communities of nodes to other hubs. In addition these hubs are organized as a "rich-club," in which densely connected nodes tend to be more connected to each other (van den Heuvel and Sporns, 2013). There are two types of rich-club hubs: connector hubs (red node **Figure 1A**), which interconnect different modules, and provincial hubs (blue nodes **Figure 1A**), which connect nodes within the same module. A study with DTI (van den Heuvel and Sporns, 2011) identified three main cortical areas (both hemispheres, near the midline) which are connector hubs: superior parietal, precuneus, and superior frontal cortex; and three subcortical regions (both hemispheres near medial regions) which are provincial hubs: putamen, hippocampus, and thalamus. Importantly, they found that attacking the rich-club connections (links between members of the rich-club) in comparison to random attacks or attacks to other hub connections caused a larger decrease in the global efficiency of the network. These hubs were defined based on structural connectivity, but there is accumulating evidence on the large overlap between brain network structure and functional connectivity especially during resting state (Cabral et al., 2014; Goni et al., 2014). Regions within the DMN, medially, contain most of the functional hubs, including most of the medial regions, including anterior cingulate cortex (ACC), precuneus/posterior cingulate gyrus. Using a measure of global functional connectivity, a study (Cole et al., 2010) found that not only the DMN regions have high functional connectivity with all other regions, but the cognitive control network (CCN) (Cole and Schneider, 2007), which comprises the dorsolateral prefrontal cortex (DLPFC), rostrolateral prefrontal cortex (RLPFC), dorsal-caudal ACC, inferior frontal junction (IFJ), posterior parietal cortex (PPC), PMC, and anterior insular cortex (AIC), has also high global connectivity. The regions in the DMN and in the CCN are among the top 5% most connected regions in the brain (Cole et al., 2010). Recently, the concept of flexible hubs (Cole et al., 2013a,b), which are brain regions (e.g., DLPFC) that quickly shift their functional connectivity patterns (become highly connected) to implement cognitive control, has been discussed as an important part of network's ability for flexible behavior. Besides, a recent theoretical work (Aguirre et al., 2014) shows that communication through heavily connected nodes facilitates synchronization between different networks. Therefore, the structural and functional hubs seem to be an essential part of the scale-free brain network organization.

Making use of its structural and functional hubs, which can flexibly adapt to different environmental demands, the scale-free configuration allows dynamical exchange of information that facilitates parallel processing and rapid changes on its own configuration (Bassett and Bullmore, 2006). There is evidence that the scale-free network characteristics, as measured by graph theory, are optimized during awake compared to sleep periods (Uehara et al., 2014), suggesting that the functional organization of the network is relevant for cognitive processing. Therefore, graph-theory can be used to investigate structural, functional and effective connectivity. Functional connectivity gives undirected edges to the network, whereas effective connectivity provides information on the direction of the interactions investigated. Moreover, the edges can be weighted according to the degree of coupling between two nodes, as estimated by the techniques mentioned previously. Knowing and estimating the changes in network properties as a result of brain stimulation, during task and resting state alike, has important implications on the understanding of its effects over behavior. In addition, the knowledge of the networks representing the target cognitive process might provide insight into optimizing stimulation protocols.

BRAIN STIMULATION AND CONNECTIVITY

There is a great deal of research analysing the impact of TMS on brain connectivity patterns during task and rest (for a review, see Shafi et al., 2012). As TMS is not covered in this paper, we only summarize four main findings on TMS-induced alterations in connectivity, which can shed light onto how connectivity changes in response to brain stimulation: (1) *state dependency:* the brain state during stimulation affects how it modifies connectivity (Massimini et al., 2005; Davare et al., 2008; Morishima et al., 2009); (2) *rich-club spreading:* stimulating areas that have more connections (rich-club nodes) will affect a larger network

(Bestmann et al., 2003, 2005; Chouinard et al., 2003); (3) *structural connectivity spreading:* stimulating one area affects other regions that are structurally connected to the main stimulated region (Pascual-Leone and Walsh, 2001; Mochizuki et al., 2004); (4) *compensatory connectivity:* inhibiting certain brain areas may trigger compensatory activity in the task related network (O'Shea et al., 2007). Although there are not many studies on the effects of tCS on brain connectivity, we will discuss some of these premises in the context of the few available ones published hitherto, which are listed in **Table 1**.

Most of the papers investigating the effect of tCS on brain connectivity analyzed the changes in the functional network during resting state (Alon et al., 2011; Keeser et al., 2011; Polania et al., 2011b, 2012a; Meinzer et al., 2012, 2013; Pena-Gomez et al., 2012). Studies vary in how they define the regions/nodes of the network. Using fMRI, some studies looked into the connectivity using M1 as a seed (Alon et al., 2011; Polania et al., 2012a; Sehm et al., 2013), while others looked into specific regions of interest (Pena-Gomez et al., 2012; Polania et al., 2012b; Chib et al., 2013; Weber et al., 2014), or into the resting state networks (Keeser et al., 2011; Pena-Gomez et al., 2012). Furthermore, graph-theory was also used for tracking connectivity changes after brain stimulation (Polania et al., 2011a).

The results on stimulating motor cortex (M1) are somehow mixed: some found increased functional connectivity within M1 (Polania et al., 2012a), whereas others found a decrease (Alon et al., 2011) or both a decrease during the stimulation but an increase afterwards (Sehm et al., 2013). One of the issues with these studies is that functional connectivity before and after stimulation was assessed during rest, yet M1 is not typically a region which is highly active during rest (Boros et al., 2008), so the impact of stimulation on brain connectivity may not be pronounced or strong as the motor network is relatively idle during rest. This possibility is supported by an EEG study on the effects of tDCS over M1 on functional connectivity during rest and during a finger tapping task (Polania et al., 2011a). These authors found that stimulation of the left motor cortex (anodal over C3/C5) with the cathodal electrode over right frontopolar electrodes (Fp2) was associated with higher connectivity of the motor areas in the gamma frequency band (60–90 Hz) during finger tapping. In addition, they found an increase in frontal connectivity in theta (4–7 Hz) and alpha (8–12 Hz) frequency bands during rest after tDCS stimulation, but this result was weaker than during task. They also found reduced coupling between frontal and occipital and areas after tDCS as compared to sham stimulation, which indicates that brain stimulation can shape connectivity not only by increasing communication between areas directly associated with the performing task, but also by reducing communication between other areas. Altogether, these results showed that the findings 1 (state-dependency) and 4 (compensatory connectivity) mentioned above can also explain some of the changes in functional connectivity following tDCS, while the aftereffects of the stimulation are still in place. The state-dependency in the cited studies is not related to the exact activity during the stimulation itself as referred in the TMS studies (Massimini et al., 2005; Davare et al., 2008; Morishima et al., 2009), but with the task conducted during the aftereffects of the stimulation. This means that the increase in coupling resulting from the stimulation is dependent on the task performed during the aftereffect period and on whether it recruits the stimulated network. In relation to finding 4 (compensatory connectivity), it seems that connectivity also changes in a zero-sum fashion, as it was suggested to be the case for most neuroenhancement interventions (Brem et al., 2014).

The state dependency seems to be important not only for tDCS, but also for tACS. By investigating how it can boost motion discrimination and lower adaptation, a study found that the method was only effective when the 10 Hz stimulation over the motion area (left hMT+) was administered during visual stimulation, but not before or after it (Kar and Krekelberg, 2014). This suggests that, differently from the tDCS, where the task conducted during the aftereffects can shape the effects of the stimulation, tACS effects on brain synchronization are dependent of the ongoing activity/task or brain state during which the stimulation is administered. In the latter study (Kar and Krekelberg, 2014), administering tACS during rest is unlikely to boost motion discrimination since the effects seem to be very dependent on the precise moment of visual perception in each trial.

The structural connections between brain areas, as in findings 2 (rich-club spreading) and 3 (structural connectivity spreading), also seem to be of importance for understanding how tCS affects the brain networks. It is possible to use the knowledge about the connectivity between areas to target deeper brain structures (Takano et al., 2011; Chib et al., 2013) which up until recently could only be targeted pharmacologically. Research with animals (Takano et al., 2011) observed an increased activation in the nucleus accumbens in rats after 10 min of stimulation over the frontal cortex. A recent study in humans (Chib et al., 2013) used tDCS to target midbrain areas (subcortical), including substantia nigra (SN) and the ventral tegmental area (VTA) by stimulating the ventral medial prefrontal cortex (VMPFC), during a face attractiveness judgment task, which is associated with the dopaminergic system for reward processing. The anodal and cathodal electrode locations were defined based on the knowledge that excitation of the VMPFC combined with inhibition of the DLPFC can bring about an increase in activity (together with dopamine release) of the midbrain (Takano et al., 2011). They found that the main stimulation groups (anodal over the VMPFC and cathodal over the DLPFC) increased their ratings of face attractiveness after the stimulation, but not the active sham group, which was stimulated for the same time, but with the opposite locations (anode over DLPFC and cathode over VMPFC). Importantly, the main stimulation elicited an increase in the BOLD signal in the midbrain areas and an increase in functional connectivity between VMPFC and the midbrain area. This increase in connectivity was correlated to the participants' ratings of attractiveness. In addition, the behavioral effect was only evident when the cathodal electrode was placed over the DLPFC, as the same effects were not found when the cathode was positioned on the vertex (Cz). This result is consistent with the idea that coordinated activity between different brain areas, in this case VMPFC and DLPFC, can influence the outcomes of the stimulation in subcortical areas. Relevantly, it also demonstrates that it is possible to exploit the brain networks structure to target

Table 1 | Studies on the effects of tCS on brain connectivity.

Study	Technique	Parameters/location	Duration	Study design	Results
Polania et al., 2011a	tDCS	1 mA 4 × 4 cm^2 Anode: left M1 Cathode: right frontopolar	10 min during rest	Within participants (two sessions) Conditions: (1) tDCS; (2) Sham	After tDCS, not sham, there was an increase in synchronization between the stimulated area with premotor and sensorimotor more pronounced in the gamma band and during the motor task
Polania et al., 2012a	tDCS	1 mA 7 × 5cm^2 Anode: left M1 Cathode: right frontopolar	10 min during rest	Within participants Conditions: (1) Anode left M1/cathode right frontopolar; (2) Anode right M1/cathode left frontopolar; (3) Sham	Anode over left M1 was associated with increased connectivity between left thalamus and the ipsilateral M1, and between left caudate and parietal association cortex. Connectivity between the caudate and regions of the default mode network (DMN) was reduced, especially with the PCC. Cathode over the left M1 resulted reduced connectivity: between right putamen and left precentral gyrus and between right thalamus and left superior frontal gyrus
Meinzer et al., 2012	tDCS	1 mA Anode: 5 × 7 cm^2 Cathode: 10 × 10 cm^2 Anode: left IFG (BA44/45) Cathode: right supraorbital	20 min of which: ~6 min during rest ~11 min during task	Within participants Conditions: (1) tDCS; (2) Sham	Anodal tDCS over the left IFG was associated with better performance in a semantic word generation task. The BOLD response reduced at stimulated areas (left ventral IFG) compared to sham during the task. An increase in connectivity in the language network areas (left IFG and anterior insula) was also observed during the tDCS compared to sham. During rest, anodal stimulation resulted in increased connectivity between the left ventral IFG and other major language network hubs which partially overlapped with the task related changes in connectivity
Meinzer et al., 2013	tDCS	1 mA Anode: 5 × 7 cm^2 Cathode: 10 × 10 cm^2 Anode: left IFG (BA44/45) Cathode: right supraorbital	20 min of which: ~6 min during rest ~11 min during task	Within participants Conditions: (1) tDCS; (2) Sham	Older participants under sham stimulation performed a semantic word generation task worse than the younger group. However, during the tDCS, there was no difference in the performance between old and young participants. During task, the stimulation was associated with lower BOLD response at the stimulated site (left IFG—anodal), but with increased connectivity between this and other areas of the language network. The differences in BOLD and connectivity between young and older were reduced during tDCS stimulation, evidencing a "youth-like" effect in the older participants' brains under stimulation
Keeser et al., 2011	tDCS	2 mA 7 × 5 cm^2 Anode: left DLPFC Cathode: right supraorbital	20 min during rest	Within participants Conditions: (1) tDCS; (2) Sham	Among four resting state networks: DMN, left and right frontal-parietal networks (FPNs) and the self-referential network, it was found that tDCS induced a change in connectivity within the DMN and the FPNs

(Continued)

Table 1 | Continued

Study	Technique	Parameters/location	Duration	Study design	Results
Pena-Gomez et al., 2012	tDCS	2 mA $7 \times 5\,cm^2$ Anode: DLPFC Cathode: right supraorbital	20 min during rest	Within participants Conditions: (1) Anodal left DLPFC; (2) Anodal right DLPFC; (3) Sham	Anodal tDCS to the DLPFC resulted in an increase in functional connectivity between prefrontal and parietal regions. There was also a decrease in the spatial configuration of the DMN following both right and left DLPFC anodal stimulation
Sehm et al., 2013	tDCS	1 mA Unilateral: Anode: right M1 Cathode: contralateral orbit; Bilateral: Anode: right M1 Cathode: left M1	20 min during rest	Within participants Conditions: (1) Unilateral; (2) Bilateral; (3) Sham	Bilateral tDCS was associated with reduced interhemispheric connectivity during stimulation and with an increase in intracortical connectivity within right M1 after the stimulation. Unilateral tDCS was associated with reduced interhemispheric connectivity, but not with increased connectivity after the stimulation as did the bilateral
Alon et al., 2011	tDCS, tPCS	tDCS: 2 mA $7 \times 4.5\,cm^2$ Anode: right M1 Cathode: left supra-orbital tPCS: Monophasic waveform with pulse duration of 33 us and interval of 33.3 us Stimulator's carrier frequency 15 kHz	12 min 48 s (split in two—STIM 1 and STIM 2 with 6 min 24 s each)	Within participants Conditions: (1) tDCS; (2) tPCS	A reduced resting functional connectivity between right and left M1 was found after stimulation in both tDCS and tPCS
Weber et al., 2014	tDCS	1.5mA $5 \times 5\,cm^2$ Anode: right DLPFC (F4) Cathode: left DLPFC (F3)	15 min rest outside scanner	Between subjects: Groups: (1) tDCS; (2) Sham	The tDCS group showed reduced connectivity between the right ACC and the rest of the brain after the stimulation during rest
Chib et al., 2013	tDCS	2 mA Anode: $3.5 \times 3.5\,cm^2$ VMPFC (Fpz) Cathode: $5 \times 5\,cm^2$ Right DLPFC (F4)	15 min during rest	Between subjects Groups*: (1) Main Stimulation; (2) Active sham group: Anode 5×5 cm over right DLPFC; and Cathode 3.5×3.5 cm over VMPFC Within-subjects: pre- vs. post-stimulation	Functional connectivity changes elicited by tDCS were evaluated during a face attractiveness judgment task, before and after stimulation. The main stimulation was associated with an increase in connectivity between the VMPFC and the midbrain area (substantia nigra and ventral tegmental area). The higher the functional connectivity between these two areas during stimulation, the better the performance in the face judgment task
Neuling et al., 2013	tACS	Individualized current around 1500 mA $5 \times 7\,cm^2$ Anode: Oz Cathode: Cz Stimulation frequency: individual alpha peak frequency (IAF)	20 min during an auditory detection task	Between subjects Experiment eyes-closed groups: (1) tACS; (2) Sham Experiment eyes-open groups: (1)tACS; (2) Sham	They found that the aftereffects of tACS were higher for the group whose stimulation was done with eyes-open, whereas it did not differ between stimulation and sham for the eyes-closed experiment. However, the coherence between right and left parietal (P4-P3) increased only for the tACS group of the eyes-closed experiment

**Other four conditions were tested behaviorally, but only the main stimulation was effective in improving attractiveness judgments, leading them to scan only this and the active sham group for comparison.*

subcortical areas and their connections. The ability to affect connections between cortical and subcortical areas by stimulating the cerebral cortex has been also demonstrated during rest (Polania et al., 2012a).

Studies looking at resting state networks (Keeser et al., 2011; Pena-Gomez et al., 2012) found changes in functional connectivity after stimulation of the DLPFC. One of these studies (Pena-Gomez et al., 2012) found that stimulating either the right or the left DLPFC resulted in robust changes in the AN and in the DMN. It was observed that anodal tDCS over DLPFC was associated with a disruption in the DMN topography, as if the anterior (medial prefrontal) and posterior components (medial posterior) of the network become temporally independent after the stimulation. On the other hand, there was an increase in functional connectivity between frontal and parietal areas, which are part of the AN. An increase in fronto-parietal connectivity related to the AN was also found by others (Keeser et al., 2011), along with an increase in connectivity between an area near the anodal electrode on the left DLPFC and the DMN regions. It may be that tDCS over the DLPFC increases the alertness for action as indicated by the networks affected by stimulation, which it was suggested by the authors of both studies (Keeser et al., 2011; Pena-Gomez et al., 2012). As we mentioned in the previous section, the DLPFC can be considered a functional "flexible hub," which plays an important role in switching from one state to the other in order to attend to the necessary task demands (Cole et al., 2013b). This might be one of the reasons why stimulating DLPFC seems to affect functional connectivity in the DMN, as it reflects the change from one to the other network. These studies support that tCS can alter the connectivity in the brain during rest. In order to improve the interpretation of the results, new studies should target specific networks and bring new hypothesis of possible behavioral correlates. For example, what does it mean to increase or decrease connectivity in certain brain networks? Would these changes, for instance, improve mood, reduce depression, increase alertness, and others? The need for behavioral correlates in these studies is crucial for understanding their functional meaning.

Hitherto, two recent studies (Meinzer et al., 2012, 2013) used fMRI to monitor the brain activity during rest as well as during a semantic word generation task while the participants received anodal tDCS over the left IFG (targeting language areas—BA 44/45—see **Table 1** for details). Both studies observed a reduction in the BOLD signal at the stimulated sites during the language task. Importantly, the connectivity between the stimulated area (left IFG) and other language-related area was increased during stimulation for both task and rest (Meinzer et al., 2012, 2013). It has been argued that these changes are related to increased neural efficiency at the stimulated site and its networks (Kar and Wright, 2014) similar to the changes observed as a result of learning (Buchel et al., 1999). These changes were found to be behaviorally relevant as the performance in the semantic word generation task improved when the participants were receiving active stimulation compared to sham. One of these studies (Meinzer et al., 2013) observed an interesting effect whereby older adults showed a pattern similar to that of their younger counterparts in terms of performance in the semantic task when receiving anodal stimulation over the left IFG, despite performing worse without stimulation. In a similar vein, the differences in BOLD activation and functional connectivity between young and older adults were reduced during anodal tDCS. In relation to the connectivity, older participants showed higher anterior (fronto-temporal, and medial frontal regions) and lower posterior (temporo-occipital, precentral, and postcentral cortices) functional connectivity than younger, which was related to worse task performance. Anodal tDCS stimulation over the left IFG seems to reverse these effects, as it reduced functional connectivity among anterior cortical areas and increased it among the posterior cortices (note that not all the age related connectivity differences were reversed though).

Considering that all but one of these studies (except Polania et al., 2011a), were conducted using tDCS in combination with fMRI, more research is needed using other tCS techniques, especially tACS and tRNS, combined with higher temporal resolution neuroimaging techniques such as EEG/MEG, as we cannot expect that all tCS techniques would impact brain connectivity in the same way. Nonetheless, there is an EEG study (Neuling et al., 2013) in which the participants' occipital cortex (anode: Oz) was stimulated in the individual alpha frequency (IAF) to compare the aftereffects of stimulating in two different conditions: eyes-closed and eyes-open. These authors found that alpha power only differs between tACS stimulation and sham in the eyes-open condition. The coherence between two parietal electrodes (P3-P4), however, was only increased after tACS stimulation with eyes-closed (not with eyes-open). Therefore, there was a difference in the aftereffects of stimulating the areas with eyes-open and eyes-closed, which support the idea that the effects of tCS are dependent on the brain state, and for tACS in particular, on the ongoing brain oscillations. Considering the time varying nature of the oscillatory brain activity, new real time protocols are being developed to adjust the stimulation frequency according to the brain oscillations in real time (Boyle and Frohlich, 2013).

CREATIVITY, BRAIN STIMULATION, AND NETWORK ANALYSIS

Creativity is a multidimensional construct that can be investigated from a number of different perspectives, from its associated processes such as convergent and divergent thinking (Sawyer, 2012), passing through the creative person, product and press or environment (Rhodes, 1961). In this paper, we borrowed the following definition of creativity from Plucker et al., 2004: *"Creativity is the interaction among aptitude, process, and environment by which an individual or group produces a perceptible product that is both novel and useful as defined within a social context" (p. 90).* In the field of Cognitive Neuroscience, the main focus of creativity research is on the processes involved in the creative thinking, including divergent and convergent thinking (Luft and Bhattacharya, 2014). Divergent thinking refers to the capacity of generating novel and original ideas to open-ended problems (e.g., think of as many unusual uses of a brick). Convergent thinking, on the other hand, refers to the process of finding a correct solution to a closed-ended problem, such as a puzzle. In the real world, however, the creative process involves both divergent and convergent thinking (Sawyer, 2012).

There are only a few studies on how we can boost creativity using tCS (Cerruti and Schlaug, 2009; Chi and Snyder, 2011, 2012; Metuki et al., 2012; Chrysikou et al., 2013), which are described in **Table 2**. On the divergent thinking study (Chrysikou et al., 2013), the authors positioned the cathodal electrode over the left or the right prefrontal cortex and the anode over the mastoid, in an attempt to inhibit the left or right DLPFC. They found that cathodal stimulation over the left DLPFC, but not over the right DLPFC, was associated with quicker responses on the uncommon uses task (the participants were asked to generate common or uncommon uses for presented objects). The authors suggested that this result is coherent with the idea that divergent thinking depends on transient hypo-frontality, but in this case, it was found to be specific to the left hemisphere.

Most of the studies cited in **Table 2** investigated creative insight, which is a convergent thinking process. In one of the insight studies (Cerruti and Schlaug, 2009) it was found that anodal stimulation over the left DLPFC increases the solution rate in a convergent thinking task, the "Remote Associate Task—RAT." In this task, the participants have to find a fourth word which makes a compound word with three words presented on the screen (e.g., food/forward/break; solution: fast). However, another study (Metuki et al., 2012) observed that anodal stimulation over the left DLPFC did not improve the solution rate when subjects were given less time to solve the problem (7 s compared to 30 s), but it did improve subjects' ability to recognize correct solutions to hard RAT problems. The authors suggested that the left DLPFC is involved in recognizing the correct solution rather than generating it, a role that has been attributed to the right hemisphere (Bowden and Jung-Beeman, 2003), especially the right anterior area (Jung-Beeman et al., 2004). A slightly different account can be suggested based on two experiments (Anderson et al., 2009) monitoring the subjects brain responses (fMRI) while they solved a compound-word RAT task (Experiment 1) and another similar paradigm which allowed faster responses (Experiment 2). They observed that while the LIPFC was associated with the word search in memory or memory retrieval, the ACC was associated with the processing of solutions. In both experiments, the LIPFC activity increased when the participants were trying to find a solution, but from the moment they reached it, the ACC activity increased and the LIPFC returned to baseline levels.

The other two insight studies (Chi and Snyder, 2011, 2012) focused on other insight problems that are less dependent on verbal processes (matchstick and 9-dot problems). In both studies (Chi and Snyder, 2011, 2012), the stimulation protocol positioned the cathodal electrode over the left anterior temporal lobe (ATL), and the anodal over the right ATL. The authors found that this protocol increased the solution rates to these problems in relation to sham stimulation (between groups).

Therefore, for insight studies, it seems that the left DLPFC, and the right ATL play a role in finding solutions for convergent thinking. Nonetheless, little is still known about how these areas communicate to generate a solution as none of these studies combined tCS with any neuroimaging techniques, making it difficult to know whether these changes in performance are indeed caused by the excited/inhibited areas (Chi and Snyder, 2011, 2012; Chrysikou et al., 2013), by a connection between the stimulated/inhibited area, or by a compensatory network mechanisms that may be triggered by inhibiting those (as in finding 4 described in the previous section). In addition, in the human motor system evidence that bilateral tDCS evokes a suppression of one hemisphere but a facilitation of the other is somewhat mixed (see Nitsche and Paulus, 2000; Mordillo-Mateos et al., 2012; Hasan et al., 2013). Thus, the biological impact of bilateral tDCS (and by virtue the mechanisms that modulate previously reported enhancements in creativity following bilateral tDCS—e.g., Chi and Snyder, 2011, 2012) remains unclear.

Previous studies on the brain activity underlying creativity found, for example, that divergent thinking is associated with higher functional connectivity between medial prefrontal cortex (mPFC) and posterior cingulate cortex (PCC), both of which are key nodes of the DMN (Takeuchi et al., 2012). It could be that inhibiting the lateral prefrontal cortex may result in higher activation of the medial prefrontal, but this can only be tested by combining tCS with neuroimaging. There are a number of studies suggesting that creativity is associated with higher connectivity, both structural (Jung et al., 2010a,b; Takeuchi et al., 2010) and functional during rest (Jaušovec and Jaušovec, 2000a; Kounios et al., 2008; Takeuchi et al., 2012) and task alike (Jaušovec and Jaušovec, 2000b; Bhattacharya and Petsche, 2002, 2005; Razumnikova and Larina, 2005). Further, there are recent suggestions that creative ideas may reside in dynamic activation patterns of spontaneous brain networks (Wiggins and Bhattacharya, 2014). On account of these works, we believe that an important step towards improving creativity through tCS would be to combine brain stimulation with neuroimaging and advanced analysis techniques, in order to find how the brain networks mediate the improvements in creative processes observed in the cited studies. Importantly, techniques such as tACS allow targeting both long range and local synchronization (Ali et al., 2013).

Based on the previous discussions, we propose a hypothetical approach for combining neuroimaging, connectivity and brain stimulation for improving creativity (**Figure 2**). In this approach, the research starts with the graph theoretical analysis of the connectivity between the regions involved in a certain process (e.g., convergent thinking—insight) as in **Figure 2A**. Using the discovered cognitive connections (**Figure 2B**), a protocol for stimulation is determined (**Figure 2C**). In **Figure 2A**, we showed a couple of regions involved in creativity. Immediately after the stimulation, the connectivity patterns (in identical conditions of the analyzed patterns in **Figures 2A,B**) are analyzed against control stimulation protocol, e.g., sham stimulation. The results are presented as a map, with the edges linking the nodes representing here the strength of the difference in connectivity between active and sham stimulation (or any other control or contrast of the experiment), as in **Figure 2D**. In **Figure 2** hypothetical example, the connectivity changed after stimulation of the left DLPFC during a RAT paradigm, especially among the temporal and frontal areas (**Figure 2D**). In the hypothetical example, there was an increase in communication between ATL and DLPFC and between the DLPFC and the ACC, which could represent coordinated (DLPFC) search of the solution in memory (ATL) and

Table 2 | Studies on tCS and creativity.

Study	Creative process	Technique	Parameters/location	Duration	Design	Paradigm	Results
Chi and Snyder, 2012	Insight	tDCS	1.6 mA (30 s raising), electrode 35 cm^2 Anode: right ATL Cathode: left ATL	10 min	Within-participants: pre-during-post Between: active vs. sham	9-dot problem	40% of the active group were able to solve the problem; none of the sham group solved it
Chi and Snyder, 2011	Insight	tDCS	1.6 mA (30 s raising) electrode 35 cm^2 Anode: right ATL Cathode: left ATL	10 min	Between participants: (1) L− R+; (2) L+ R−; (3) Sham stimulation	Matchstick problems	60% of the participants in the L-R+ group were able to solve the difficult problems whereas lower than 20% in the other groups solved it
Metuki et al., 2012	Insight	tDCS	1 mA (30 s raising) electrode 35 cm^2 Unilateral active Anode: left DLPFC (F3); Cathode: right OFC (Fp2)	11 min (5 min pre + 6 online)	2 × 2Within-participants: (1) Active vs. sham (sessions separated by a week); (2) Easy vs. Hard	RAT (CRA) with limited time (to investigate solution identification rather than generation)	They found that stimulation did not affect the rate of solution for either hard or easy problems. However, they found an interaction between stimulation and difficulty for solution recognition, as the participants in the active stimulation group were more able to recognize correct solutions for hard problems
Cerruti and Schlaug, 2009	Insight	tDCS	1 mA Anode: 16.3 cm^2 Cathode: 30 cm^2 Experiment 1 Anode: left DLPFC Cathode: right OFC Experiment 2 Anode: left DLPFC Cathode: right DLPFC	20 min 16 min stimulation + 4 min stimulation during the verbal fluency task	Within-participants design with (3 h session): (1) Anodal electrode location: F3 vs. right supraorbital region (Experiment 1); F3 vs. F4 (Experiment 2); (2) Condition: active anodal, active cathodal, sham	Verbal Fluency (VF) + RAT (CRA) with 30 s to solve	They found that the stimulation did not improve VF, but was associated with higher solution rates when the stimulated area was above the left DLPFC. The two experiments showed the same result, with higher solution rates for anodal on the left DLPFC
Chrysikou et al., 2013	Divergent thinking (flexible tool use)	tDCS	1.5 mA 25 cm^2 electrodes Cathode: F7 or F8 Anode: on the contralateral mastoid (the main purpose was to cause inhibition of PFC)	20 min (including 10 s ramp-up + 10 s ramp down). Stimulation began for 180 s prior to the tasks	Between-subjects design with two factors: Stimulation protocol (groups): (1) Cathodal Left (F7) and anodal on mastoid; (2) Cathodal Right (F8) and anodal on mastoid; (3) Sham Task (groups): (1) Common uses; (2) Uncommon uses	Div. Thinking: participants were asked to generate either (1) common vs. (2) uncommon uses for the objects presented on the screen (60 grayscale pictures). Each participant was assigned to only one of these two conditions. The performance was measure to response onset time	There was a significant interaction between stimulation protocol and task condition, since cathodal over the left PFC was associated with in an decrease in the response times for the uncommon uses task. There was no difference in performance between stimulation conditions in the common uses task. In addition, cathodal stimulation over the left PFC was associated with lower number of response omissions in the uncommon uses task only (no difference in the common uses task)

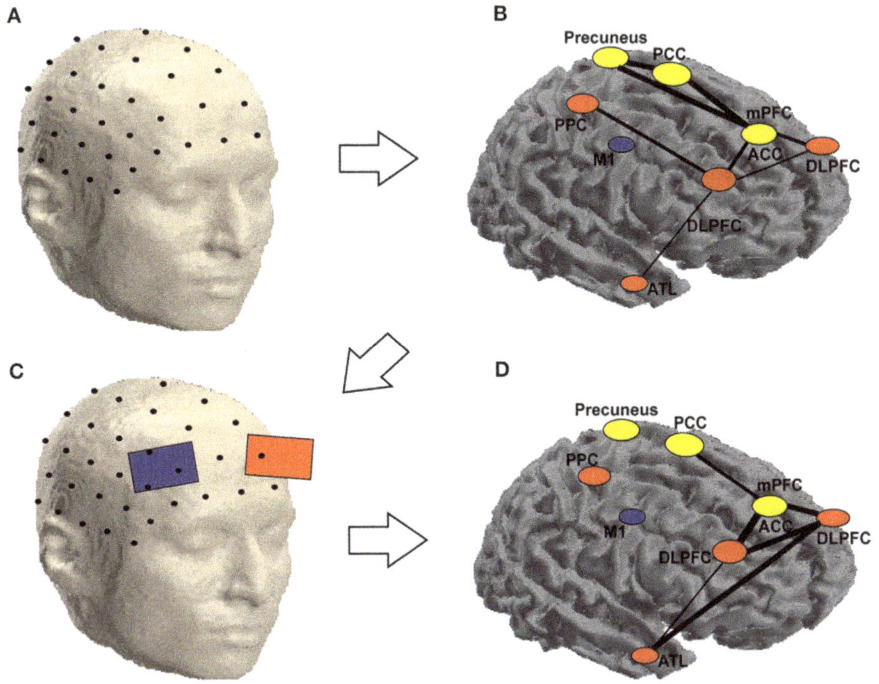

FIGURE 2 | Schematic representation of the possible combination of tCS and functional (EEG) brain connectivity to enhance creativity. An array of scalp electrodes, a subset of which is depicted in **(A)**, is recorded. In **(B)** is possible to identify ROIs which are highly connected (yellow) and the ones that are flexible hubs (red) or less connected areas (blue) during a solution vs. non-solution RAT task. This helps identifying the target electrodes to stimulate as in **(C)**. Stimulating these electrodes may not only eliminate the differences for the corresponding nodes, but also reduce them for areas in the same network, which are not stimulated but functionally connected to the targeted ones as depicted in **(D)**. It is worth noting that the labels and the networks drawn in the figure are only for demonstration, as they are not precisely equivalent to their anatomical locations (they are only approximate locations on a surface, the areas in yellow are located in the medial area of the brain, which cannot be seen in a cortical mesh). The areas are abbreviated as follows: PCC, posterior cingulate cortex; PPC, posterior parietal cortex; M1, primary motor cortex; mPFC, medial prefrontal cortex; ACC, anterior cingulate cortex; DLPFC, dorsolateral prefrontal cortex; ATL, anterior temporal lobe.

the recognition of the correct solution (ACC), from DLPFC to ACC. Note that this approach does not account for the direction of the interactions, which could be also tested using effective connectivity analysis techniques such as dynamic causal modeling or Granger causality. In divergent thinking, the approach would probably result in a higher change over the posterior rather than anterior regions.

LIMITATIONS OF GRAPH-THEORY AND BRAIN STIMULATION

Notwithstanding the advances emerging from the combination of tCS and neuroimaging for the understanding of the connectivity changes in response to brain stimulation, there are many limitations of both methods which can be thought as new challenges for this enterprise. First, despite its usefulness in characterizing brain network during cognitive functions (Sporns, 2014), the application of graph theory is not problem-free (Fornito et al., 2013). The approach, after all, is based on sophisticated mathematical techniques that require judicious choices at various steps of the analysis. Perhaps the most obvious one is the need to choose among a number of possible strategies to reconstruct the networks, which do not always lead to a convergent or consistent outcome. For instance, one has to decide whether the links will be weighted or unweighted, directed or not, whether to use a fixed value or a fixed link density across participants as a threshold or to use statistical controls such as surrogate data analysis in order to determine the significance in a per-link basis. Further, especially in the case of EEG/MEG, many different bivariate indices of functional/effective connectivity are available (e.g., Niso et al., 2013). Besides, spurious characterization of a network could result from an inappropriate temporal and/or spatial sampling of the underlying systems (Bialonski et al., 2010, 2011). Last, but not least, the relationship between connectivity at the sensor/electrode level and connectivity at the neural source level is more complicated than traditionally assumed (Ewald et al., 2012). Nevertheless, we argue that graph theory is a very useful tool to study the synchronized activity between different brain areas underlying most cognitive functions, as it can be used to characterize these patterns of brain connectivity. Moreover, it can be also used to understand how local changes (whether internally or externally generated) are able to affect other distant brain areas. For instance, in focal epilepsy research a paradigm shift is currently taking place whereby attention is increasingly not toward the epileptic focus itself, the classical and obvious target area of the neuroscientific research on epilepsy, but the epileptic network and its characteristics (Lehnertz et al., 2014), offering a tremendous potential in minimizing the extent of surgical intervention.

The tCS methods also face limitations that have to be considered when attempting to develop protocols to boost specific cognitive functions. Currently, there are many issues related to our lack of understanding of how tCS, in its different modalities, shapes neural activity. First, as tCS methods in humans are non-invasive, the stimulation is applied to the skull rather than directly to the brain, meaning that the spatial resolution of tCS is diffuse due to skull dispersion. The spatial resolution can be improved with small stimulation electrodes (Datta et al., 2009), but it still does not overcome the problem that the stimulation is indirect and the electrodes often too large for such focal stimulation of a small cortical area. The second limitation, which is closely related to the first, is the lack of control of the stimulation current reaching the brain as the current is altered as it passes through the skull to be then conducted by the cerebrospinal fluid to the brain. Individual differences in skull thickness and shape may interact with how much current is actually reaching the brain (Datta et al., 2009). Therefore, even with advanced modeling of the current (Wagner et al., 2007; Shahid et al., 2014), it is difficult to predict how much current is actually reaching the brain. Third, the stimulation effects, as stated earlier in the Introduction, are not straightforward. For example, anodal stimulation does not always cause increase excitability, and vice versa for cathodal (Nitsche and Paulus, 2000; Antal et al., 2004; Moliadze et al., 2010). Further, other factors such as increasing the intensity (Batsikadze et al., 2013) or including a task during stimulation (Antal et al., 2007) can also change the effects in a complicated fashion. Therefore, it is important for these factors to be controlled carefully in tCS studies. Moreover, when one considers these limitations in conjunction with the fact that stimulating one area of the brain can affect a network of regions, it hampers the possibility of claiming "cause-effects" relations between a single stimulated brain region and specific cognitive functions as the stimulation effects are not entirely known.

CONCLUSION

In this paper, we discussed the possibility of combining tCS with neuroimaging and graph theory for analysing the impact of brain stimulation on brain connectivity. In doing so, we highlight how graph theoretical analysis can help in understanding how the brain networks are affected by tCS in specific locations. In addition, we suggest that the knowledge of structural connectivity pathways can be used to target a network of brain areas rather than a single area and that ongoing brain connectivity during and just after (during the aftereffects period) tCS is an important factor in determining the connectivity changes in response to stimulation. In the future, we suggest using graph theory not only to understand the network effects of stimulating different brain areas, but also to develop tCS protocols that can target connectivity rather than individual brain areas.

ACKNOWLEDGMENTS

The authors are supported by the CREAM project that has been funded by the European Commission under Grant Agreement no 612022. This publication reflects the views only of the authors, and the European Commission cannot be held responsible for any use which may be made of the information contained therein. Michael J. Banissy is also supported by the Economic and Social Research Council (ES/K00882X/1).

REFERENCES

Aguirre, J., Sevilla-Escoboza, R., Gutiérrez, R., Papo, D., and Buldú, J. M. (2014). Synchronization of interconnected networks: the role of connector nodes. *Phys. Rev. Lett.* 112:248701. doi: 10.1103/PhysRevLett.112.248701

Ali, M. M., Sellers, K. K., and Frohlich, F. (2013). Transcranial alternating current stimulation modulates large-scale cortical network activity by network resonance. *J. Neurosci.* 33, 11262–11275. doi: 10.1523/JNEUROSCI.5867-12.2013

Alon, G., Roys, S. R., Gullapalli, R. P., and Greenspan, J. D. (2011). Non-invasive electrical stimulation of the brain (ESB) modifies the resting-state network connectivity of the primary motor cortex: a proof of concept fMRI study. *Brain Res.* 1403, 37–44. doi: 10.1016/j.brainres.2011.06.013

Amadi, U., Ilie, A., Johansen-Berg, H., and Stagg, C. J. (2014). Polarity-specific effects of motor transcranial direct current stimulation on fMRI resting state networks. *Neuroimage* 88, 155–161. doi: 10.1016/j.neuroimage.2013.11.037

Anderson, J. R., Anderson, J. F., Ferris, J. L., Fincham, J. M., and Jung, K. J. (2009). Lateral inferior prefrontal cortex and anterior cingulate cortex are engaged at different stages in the solution of insight problems. *Proc. Natl. Acad. Sci. U.S.A.* 106, 10799–10804. doi: 10.1073/pnas.0903953106

Antal, A., Boros, K., Poreisz, C., Chaieb, L., Terney, D., and Paulus, W. (2008). Comparatively weak after-effects of transcranial alternating current stimulation (tACS) on cortical excitability in humans. *Brain Stimul.* 1, 97–105. doi: 10.1016/j.brs.2007.10.001

Antal, A., Kincses, T. Z., Nitsche, M. A., Bartfai, O., and Paulus, W. (2004). Excitability changes induced in the human primary visual cortex by transcranial direct current stimulation: direct electrophysiological evidence. *Invest. Ophthalmol. Vis. Sci.* 45, 702–707. doi: 10.1167/iovs.03-0688

Antal, A., Terney, D., Poreisz, C., and Paulus, W. (2007). Towards unravelling task-related modulations of neuroplastic changes induced in the human motor cortex. *Eur. J. Neurosci.* 26, 2687–2691. doi: 10.1111/j.1460-9568.2007.05896.x

Barabasi, A. L., and Albert, R. (1999). Emergence of scaling in random networks. *Science* 286, 509–512. doi: 10.1126/science.286.5439.509

Barttfeld, P., Wicker, B., Cukier, S., Navarta, S., Lew, S., and Sigman, M. (2011). A big-world network in ASD: dynamical connectivity analysis reflects a deficit in long-range connections and an excess of short-range connections. *Neuropsychologia* 49, 254–263. doi: 10.1016/j.neuropsychologia.2010.11.024

Bassett, D. S., and Bullmore, E. (2006). Small-world brain networks. *Neuroscientist* 12, 512–523. doi: 10.1177/1073858406293182

Batsikadze, G., Moliadze, V., Paulus, W., Kuo, M. F., and Nitsche, M. A. (2013). Partially non-linear stimulation intensity-dependent effects of direct current stimulation on motor cortex excitability in humans. *J. Physiol.* 591, 1987–2000. doi: 10.1113/jphysiol.2012.249730

Bestmann, S., Baudewig, J., Siebner, H. R., Rothwell, J. C., and Frahm, J. (2003). Subthreshold high-frequency TMS of human primary motor cortex modulates interconnected frontal motor areas as detected by interleaved fMRI-TMS. *Neuroimage* 20, 1685–1696. doi: 10.1016/j.neuroimage.2003.07.028

Bestmann, S., Baudewig, J., Siebner, H. R., Rothwell, J. C., and Frahm, J. (2005). BOLD MRI responses to repetitive TMS over human dorsal premotor cortex. *Neuroimage* 28, 22–29. doi: 10.1016/j.neuroimage.2005.05.027

Bettus, G., Wendling, F., Guye, M., Valton, L., Regis, J., Chauvel, P., et al. (2008). Enhanced EEG functional connectivity in mesial temporal lobe epilepsy. *Epilepsy Res.* 81, 58–68. doi: 10.1016/j.eplepsyres.2008.04.020

Bhattacharya, J., and Petsche, H. (2002). Shadows of artistry: cortical synchrony during perception and imagery of visual art. *Brain Res. Cogn. Brain Res.* 13, 179–186. doi: 10.1016/S0926-6410(01)00110-0

Bhattacharya, J., and Petsche, H. (2005). Drawing on mind's canvas: differences in cortical integration patterns between artists and non-artists. *Hum. Brain Mapp.* 26, 1–14. doi: 10.1002/hbm.20104

Bialonski, S., Horstmann, M. T., and Lehnertz, K. (2010). From brain to earth and climate systems: small-world interaction networks or not? *Chaos* 20, 013134. doi: 10.1063/1.3360561

Bialonski, S., Wendler, M., and Lehnertz, K. (2011). Unraveling spurious properties of interaction networks with tailored random networks. *PLoS ONE* 6:e22826. doi: 10.1371/journal.pone.0022826

Bikson, M., Inoue, M., Akiyama, H., Deans, J. K., Fox, J. E., Miyakawa, H., et al. (2004). Effects of uniform extracellular DC electric fields on excitability in rat hippocampal slices *in vitro*. *J. Physiol.* 557, 175–190. doi: 10.1113/jphysiol.2003.055772

Bindman, L. J., Lippold, O. C., and Redfearn, J. W. (1962). Long-lasting changes in the level of the electrical activity of the cerebral cortex produced bypolarizing currents. *Nature* 196, 584–585. doi: 10.1038/196584a0

Bindman, L. J., Lippold, O. C., and Redfearn, J. W. (1964). The action of brief polarizing currents on the cerebral cortex of the rat (1) during current flow and (2) in the production of long-lasting after-effects. *J. Physiol.* 172, 369–382.

Bliss, T. V., and Lomo, T. (1973). Long-lasting potentiation of synaptic transmission in the dentate area of the anaesthetized rabbit following stimulation of the perforant path. *J. Physiol.* 232, 331–356.

Boets, B., Op De Beeck, H. P., Vandermosten, M., Scott, S. K., Gillebert, C. R., Mantini, D., et al. (2013). Intact but less accessible phonetic representations in adults with dyslexia. *Science* 342, 1251–1254. doi: 10.1126/science.1244333

Boggio, P. S., Nunes, A., Rigonatti, S. P., Nitsche, M. A., Pascual-Leone, A., and Fregni, F. (2007). Repeated sessions of noninvasive brain DC stimulation is associated with motor function improvement in stroke patients. *Restor. Neurol. Neurosci.* 25, 123–129.

Boggio, P. S., Rigonatti, S. P., Ribeiro, R. B., Myczkowski, M. L., Nitsche, M. A., Pascual-Leone, A., et al. (2008). A randomized, double-blind clinical trial on the efficacy of cortical direct current stimulation for the treatment of major depression. *Int. J. Neuropsychopharmacol.* 11, 249–254. doi: 10.1017/S1461145707007833

Boros, K., Poreisz, C., Munchau, A., Paulus, W., and Nitsche, M. A. (2008). Premotor transcranial direct current stimulation (tDCS) affects primary motor excitability in humans. *Eur. J. Neurosci.* 27, 1292–1300. doi: 10.1111/j.1460-9568.2008.06090.x

Bowden, E. M., and Jung-Beeman, M. (2003). Aha! Insight experience correlates with solution activation in the right hemisphere. *Psychon. Bull. Rev.* 10, 730–737. doi: 10.3758/BF03196539

Boyle, M. R., and Frohlich, F. (2013). "EEG feedback-controlled transcranial alternating current stimulation," in *2013 6th International IEEE/EMBS Conference on Neural Engineering* (San Diego, CA: NER), 140–143. doi: 10.1109/NER.2013.6695891

Brem, A. K., Fried, P. J., Horvath, J. C., Robertson, E. M., and Pascual-Leone, A. (2014). Is neuroenhancement by noninvasive brain stimulation a net zero-sum proposition? *Neuroimage* 85(pt 3), 1058–1068. doi: 10.1016/j.neuroimage.2013.07.038

Bressler, S. L., and Menon, V. (2010). Large-scale brain networks in cognition: emerging methods and principles. *Trends Cogn. Sci.* 14, 277–290. doi: 10.1016/j.tics.2010.04.004

Buchel, C., Coull, J. T., and Friston, K. J. (1999). The predictive value of changes in effective connectivity for human learning. *Science* 283, 1538–1541. doi: 10.1126/science.283.5407.1538

Cabral, J., Luckhoo, H., Woolrich, M., Joensson, M., Mohseni, H., Baker, A., et al. (2014). Exploring mechanisms of spontaneous functional connectivity in MEG: how delayed network interactions lead to structured amplitude envelopes of band-pass filtered oscillations. *Neuroimage* 90, 423–435. doi: 10.1016/j.neuroimage.2013.11.047

Cerruti, C., and Schlaug, G. (2009). Anodal transcranial direct current stimulation of the prefrontal cortex enhances complex verbal associative thought. *J. Cogn. Neurosci.* 21, 1980–1987. doi: 10.1162/jocn.2008.21143

Chi, R. P., and Snyder, A. W. (2011). Facilitate insight by non-invasive brain stimulation. *PLoS ONE* 6:e16655. doi: 10.1371/journal.pone.0016655

Chi, R. P., and Snyder, A. W. (2012). Brain stimulation enables the solution of an inherently difficult problem. *Neurosci. Lett.* 515, 121–124. doi: 10.1016/j.neulet.2012.03.012

Chib, V. S., Yun, K., Takahashi, H., and Shimojo, S. (2013). Noninvasive remote activation of the ventral midbrain by transcranial direct current stimulation of prefrontal cortex. *Transl. Psychiatry* 3, e268. doi: 10.1038/tp.2013.44

Chouinard, P. A., Van Der Werf, Y. D., Leonard, G., and Paus, T. (2003). Modulating neural networks with transcranial magnetic stimulation applied over the dorsal premotor and primary motor cortices. *J. Neurophysiol.* 90, 1071–1083. doi: 10.1152/jn.01105.2002

Chrysikou, E. G., Hamilton, R. H., Coslett, H. B., Datta, A., Bikson, M., and Thompson-Schill, S. L. (2013). Noninvasive transcranial direct current stimulation over the left prefrontal cortex facilitates cognitive flexibility in tool use. *Cogn. Neurosci.* 4, 81–89. doi: 10.1080/17588928.2013.768221

Cole, M. W., Laurent, P., and Stocco, A. (2013a). Rapid instructed task learning: a new window into the human brain's unique capacity for flexible cognitive control. *Cogn. Affect. Behav. Neurosci.* 13, 1–22. doi: 10.3758/s13415-012-0125-7

Cole, M. W., Pathak, S., and Schneider, W. (2010). Identifying the brain's most globally connected regions. *Neuroimage* 49, 3132–3148. doi: 10.1016/j.neuroimage.2009.11.001

Cole, M. W., Reynolds, J. R., Power, J. D., Repovs, G., Anticevic, A., and Braver, T. S. (2013b). Multi-task connectivity reveals flexible hubs for adaptive task control. *Nat. Neurosci.* 16, 1348–1355. doi: 10.1038/nn.3470

Cole, M. W., and Schneider, W. (2007). The cognitive control network: integrated cortical regions with dissociable functions. *Neuroimage* 37, 343–360. doi: 10.1016/j.neuroimage.2007.03.071

Datta, A., Bansal, V., Diaz, J., Patel, J., Reato, D., and Bikson, M. (2009). Gyri-precise head model of transcranial direct current stimulation: improved spatial focality using a ring electrode versus conventional rectangular pad. *Brain Stimul.* 2, 201–207, 207.e1. doi: 10.1016/j.brs.2009.03.005

Davare, M., Lemon, R., and Olivier, E. (2008). Selective modulation of interactions between ventral premotor cortex and primary motor cortex during precision grasping in humans. *J. Physiol.* 586, 2735–2742. doi: 10.1113/jphysiol.2008.152603

Deans, J. K., Powell, A. D., and Jefferys, J. G. (2007). Sensitivity of coherent oscillations in rat hippocampus to AC electric fields. *J. Physiol.* 583, 555–565. doi: 10.1113/jphysiol.2007.137711

Delorme, A., and Makeig, S. (2004). EEGLAB: an open source toolbox for analysis of single-trial EEG dynamics including independent component analysis. *J. Neurosci. Methods* 134, 9–21. doi: 10.1016/j.jneumeth.2003.10.009

Ewald, A., Marzetti, L., Zappasodi, F., Meinecke, F. C., and Nolte, G. (2012). Estimating true brain connectivity from EEG/MEG data invariant to linear and static transformations in sensor space. *Neuroimage* 60, 476–488. doi: 10.1016/j.neuroimage.2011.11.084

Faria, P., Hallett, M., and Miranda, P. C. (2011). A finite element analysis of the effect of electrode area and inter-electrode distance on the spatial distribution of the current density in tDCS. *J. Neural Eng.* 8:066017. doi: 10.1088/1741-2560/8/6/066017

Fornito, A., Zalesky, A., and Breakspear, M. (2013). Graph analysis of the human connectome: promise, progress, and pitfalls. *Neuroimage* 80, 426–444. doi: 10.1016/j.neuroimage.2013.04.087

Fregni, F., Boggio, P. S., Nitsche, M., Bermpohl, F., Antal, A., Feredoes, E., et al. (2005). Anodal transcranial direct current stimulation of prefrontal cortex enhances working memory. *Exp. Brain Res.* 166, 23–30. doi: 10.1007/s00221-005-2334-6

Friston, K. J. (2011). Functional and effective connectivity: a review. *Brain Connect.* 1, 13–36. doi: 10.1089/brain.2011.0008

Frohlich, F., and McCormick, D. A. (2010). Endogenous electric fields may guide neocortical network activity. *Neuron* 67, 129–143. doi: 10.1016/j.neuron.2010.06.005

Frohlich, F., and Schmidt, S. L. (2013). Rational design of transcranial current stimulation (TCS) through mechanistic insights into cortical network dynamics. *Front. Hum. Neurosci.* 7:804. doi: 10.3389/fnhum.2013.00804

Fuster, J. M. (2000). The module: crisis of a paradigm. *Neuron* 26, 51–53. doi: 10.1016/S0896-6273(00)81137-X

Gartside, I. B. (1968). Mechanisms of sustained increases of firing rate of neurons in the rat cerebral cortex after polarization: reverberating circuits or modification of synaptic conductance? *Nature* 220, 382–383. doi: 10.1038/220382a0

Goni, J., van den Heuvel, M. P., Avena-Koenigsberger, A., Velez De Mendizabal, N., Betzel, R. F., Griffa, A., et al. (2014). Resting-brain functional connectivity predicted by analytic measures of network communication. *Proc. Natl. Acad. Sci. U.S.A.* 111, 833–838. doi: 10.1073/pnas.1315529111

Goswami, U. (2000). Phonological representations, reading development and dyslexia: towards a cross-linguistic theoretical framework. *Dyslexia* 6, 133–151. doi: 10.1002/(sici)1099-0909(200004/06)6:2<133::aid-dys160>3.0.co;2-a

Hasan, A., Bergener, T., Nitsche, M. A., Strube, W., Bunse, T., Falkai, P., et al. (2013). Impairments of motor-cortex responses to unilateral and bilateral direct current stimulation in schizophrenia. *Front. Psychiatry* 4:121. doi: 10.3389/fpsyt.2013.00121

Horwitz, B. (2003). The elusive concept of brain connectivity. *Neuroimage* 19, 466–470. doi: 10.1016/S1053-8119(03)00112-5

Jaušovec, N., and Jaušovec, K. (2000a). Differences in resting EEG related to ability. *Brain Topogr.* 12, 229–240. doi: 10.1023/A:1023446024923

Jaušovec, N., and Jaušovec, K. (2000b). EEG activity during the performance of complex mental problems. *Int. J. Psychophysiol.* 36, 73–88. doi: 10.1016/S0167-8760(99)00113-0

Jung, R. E., Grazioplene, R., Caprihan, A., Chavez, R. S., and Haier, R. J. (2010a). White matter integrity, creativity, and psychopathology: disentangling constructs with diffusion tensor imaging. *PLoS ONE* 5:e9818. doi: 10.1371/journal.pone.0009818

Jung, R. E., Segall, J. M., Jeremy Bockholt, H., Flores, R. A., Smith, S. M., Chavez, R. S., et al. (2010b). Neuroanatomy of creativity. *Hum. Brain Mapp.* 31, 398–409. doi: 10.1002/hbm.20874

Jung-Beeman, M., Bowden, E. M., Haberman, J., Frymiare, J. L., Arambel-Liu, S., Greenblatt, R., et al. (2004). Neural activity when people solve verbal problems with insight. *PLoS Biol.* 2:E97. doi: 10.1371/journal.pbio.0020097

Kanai, R., Paulus, W., and Walsh, V. (2010). Transcranial alternating current stimulation (tACS) modulates cortical excitability as assessed by TMS-induced phosphene thresholds. *Clin. Neurophysiol.* 121, 1551–1554. doi: 10.1016/j.clinph.2010.03.022

Kanwisher, N., McDermott, J., and Chun, M. M. (1997). The fusiform face area: a module in human extrastriate cortex specialized for face perception. *J. Neurosci.* 17, 4302–4311.

Kar, K., and Krekelberg, B. (2014). Transcranial alternating current stimulation attenuates visual motion adaptation. *J. Neurosci.* 34, 7334–7340. doi: 10.1523/JNEUROSCI.5248-13.2014

Kar, K., and Wright, J. (2014). Probing the mechanisms underlying the mitigation of cognitive aging with anodal transcranial direct current stimulation. *J. Neurophysiol.* 111, 1397–1399. doi: 10.1152/jn.00736.2013

Keeser, D., Meindl, T., Bor, J., Palm, U., Pogarell, O., Mulert, C., et al. (2011). Prefrontal transcranial direct current stimulation changes connectivity of resting-state networks during fMRI. *J. Neurosci.* 31, 15284–15293. doi: 10.1523/JNEUROSCI.0542-11.2011

Kounios, J., Fleck, J., Green, D., Payne, L., Stevenson, J. L., Bowden, E. M., et al. (2008). The origins of insight in resting-state brain activity. *Neuropsychologia* 46, 281–291. doi: 10.1016/j.neuropsychologia.2007.07.013

Kwon, Y. H., Ko, M. H., Ahn, S. H., Kim, Y. H., Song, J. C., Lee, C. H., et al. (2008). Primary motor cortex activation by transcranial direct current stimulation in the human brain. *Neurosci. Lett.* 435, 56–59. doi: 10.1016/j.neulet.2008.02.012

Lang, N., Siebner, H. R., Ward, N. S., Lee, L., Nitsche, M. A., Paulus, W., et al. (2005). How does transcranial DC stimulation of the primary motor cortex alter regional neuronal activity in the human brain? *Eur. J. Neurosci.* 22, 495–504. doi: 10.1111/j.1460-9568.2005.04233.x

Lehnertz, K., Ansmann, G., Bialonski, S., Dickten, H., Geier, C., and Porz, S. (2014). Evolving networks in the human epileptic brain. *Physica D Nonlin. Phenom.* 267, 7–15. doi: 10.1016/j.physd.2013.06.009

Liebetanz, D., Nitsche, M. A., Tergau, F., and Paulus, W. (2002). Pharmacological approach to the mechanisms of transcranial DC-stimulation-induced after-effects of human motor cortex excitability. *Brain* 125, 2238–2247. doi: 10.1093/brain/awf238

Luft, C. D. B., and Bhattacharya, J. (2014). "Correlatos neurales de la creatividad," in *Conectividad Funcional y Anatómica en el Crebro Humano: Análisis De Señales y Aplicaciones en Ciencias de la Salud*, eds F. Maestú, E. Pereda, and F. Del Pozo (Madrid: Elsevier), (in press).

Malenka, R. C., and Bear, M. F. (2004). LTP and LTD: an embarrassment of riches. *Neuron* 44, 5–21. doi: 10.1016/j.neuron.2004.09.012

Massimini, M., Ferrarelli, F., Huber, R., Esser, S. K., Singh, H., and Tononi, G. (2005). Breakdown of cortical effective connectivity during sleep. *Science* 309, 2228–2232. doi: 10.1126/science.1117256

Meinzer, M., Antonenko, D., Lindenberg, R., Hetzer, S., Ulm, L., Avirame, K., et al. (2012). Electrical brain stimulation improves cognitive performance by modulating functional connectivity and task-specific activation. *J. Neurosci.* 32, 1859–1866. doi: 10.1523/JNEUROSCI.4812-11.2012

Meinzer, M., Lindenberg, R., Antonenko, D., Flaisch, T., and Floel, A. (2013). Anodal transcranial direct current stimulation temporarily reverses age-associated cognitive decline and functional brain activity changes. *J. Neurosci.* 33, 12470–12478. doi: 10.1523/JNEUROSCI.5743-12.2013

Metuki, N., Sela, T., and Lavidor, M. (2012). Enhancing cognitive control components of insight problems solving by anodal tDCS of the left dorsolateral prefrontal cortex. *Brain Stimul.* 5, 110–115. doi: 10.1016/j.brs.2012.03.002

Mochizuki, H., Huang, Y. Z., and Rothwell, J. C. (2004). Interhemispheric interaction between human dorsal premotor and contralateral primary motor cortex. *J. Physiol.* 561, 331–338. doi: 10.1113/jphysiol.2004.072843

Moliadze, V., Antal, A., and Paulus, W. (2010). Electrode-distance dependent after-effects of transcranial direct and random noise stimulation with extracephalic reference electrodes. *Clin. Neurophysiol.* 121, 2165–2171. doi: 10.1016/j.clinph.2010.04.033

Monte-Silva, K., Kuo, M. F., Hessenthaler, S., Fresnoza, S., Liebetanz, D., Paulus, W., et al. (2013). Induction of late LTP-like plasticity in the human motor cortex by repeated non-invasive brain stimulation. *Brain Stimul.* 6, 424–432. doi: 10.1016/j.brs.2012.04.011

Mordillo-Mateos, L., Turpin-Fenoll, L., Millan-Pascual, J., Nunez-Perez, N., Panyavin, I., Gomez-Arguelles, J. M., et al. (2012). Effects of simultaneous bilateral tDCS of the human motor cortex. *Brain Stimul.* 5, 214–222. doi: 10.1016/j.brs.2011.05.001

Morishima, Y., Akaishi, R., Yamada, Y., Okuda, J., Toma, K., and Sakai, K. (2009). Task-specific signal transmission from prefrontal cortex in visual selective attention. *Nat. Neurosci.* 12, 85–91. doi: 10.1038/nn.2237

Neuling, T., Rach, S., and Herrmann, C. S. (2013). Orchestrating neuronal networks: sustained after-effects of transcranial alternating current stimulation depend upon brain states. *Front. Hum. Neurosci.* 7:161. doi: 10.3389/fnhum.2013.00161

Niso, G., Bruna, R., Pereda, E., Gutierrez, R., Bajo, R., Maestu, F., et al. (2013). HERMES: towards an integrated toolbox to characterize functional and effective brain connectivity. *Neuroinformatics* 11, 405–434. doi: 10.1007/s12021-013-9186-1

Nitsche, M. A., Boggio, P. S., Fregni, F., and Pascual-Leone, A. (2009). Treatment of depression with transcranial direct current stimulation (tDCS): a review. *Exp. Neurol.* 219, 14–19. doi: 10.1016/j.expneurol.2009.03.038

Nitsche, M. A., Cohen, L. G., Wassermann, E. M., Priori, A., Lang, N., Antal, A., et al. (2008). Transcranial direct current stimulation: state of the art 2008. *Brain Stimul.* 1, 206–223. doi: 10.1016/j.brs.2008.06.004

Nitsche, M. A., Fricke, K., Henschke, U., Schlitterlau, A., Liebetanz, D., Lang, N., et al. (2003). Pharmacological modulation of cortical excitability shifts induced by transcranial direct current stimulation in humans. *J. Physiol.* 553, 293–301. doi: 10.1113/jphysiol.2003.049916

Nitsche, M. A., and Paulus, W. (2000). Excitability changes induced in the human motor cortex by weak transcranial direct current stimulation. *J. Physiol.* 527(pt 3), 633–639. doi: 10.1111/j.1469-7793.2000.t01-1-00633.x

Nitsche, M. A., and Paulus, W. (2001). Sustained excitability elevations induced by transcranial DC motor cortex stimulation in humans. *Neurology* 57, 1899–1901. doi: 10.1212/WNL.57.10.1899

Oostenveld, R., Fries, P., Maris, E., and Schoffelen, J. M. (2011). FieldTrip: open source software for advanced analysis of MEG, EEG, and invasive electrophysiological data. *Comput. Intell. Neurosci.* 2011:156869. doi: 10.1155/2011/156869

O'Shea, J., Johansen-Berg, H., Trief, D., Gobel, S., and Rushworth, M. F. (2007). Functionally specific reorganization in human premotor cortex. *Neuron* 54, 479–490. doi: 10.1016/j.neuron.2007.04.021

Parra, L. C., and Bikson, M. (2004). Model of the effect of extracellular fields on spike time coherence. *Conf. Proc. IEEE Eng. Med. Biol. Soc.* 6, 4584–4587. doi: 10.1109/IEMBS.2004.1404271

Pascual-Leone, A., and Walsh, V. (2001). Fast backprojections from the motion to the primary visual area necessary for visual awareness. *Science* 292, 510–512. doi: 10.1126/science.1057099

Pena-Gomez, C., Sala-Lonch, R., Junque, C., Clemente, I. C., Vidal, D., Bargallo, N., et al. (2012). Modulation of large-scale brain networks by transcranial direct current stimulation evidenced by resting-state functional MRI. *Brain Stimul.* 5, 252–263. doi: 10.1016/j.brs.2011.08.006

Pereda, E., Quiroga, R. Q., and Bhattacharya, J. (2005). Nonlinear multivariate analysis of neurophysiological signals. *Prog. Neurobiol.* 77, 1–37. doi: 10.1016/j.pneurobio.2005.10.003

Plucker, J. A., Beghetto, R. A., and Dow, G. T. (2004). Why isn't creativity more important to educational psychologists? Potentials, pitfalls, and future directions in creativity research. *Educ. Psychol.* 39, 83–96. doi: 10.1207/s15326985ep3902_1

Polania, R., Nitsche, M. A., and Paulus, W. (2011a). Modulating functional connectivity patterns and topological functional organization of the human brain with transcranial direct current stimulation. *Hum. Brain Mapp.* 32, 1236–1249. doi: 10.1002/hbm.21104

Polania, R., Paulus, W., Antal, A., and Nitsche, M. A. (2011b). Introducing graph theory to track for neuroplastic alterations in the resting human brain: a transcranial direct current stimulation study. *Neuroimage* 54, 2287–2296. doi: 10.1016/j.neuroimage.2010.09.085

Polania, R., Paulus, W., and Nitsche, M. A. (2012a). Modulating cortico-striatal and thalamo-cortical functional connectivity with transcranial direct current stimulation. *Hum. Brain Mapp.* 33, 2499–2508. doi: 10.1002/hbm.21380

Polania, R., Paulus, W., and Nitsche, M. A. (2012b). Reorganizing the intrinsic functional architecture of the human primary motor cortex during rest with non-invasive cortical stimulation. *PLoS ONE* 7:e30971. doi: 10.1371/journal.pone.0030971

Purpura, D. P., and McMurtry, J. G. (1965). Intracellular activities and evoked potential changes during polarization of motor cortex. *J. Neurophysiol.* 28, 166–185.

Radman, T., Ramos, R. L., Brumberg, J. C., and Bikson, M. (2009). Role of cortical cell type and morphology in subthreshold and suprathreshold uniform electric field stimulation *in vitro*. *Brain Stimul.* 2, 215–228, 228. e1–e3. doi: 10.1016/j.brs.2009.03.007

Rahman, A., Reato, D., Arlotti, M., Gasca, F., Datta, A., Parra, L. C., et al. (2013). Cellular effects of acute direct current stimulation: somatic and synaptic terminal effects. *J. Physiol.* 591, 2563–2578. doi: 10.1113/jphysiol.2012.247171

Razumnikova, O. M., and Larina, E. N. (2005). Hemispheric interactions during a search of original verbal associations: EEG coherence in creative men and women. *Zh. Vyssh. Nerv. Deiat. Im. I P Pavlova* 55, 777–787.

Reato, D., Rahman, A., Bikson, M., and Parra, L. C. (2010). Low-intensity electrical stimulation affects network dynamics by modulating population rate and spike timing. *J. Neurosci.* 30, 15067–15079. doi: 10.1523/JNEUROSCI.2059-10.2010

Rhodes, M. (1961). An analysis of creativity. *Phi Delta Kappan* 42, 305–310.

Rigonatti, S. P., Boggio, P. S., Myczkowski, M. L., Otta, E., Fiquer, J. T., Ribeiro, R. B., et al. (2008). Transcranial direct stimulation and fluoxetine for the treatment of depression. *Eur. Psychiatry* 23, 74–76. doi: 10.1016/j.eurpsy.2007.09.006

Rioult-Pedotti, M. S., Friedman, D., and Donoghue, J. P. (2000). Learning-induced LTP in neocortex. *Science* 290, 533–536. doi: 10.1126/science.290.5491.533

Rubinov, M., and Sporns, O. (2010). Complex network measures of brain connectivity: uses and interpretations. *Neuroimage* 52, 1059–1069. doi: 10.1016/j.neuroimage.2009.10.003

Ruffini, G., Wendling, F., Merlet, I., Molaee-Ardekani, B., Mekonnen, A., Salvador, R., et al. (2013). Transcranial current brain stimulation (tCS): models and technologies. *IEEE Trans. Neural Syst. Rehabil. Eng.* 21, 333–345. doi: 10.1109/TNSRE.2012.2200046

Santiesteban, I., Banissy, M. J., Catmur, C., and Bird, G. (2012). Enhancing social ability by stimulating right temporoparietal junction. *Curr. Biol.* 22, 2274–2277. doi: 10.1016/j.cub.2012.10.018

Sawyer, K. (2012). *Explaining Creativity: The Science of Human Innovation.* New York, NY: Oxford University Press, Inc.

Schaal, N. K., Williamson, V. J., and Banissy, M. J. (2013). Anodal transcranial direct current stimulation over the supramarginal gyrus facilitates pitch memory. *Eur. J. Neurosci.* 38, 3513–3518. doi: 10.1111/ejn.12344

Sehm, B., Kipping, J., Schafer, A., Villringer, A., and Ragert, P. (2013). A comparison between uni- and bilateral tDCS effects on functional connectivity of the human motor cortex. *Front. Hum. Neurosci.* 7:183. doi: 10.3389/fnhum.2013.00183

Shafi, M. M., Westover, M. B., Fox, M. D., and Pascual-Leone, A. (2012). Exploration and modulation of brain network interactions with noninvasive brain stimulation in combination with neuroimaging. *Eur. J. Neurosci.* 35, 805–825. doi: 10.1111/j.1460-9568.2012.08035.x

Shahid, S. S., Bikson, M., Salman, H., Wen, P., and Ahfock, T. (2014). The value and cost of complexity in predictive modelling: role of tissue anisotropic conductivity and fibre tracts in neuromodulation. *J. Neural Eng.* 11:036002. doi: 10.1088/1741-2560/11/3/036002

Snowball, A., Tachtsidis, I., Popescu, T., Thompson, J., Delazer, M., Zamarian, L., et al. (2013). Long-term enhancement of brain function and cognition using cognitive training and brain stimulation. *Curr. Biol.* 23, 987–992. doi: 10.1016/j.cub.2013.04.045

Sporns, O. (2011). *Networks of the Brain.* Cambridge, MA: MIT Press.

Sporns, O. (2014). Contributions and challenges for network models in cognitive neuroscience. *Nat. Neurosci.* 17, 652–660. doi: 10.1038/nn.3690

Sporns, O., Chialvo, D. R., Kaiser, M., and Hilgetag, C. C. (2004). Organization, development and function of complex brain networks. *Trends Cogn. Sci.* 8, 418–425. doi: 10.1016/j.tics.2004.07.008

Takano, Y., Yokawa, T., Masuda, A., Niimi, J., Tanaka, S., and Hironaka, N. (2011). A rat model for measuring the effectiveness of transcranial direct current stimulation using fMRI. *Neurosci. Lett.* 491, 40–43. doi: 10.1016/j.neulet.2011.01.004

Takeuchi, H., Taki, Y., Hashizume, H., Sassa, Y., Nagase, T., Nouchi, R., et al. (2012). The association between resting functional connectivity and creativity. *Cereb. Cortex* 22, 2921–2929. doi: 10.1093/cercor/bhr371

Takeuchi, H., Taki, Y., Sassa, Y., Hashizume, H., Sekiguchi, A., Fukushima, A., et al. (2010). White matter structures associated with creativity: evidence from diffusion tensor imaging. *Neuroimage* 51, 11–18. doi: 10.1016/j.neuroimage.2010.02.035

Terao, Y., and Ugawa, Y. (2002). Basic mechanisms of TMS. *J. Clin. Neurophysiol.* 19, 322–343. doi: 10.1097/00004691-200208000-00006

Terhune, D. B., and Cohen Kadosh, R. (2013). Modulating cognitive control in major depression with transcranial electrical stimulation. *Biol. Psychiatry* 73, 595–596. doi: 10.1016/j.biopsych.2013.01.006

Terney, D., Chaieb, L., Moliadze, V., Antal, A., and Paulus, W. (2008). Increasing human brain excitability by transcranial high-frequency random noise stimulation. *J. Neurosci.* 28, 14147–14155. doi: 10.1523/JNEUROSCI.4248-08.2008

Uehara, T., Yamasaki, T., Okamoto, T., Koike, T., Kan, S., Miyauchi, S., et al. (2014). Efficiency of a "small-world" brain network depends on consciousness level: a resting-state FMRI study. *Cereb. Cortex* 24, 1529–1539. doi: 10.1093/cercor/bht004

van den Heuvel, M. P., and Sporns, O. (2011). Rich-club organization of the human connectome. *J. Neurosci.* 31, 15775–15786. doi: 10.1523/JNEUROSCI.3539-11.2011

van den Heuvel, M. P., and Sporns, O. (2013). Network hubs in the human brain. *Trends Cogn. Sci.* 17, 683–696. doi: 10.1016/j.tics.2013.09.012

van den Heuvel, M. P., Sporns, O., Collin, G., Scheewe, T., Mandl, R. C., Cahn, W., et al. (2013). Abnormal rich club organization and functional brain dynamics in schizophrenia. *JAMA Psychiatry* 70, 783–792. doi: 10.1001/jamapsychiatry.2013.1328

Wagner, T., Fregni, F., Fecteau, S., Grodzinsky, A., Zahn, M., and Pascual-Leone, A. (2007). Transcranial direct current stimulation: a computer-based human model study. *Neuroimage* 35, 1113–1124. doi: 10.1016/j.neuroimage.2007.01.027

Watts, D. J., and Strogatz, S. H. (1998). Collective dynamics of 'small-world' networks. *Nature* 393, 440–442. doi: 10.1038/30918

Weber, M. J., Messing, S. B., Rao, H., Detre, J. A., and Thompson-Schill, S. L. (2014). Prefrontal transcranial direct current stimulation alters activation and connectivity in cortical and subcortical reward systems: a tDCS-fMRI study. *Hum. Brain Mapp.* 35, 3673–3686. doi: 10.1002/hbm.22429

Wiggins, G., and Bhattacharya, J. (2014). Mind the gap: an attempt to bridge computational and neuroscientific approaches to study creativity. *Front. Hum. Neurosci.* 8:540. doi: 10.3389/fnhum.2014.00540

4

Selective visual attention to drive cognitive brain–machine interfaces: from concepts to neurofeedback and rehabilitation applications

Elaine Astrand, Claire Wardak and Suliann Ben Hamed*

CNRS, Cognitive Neuroscience Center, UMR 5229, University of Lyon 1, Bron Cedex, France

Edited by:
Mikhail Lebedev, Duke University, USA

Reviewed by:
Guilherme Wood, Karl-Franzens-University of Graz, Austria
Georgia Gregoriou, University of Crete, Greece

***Correspondence:**
Suliann Ben Hamed, CNRS, Cognitive Neuroscience Center, UMR 5229, University of Lyon 1, 67 Boulevard Pinel, 69675 Bron Cedex, France
e-mail: benhamed@isc.cnrs.fr

Brain–machine interfaces (BMIs) using motor cortical activity to drive an external effector like a screen cursor or a robotic arm have seen enormous success and proven their great rehabilitation potential. An emerging parallel effort is now directed to BMIs controlled by endogenous cognitive activity, also called cognitive BMIs. While more challenging, this approach opens new dimensions to the rehabilitation of cognitive disorders. In the present work, we focus on BMIs driven by visuospatial attention signals and we provide a critical review of these studies in the light of the accumulated knowledge about the psychophysics, anatomy, and neurophysiology of visual spatial attention. Importantly, we provide a unique comparative overview of the several studies, ranging from non-invasive to invasive human and non-human primates studies, that decode attention-related information from ongoing neuronal activity. We discuss these studies in the light of the challenges attention-driven cognitive BMIs have to face. In a second part of the review, we discuss past and current attention-based neurofeedback studies, describing both the covert effects of neurofeedback onto neuronal activity and its overt behavioral effects. Importantly, we compare neurofeedback studies based on the amplitude of cortical activity to studies based on the enhancement of cortical information content. Last, we discuss several lines of future research and applications for attention-driven cognitive brain-computer interfaces (BCIs), including the rehabilitation of cognitive deficits, restored communication in locked-in patients, and open-field applications for enhanced cognition in normal subjects. The core motivation of this work is the key idea that the improvement of current cognitive BMIs for therapeutic and open field applications needs to be grounded in a proper interdisciplinary understanding of the physiology of the cognitive function of interest, be it spatial attention, working memory or any other cognitive signal.

Keywords: brain–machine interfaces, brain–computer interfaces, cognition, spatial attention, neurofeedback, neural training, frontal eye field, prefrontal cortex

INTRODUCTION

Only a couple of decades ago imagining an interface between the human brain and a machine was more of a science fiction than of a scientific endeavor. Chapin et al. (1999) pioneered the field with the first demonstration of a real time motor brain–machine interface (BMI) that is the demonstration that brain activity from the rat motor cortex can be used to control a robotic arm. This achievement brought about the realization of the enormous potential of the field, which up to this day has not ceased to expand.

The main objective of motor BMIs is the rehabilitation of patients with major motor deficits yet preserved cortical motor functions. Applications involve for example controlling a screen cursor using motor or premotor cortex brain activity in monkeys (Serruya et al., 2002; Taylor et al., 2002; Santhanam et al., 2006; Kim et al., 2011) and in tetraplegic human patients (Hochberg et al., 2006) which has been proven feasible with a remarkable spatial accuracy. As computer-assisted aids continue to permeate our everyday life environments, this approach is expected to grant patients who have difficulties moving their arms or hands an increased autonomy and freedom of action. Pushing BMIs yet a step further, several studies show that motor cortical activities can also be used to control robotic arms in their reaching and grasping components with an impressive degree of precision, both in monkeys (Carmena et al., 2003; Tillery et al., 2003; Lebedev et al., 2005; Velliste et al., 2008; Ifft et al., 2013) and in humans. This has for example allowed a tetraplegic patient to help herself with a drink with the aid of an artificial arm controlled by her motor cortex activity (Hochberg et al., 2012).

Several new directions are currently being explored by BMI research. For example, a recent study demonstrates that incorporating sensory feedback to a motor brain-computer interface (BCI) improves its performance (Suminski et al., 2010). Along another line, Shanechi et al. (2014) demonstrate that the signals decoded from the motor cortical activity recorded in a monkey performing a sensorimotor task can be used to stimulate the spinal cord and muscles of a second anesthetized monkey giving rise to directed movements of its limb toward distinct targets. This study opens new rehabilitation perspectives for paralyzed patients. The exhaustive review of the major advances in motor BMIs and their novel perspectives is however beyond the scope of the present review.

BASIC PRINCIPLES UNDERLYING BRAIN–MACHINE INTERFACES

The basic concept behind BMIs is the interpretation, in real time, of cortical neuronal population activities and their translation into a goal directed action through a diversity of external effectors (**Figure 1A**). Developing a BMI includes two distinct phases (**Figure 1B**): (1) a learning or training phase during which a classifier learns to associate the observed instantaneous simultaneous activity of a neuronal population with the actual state of the variable of interest (the position of a stimulus in space, the direction of an intended motor plan, the spatial location of visuospatial attention, or the content of short term memory etc.); (2) a testing phase during which the classifier defined in the learning phase is used to define the most probable state of the variable of interest, given the observed instantaneous simultaneous activity of the recorded neuronal population. Above-chance decoding accuracy indicates that the neuronal population contains reliable information about the variable of interest.

In its simplest form, the mapping between the neuronal code and the desired output relies on the interpretation of the subject's endogenous neuronal codes. For example identifying the neuronal codes with which a set of movements is encoded in the motor cortex allows to associate a given neuronal population activity

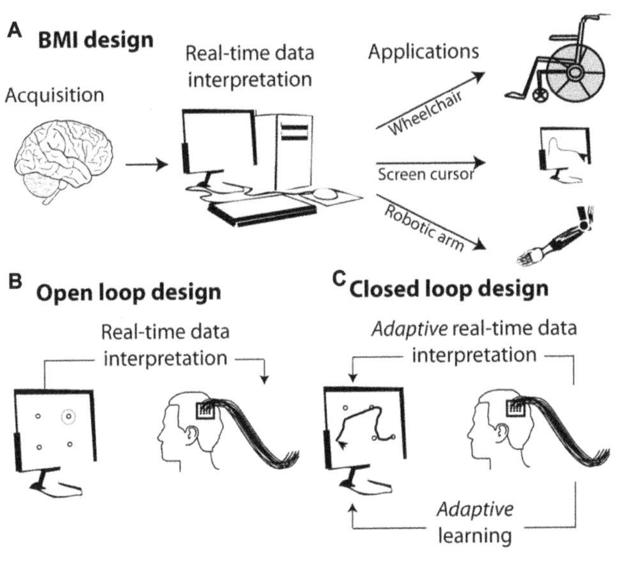

FIGURE 1 | From brain signals to controlled external effectors. **(A)** Schematic representation of the workings behind brain–machine interfaces (BMI). **(B)** Open loop BMI. The subject is here implanted with intracortical electrodes in the primary motor cortex. The activity of this cortical region is used to select a target on the screen without the subject being required to adjust his or her neuronal activity. **(C)** Closed loop design. The activity of the motor cortex is used to guide a cursor on the screen. The subject sees the screen cursor in real time and is required to adapt his or her brain activity in order to increase the precision of the cursor's trajectory.

(e.g., corresponding to moving one's arm left) with a specific spatially congruent external effector output (e.g., moving a cursor left, **Figure 1B**). More complex designs are further based on the adaptive capabilities of the primate cortex and rely on learning and positive reinforcement procedures. In these designs, subjects learn to produce the neuronal population activities that best control the effector output, thanks to a sensory feedback (e.g., seeing the cursor's trajectory) that allows them to assess how well they are successful at controlling the external effector (**Figure 1C**).

COGNITIVE BRAIN–MACHINE INTERFACES (cBMI)

While most of the research effort in neural prosthetics has concentrated on the use of motor signals to drive external devices, new directions in the field of BMIs are also emerging. For example, Musallam et al. (2004) have shown, in the context of motor behavior, that cognitive signals such as the expected value of a reward, i.e., the subject's motivation, can be decoded, at the single trial time scale, from parietal neural activity. Jerbi et al. (2009) show that such signals as attention orientation signals and mental calculation signals can be used to drive a cognitive BCI. Instead of decoding movement-related signals from motor specific cortical activity, these cognitive BMIs (cBMIs) seek to access the content of cognitive processes. One of their principal long-term goals is to develop therapeutic tools for the treatment of cognitive disorders.

In healthy subjects, motor cortical commands can be objectified and time-locked to overt limb displacements. In contrast, cognitive processes, such as planning, holding information in short-term memory or orienting one's attention in the environment, are essentially internal subjective processes. From a behavioral point of view, their content is covert and can be inferred only indirectly from their effects on other overt measures (e.g., oral report, reaction time measures, detection rates etc.). From a neurophysiological point of view, their neural bases are increasingly understood and clear neuronal signatures can be assigned to them. However, unlike sensory or motor processes, these cognitive processes cannot be precisely time-locked to objective external events. In addition, they are often multiplexed with sensory, motor as well as other cognitive signals. As a result, cBMIs currently appear as more challenging than motor BMIs. The present review focuses on a major cognitive function, namely visuospatial attention (**Figure 2A**), which is known to enhance visual processing both at the behavioral (**Figure 2B**) and neurophysiological levels (**Figure 2C**, see below). It proposes a precisely quantified comparative overview of the different cBMI approaches that have been developed to decode this cognitive signal at the scale of the single trial (**Figure 2D**). It also explores the initial steps at using such cBMIs for cognitive rehabilitation purposes. These studies are discussed in the light of the accumulated knowledge about the psychophysics, anatomy, and neurophysiology of visual spatial attention. The core motivation of the present review is the key idea that the improvement of current cBMIs for therapeutic and open field applications needs to be grounded in a proper interdisciplinary understanding of the physiology of the cognitive function of interest, be it spatial attention, working memory or any other cognitive signal.

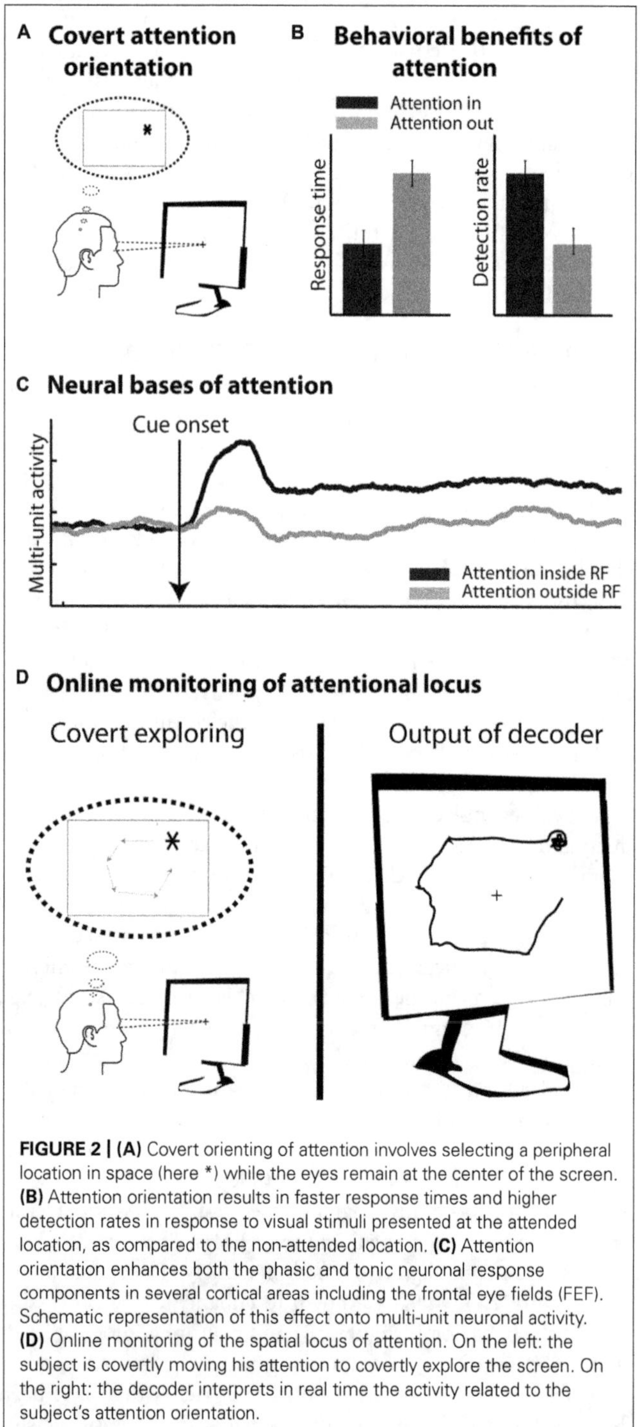

FIGURE 2 | (A) Covert orienting of attention involves selecting a peripheral location in space (here *) while the eyes remain at the center of the screen. **(B)** Attention orientation results in faster response times and higher detection rates in response to visual stimuli presented at the attended location, as compared to the non-attended location. **(C)** Attention orientation enhances both the phasic and tonic neuronal response components in several cortical areas including the frontal eye fields (FEF). Schematic representation of this effect onto multi-unit neuronal activity. **(D)** Online monitoring of the spatial locus of attention. On the left: the subject is covertly moving his attention to covertly explore the screen. On the right: the decoder interprets in real time the activity related to the subject's attention orientation.

VISUOSPATIAL ATTENTION AND ITS NEURAL CORRELATES

Orienting one's attention toward a given location in space enhances visual processing at that location (**Figure 2B**). Reaction times are faster (Posner et al., 1980, but see also Albares et al., 2011), spatial processing (Bashinski and Bacharach, 1980; Prinzmetal et al., 2005; Ibos et al., 2009) and spatial resolution are enhanced at the attended location (Yeshurun and Carrasco, 1998; Gobell and Carrasco, 2005; Carrasco and Yeshurun, 2009; Anton-Erxleben and Carrasco, 2013) and spatial representation is distorted up to several degrees away from the attended location (Wardak et al., 2011a). At the neuronal level, attention is described to modulate both the baseline (e.g., Armstrong et al., 2009; Ibos et al., 2013) and the visual responses (e.g., McAdams and Maunsell, 1999), to decrease neuronal response latency (Lee et al., 2007), as well as to modify the neurons' spatial selectivity profiles (Ben Hamed et al., 1997, 2002; Anton-Erxleben et al., 2009). At the neuronal population level, attention is also thought to decrease interneuronal correlations (Cohen and Maunsell, 2009).

Spatial orienting of attention can be achieved through two different mechanisms. It can either be driven by external stimuli that capture attention. This mechanism is referred to as exogenous, bottom-up or involuntary attention. Alternatively, attention can be voluntarily driven by internal goals. This mechanism is referred to as endogenous, top-down or voluntary attention. Early on, Posner et al. (1980) and Jonides (1981) suggested that a single cortical system controls both the endogenous and the exogenous orientation of attention. In contrast with this proposal, Müller and Rabbitt (1989) postulated that the endogenous and exogenous orienting of attention are functionally distinct and constitute separate mechanisms in constant competition with each other (e.g., Zénon et al., 2008, 2009). Confirming this view, recent functional magnetic resonance imaging (fMRI)-studies demonstrate the co-existence of two distinct frontoparietal networks involved in orienting attention (Corbetta and Shulman, 2002): a dorsal network that is active during top-down attentional control, i.e., when attention is internally maintained or voluntarily driven (Kastner et al., 1999; Shulman et al., 1999; Corbetta et al., 2000; Hopfinger et al., 2000; Kincade et al., 2005), and a ventral network that is activated when attention is reoriented both voluntarily and by relevant but unexpected stimuli (Arrington et al., 2000; Corbetta et al., 2000; Macaluso et al., 2002; Kincade et al., 2005; Vossel et al., 2006). In the non-human primate, a bilateral frontoparietal attentional network involving the frontal eye fields (FEF; Bruce and Goldberg, 1985) and the lateral intraparietal area (LIP; Barash et al., 1991; Ben Hamed et al., 2001) is described. These areas are activated by both endogenously driven attention and exogenously driven attention to task-relevant stimuli (Gottlieb et al., 1998; Armstrong et al., 2009; Gregoriou et al., 2009; Suzuki and Gottlieb, 2013). Interestingly, during endogenous top-down driven attention, FEF neurons tend to respond earlier than LIP neurons whereas during exogenous bottom-up driven attention, the inverse is observed (Buschman and Miller, 2007; Ibos et al., 2013). The distinction between a dorsal and a ventral frontoparietal network is still unclear in the macaque monkey. The FEF possibly belongs to a putative monkey dorsal attentional network while area 45, ventral to area FEF, possibly belongs to a putative monkey ventral attentional network (Wardak et al., 2011b).

VISUOSPATIAL ATTENTIONAL SIGNALS FROM A cBMI PERSPECTIVE

TIME-LOCKING

The feasibility of cBMIs based on visuospatial attention signals as compared to motor or sensory BMIs depends on the existence of neuronal population activity patterns that distinguish between whether the subject is orienting its attention say to the left or to the right of the visual field. The P300 speller is an example of a successful non-invasive cBMI driven by the decoding of visuospatial attentional locus as inferred from the modulation of neuronal responses to a visual stimulus presented at the specific locus of attention. Another approach is to decode sustained attentional brain correlates toward different spatial positions from neuronal population activities. This approach is different because decoding such sustained information cannot be precisely time-locked to an external event. As a result, identifying its precise neuronal activation pattern during the training phase of the decoding is in itself a challenge.

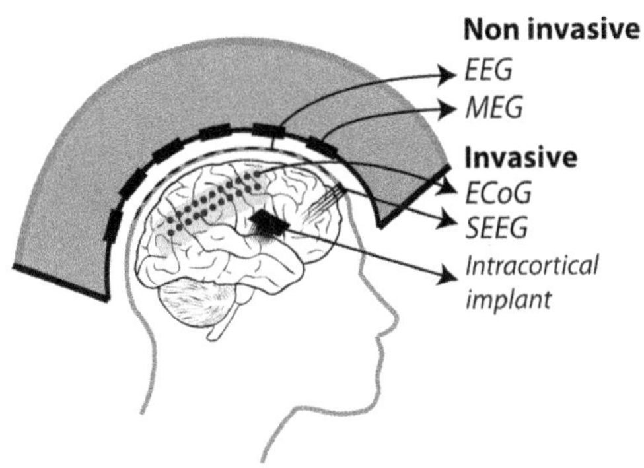

FIGURE 3 | Different recording methods used to control BMIs. Invasive methods includes: ECoG electrodes placed on the dura, SEEG electrodes placed through the skull into the cortex and intracortical electrodes implanted in the cortex. Non-invasive methods include: EEG electrodes placed on the scalp and MEG squids placed around the head.

DECODING ATTENTION-RELATED CORTICAL INFORMATION

One important question is whether such attentional information, because of its self-initiated endogenous nature, can be decoded with an accuracy that is comparable to that obtained from sensory and motor related activities. Two studies are interesting in this respect. Armstrong et al. (2009) recorded neuronal responses from the macaque FEF while the animals were involved in a cued target detection task. The cue was an exogenous cue, having the same spatial location as the target. Astrand et al. (2014a) also recorded neuronal responses from the macaque FEF while the animals were involved in a cued target detection task, except that in this case, the cue was calling for an endogenous orienting of attention toward the cued location (FarbodKia et al., 2011; Astrand et al., 2014a). An exogenous cue is thought to involuntarily shift the subject's attention to its location whereas to shift attention to a location indicated by an endogenous cue, the subject needs to voluntarily orient its attention toward it (Jonides, 1981). Both studies thus manipulate spatial attention but the cue that was used called for different orientation processes. Armstrong et al. (2009) show that both visual and sustained attention information can be decoded from a macaque FEF population of neurons modulated both by visual stimuli and attention orientation. Specifically, they report 100% accuracy for the decoding of the spatial location of a visual peripheral stimulus and up to 90% accuracy for the decoding of the spatial locus of sustained attention. They also describe a lower decoding variability for a visual stimulus than for sustained attention. Astrand et al. (2014a) report a similar trend on a random neuronal population selection including both attention-selective neurons and attention non-selective neurons. They further quantify the sensitivity of decoding accuracy to neuronal population size and trial number. In addition, they show that, using populations of visual-selective and attention-related neurons of the exact same size, comparable decoding accuracies are obtained for both variables. This is a strong indication that both exogenous (visual) and endogenous (attention-related) information are encoded in the cortex with a similar reliability. As a result, cognitive variables such as attention can be expected to be decoded from neuronal population activities with similar accuracies as those achieved when decoding sensory or motor variables (for example, see Ben Hamed et al., 2003, 2007).

USING ATTENTION-RELATED SIGNALS TO CONTROL A BRAIN–MACHINE INTERFACE

In the following, we will present an overview of recent studies evaluating the accuracy with which attention-related cortical information can be decoded. These range from non-invasive recording studies in humans [MagnetoEncephaloGraphic recordings (MEG), Electroencephalographic (EEG) recordings and fMRI] to invasive recording studies in human (ECoG) and non-human primate [ECoG, multi-unit neuronal activity (MUA) recordings and single-unit neuronal activity (SUA) recordings] subjects (**Figure 3**). Whenever possible, we document for each study the following information (**Table 1**): (1) the type of signal component each study relies on, (2), whether attention is driven endogenously or exogenously, (3) how well each method succeeds at decoding attentional engagement signals (i.e., the fact that the subject is focusing its attention as compared to no attentional focus), (4) how well each method allows to distinguish between left and right attentional orientation, (5) how well each method allows to distinguish between attentional loci situated in the same visual hemifield, and (6) how visual distractors interfere with the decoding of attention. Points 4 and 5 reflect the spatial resolution with which attention-related signals can be accessed. All this comparative information is presented in **Table 1**. Importantly, to be considered as robust, it has been proposed that BCI performance needs to be above 70% (Kübler et al., 2004, 2006), a threshold accuracy to keep in mind while analyzing **Table 1**.

NON-INVASIVE STUDIES IN HUMANS (MEG, EEG, AND fMRI)

The first attempt at decoding attention orientation at the single trial level is that of van Gerven and Jensen (2009). The authors recorded the cortical activity using MEG while subjects were covertly attending to one amongst four possible locations in space, previously indicated by an endogenous central cue. Analyzing these signals offline, and specifically the alpha-band power (8–14 Hz) of the parieto-occipital captors, they report an average decoding performance of 69% when discriminating between two possible spatial locations (chance being at 50%). They observe better decoding performances at discriminating *left/right* locations (78%, average calculated over their best subjects) than *up/down* locations (58%, *ibid*). They additionally report an average decoding performance of 41% when discriminating between four possible spatial locations (chance being at 25%). This study

Table 1 | Comparative overview of the non-invasive EEG and MEG and invasive ECoG, SEEG and neuronal recording studies, in humans and non-human primates, that have aimed at decoding attention-related information from the ongoing neuronal activity in a perspective of using these signals to drive BMIs.

	Study	Signal	Attention	Atentional engagement	Average decoding performance	Left/right attention	Up/down attention	Distracters
Non-invasive	van Gerven and Jensen (2009)	MEG/Alpha power (8–14 Hz) occipito-parietal channels	Endogenous	–	*2 positions*: 69% ($n = 15$ subjects, chance at 50%) *4 positions*: 41% ($n = 15$ subjects, chance at 25%)	Five best subjects: 78%	Five best subjects: 58%	–
	Treder et al. (2011)	EEG/Alpha power	Endogenous	–	*2 positions*: 75% ($n = 8$ subjects, chance at 50%)	–	–	–
	Morioka et al. (2014)	EEG/Alpha and Beta Power guided by NIRS	*Exogenous*	–	*2 positions*: 79% ($n = 8$ subjects, chance at 50%)	79%	–	–
	Andersson et al. (2011)	fMRI/7T	Endogenous	–	–	*Online fixed threshold:* L: 41%/R: 25% ($n = 7$) *Offline fixed threshold*: L: 89%/R: 88% ($n = 7$) *Online adaptive threshold*: L: 75%/R: 85% ($n = 2$)	–	–
	Andersson et al. (2012)	fMRI	Endogenous	–	*2 positions*: 79% ($n = 9$ subjects, chance at 50%)	77%	82%	–
Invasive in humans	Gunduz et al. (2012)	ECoG/Power from all frequency bands	Endogenous	84% (chance 50%)	*3 positions*: 48% (35% during motor engagement) (chance at 33%)	–	–	–
	Andersson et al. (2011)	ECoG/High gamma power	Endogenous	–	*3 positions*: 70% (chance at 33%)	Left: 55%/Right: 60%/Center: 82%	–	–
Invasive in non-human primates	Rotermund et al. (2013)	ECoG/Power, phase coherence and difference	*Exogenous*	–	*2 positions*: 96% (chance at 50%)	94%	99%	Present but not quantified
	Astrand et al. (2014a)	SUA/average spiking rate	Endogenous	–	–	82%	–	Present but not quantified
	Astrand et al. (2014b)	MUA/average spiking rate	Endogenous/ *Exogenous*	90–100%	*4 positions*: 67%/79% (chance at 25%)	–	–	–
	Armstrong et al. (2009)	SUA/average spiking rate	*Exogenous*	–	*2 positions*: 90% (chance at 50%)	–	–	20% drop in performance
	Zhang et al. (2011)	SUA/average spiking rate	Endogenous	–	*3 positions*: 56% (chance at 33%)	–	*3 positions* 56%	10% drop in performance

thus provided the first evidence that endogenous spatial orientation of attention can potentially be monitored in real time. A subsequent EEG study, using a very similar experimental design reports an average performance of 75% (chance being at 50%) based on the alpha power of the recorded signals (Treder et al., 2011). Morioka et al. (2014), report a slightly higher average decoding performance (79%) using near-infrared spectroscopy (NIRS) as prior information for the analysis of the EEG signals. It is however not clear if this improved performance results from using the NIRS prior information or is due to the fact that an exogenous cue was used instead of an endogenous cue. Using fMRI, Andersson et al. (2011, 2012) take the field one step further by decoding, in real time, the spatial orientation of attention between three endogenously cued locations (one central and two peripheral locations, 2011) and five endogenously cued locations (one central and four peripheral locations, 2012).When using an adaptive threshold on the classification of the real-time BOLD signal, thanks to a real-time design, they obtain a decoding performance of attention orientation (79, 75% at decoding attention to the left and 85% at decoding attention to the right) equal to that obtained with EEG. In contrast with van Gerven and Jensen (2009), they demonstrate a slightly better performance at discriminating between up/down attention (82%) than between left/right attention (77%). When reprocessed offline the average decoding performances reported by Andersson et al. (2011, 2012) reaches 88% (89% at decoding attention to the left and 88% at decoding attention to the right).This sets the ground for a promising future in the field of attention cBMI. Importantly, it is to be noted that all of these non-invasive studies aiming at decoding spatial attention signals from human cortical activities report an important intersubject variability, overall attention orientation decoding performance being high in some subjects and almost at chance in other subjects. See **Table 1** for comparison of the above studies.

INVASIVE STUDIES IN HUMANS (ECoG)

Drawing nearer to the source of the cortical signals, ECoG studies in patients implanted for clinical purposes predicted higher performances for decoding spatial attention than non-invasive techniques. Gunduz et al. (2012) report a performance of 84% at decoding whether a subject is engaging its spatial attention or not using the spectral power amplitude from all frequency bands and a performance of only 48% at decoding the location of attention amongst three possible spatial positions (chance at 33%). Andersson et al. (2011) focus on the high gamma power and report an average of performance of 70% in a similar design (chance at 33%). The discrepancy between these two studies most probably reflects the dependence of the decoding performance upon the exact localization of the ECoG electrode arrays in each subject. Interestingly, Andersson et al. (2011) used the exact same design to decode spatial attention both from ECoG implanted patients and from subjects included in the fMRI experiment described in the previous section. Surprisingly enough, the average decoding performance is higher in the fMRI-based non-invasive approach than in the ECoG implanted patient. This is most probably due to the fact that the fMRI-based protocol specifically relies on the analysis of the regions of interest (ROIs) that are specifically activated by attention orientation, while the ECoG recording correspond to an averaged smoothed analog of these signals. See **Table 1** for comparison of the above studies.

INVASIVE STUDIES IN NON-HUMAN PRIMATES (ECoG, SUA, MUA)

These approaches are expected to yield the highest decoding performances as compared to the two previous approaches, due to the fact that the recording are specifically targeted to the cortical regions involved in attention processing (closest to these regions, on the cortical surface for ECoG, and right within these regions for MUA and SUA recordings), though the number of simultaneously recorded signal sources is also a variable to take into account (the higher the number of recording contacts, the higher the expected decoding performance). MUA can be considered as averaged SUA, as MUA represents several neurons at the same time while SUA represents well identified individual neurons. In a very elegant study, Rotermund et al. (2013) demonstrate extremely high accuracies in discriminating between two exogenously driven attentional loci (average 96%), with slightly better performance for two attentional loci situated in the same visual hemifield (99%) as compared to two attentional loci situated in different visual hemifields (94%), in agreement with the non-invasive fMRI driven study by Andersson et al. (2012). Importantly, Rotermund et al. (2013) placed the ECoG array onto the visual areas V1 and V4 the activity of which is known to be strongly modulated by attention, according to a strict topography matching attention allocation. While these areas can functionally be considered as downstream from the parietofrontal network described above, the fact that attention can be decoded with such high performances from these regions is noteworthy given that these areas are not expected to be subjected to eye-movement or motor planning interferences that can possibly degrade the decoding of spatial attention in other cortical regions (see below). This performance is to be compared with the performance of 90% at predicting the location of attentional locus amongst two possible locations (inside or outside the receptive field) following an endogenous cue (Armstrong et al., 2009), when using the SUA of attention-selective cells recorded in the monkey prefrontal cortex (FEF). Astrand et al. (2014a) report that it is possible to predict whether a monkey was orienting its attention to the right or to the left visual field from the activity of a cortical population of mixed selectivities (attentional and non-attentional) with a performance of 82%. Both these studies (Armstrong et al., 2009; Astrand et al., 2014a) correspond to a coarse approximation of real-time decoding of attention orientation, as they involve the artificial concatenation of cells recorded in independent sessions and having different spatial selectivities. More recently, Astrand et al. (2014b) report, in a real-time decoding design, a 67% performance at discriminating between four possible attentional locations from MUA recordings in the FEF, following an endogenous cue (79% when attention is oriented exogenously). The performance with which they can predict whether the monkey has engaged its attention or not is around 90% for endogenous cueing (98% when attention is oriented exogenously).

DEPENDENCE OF DECODING PERFORMANCE ON THE EXPERIMENTAL DESIGN

Classification accuracy increases as a function of the number of recorded signals and as a function of the number of available training trials (e.g., Armstrong et al., 2009; Astrand et al., 2014a). The impact of these two parameters on classification accuracy depends on the classification algorithm being used. Indeed, regularized linear regression classifiers appear to be more resilient to low number of recorded signals and low number of trials than other decoders (e.g., support vector machine, reservoir, linear regression, see Astrand et al., 2014a). The impact of these two parameters on classification accuracy also depends on how much information about the variable of interest is present in each recorded signal. For example, a 75% decoding performance of spatial attention can be achieved with as few as 15 trials per condition when each recorded signal has been selected on the basis of its high attention-related content (e.g., attention-related cells in SUA decoding studies). When no prior selection is exerted onto the recorded signals, up to 80 trials are required to reach this 75% decoding performance (Astrand et al., 2014a). As the number of recorded signals and/or the number of trials increases, the impact of further increasing any of these two parameters onto the decoding performance decreases (Astrand et al., 2014a). **Table 2** summarizes, for each of the different studies decoding spatial attention discussed above, the number of recorded signals and how they are placed with respect to the brain, the classifier being used as well as the number of available trials for the classification analysis. In general, there appears to be a trade-off between the number of recorded signals and the number of trials required to achieve a high decoding performance (Astrand et al., 2014a). A precise quantification of this trade-off per type of recorded signal, from non-invasive to invasive, is unfortunately missing and would be extremely useful. This would allow a more direct comparison between the different types of studies. But most importantly, this would allow to better adjust the experimental design to the constraints of the method being used. One expects for example that a higher number of trials will significantly improve the decoding performance achieved in implanted patients. Quantifying this trade-off is all the more important if we want to move from a two-class decoding design (e.g., left/right) to a multi-class (e.g., upper left/upper right/lower right/lower left) or to a 2D continuous decoding design (e.g., x, y), in which case, the number of available trials per condition clearly becomes a limitative parameter.

Overall, most of these studies report a decoding performance above the 70% criteria for a robust BMI (Kübler et al., 2004, 2006). However, in spite of the fact that several experimental parameters contribute to the final decoding performance, invasive attention-based approaches in the non-human primate produce the highest decoding performances as compared to both invasive and non-invasive recording approaches in humans. This provides grounds of improvement for the latter. This is most probably due to the fact that the recordings can be performed closest to the source of the attention-related signals. Supporting this hypothesis, fMRI decoding of spatial attention (driven by activations in ROIs specifically identified based on their contribution to spatial attention processes) outperforms all other non-invasive decoding approaches.

CHALLENGES OF ATTENTION-DRIVEN COGNITIVE BRAIN–MACHINE INTERFACES

ENDOGENOUS VERSUS EXOGENOUS ATTENTION

As seen above, attention can be voluntarily controlled by the subject or involuntarily oriented by an external event. An efficient cBMI is expected to be able to infer spatial attention signals independently of how attention has been driven. Given the functionally partially distinct neural bases of endogenous and exogenous attention orientation, it is thus crucial to quantify, from a cBMI perspective, (1) whether both types of attention orientation modes lead to comparable decoding accuracies, i.e., whether the performance of a cBMI driven by endogenous attention signals is comparable to that of a cBMI driven by exogenous attention signals; and (2) whether a cBMI driven by say endogenous attention signals can generalize and also be driven by exogenous attention signals and vice versa. As discussed above, a recent study shows that the decoding of spatial attention during a cued target detection task from MUA recordings in the non-human primate FEF is partially dependent on whether attention is oriented endogenously or exogenously (Astrand et al., 2014b). Importantly, the decoding performance of exogenous attention signals (79%) is higher than that obtained when decoding endogenous attention signals (67%). Most interestingly, they additionally show that a classifier trained at decoding endogenous attention successfully reads out exogenous spatial attention neuronal signals (54%), though significantly less than if the classifier is directly trained on exogenous attention (drop of 13%). The relationship is not symmetrical as a classifier trained at decoding exogenous attention successfully reads out endogenous spatial attention neuronal signals with a performance of 62%, again slightly lower than if the classifier is directly trained on endogenous attention (drop of 5%).

SUSCEPTIBILITY OF ATTENTION-DRIVEN COGNITIVE BRAIN–MACHINE INTERFACES TO SENSORY AND COGNITIVE FACTORS

Neuronal signals collected from the primary motor cortex are only marginally affected by changes in the sensory environment (e.g., changes in the visual or somatosensory information) or by changes in the cognitive context (e.g., changes in what the subject is thinking about or planning to do). As a result, the generalization capabilities of motor BMIs are unaffected by such varying circumstances. It is still unclear whether this is also the case for cBMIs. While the several studies cited above quantified how well a cognitive variable, namely spatial attention, can be predicted from cortical activity response patterns, none directly tested whether and how this prediction was affected by either a change in the sensory environment or in the cognitive context. A recent report by Astrand et al. (2013) shows that the decoding of spatial attention orientation during the delay period of a memory-guided saccade task is affected by the presence of visual noise. Precisely, they report a 62% performance at decoding spatial attention orientation and spatial short-term memory information from MUA activities recorded in the non-human primate FEF during the delay period of a memory-guided saccade task in the absence of any visual noise and a performance of 63% in the presence of visual noise. When a classifier is trained at decoding this spatial attention orientation in the absence of visual noise and is tested

Table 2 | Comparative overview of the type of signals used for the decoding of spatial attention in the studies discussed in Table 1.

	Study	Signal	# Recorded signals	Coverage	Classification	Available trials
Non-invasive	van Gerven and Jensen (2009)	MEG/Alpha power (8–14 Hz) occipito-parietal channels	275 DC Squid axial gradiometers	Full head	Support Vector Machine w. linear kernel	128 trials per condition
	Treder et al. (2011)	EEG/Alpha power	64 channels	Full head	Logistic regression with L2 regularizer	40 trials per position
	Morioka et al. (2014)	EEG/Alpha and Beta Power guided by NIRS	EEG: 64 channels. NIRS: 49 channels.	Full head EEG. Parietal and occipital NIRS	Sparse logistic regression	88 trials per position
	Andersson et al. (2011)	fMRI/7T	Two ROIs: right vs. left and left vs. right	Full head		8 trials (13s) per condition
	Andersson et al. (2012)	fMRI		Full head		9 trials (13s) per position
Invasive in humans	Gunduz et al. (2012)	ECoG/Power from all frequency bands	86, 78, 64, 103, and 88 electrodes	Left hemisphere, 1 subject right hemisphere. No occipital lobe	Stepwise regression and Bayesian classification	40 trials per position (except for one subject: 80)
	Andersson et al. (2011)	ECoG/High gamma power	64 electrodes	Left parietal-occipital cortex		20 left/20 right/39 center
Invasive in non-human primates	Rotermund et al. (2013)	ECoG/Power, phase coherence and difference	36 and 37 electrodes	Extrastriate area V4 and portions of V1/V2 along lunate sulcus	Support Vector Machine w. Gaussian kernel	~several hundred trials
	Astrand et al. (2014a)	SUA/average spiking rate	131 neurons	Single hemisphere, Right or Left Frontal Eye Fields	Linear Regression with regularization	60 trials per condition
	Astrand et al. (2014b)	MUA/average spiking rate	48 channels	Both hemispheres, Frontal Eye Fields	Linear Regression with regularization	60 trials per position
	Armstrong et al. (2009)	SUA/average spiking rate	40 neurons	Right Frontal Eye Field	Support Vector Machine w. linear kernel	>10 trials per condition (leave-one out procedure)
	Zhang et al. (2011)	SUA/average spiking rate	187 neurons	Anterior Inferior Temporal cortex, single hemisphere	Correlation Coefficient Classifier	12 trials per stimulus (leave-one-out procedure)

This includes the type of recording method, the number of recorded signals, brain coverage, the type of classifier used for the decoding, the available number of trials per condition.

on MUA activities collected in the presence of visual noise (or vice versa) performance drops by 12%, though it remains well above chance. The decoding of spatial attention signals are thus affected by changes in the sensory environment. Astrand et al. (2013) similarly show that the decoding of the spatial position of a visual stimulus from MUA activities recorded in the non-human primate FEF depends on whether the monkey is for example performing a memory-guided saccade task or a simple target detection task (decoding performance across contexts leads to a drop in 18%, Astrand et al., 2013). Last, as described above, the authors also show that the decoding performance of spatial attention depends on whether attention is oriented endogenously or exogenously, a situation that can be seen as a change in the cognitive context (Astrand et al., 2014b).

SUSCEPTIBILITY OF ATTENTION-DRIVEN COGNITIVE BRAIN–MACHINE INTERFACES TO DISTRACTERS

Another important aspect to consider is how distracters affect the spatial location of attention and hence the stability of a cBMI based on spatial attention signals. Such distracters can be considered as a specific case of a sensory change in the subject's environment (cf. above).In an urban environment where we are constantly exposed to salient stimuli, the endogenous attention that corresponds to an internal objective that the subject wishes to achieve will be continually interrupted by a diversity of external stimuli, both relevant (traffic lights, car horns, your children's voice etc.) or irrelevant (christmas lights, traffic flow, strangers passing by etc.).Several behavioral studies show that peripheral cues automatically capture attention (Jonides and Irwing, 1981; Christ and Abrams, 2006; Neo and Chua, 2006; Schreij et al., 2008). However, attentional capture is not constant. For example, when subjects are explicitly instructed to ignore a peripheral cue, attentional capture is reduced, though not completely abolished (Lambert et al., 1987). Similarly, if attention is highly focused, for example when the subject strongly expects a visual event at a certain location (e.g., following a 100% validity cue), the attentional capture as measured from reaction times is extremely weak (Yantis and Jonides, 1990). In contrast, if the subject is expecting a visual event that can take place at an undefined location (its attention is thus diffuse, e.g., following a 25% validity cue), the attentional capture is much stronger (Yantis and Jonides, 1990). The same reduction in attentional capture can also be observed in visual search experiments where subjects need to distribute their attention over the whole search display in order to scan the scene efficiently (Schreij et al., 2008). Last, attentional capture also depends on the complexity of the visual scene (which is the case of our everyday environment). Cosman and Vecera (2009) show that, when subjects need to search for an item in a complex environment, attentional capture declines as the complexity of the visual scene increases.

These behavioral observations are in agreement with single cell recordings in the monkey parietal cortex. For example, the neurons of the LIP (Ben Hamed et al., 2001), an area functionally associated with attentional processes (Wardak et al., 2002, 2004), are specifically activated by behaviorally relevant visual events independently of whether relevance is due to the intrinsic properties of the stimuli (e.g., an abrupt onset high contrast stimulus) or to its extrinsic properties (e.g., a low contrast stimulus, the processing of which is important to the ongoing task, Gottlieb et al., 1998; Kusunoki et al., 2000). Spatial attentional priority is suggested to be encoded by the differential response between the neurons encoding a specific spatial location against the response of the entire LIP population (Bisley and Goldberg, 2003). Consequently, the selection of a spatial location by attention can be biased by focal LIP optogenetic or electrical microstimulation, mimicking an attention interference or capture (Dai et al., 2014). A recent study by Suzuki and Gottlieb (2013) further suggests that these suppression mechanisms might differ between the prefrontal and parietal nodes of the parietofrontal attentional network. Specifically, the neuronal response to distractors is weaker in the prefrontal cortex than in parietal cortex, indicating a stronger suppression. Additionally, the degree of this suppression with behavioral suppression markers is stronger in the prefrontal cortex. Last, reversible inactivation of the prefrontal cortex leads to a more severe distractability than observed following inactivation of the parietal cortex.

From a decoding perspective, Astrand et al. (2014b) show that a distracter interferes with the performance with which spatial attention can be decoded from FEF MUA recordings in the non-human primates performing a cued target detection task. As observed by others (Armstrong et al., 2009; Zhang et al., 2011), distractors interfere with the accuracy with which spatial attention can be decoded on correct trials. Astrand et al. (2014b) further show that this interference is maximal on false alarm trials, i.e., on trials in which the monkey erroneously responded to the distractor instead of waiting for the target. The distractor interference is similar between correct trials and trials on which the monkey missed the target. Remarkably, the accuracy with which spatial attention can be decoded is much lower on incorrect trials than on correct trials, whether attention has been oriented endogenously (25%) or exogenously (40%), a trend also reported by Armstrong et al. (2009).

SUSCEPTIBILITY OF ATTENTION-DRIVEN COGNITIVE BRAIN–MACHINE INTERFACES TO EYE MOVEMENTS

The last constraint that needs to be discussed in the context of attention-driven BMIs is eye movements. Indeed, the attentional frontoparietal network described above is highly overlapping with, though distinct from, the cortical oculomotor network (Corbetta et al., 1998; Wardak et al., 2006). In all of the studies considered above, the subjects are required to maintain eye fixation during the decoding procedure. As a result, they are behaviorally constrained to suppress an oculomotor-related signal. Studies evaluating the impact of eye movements on cBMIs are yet missing. Treder et al. (2011) demonstrate that high accuracy for EEG-based classification is often associated with low accuracy for eye movement electrooculography (EOG)-based classification, and vice versa. This suggests a dissociation between EEG- and EOG-based classification. It also indicates that eye movements disturb the decoding of attention orientation if not taken into account. Gunduz et al. (2012) further show that, in the absence of any prior processing, the performance with which attention orientation can be decoded in ECoG-implanted patients drops from 48 to 35% when the subjects are planning their motor response (i.e., hardly above the

33% chance level). This suggests that a "naïve" attention decoding performance is most probably disrupted by other signals than just eye-movements, including motor planning. The exact location of the recording sensors is expected to highly impact on such interferences. However, generally speaking, real-time denoising algorithms minimizing the impact of eye movement signals over the attention-related signals are potentially promising. Extremely simple strategies such as analyzing cortical signals only at a distance from eye movements might also prove sufficient.

Overall, in spite of the notable progress in the field of attention-driven cBMIs, several challenges need to be faced before large field therapeutical applications can be considered. A tight interaction between the field of real-time decoding of cortical activity and cognitive neurosciences is expected to have a major impact on facing these challenges, the growing understanding of how the brain functions playing a crucial role toward refined machine learning strategies to handle and analyze massive cortical recordings. This being said, prospective therapeutical application for such cBMIs can already be foreseen, as will be described below.

NEUROFEEDBACK AND COGNITIVE CONTROL

The capacity of the brain to restore and ameliorate its functioning after a major trauma or disease is still poorly understood. It is known that after a CNS disease or trauma (such as a stroke), the brain undergoes extensive functional reorganization (Murase et al., 2004; Nudo, 2006; He et al., 2007; Grefkes et al., 2008; Wang et al., 2010). Building on these impressive adaptive capabilities of the brain, researchers have, in the last 50 years, investigated the ability of the brain to modulate its activity and improve overt behavioral performance thanks to neurofeedback techniques. Initially, this technique consisted in continuously providing the patient with a feedback on the level of activity of a specific cortical region (e.g., thanks to an auditory or visual feedback correlating with the intensity of this cortical activity) and instructing the patient to increase or decrease this activity by their own volition. It has been proven efficient in treating patients with attention disorders and in reducing seizures in epileptic patients (reviewed below). More recent feedback techniques are not based on the raw cortical signals but rather use decoding procedures as described above in order to quantify the exact information of interest contained in the neuronal signals and provide this information as a feedback to the subjects. The subject's goal is then to improve this specific information through cognitive control. This is a very promising tool that could be used to target specific functions in order to enhance the activity in the brain, both in patients with cognitive deficits arising from acute brain damage or neurodegenerative or neurodevelopmental conditions, as well as in normal subjects seeking to enhance their own cognitive functions.

NEUROFEEDBACK AND COVERT NEURONAL ACTIVITY

When we are trained on a specific task, our performance often becomes better. Several studies have investigated the underlying neural bases that account for this behavioral improvement. In visual perceptual tasks that involve difficult discriminations, it has been observed that a behavioral improvement in perceptual sensitivity is strongly coupled with improved neural sensitivity in early and intermediate visual areas (Schoups et al., 2001; Yang and Maunsell, 2004; Hua et al., 2010) as well as in higher visual decision areas (Law and Gold, 2008). The idea behind neurofeedback is precisely grounded on such observations. Indeed, if the brain is capable of modulating its activity through learning, why not by voluntary control of the neuronal activity of specific brain areas? Several fMRI studies have approached this question by providing participants with a visual feedback of the level of activity (BOLD signal) in a specific area of the brain and asking them to increase or decrease this level. These studies have all come to the conclusion that brain activity can be regulated and enhanced volitionally by the subject (Weiskopf et al., 2003; deCharms et al., 2004, 2005; Caria et al., 2007; Scharnowski et al., 2014), even when trading the continuous visual feedback for a monetary reward feedback the value of which correlated with the level of activity of the cortical area of interest (Bray et al., 2007). On a neuronal level, electrophysiological studies not only confirm the above results but reveal a remarkable plasticity of individual neurons to modulate their activity under volitional control (Fetz, 1969, 2007; Cerf et al., 2010; Kobayashi et al., 2010; Schafer and Moore, 2011). For example, Fetz performed, in 1969, a visual and auditory feedback experiment where monkeys were rewarded for increasing the activity of newly isolated neurons in the precentral motor cortex. They observe that the activity could be increased with as much as 50–500% above the initial spike rates.

NEUROFEEDBACK AND OVERT BEHAVIORAL PERFORMANCE

The above studies demonstrate the feasibility of modulating the activity of our own brain by voluntary control. The next question is thus whether this neuronal modulation has an impact on overt behavior? Being able to increase or decrease the activity in the brain is amazing but quite useless if it does not lead to a measurable change in cognitive performance. In the field of EEG neurofeedback, it has actually been known for a long time that a voluntary change in the EEG rhythm, i.e., in the frequency content of the scalp EEG signals, can improve behavior (Wyrwicka and Sterman, 1968; Sterman et al., 1969). For example, Sterman and colleagues highlighted the specific impact of the *sensorimotor rhythm* (SMR: 12–14 Hz) on the capacity to inhibit ongoing behavior. They used neurofeedback to regulate this electrophysiological signature and thereby the frequency of the refractory seizures of a female patient. Specifically, after several months of EEG neurofeedback training to enhance the SMR, the authors noted that the seizures essentially ceased at the same time that a significant increase in the 11–15 Hz frequency band and a corresponding decrease in lower frequencies were observed (Sterman and Friar, 1972). This initial study was followed by a wave of studies describing the clinical benefits of using EEG driven neurofeedback over placebo experimental designs on patients with seizure disorders refractory to pharmacological treatments (Sterman et al., 1974; Kaplan, 1975; Seifert and Lubar, 1975; Kuhlman and Allison, 1977; Kuhlman, 1978; Sterman and Macdonald, 1978; Lantz and Sterman, 1988; Andrews and Schonfeld, 1992; Hansen et al., 1996). A different line of research using the same technique has tried to treat attention disorders such as attention deficit/hyperactivity disorder (ADHD). The first study conducted by Lubar and Shouse (1976), showed that SMR training improved inattentive symptoms in an

11-year old boy with hyperactivity. Further studies confirm that neurofeedback training has a significant effect on reducing hyperactivity or impulsivity symptoms in ADHD (Lubar, 1991; Lubar et al., 1995; Lindén et al., 1996; Thompson and Thompson, 1998; Kaiser and Othmer, 2000). Remarkably, this SMR-driven neurofeedback has further been proven as equally effective as medication (Rossiter and La Vaque, 1995).

Several recent fMRI-based neurofeedback studies show that the operant control of cortical activity can also lead to changes in behavior and to interesting therapeutical applications. For example, Rota et al. (2009) show that the self-regulation of the activity of the right inferior frontal gyrus improves the identification of emotional prosodic intonations. Haller et al. (2010) show that the operant control of the activity of the auditory cortex allows to improve chronic tinnitus, a condition in which subjects perceive more or less constantly an aversive tone or noise, in the absence of any objective external sound source. More recently, Subramanian et al. (2011) show that the clinical motor symptoms of Parkinson disease patients can be improved thanks to neurofeedback driven by the fMRI activity of their supplementary motor area.

In a single-cell recording study in the non-human primates, Schafer and Moore (2011) show that monkeys can learn to modulate the firing rate of individual prefrontal neurons (specifically recorded in the FEF). Importantly, they show that during up-regulation sessions (as compared to down-regulation), an increased firing rate leads to enhanced target discrimination in the receptive field of that neuron. This is a nice demonstration that the voluntary control of FEF neuronal activity is specifically associated with an enhancement of selective spatial attention. It is interesting to compare the finding to Schafer and Moore (2011) in the non-human primate to those obtained by Scharnowski et al. (2012) using fMRI-driven neurofeedback in human subjects. In this study, Scharnowski et al. (2014) demonstrate that the control of the ongoing spontaneous activity as estimated by the BOLD fMRI signal in the visual cortex results in improved visual perception. The authors further show that these observations correlated with increased effective connectivity between the visual cortex and the superior parietal lobe, suggesting that the improved visual perception resulted from enhanced top-down attentional control processes. Top-down attention has been repeatedly shown to modulate the activity of early visual areas (Brefczynski and DeYoe, 1999; Kastner et al., 1999; Li et al., 2008; Gregoriou et al., 2009). The fact that operant control of the activity of visual cortex did not exclusively involve local processes restricted to this cortical region but also involved long-distance and large-scale networks is an indication that the behavioral effects of neurofeedback are maximized by the involvement of the adaptive capabilities of higher level associative cortical regions such as the parietal or the prefrontal cortex.

The above studies all have in common to require the subjects to either increase or decrease the cortical activity being recorded. Cerf et al. (2010) use a concept that is completely different. Instead of just modulating the level of activity, they ask the subjects to actually enhance the information content of the recorded population activity. Specifically, they show that by focusing attention on a concept represented by a target image, neurons in the medial temporal lobe (MTL), an area involved in generating memories of fact and events (Squire and Zola-Morgan, 1991), increase their activity. In this study twelve patients implanted with intracranial electrodes were instructed to manipulate the display of two superimposed images by modulating the firing rate of four MTL units in their brain. The initial visibility of the two images was 50% and the patients were instructed to enhance a target image so as to make it 100% visible. The visibility of the two images was continuously updated via a real-time decoding procedure reflecting the information contained in the spiking activity of these four neurons about either images. This nicely designed experiment is yet limited because the authors only used four units in the decoder which leads to a straightforward interpretation of the decoding performance. Indeed, in this configuration, an increased decoding performance directly translates into an increase in the activity of the unit specifically tuned to the target image and/or decreased activity for the other units. A decoding performance based on the increases or decreases in the information content of hundreds of neurons would result in a much more complex pattern of neuronal changes, possibly more based on functional population synergies than on the mere increase in the activity of selective cells associated with a decrease in the activity of the non-selective cells. Shibata et al. (2011) demonstrate the feasibility of such an experimental design. Participants were given feedback based on the real-time decoding of BOLD fMRI activity. The decoder was configured to discriminate between different angles of a Gabor patch (10°/70°/130°) based on the fMRI BOLD signal recorded from V1 and V2 prior to the neurofeedback procedure. During the neurofeedback sessions, the participants were instructed to enlarge a green circle presented on the screen. For each subject, the size of the green circle was manipulated by how well they could encode a given Gabor patch orientation in their fMRI BOLD activity. The specific angle driving the change in the circle's size changed from one subject to the other. All participants succeeded in increasing the circle. They were therefore all able to increase the information content related to the assigned specific angle even though the strategies they overtly reported were far from the true workings of the experiment. Importantly, this led to an increased perceptual sensitivity specific to the angle used during feedback in contrast with the two other angles. The results of this experiment are important in several aspects. First, they prove the feasibility of human subjects voluntarily increasing their cortical information content relative to a specific visual feature. Second, they suggest that training the brain to increase its information content directly leads to an improvement in overt behavior. Third, they indicate that the improvements are specific to the exact feature that is being trained, similarly to what can be obtained through perceptual learning.

FUTURE DIRECTIONS

COGNITIVE BRAIN–MACHINE INTERFACES FOR COGNITIVE REHABILITATION

As covered in the previous section, neurofeedback applications based on the raw or interpreted (decoded) cognitive information have already been proven efficient for several rehabilitation applications ranging from auditory tinnitus to Parkinson's disease, seizures, ADHD. These applications are progressively infusing off the laboratory patient care protocols. For example, several start-ups are now providing ADHD EEG-based neurofeedback game platforms integrating enriched immersive virtual 3D environment technologies with neurofeedback training. A challenge facing these future directions is constructing neurofeedback environments that are optimally targeted to specific pathologies. In the above discussed examples, Parkinson's disease clinical symptoms were improved using the activity of the supplementary motor area. ADHD was improved using the sensory motor rhythm involved in overt behavior inhibition. These conditions were thus critically improved by targeting the specific cortical nodes of the dysfunction which have been associated with the overt clinical symptoms. The further development of such rehabilitation methods based on neurofeedback will require a tight interaction between fundamental neuroscience research providing an ever growing understanding of the neural bases of cognition and its deficits and clinical neuroscience research evaluating the impact of specific neurofeedback designs on well identified groups of patients (as defined by clear-cut genotypes, functional deficits or behavioral deficits). For example, while SMR-based neurofeedback has been shown to reduce impulsivity in hyperactive ADHD patients, it is expected that ADHD patients with low hyperactivity symptoms but high inattention symptoms will not benefit by this approach, due to a different functional deficit underlying their symptoms.

COGNITIVE BRAIN–MACHINE INTERFACES TO PALLIATE FOR A DEFICIT IN COMMUNICATION

Most of these above foreseen applications will rely on non-invasive cBMI designs. However, in the case of extremely severe cognitive deficits, cost–benefit recommendations will be needed to evaluate whether invasive cBMIs are ethically acceptable. Two such conditions come to mind. The first condition is the case of total locked-in patients, who are unable to move any muscle of their body including their eyes, while they are otherwise aware and awake. The motor recovery is extremely rare and often very minimal. In a recent report, a locked-in patient was able to communicate via sniffing (Plotkin et al., 2010). Using a direct brain-interface, another total locked-in patient was able to answer yes-or-no questions (Parker, 2003; Keiper, 2006).The second condition that could justify invasive cBMIs corresponds to minimally conscious patients. Unlike patients in a persistent vegetative state, these patients have partially preserved conscious awareness. Recent studies indicate that the overall brain metabolism of these patients is 20–40% lower than that of normal subjects, though slightly higher than that of patients in a vegetative state (Schiff et al., 2005). In addition, several studies indicate some degree of preserved cognitive functions. For example, sounds result in a more widespread activation of the primary auditory and prefrontal associative areas in minimally conscious patients than in vegetative state patients (Laureys et al., 2004), more so when narratives were presented as compared to meaningless narratives played backward (Schiff et al., 2002; Coleman et al., 2007). More recently, and in tight relation with the attention-driven cBMIs discussed above, preserved exogenous attention functions and preserved underlying brain processes have been described in these patients, in association with a marked deficit in endogenous attention processes (Chennu et al., 2013). From a therapeutical perspective, deep brain thalamic stimulation has been described to improve the condition of minimally conscious patients (Laureys et al., 2007). Invasive cBMIs are also potentially interesting in this respect. In a first step, cBMIs can serve to assess and quantify the information content of the baseline or stimulus-induced cortical activity of these patients, and possibly serve to interpret part of their phenomenological experience (pain, surprise, attention, etc.). In a second step, cBMIs associated with focal stimulation approaches such as electric or optogenetic stimulations can help increase the information content of specific cortical regions. As soon as consciousness is high enough for the subject to express a preference (e.g., hearing the name of her loved ones instead of the names of strangers), this activity can be used for feedback-cBMI designs that can further help reinforce the weak yet meaningful endogenous cortical activities of minimally conscious patients. While this can seem like science fiction, all the theoretical and experimental grounds are set to make this possible.

OPEN FIELD COGNITIVE BRAIN–MACHINE INTERFACES FOR ENHANCED COGNITION

In addition to rehabilitation, there is a growing social pressure for healthy individuals to increase their cognitive performance or preserve it from aging. Several tools are already being used to this goal, ranging from cognitive training (through a growing range of enriched video game applications, see for example Cardoso-Leite and Bavelier, 2014), to cognitive pharmacological enhancers (i.e., drugs primarily developed to treat people with cognitive or motor function difficulties that are used by healthy subjects to improve memory, attention, concentration, and planning, see for example Greely et al., 2008), to off-the-laboratory brain stimulation (transcranial direct current stimulation – tDCS-kits are now commercially available). In this context, given its consequences on behavioral performance as described above, non-invasive neurofeedback applications can be considered as a safe improved alternative to cognitive training, as compared to cognitive enhancers or brain stimulation.

SHARED COGNITION

In a recent report, Pais-Vieira et al. (2013) describe an astounding brain-to-brain interface (BTBI). The cortical activity of an "encoder" rat, performing a learned sensorimotor task was injected, using intracortical microstimulations, into the matching cortical area of a "decoder" rat that was able to learn to use these alien activity patterns to perform the sensorimotor choices as the "encoder" rat. This opens amazing perspectives. From a rehabilitation point of view, one can think of injecting in target cortical regions of the brain of a patient suffering from a severe cognitive deficit the activity patterns recorded from healthy subjects in well-defined contexts. This is not very different from deep brain stimulation procedures now classically used in Parkinson Disease patients for example or from trans-cranial direct current stimulation applied in severe refractory depression, except that the stimulations would in this case correspond to the cognitive information content of healthy subjects.

CLOSING THE LOOP

Overall, this review brings together several studies that not only demonstrate the feasibility of decoding spatial attention in real time using a diversity of experimental set-ups, but that also show that this real-time decoding can further be used for rehabilitation purposes. As a concluding note, we would like to highlight the fact that this field of cBMIs, and specifically attention-driven BMIs, is still young and that the reviewed studies mostly represent proofs of concept. We believe that the real-time access to spatial attention signals (and other cognitive information) also has the potential to bring about a novel understanding of the neural bases of these cognitive processes that cannot be accessed by more classical investigation methods. Taking this fundamental neuroscience perspective on cBMI research will also provide a better understanding of why and how neurofeedback improves cognition. These are the crucial challenges the field will need to face in the coming years.

ACKNOWLEDGMENTS

Elaine Astrand was funded by the Fondation pour la recherché médicale (FRM) and the Direction générale des armées (DGA). Suliann Ben Hamed was funded by the French Agence nationale de la recherche (Grant #ANR-05-JCJC-0230-01 and Grant # ANR-11-BSV4-0011), as well as by a CNRS bioinformatics grant.

REFERENCES

Albares, M., Criaud, M., Wardak, C., Nguyen, S. C. T., Ben Hamed, S., and Boulinguez, P. (2011). Attention to baseline: does orienting visuospatial attention really facilitate target detection? *J. Neurophysiol.* 106, 809–816. doi: 10.1152/jn.00206.2011

Andersson, P., Pluim, J. P. W., Siero, J. C. W., Klein, S., Viergever, M. A., and Ramsey, N. F. (2011). Real-time decoding of brain responses to visuospatial attention using 7T fMRI. *PLoS ONE* 6:e27638. doi: 10.1371/journal.pone.0027638

Andersson, P., Ramsey, N. F., Raemaekers, M., Viergever, M. A., and Pluim, J. P. W. (2012). Real-time decoding of the direction of covert visuospatial attention. *J. Neural Eng.* 9:045004. doi: 10.1088/1741-2560/9/4/045004

Andrews, D. J., and Schonfeld, W. H. (1992). Predictive factors for controlling seizures using a behavioural approach. *Seizure* 1, 111–116. doi: 10.1016/1059-1311(92)90008-O

Anton-Erxleben, K., and Carrasco, M. (2013). Attentional enhancement of spatial resolution: linking behavioural and neurophysiological evidence. *Nat. Rev. Neurosci.* 14, 188–200. doi: 10.1038/nrn3443

Anton-Erxleben, K., Stephan, V. M., and Treue, S. (2009). Attention reshapes center-surround receptive field structure in macaque cortical area MT. *Cereb. Cortex* 19, 2466–2478. doi: 10.1093/cercor/bhp002

Armstrong, K. M., Chang, M. H., and Moore, T. (2009). Selection and maintenance of spatial information by frontal eye field neurons. *J. Neurosci.* 29, 15621–15629. doi: 10.1523/JNEUROSCI.4465-09.2009

Arrington, C. M., Carr, T. H., Mayer, A. R., and Rao, S. M. (2000). Neural mechanisms of visual attention: object-based selection of a region in space. *J. Cogn. Neurosci.* 12, 106–117. doi: 10.1162/089892900563975

Astrand, E., Enel, P., Ibos, G., Dominey, P. F., Baraduc, P., and Ben Hamed, S. (2014a). Comparison of classifiers for decoding sensory and cognitive information from prefrontal neuronal populations. *PLoS ONE* 9:e86314. doi: 10.1371/journal.pone.0086314

Astrand, E., Wardak, C., and Ben Hamed, S. (2014b). "Real-time decoding of visual attention from monkey prefrontal population activities: towards context independent high performance cognitive brain computer interfaces," in *FENS Meeting*, Milan.

Astrand, E., Huguet, N., Wardak, C., and Ben Hamed, S. (2013). "Real-time decoding from prefrontal neuronal population activities: how flexible is the decoding?," in *Annual Meeting of the Sociétéfrançaise des neurosciences*, Lyon.

Barash, S., Bracewell, R. M., Fogassi, L., Gnadt, J. W., and Andersen, R. A. (1991). Saccade-related activity in the lateral intraparietal area. II. Spatial properties. *J. Neurophysiol.* 66, 1109–1124.

Bashinski, H. S., and Bacharach, V. R. (1980). Enhancement of perceptual sensitivity as the result of selectively attending to spatial locations. *Percept. Psychophys.* 28, 241–248. doi: 10.3758/BF03204380

Ben Hamed, S., Duhamel, J.-R., Bremmer, F., and Graf, W. (1997). Attentional modulation of visual receptive fields in the posterior parietal cortex of the behaving macaque. *Exp. Brain Res. Series* 25, 371–384.

Ben Hamed, S., Duhamel, J.-R., Bremmer, F., and Graf, W. (2001). Representation of the visual field in the lateral intraparietal area of macaque monkeys: a quantitative receptive field analysis. *Exp. Brain Res.* 140, 127–144. doi: 10.1007/s002210100785

Ben Hamed, S., Duhamel, J.-R., Bremmer, F., and Graf, W. (2002). Visual receptive field modulation in the lateral intraparietal area during attentive fixation and free gaze. *Cereb. Cortex* 12, 234–245. doi: 10.1093/cercor/12.3.234

Ben Hamed, S., Page, W., Duffy, C., and Pouget, A. (2003). MSTd neuronal basis functions for the population encoding of heading direction. *J. Neurophysiol.* 90, 549–558. doi: 10.1152/jn.00639.2002

Ben Hamed, S., Schieber, M. H., and Pouget, A. (2007). Decoding M1 neurons during multiple finger movements. *J. Neurophysiol.* 98, 327–333. doi: 10.1152/jn.00760.2006

Bisley, J. W., and Goldberg, M. E. (2003). Neuronal activity in the lateral intraparietal area and spatial attention. *Science* 299, 81–86. doi: 10.1126/science.1077395

Bray, S., Shimojo, S., and O'Doherty, J. P. (2007). Direct instrumental conditioning of neural activity using functional magnetic resonance imaging-derived reward feedback. *J. Neurosci.* 27, 7498–7507. doi: 10.1523/JNEUROSCI.2118-07.2007

Brefczynski, J. A., and DeYoe, E. A. (1999). A physiological correlate of the "spotlight" of visual attention. *Nat. Neurosci.* 2, 370–374. doi: 10.1038/7280

Bruce, C. J., and Goldberg, M. E. (1985). Primate frontal eye fields. I. Single neurons discharging before saccades. *J. Neurophysiol.* 53, 603–635.

Buschman, T. J., and Miller, E. K. (2007). Top-down versus bottom-up control of attention in the prefrontal and posterior parietal cortices. *Science* 315, 1860–1862. doi: 10.1126/science.1138071

Cardoso-Leite, P., and Bavelier, D. (2014). Video game play, attention, and learning: how to shape the development of attention and influence learning? *Curr. Opin. Neurol.* 27, 185–191. doi: 10.1097/WCO.0000000000000077

Caria, A., Veit, R., Sitaram, R., Lotze, M., Weiskopf, N., Grodd, W., et al. (2007). Regulation of anterior insular cortex activity using real-time fMRI. *Neuroimage* 35, 1238–1246. doi: 10.1016/j.neuroimage.2007.01.018

Carmena, J. M., Lebedev, M. A., Crist, R. E., O'Doherty, J. E., Santucci, D. M., Dimitrov, D. F., et al. (2003). Learning to control a brain–machine interface for reaching and grasping by primates. *PLoS Biol.* 1:E42. doi: 10.1371/journal.pbio.0000042

Carrasco, M., and Yeshurun, Y. (2009). Covert attention effects on spatial resolution. *Prog. Brain Res.* 176, 65–86. doi: 10.1016/S0079-6123(09)17605-7

Cerf, M., Thiruvengadam, N., Mormann, F., Kraskov, A., Quiroga, R. Q., Koch, C., et al. (2010). On-line, voluntary control of human temporal lobe neurons. *Nature* 467, 1104–1108. doi: 10.1038/nature09510

Chapin, J. K., Moxon, K. A., Markowitz, R. S., and Nicolelis, M. A. (1999). Real-time control of a robot arm using simultaneously recorded neurons in the motor cortex. *Nat. Neurosci.* 2, 664–670. doi: 10.1038/10223

Chennu, S., Finoia, P., Kamau, E., Monti, M. M., Allanson, J., Pickard, J. D., et al. (2013). Dissociable endogenous and exogenous attention in disorders of consciousness. *Neuroimage Clin.* 3, 450–461. doi: 10.1016/j.nicl.2013.10.008

Christ, S. E., and Abrams, R. A. (2006). Abrupt onsets cannot be ignored. *Psychon. Bull. Rev.* 13, 875–880. doi: 10.3758/BF03194012

Cohen, M. R., and Maunsell, J. H. R. (2009). Attention improves performance primarily by reducing interneuronal correlations. *Nat. Neurosci.* 12, 1594–1600. doi: 10.1038/nn.2439

Coleman, M. R., Rodd, J. M., Davis, M. H., Johnsrude, I. S., Menon, D. K., Pickard, J. D., et al. (2007). Do vegetative patients retain aspects of language comprehension? Evidence from fMRI. *Brain* 130, 2494–2507. doi: 10.1093/brain/awm170

Corbetta, M., Akbudak, E., Conturo, T. E., Snyder, A. Z., Ollinger, J. M., Drury, H. A., et al. (1998). A common network of functional areas for attention and eye movements. *Neuron* 21, 761–773. doi: 10.1016/S0896-6273(00)80593-0

Corbetta, M., Kincade, J. M., Ollinger, J. M., McAvoy, M. P., and Shulman, G. L. (2000). Voluntary orienting is dissociated from target detection in human posterior parietal cortex. *Nat. Neurosci.* 3, 292–297. doi: 10.1038/73009

Corbetta, M., and Shulman, G. L. (2002). Control of goal-directed and stimulus-driven attention in the brain. *Nat. Rev. Neurosci.* 3, 201–215. doi: 10.1038/nrn755

Cosman, J. D., and Vecera, S. P. (2009). Perceptual load modulates attentional capture by abrupt onsets. *Psychon. Bull. Rev.* 16, 404–410. doi: 10.3758/PBR.16.2.404

Dai, J., Brooks, D. I., and Sheinberg, D. L. (2014). Optogenetic and electrical microstimulation systematically bias visuospatial choice in primates. *Curr. Biol.* 24, 63–69. doi: 10.1016/j.cub.2013.11.011

deCharms, R. C., Christoff, K., Glover, G. H., Pauly, J. M., Whitfield, S., and Gabrieli, J. D. E. (2004). Learned regulation of spatially localized brain activation using real-time fMRI. *Neuroimage* 21, 436–443. doi: 10.1016/j.neuroimage.2003.08.041

deCharms, R. C., Maeda, F., Glover, G. H., Ludlow, D., Pauly, J. M., Soneji, D., et al. (2005). Control over brain activation and pain learned by using real-time functional MRI. *Proc. Natl. Acad. Sci. U.S.A.* 102, 18626–18631. doi: 10.1073/pnas.0505210102

FarbodKia, S., Åstrand, E., Ibos, G., and Ben Hamed, S. (2011). Readout of the intrinsic and extrinsic properties of a stimulus from un-experienced neuronal activities: towards cognitive neuroprostheses. *J. Physiol. Paris* 105, 115–122. doi: 10.1016/j.jphysparis.2011.07.015

Fetz, E. E. (1969). Operant conditioning of cortical unit activity. *Science* 163, 955–958. doi: 10.1126/science.163.3870.955

Fetz, E. E. (2007). Volitional control of neural activity: implications for brain–computer interfaces. *J. Physiol.* 579, 571–579. doi: 10.1113/jphysiol.2006.127142

Gobell, J., and Carrasco, M. (2005). Attention alters the appearance of spatial frequency and gap size. *Psychol. Sci.* 16, 644–651. doi: 10.1111/j.1467-9280.2005.01588.x

Gottlieb, J. P., Kusunoki, M., and Goldberg, M. E. (1998). The representation of visual salience in monkey parietal cortex. *Nature* 391, 481–484. doi: 10.1038/35135

Greely, H., Sahakian, B., Harris, J., Kessler, R. C., Gazzaniga, M., Campbell, P., et al. (2008). Towards responsible use of cognitive-enhancing drugs by the healthy. *Nature* 456, 702–705. doi: 10.1038/456702a

Grefkes, C., Nowak, D. A., Eickhoff, S. B., Dafotakis, M., Küst, J., Karbe, H., et al. (2008). Cortical connectivity after subcortical stroke assessed with functional magnetic resonance imaging. *Ann. Neurol.* 63, 236–246. doi: 10.1002/ana.21228

Gregoriou, G. G., Gotts, S. J., Zhou, H., and Desimone, R. (2009). High-frequency, long-range coupling between prefrontal and visual cortex during attention. *Science* 324, 1207–1210. doi: 10.1126/science.1171402

Gunduz, A., Brunner, P., Daitch, A., Leuthardt, E. C., Ritaccio, A. L., Pesaran, B., et al. (2012). Decoding covert spatial attention using electrocorticographic (ECoG) signals in humans. *Neuroimage* 60, 2285–2293. doi: 10.1016/j.neuroimage.2012.02.017

Haller, S., Birbaumer, N., and Veit, R. (2010). Real-time fMRI feedback training may improve chronic tinnitus. *Eur. Radiol.* 20, 696–703. doi: 10.1007/s00330-009-1595-z

Hansen, L. M., Trudeau, D. L., and Grace, D. L. (1996). Neurotherapy and drug therapy in combination for adult ADHD, personality disorder, and seizure disorder. *J. Neurother.* 2, 6–14. doi: 10.1300/J184v02n01_02

He, B. J., Snyder, A. Z., Vincent, J. L., Epstein, A., Shulman, G. L., and Corbetta, M. (2007). Breakdown of functional connectivity in frontoparietal networks underlies behavioral deficits in spatial neglect. *Neuron* 53, 905–918. doi: 10.1016/j.neuron.2007.02.013

Hochberg, L. R., Bacher, D., Jarosiewicz, B., Masse, N. Y., Simeral, J. D., Vogel, J., et al. (2012). Reach and grasp by people with tetraplegia using a neurally controlled robotic arm. *Nature* 485, 372–375. doi: 10.1038/nature11076

Hochberg, L. R., Serruya, M. D., Friehs, G. M., Mukand, J. A., Saleh, M., Caplan, A. H., et al. (2006). Neuronal ensemble control of prosthetic devices by a human with tetraplegia. *Nature* 442, 164–171. doi: 10.1038/nature04970

Hopfinger, J. B., Buonocore, M. H., and Mangun, G. R. (2000). The neural mechanisms of top-down attentional control. *Nat. Neurosci.* 3, 284–291. doi: 10.1038/72999

Hua, T., Bao, P., Huang, C.-B., Wang, Z., Xu, J., Zhou, Y., et al. (2010). Perceptual learning improves contrast sensitivity of V1 neurons in cats. *Curr. Biol.* 20, 887–894. doi: 10.1016/j.cub.2010.03.066

Ibos, G., Duhamel, J.-R., and Ben Hamed, S. (2009). The spatial and temporal deployment of voluntary attention across the visual field. *PLoS ONE* 4:e6716. doi: 10.1371/journal.pone.0006716

Ibos, G., Duhamel, J.-R., and Ben Hamed, S. (2013). A functional hierarchy within the parietofrontal network in stimulus selection and attention control. *J. Neurosci.* 33, 8359–8369. doi: 10.1523/JNEUROSCI.4058-12.2013

Ifft, P. J., Shokur, S., Li, Z., Lebedev, M. A., and Nicolelis, M. A. L. (2013). A brain–machine interface enables bimanual arm movements in monkeys. *Sci. Transl. Med.* 5:210ra154. doi: 10.1126/scitranslmed.3006159

Jerbi, K., Freyermuth, S., Minotti, L., Kahane, P., Berthoz, A., and Lachaux, J.-P. (2009). Watching brain TV and playing brain ball exploring novel BCI strategies using real-time analysis of human intracranial data. *Int. Rev. Neurobiol.* 86, 159–168. doi: 10.1016/S0074-7742(09)86012-1

Jonides, J. (1981). "Voluntary vs. automatic control over the mind's eye's movement," in *Attention and performance IX*, eds J. B. Long and A. D. Baddely (Hillsdale, NJ: Lawrence Erlbaum Associates), 187–203.

Jonides, J., and Irwing, D. E. (1981). Capturing attention. *Cognition* 145–150. doi: 10.1016/0010-0277(81)90038-X

Kaiser, D. A., and Othmer, S. (2000). Effect of neurofeedback on variables of attention in a large multi-center trial. *J. Neurother.* 4, 5–15. doi: 10.1300/J184v04n01_02

Kaplan, B. J. (1975). Biofeedback in epileptics: equivocal relationship of reinforced EEG frequency to seizure reduction. *Epilepsia* 16, 477–485. doi: 10.1111/j.1528-1157.1975.tb06076.x

Kastner, S., Pinsk, M. A., De Weerd, P., Desimone, R., and Ungerleider, L. G. (1999). Increased activity in human visual cortex during directed attention in the absence of visual stimulation. *Neuron* 22, 751–761. doi: 10.1016/S0896-6273(00)80734-5

Keiper, A. (2006). The age of neuroelectronics. *New Atlantis* 11, 4–41.

Kim, S.-P., Simeral, J. D., Hochberg, L. R., Donoghue, J. P., Friehs, G. M., and Black, M. J. (2011). Point- and-click cursor control with an intracortical neural interface system by humans with tetraplegia. *IEEE Trans. Neural Syst. Rehabil. Eng.* 19, 193–203. doi: 10.1109/TNSRE.2011.2107750

Kincade, J. M., Abrams, R. A., Astafiev, S. V., Shulman, G. L., and Corbetta, M. (2005). An event-related functional magnetic resonance imaging study of voluntary and stimulus-driven orienting of attention. *J. Neurosci.* 25, 4593–4604. doi: 10.1523/JNEUROSCI.0236-05.2005

Kobayashi, S., Schultz, W., and Sakagami, M. (2010). Operant conditioning of primate prefrontal neurons. *J. Neurophysiol.* 103, 1843–1855. doi: 10.1152/jn.00173.2009

Kübler, A., Mushahwar, V. K., Hochberg, L. R., and Donoghue, J. P. (2006). BCI meeting 2005 – workshop on clinical issues and applications. *IEEE Trans. Neural Syst. Rehabil. Eng.* 14, 131–134. doi: 10.1109/TNSRE.2006.875585

Kübler, A., Neumann, N., Wilhelm, B., Hinterberger, T., and Birbaumer, N. (2004). Predictability of brain – computer communication. *J. Psychophysiol.* 18, 121–129. doi: 10.1027/0269-8803.18.23.121

Kuhlman, W. N. (1978). EEG feedback training of epileptic patients: clinical and electroencephalographic analysis. *Electroencephalogr. Clin. Neurophysiol.* 45, 699–710. doi: 10.1016/0013-4694(78)90138-4

Kuhlman, W. N., and Allison, T. (1977). EEG feedback training in the treatment of epilepsy: some questions and some answers. *Pavlov. J. Biol. Sci.* 12, 112–122. doi: 10.1007/BF03004498

Kusunoki, M., Gottlieb, J., and Goldberg, M. E. (2000). The lateral intraparietal area as a salience map: the representation of abrupt onset, stimulus motion, and task relevance. *Vision Res.* 40, 1459–1468. doi: 10.1016/S0042-6989(99)00212-6

Lambert, A., Spencer, E., and Mohindra, N. (1987). Automaticity and the capture of attention by a peripheral display change. *Curr. Psychol.* 6, 136–147. doi: 10.1007/BF02686618

Lantz, D. L., and Sterman, M. B. (1988). Neuropsychological assessment of subjects with uncontrolled epilepsy: effects of EEG feedback training. *Epilepsia* 29, 163–171. doi: 10.1111/j.1528-1157.1988.tb04414.x

Laureys, S., Owen, A. M., and Schiff, N. D. (2004). Brain function in coma, vegetative state, and related disorders. *Lancet Neurol.* 3, 537–546. doi: 10.1016/S1474-4422(04)00852-X

Laureys, S., Perrin, F., and Brédart, S. (2007). Self-consciousness in non-communicative patients. *Conscious. Cogn.* 16, 722–741; discussion 742–745. doi: 10.1016/j.concog.2007.04.004

Law, C.-T., and Gold, J. I. (2008). Neural correlates of perceptual learning in a sensory-motor, but not a sensory, cortical area. *Nat. Neurosci.* 11, 505–513. doi: 10.1038/nn2070

Lebedev, M. A., Carmena, J. M., O'Doherty, J. E., Zacksenhouse, M., Henriquez, C. S., Principe, J. C., et al. (2005). Cortical ensemble adaptation to represent velocity of an artificial actuator controlled by a brain – machine interface. *J. Neurosci.* 25, 4681–4693. doi: 10.1523/JNEUROSCI.4088-04.2005

Lee, J., Williford, T., and Maunsell, J. H. R. (2007). Spatial attention and the latency of neuronal responses in macaque area V4. *J. Neurosci.* 27, 9632–9637. doi: 10.1523/JNEUROSCI.2734-07.2007

Li, X., Lu, Z.-L., Tjan, B. S., Dosher, B. A., and Chu, W. (2008). Blood oxygenation level-dependent contrast response functions identify mechanisms of covert attention in early visual areas. *Proc. Natl. Acad. Sci. U.S.A.* 105, 6202–6207. doi: 10.1073/pnas.0801390105

Lindén, M., Habib, T., and Radojevic, V. (1996). A controlled study of the effects of EEG biofeedback on cognition and behavior of children with attention deficit disorder and learning disabilities. *Biofeedback Self Regul.* 21, 35–49. doi: 10.1007/BF02214148

Lubar, J. F. (1991). Discourse on the development of EEG diagnostics and biofeedback for attention-deficit/hyperactivity disorders. *Biofeedback Self Regul.* 16, 201–225. doi: 10.1007/BF01000016

Lubar, J. F., and Shouse, M. N. (1976). EEG and behavioral changes in a hyperkinetic child concurrent with training of the sensorimotor rhythm (SMR): a preliminary report. *Biofeedback Self Regul.* 1, 293–306. doi: 10.1007/BF01001170

Lubar, J. F., Swartwood, M. O., Swartwood, J. N., and O'Donnell, P. H. (1995). Evaluation of the effectiveness of EEG neurofeedback training for ADHD in a clinical setting as measured by changes in T.O.V.A. scores, behavioral ratings, and WISC-R performance. *Biofeedback Self Regul.* 20, 83–99. doi: 10.1007/BF01712768

Macaluso, E., Frith, C. D., and Driver, J. (2002). Supramodal effects of covert spatial orienting triggered by visual or tactile events. *J. Cogn. Neurosci.* 14, 389–401. doi: 10.1162/089892902317361912

McAdams, C. J., and Maunsell, J. H. (1999). Effects of attention on the reliability of individual neurons in monkey visual cortex. *Neuron* 23, 765–773. doi: 10.1016/S0896-6273(01)80034-9

Morioka, H., Kanemura, A., Morimoto, S., Yoshioka, T., Oba, S., Kawanabe, M., et al. (2014). Decoding spatial attention by using cortical currents estimated from electroencephalography with near-infrared spectroscopy prior information. *Neuroimage* 90, 128–139. doi: 10.1016/j.neuroimage.2013.12.035

Müller, H. J., and Rabbitt, P. M. (1989). Reflexive and voluntary orienting of visual attention: time course of activation and resistance to interruption. *J. Exp. Psychol. Hum. Percept. Perform.* 15, 315–330. doi: 10.1037/0096-1523.15.2.315

Murase, N., Duque, J., Mazzocchio, R., and Cohen, L. G. (2004). Influence of interhemispheric interactions on motor function in chronic stroke. *Ann. Neurol.* 55, 400–409. doi: 10.1002/ana.10848

Musallam, S., Corneil, B. D., Greger, B., Scherberger, H., and Andersen, R. A. (2004). Cognitive control signals for neural prosthetics. *Science* 305, 258–262. doi: 10.1126/science.1097938

Neo, G., and Chua, F. K. (2006). Capturing focused attention. *Percept. Psychophys.* 68, 1286–1296. doi: 10.3758/BF03193728

Nudo, R. J. (2006). Mechanisms for recovery of motor function following cortical damage. *Curr. Opin. Neurobiol.* 16, 638–644. doi: 10.1016/j.conb.2006.10.004

Pais-Vieira, M., Lebedev, M., Kunicki, C., Wang, J., and Nicolelis, M. A. L. (2013). A brain-to-brain interface for real-time sharing of sensorimotor information. *Sci. Rep.* 3:1319. doi: 10.1038/srep01319

Parker, I. (2003). Reading minds. *The New Yorker*, 52–63.

Plotkin, A., Sela, L., Weissbrod, A., Kahana, R., Haviv, L., Yeshurun, Y., et al. (2010). Sniffing enables communication and environmental control for the severely disabled. *Proc. Natl. Acad. Sci. U.S.A.* 107, 14413–14418. doi: 10.1073/pnas.1006746107

Posner, M. I., Snyder, C. R., and Davidson, B. J. (1980). Attention and the detection of signals. *J. Exp. Psychol.* 109, 160–174. doi: 10.1037/0096-3445.109.2.160

Prinzmetal, W., McCool, C., and Park, S. (2005). Attention: reaction time and accuracy reveal different mechanisms. *J. Exp. Psychol. Gen.* 134, 73–92. doi: 10.1037/0096-3445.134.1.73

Rossiter, D. T. R., and La Vaque, T. J. (1995). A comparison of EEG biofeedback and psychostimulants in treating attention deficit/hyperactivity disorders. *J. Neurother.* 1, 48–59. doi: 10.1300/J184v01n01_07

Rota, G., Sitaram, R., Veit, R., Erb, M., Weiskopf, N., Dogil, G., et al. (2009). Self-regulation of regional cortical activity using real-time fMRI: the right inferior frontal gyrus and linguistic processing. *Hum. Brain Mapp.* 30, 1605–1614. doi: 10.1002/hbm.20621

Rotermund, D., Ernst, U., Mandon, S., Taylor, K., Smiyukha, Y., Kreiter, A., et al. (2013). Toward high performance, weakly invasive brain computer interfaces using selective visual attention. *J. Neurosci.* 33, 6001–6011. doi: 10.1523/JNEUROSCI.4225-12.2013

Santhanam, G., Ryu, S. I., Yu, B. M., Afshar, A., and Shenoy, K. V. (2006). A high-performance brain – computer interface. *Nature* 442, 195–198. doi: 10.1038/nature04968

Schafer, R. J., and Moore, T. (2011). Selective attention from voluntary control of neurons in prefrontal cortex. *Science* 332, 1568–1571. doi: 10.1126/science.1199892

Scharnowski, F., Hutton, C., Josephs, O., Weiskopf, N., and Rees, G. (2012). Improving visual perception through neurofeedback. *J. Neurosci.* 32, 17830–17841. doi: 10.1523/JNEUROSCI.6334-11.2012

Scharnowski, F., Rosa, M. J., Golestani, N., Hutton, C., Josephs, O., Weiskopf, N., et al. (2014). Connectivity changes underlying neurofeedback training of visual cortex activity. *PLoS ONE* 9:e91090. doi: 10.1371/journal.pone.0091090

Schiff, N. D., Plum, F., and Rezai, A. R. (2002). Developing prosthetics to treat cognitive disabilities resulting from acquired brain injuries. *Neurol. Res.* 24, 116–124. doi: 10.1179/016164102101199576

Schiff, N. D., Rodriguez-Moreno, D., Kamal, A., Kim, K. H. S., Giacino, J. T., Plum, F., et al. (2005). fMRI reveals large-scale network activation in minimally conscious patients. *Neurology* 64, 514–523. doi: 10.1212/01.WNL.0000150883.10285.44

Schoups, A., Vogels, R., Qian, N., and Orban, G. (2001). Practising orientation identification improves orientation coding in V1 neurons. *Nature* 412, 549–553. doi: 10.1038/35087601

Schreij, D., Owens, C., and Theeuwes, J. (2008). Abrupt onsets capture attention independent of top-down control settings. *Percept. Psychophys.* 70, 208–218. doi: 10.3758/PP.70.2.208

Seifert, A. R., and Lubar, J. F. (1975). Reduction of epileptic seizures through EEG biofeedback training. *Biol. Psychol.* 3, 157–184. doi: 10.1016/0301-0511(75)90033-2

Serruya, M. D., Hatsopoulos, N. G., Paninski, L., Fellows, M. R., and Donoghue, J. P. (2002). Instant neural control of a movement signal. *Nature* 416, 141–142. doi: 10.1038/416141a

Shanechi, M. M., Hu, R. C., and Williams, Z. M. (2014). A cortical–spinal prosthesis for targeted limb movement in paralysed primate avatars. *Nat. Commun.* 5:3237. doi: 10.1038/ncomms4237

Shibata, K., Watanabe, T., Sasaki, Y., and Kawato, M. (2011). Perceptual learning incepted by decoded fMRI neurofeedback without stimulus presentation. *Science* 334, 1413–1415. doi: 10.1126/science.1212003

Shulman, G. L., Ollinger, J. M., Akbudak, E., Conturo, T. E., Snyder, A. Z., Petersen, S. E., et al. (1999). Areas involved in encoding and applying directional expectations to moving objects. *J. Neurosci.* 19, 9480–9496.

Squire, L. R., and Zola-Morgan, S. (1991). The medial temporal lobe memory system. *Science* 253, 1380–1386. doi: 10.1126/science.1896849

Sterman, M. B., and Friar, L. (1972). Suppression of seizures in an epileptic following sensorimotor EEG feedback training. *Electroencephalogr. Clin. Neurophysiol.* 33, 89–95. doi: 10.1016/0013-4694(72)90028-4

Sterman, M. B., and Macdonald, L. R. (1978). Effects of central cortical EEG feedback training on incidence of poorly controlled seizures. *Epilepsia* 19, 207–222. doi: 10.1111/j.1528-1157.1978.tb04483.x

Sterman, M. B., Macdonald, L. R., and Stone, R. K. (1974). Biofeedback training of the sensorimotor electroencephalogram rhythm in man: effects on epilepsy. *Epilepsia* 15, 395–416. doi: 10.1111/j.1528-1157.1974.tb04016.x

Sterman, M. B., Wyrwicka, W., and Roth, S. (1969). Electrophysiological correlates and neural substrates of alimentary behavior in the cat. *Ann. N. Y. Acad. Sci.* 157, 723–739. doi: 10.1111/j.1749-6632.1969.tb12916.x

Subramanian, L., Hindle, J. V., Johnston, S., Roberts, M. V., Husain, M., Goebel, R., et al. (2011). Real-time functional magnetic resonance imaging neurofeedback for treatment of Parkinson's disease. *J. Neurosci.* 31, 16309–16317. doi: 10.1523/JNEUROSCI.3498-11.2011

Suminski, A. J., Tkach, D. C., Fagg, A. H., and Hatsopoulos, N. G. (2010). Incorporating feedback from multiple sensory modalities enhances brain–machine interface control. *J. Neurosci.* 30, 16777–16787. doi: 10.1523/JNEUROSCI.3967-10.2010

Suzuki, M., and Gottlieb, J. (2013). Distinct neural mechanisms of distractor suppression in the frontal and parietal lobe. *Nat. Neurosci.* 16, 98–104. doi: 10.1038/nn.3282

Taylor, D. M., Tillery, S. I. H., and Schwartz, A. B. (2002). Direct cortical control of 3D neuroprosthetic devices. *Science* 296, 1829–1832. doi: 10.1126/science.1070291

Thompson, L., and Thompson, M. (1998). Neurofeedback combined with training in metacognitive strategies: effectiveness in students with ADD. *Appl. Psychophysiol. Biofeedback* 23, 243–263. doi: 10.1023/A:1022213731956

Tillery, S. I. H., Taylor, D. M., and Schwartz, A. B. (2003). "The general utility of a neuroprosthetic device under direct cortical control," in *Proceedings of the 25th Annual International Conference of the IEEE Engineering in Medicine and Biology Society*, Vol. 3, Cancun, 2043–2046.

Treder, M. S., Bahramisharif, A., Schmidt, N. M., van Gerven, M. A., and Blankertz, B. (2011). Brain – computer interfacing using modulations of alpha activity induced by covert shifts of attention. *J. Neuroeng. Rehabil.* 8:24. doi: 10.1186/1743-0003-8-24

van Gerven, M., and Jensen, O. (2009). Attention modulations of posterior alpha as a control signal for two-dimensional brain – computer interfaces. *J. Neurosci. Methods* 179, 78–84. doi: 10.1016/j.jneumeth.2009.01.016

Velliste, M., Perel, S., Spalding, M. C., Whitford, A. S., and Schwartz, A. B. (2008). Cortical control of a prosthetic arm for self-feeding. *Nature* 453, 1098–1101. doi: 10.1038/nature06996

Vossel, S., Thiel, C. M., and Fink, G. R. (2006). Cue validity modulates the neural correlates of covert endogenous orienting of attention in parietal and frontal cortex. *Neuroimage* 32, 1257–1264. doi: 10.1016/j.neuroimage.2006.05.019

Wang, L., Yu, C., Chen, H., Qin, W., He, Y., Fan, F., et al. (2010). Dynamic functional reorganization of the motor execution network after stroke. *Brain* 133, 1224–1238. doi: 10.1093/brain/awq043

Wardak, C., Denève, S., and Ben Hamed, S. (2011a). Focused visual attention distorts distance perception away from the attentional locus. *Neuropsychologia* 49, 535–545. doi: 10.1016/j.neuropsychologia.2010.12.008

Wardak, C., Olivier, E., and Duhamel, J.-R. (2011b). The relationship between spatial attention and saccades in the frontoparietal network of the monkey. *Eur. J. Neurosci.* 33, 1973–1981. doi: 10.1111/j.1460-9568.2011.07710.x

Wardak, C., Ibos, G., Duhamel, J.-R., and Olivier, E. (2006). Contribution of the monkey frontal eye field to covert visual attention. *J. Neurosci.* 26, 4228–4235. doi: 10.1523/JNEUROSCI.3336-05.2006

Wardak, C., Olivier, E., and Duhamel, J.-R. (2002). Saccadic target selection deficits after lateral intraparietal area inactivation in monkeys. *J. Neurosci.* 22, 9877–9884.

Wardak, C., Olivier, E., and Duhamel, J.-R. (2004). A deficit in covert attention after parietal cortex inactivation in the monkey. *Neuron* 42, 501–508. doi: 10.1016/S0896-6273(04)00185-0

Weiskopf, N., Veit, R., Erb, M., Mathiak, K., Grodd, W., Goebel, R., et al. (2003). Physiological self-regulation of regional brain activity using real-time functional magnetic resonance imaging (fMRI): methodology and exemplary data. *Neuroimage* 19, 577–586. doi: 10.1016/S1053-8119(03)00145-9

Wyrwicka, W., and Sterman, M. B. (1968). Instrumental conditioning of sensorimotor cortex EEG spindles in the waking cat. *Physiol. Behav.* 3, 703–707. doi: 10.1016/0031-9384(68)90139-X

Yang, T., and Maunsell, J. H. R. (2004). The effect of perceptual learning on neuronal responses in monkey visual area V4. *J. Neurosci.* 24, 1617–1626. doi: 10.1523/JNEUROSCI.4442-03.2004

Yantis, S., and Jonides, J. (1990). Abrupt visual onsets and selective attention: voluntary versus automatic allocation. *J. Exp. Psychol. Hum. Percept. Perform.* 16, 121–134. doi: 10.1037/0096-1523.16.1.121

Yeshurun, Y., and Carrasco, M. (1998). Attention improves or impairs visual performance by enhancing spatial resolution. *Nature* 396, 72–75. doi: 10.1038/23936

Zénon, A., Ben Hamed, S., Duhamel, J.-R., and Olivier, E. (2008). Spatial and temporal dynamics of attentional guidance during inefficient visual search. *PLoS ONE* 3:e2219. doi: 10.1371/journal.pone.0002219

Zénon, A., Ben Hamed, S., Duhamel, J.-R., and Olivier, E. (2009). Attentional guidance relies on a winner-take-all mechanism. *Vision Res.* 49, 1522–1531. doi: 10.1016/j.visres.2009.03.010

Zhang, Y., Meyers, E. M., Bichot, N. P., Serre, T., Poggio, T. A., and Desimone, R. (2011). Object decoding with attention in inferior temporal cortex. *Proc. Natl. Acad. Sci. U.S.A.* 108, 8850–8855. doi: 10.1073/pnas.1100999108

5

Thinking caps for everyone? The role of neuro-enhancement by non-invasive brain stimulation in neuroscience and beyond

Felix Duecker[1,2]*, Tom A. de Graaf[1,2] and Alexander T. Sack[1,2]

[1] Department of Cognitive Neuroscience, Faculty of Psychology and Neuroscience, Maastricht University, Maastricht, Netherlands
[2] Maastricht Brain Imaging Center, Maastricht University, Maastricht, Netherlands

Edited by:
Manuel Casanova, University of Louisville, USA

Reviewed by:
Casto Rivadulla, Universty of Coruna, Spain
Victor De Lafuente, Universidad Nacional Autónoma de México, Mexico

***Correspondence:**
Felix Duecker, Department of Cognitive Neuroscience, Faculty of Psychology and Neuroscience, Maastricht University, P.O. Box 616, 6200 MD, Maastricht, Netherlands
e-mail:
felix.duecker@maastrichtuniversity.nl

Neuro-enhancement by non-invasive brain stimulation (NIBS) has recently made considerable progress, triggering discussions regarding future applications to enhance human performance. We show that neuroscientific research does not aim at improving brain functions *per se*. Instead, neuro-enhancement is a research tool that has great potential to reveal the neural mechanisms underlying perception, cognition, and behavior. We provide instructive examples that showcase the relevance of neuro-enhancement by NIBS in neuroscience. Importantly, we argue that the scientific value of neuro-enhancement critically depends on our understanding of why enhancing effects occur. This is in contrast to applications of neuro-enhancement in other domains, where such knowledge may not be required. We conclude that neuro-enhancement as a therapeutic tool or in healthy people outside of neuroscience should be kept conceptually distinct, as these are separate domains with entirely different motives for enhancing human performance. Consequently, the underlying principles that justify the application of NIBS will be different in each domain and arguments for or against neuro-enhancement in one domain do not necessarily generalize to other domains.

Keywords: neuro-enhancement, mechanisms of enhancement, non-invasive brain stimulation, transcranial magnetic stimulation, transcranial current stimulation

The suggestion to "put on your thinking cap" is generally seen as purely metaphorical. Recent advances of non-invasive brain stimulation (NIBS) techniques have created the prospect of real "thinking caps" that might have the potential to improve perception, cognition, and behavior. Outside the scientific community, these developments have been often interpreted as reflecting the ambition to enhance human performance *per se*, leading to heated debates on applicability, desirability and morality of neuro-enhancement. And indeed, people should carefully consider whether, how, and when the application of NIBS to enhance brain function is appropriate (Farah et al., 2004; Cohen Kadosh et al., 2012). We here argue that in neuroscientific research, the enhancement of brain function serves as a means to an end, that is, it aims at gaining insights into brain function. The scientific value of neuro-enhancement therefore critically depends not on the fact *that* enhancing effects occur, but on our understanding of *why* they occur. This is in contrast to applications of neuro-enhancement in other (non-academic) domains where such knowledge may be not required. In this article, we first explain the relevance of neuro-enhancement by NIBS for neuroscience and showcase how it has produced valuable insights into how the brain works. Then, we outline the different domains that neuro-enhancement by NIBS could be considered for. Rather than making any judgments on the moral or ethical justifications of neuro-enhancement here, we argue that the debate on such matters should be held separately for each of these domains. From this follows that arguments against neuro-enhancement in one domain do not necessarily apply to other domains.

EFFECTS OF NIBS

The growing popularity of NIBS is due to the fact that induced brain changes have been shown to be perceptually, cognitively, and behaviorally relevant. In other words, NIBS can affect everything from low-level vision (Amassian et al., 1989) to attention (Duecker et al., 2013) to social-economic behavior (Knoch et al., 2006). The most common NIBS techniques are transcranial magnetic stimulation (TMS), transcranial current stimulation (tCS) with either direct (tDCS) or alternating (tACS) currents, and transcranial static magnetic stimulation (tSMS). TMS involves the administration of magnetic pulses to localized brain areas. The effects of single pulse TMS are short-lasting and can affect ongoing neuronal processes whereas rhythmic pulse sequences can yield long-lasting effects on the human brain (see e.g., Hallett, 2007 for a TMS primer). In contrast, tCS is applied over larger areas of cortex to send an electrical current through brain matter (see e.g., Paulus, 2011a for a tCS primer). Finally, tSMS exposes the brain to a static magnetic field by positioning a magnet on the head (Oliviero et al., 2011; Paulus, 2011b). Simply speaking, these techniques produce a combination of excitatory and inhibitory effects at the neuronal level. The polarization of neurons is changed and, depending on the stimulation parameters, regional cortical excitability either increases or decreases. Many different stimulation protocols have been developed over the years and it is common practice to label protocols as either inhibitory or excitatory. It is very tempting to directly relate these effects on cortical excitability to changes in brain function such that excitatory protocols necessarily lead to neuro-enhancement. However, this would be an oversimplification. Whether a particular NIBS protocol will have enhancing or impairing effects on the perceptual, cognitive, or behavioral level will depend not only on excitability changes but also on the functional properties and underlying mechanisms of all brain areas involved, as well as the interactions between them. This is exactly why both neuro-disruption and neuro-enhancement effects are scientifically valuable; because in the proper theoretical framework they allow us to begin teasing apart this functional neuronal architecture. Due to this complexity, we will here not provide an overview of all available NIBS protocols but will instead present mechanisms of neuro-enhancement with instructive examples mostly drawn from the attention literature.

ACCIDENTAL NEURO-ENHANCEMENT

Interestingly, NIBS was initially rarely conceptualized as a neuro-enhancing method but was instead applied with the aim to disrupt brain activity. The idea was to reveal a causal structure-function relationship through a NIBS-induced behavioral deficit, indicating the functional necessity of the stimulated brain area for normal task performance (Sack, 2006). Enhancing effects were very uncommon and their occurrence was rather incidental than purposefully induced. For example, Walsh et al. (1998) showed that TMS over hMT+/V5 lead to perceptual enhancements as reflected by improved performance on a visual search task when motion was either absent or task-irrelevant. Similarly, improvements in cognitive performance have been found in the context of picture naming (Mottaghy et al., 1999) and other language-related processes (Epstein, 1998). As most authors acknowledged, interpretation of these results was difficult because a theoretical framework to explain such findings was often lacking.

PURPOSEFUL NEURO-ENHANCEMENT

Once the potential to enhance brain function by NIBS was recognized, the effects of many different NIBS protocols were explored and, unsurprisingly, excitatory protocols often led to improved performance (Coffman et al., 2014; Luber and Lisanby, 2014). This research line has clearly shown that NIBS is capable of improving various brain functions including perception, attention, memory, and even acquisition of skills that are highly relevant for everyday life such as numerical abilities (Cohen Kadosh et al., 2013) and arithmetic (Snowball et al., 2013). In some sense, this is very similar to the original approach of revealing causal structure-function relationships outlined above. After all, also enhancing effects do imply a functional role of the stimulated brain area in a particular process. However, when the underlying mechanisms that cause an enhancement remain unknown, enhancement results, as exciting as they may be, can be of limited scientific value when not followed-up by further investigations. As will be argued below, NIBS primarily delivers its full potential when embedded in scientific theory. It then produces strong direct evidence regarding the mechanisms underlying brain functions.

INTER-HEMISPHERIC COMPETITION REVEALED WITH NIBS

The application of NIBS has been particularly successful in the context of attention research. Neuroimaging studies had already produced detailed knowledge regarding the brain networks involved in attentional control (Corbetta and Shulman, 2002) but struggled to differentiate between several competing models that were based on lesion studies in neglect patients (Kinsbourne, 1977; Heilman and Abell, 1980; Mesulam, 1981). Because these models were originally developed to explain attentional deficits after brain damage, it was relatively easy to derive hypotheses regarding the consequences of NIBS on attention in healthy people. Interestingly, one of these models also predicted enhancing effects of NIBS, namely Kinsbourne's (1977) "opponent processor" model. It stated that each hemisphere has a natural attention bias to the contralateral side of space. Under normal conditions, the two hemispheres are kept in balance due to inter-hemispheric competition. Whenever an imbalance between the hemispheres occurs, attention will be biased towards one side of space. In the context of neuro-enhancement, there are two important aspects to this model. First, in a situation of inter-hemispheric competition, behavioral enhancement and impairment are predicted to be two sides of the same coin. When the overall attention bias is directed towards one hemifield, processing for stimuli on that side of space will be improved at the expense of impaired processing for stimuli on the other side of space. Specifically, any change in excitability of one hemisphere will always affect its inhibitory influence on the other hemisphere as well, so that the final imbalance between the hemispheres is determined by the interaction between them. Second, such an imbalance can be induced in different ways, either by facilitating or inhibiting one hemisphere. As already explained above, this local excitability change then also affects the other hemisphere where the opposite effect occurs. Thus, this model lends itself perfectly for being tested with NIBS. Hilgetag et al. (2001) were among the first to directly test Kinsbourne's "opponent processor" model. They applied 1 Hz repetitive TMS over right or left parietal cortex and assessed performance on a target detection task. As one might expect with a protocol that decreases cortical excitability, target detection was impaired in the contralateral hemifield. In addition, however, they also observed enhanced target detection in the ipsilateral hemifield, strongly supporting the notion of inter-hemispheric competition. Importantly, these results make perfect sense in the light of Kinsbourne's "opponent processor" model but would be puzzling and less informative if this model did not exist. In other words, in and of itself the enhancement of ipsilateral processing was an interesting trivia. But in the appropriate theoretical framework, the enhancement result became neuro-scientifically valuable. Similarly, and corroborating this finding, Dambeck et al. (2006) found a contralateral impairment of target detection with single-pulse TMS over right or left parietal cortex. Strikingly, when applying TMS over both hemispheres simultaneously, the behavioral effects of unilateral TMS disappeared and performance was back to normal because the balance between hemispheres remained unchanged. Again, this seemingly paradoxical result is turned into meaningful insights into the mechanisms underlying attention control when linked to the appropriate theoretical framework. As pointed out before, the effects of NIBS are not simply determined by the stimulation protocol but are also a consequence of the functional architecture of the brain. In this sense, these findings are extremely valuable as they can be directly related to competing models of attentional control.

ENTRAINMENT AND PHASE-COUPLING

Thus far, NIBS-induced changes of cortical excitability have been conceptualized as rather static effects. However, it is well-established that rhythmic patterns of neural activity are an essential aspect of information processing in the brain. In the context of attention, the power and phase of alpha-band activity in occipito-parietal regions has repeatedly been related to attentional/perceptual performance (Jensen and Mazaheri, 2010; Klimesch, 2012). Alpha power is negatively correlated with perceptual performance (van Dijk et al., 2008) and lateralized when shifting attention to one hemifield (Händel et al., 2011). It is possible to "entrain" alpha-band activity in the brain using rhythmic sensory stimulation (e.g., de Graaf et al., 2013), but also directly and locally, using non-invasive brain stimulation (e.g., Romei et al., 2010; Thut et al., 2011), in order to investigate frequency-dependent modulations of task performance. Romei et al. (2010) applied a short burst of rhythmic TMS at alpha frequency, or flanker frequencies (theta or beta), prior to stimulus presentation. Only for alpha-frequency stimulation, target visibility in the contralateral visual field was reduced, while it was enhanced in the ipsilateral hemifield. So as above, impairment and enhancement co-occurred due to inter-hemispheric competition, but this time in a frequency-dependent way. Recent studies have pushed even further, demonstrating that not only the frequency of oscillations but also their phase can be essential for neural processing. Polanía et al. (2012) used tACS with electrode patches on frontal and parietal cortex both connected to a third reference electrode on the vertex. Previously acquired EEG results revealed a 0-degree phase lag in synchronized activity in the theta band between frontal and parietal cortex during a working memory task. When frontal and parietal regions were stimulated with an oscillating current pattern at a similar frequency, the phase lag between the frontal and parietal stimulation determined working memory performance. This highly advanced NIBS protocol yielded a fairly simple finding: stimulation of the fronto-parietal network in sync enhanced working memory performance whereas out of sync stimulation impaired working memory performance. This has deep and intriguing implications for our understanding of brain function and, together with the other examples described above, demonstrates how far NIBS has come as a research tool. It can produce neuro-enhancing effects, but its scientific power lies in revealing the neural mechanisms underlying perception, cognition, and behavior. And the growing complexity of NIBS approaches enables increasingly meaningful results, increasingly strong conclusions, and increasingly specific hypotheses about functional brain architecture.

NEURO-ENHANCEMENT BEYOND NEUROSCIENCE

The overview we presented in this article has focused on neuro-enhancement as a research tool, mainly taking brain mechanisms underlying attention as an example, and illustrated how it can produce valuable insights into the neural mechanisms underlying human behavior and cognition. We outlined the various forms neuro-enhancement can take, the various experimental settings underlying them, and the many valuable neuroscientific insights one could gleam from it. Importantly, in the neuroscientific domain neuro-enhancement by NIBS mainly serves its purpose when embedded in theoretical models of the brain. Enhancing effects that lack any explanation are of very limited scientific value and require further attempts to unravel the underlying mechanisms.

Beyond neuroscience, however, the application of NIBS for neuro-enhancement is not necessarily motivated by its scientific value. Instead, enhancing perception, cognition, and behavior could, for some, be considered a goal in itself *irrespective of the underlying mechanisms* that produce such effects. That would be neuro-enhancement as an endgoal, rather than as a means to an end. We therefore suggest that the current debate concerning application of neuro-enhancement should be distinguished for different domains. Specifically, we propose three domains that should be kept separate, at least to some extent, namely neuro-enhancement (a) as a research tool; (b) as a therapeutic tool and (c) applied in healthy people outside of neuroscience.

Note that we certainly do not argue for a "hands-off" approach of scientists to the larger debate on desirability of neuro-enhancement in general. After all, it is undeniable that clinical or non-academic applications of neuro-enhancement stem directly from the efforts in the academic domain. If the science doesn't first develop the tool, there is no tool to be applied outside the scientific setting. What we argue for instead is to have the debate in all domains, but to keep in mind clearly which domain we are discussing. We should keep an open mind to the possibility that the ethical, moral, and practical conclusions that may flow from the larger neuro-enhancement debate will be different for each of the three domains. At present, some neuro-enhancing approaches of NIBS have the potential to be applied as a therapeutic tool in patients, and results so far are promising (Hummel and Cohen, 2006; Miniussi et al., 2008). Still, most neuro-enhancing effects of NIBS appear to be of very limited practical relevance in everyday life. But as the field progresses the possible applications of NIBS will increase. People may have serious concerns about such possible future application of NIBS to healthy human brains in schools, universities, or the workplace. A debate would ensue whether or not society should desire, or even allow, such practices. Should companies be allowed to have their employees wear "thinking caps" to boost performance? Would they even be allowed to demand it from their workers? These are relevant questions that should be discussed by laypeople, government, and scientists. They are extreme examples in a sense, but they allow us to highlight the key point here, which is that the different domains where neuro-enhancement is now or in the future applicable should be considered separately in discussions about neuro-enhancement, its value, its risks, its desirability, its development and its general pursuit. Neuroscientists should participate in this discussion, contributing their expertise. But laypeople should participate as well, since law- and policy-makers need to develop rules and regulations on the basis of both expert opinion and societal support. But such rules and regulations should, in our view, be specific to the different domains. If the debate takes shape according to these lines, we believe that neuro-enhancement can continue to be of great value for our understanding of the brain, of potential use in clinical and therapeutic environments, and perhaps in the future applied responsibly in non-academic settings.

ACKNOWLEDGMENTS

This work was supported by the European Research Council under the European Union's Seventh Framework Programme (FP7/2007–2013)/ERC Grant agreement (263472, awarded to Alexander T. Sack), and the Netherlands Organization for Scientific Research (451-13-024 to Tom A. de Graaf).

REFERENCES

Amassian, V. E., Cracco, R. Q., Maccabee, P. J., Cracco, J. B., Rudell, A., and Eberle, L. (1989). Suppression of visual perception by magnetic coil stimulation of human occipital cortex. *Electroencephalogr. Clin. Neurophysiol.* 74, 458–462. doi: 10.1016/0168-5597(89)90036-1

Coffman, B. A., Clark, V. P., and Parasuraman, R. (2014). Battery powered thought: enhancement of attention, learning, and memory in healthy adults using transcranial direct current stimulation. *Neuroimage* 85(Pt. 3), 895–908. doi: 10.1016/j.neuroimage.2013.07.083

Cohen Kadosh, R., Dowker, A., Heine, A., Kaufmann, L., and Kucian, K. (2013). Interventions for improving numerical abilities: present and future. *Trends Neurosci. Educ.* 2, 85–93. doi: 10.1016/j.tine.2013.04.001

Corbetta, M., and Shulman, G. L. (2002). Control of goal-directed and stimulus-driven attention in the brain. *Nat. Rev. Neurosci.* 3, 201–215. doi: 10.1038/nrn755

Dambeck, N., Sparing, R., Meister, I. G., Wienemann, M., Weidemann, J., Topper, R., et al. (2006). Interhemispheric imbalance during visuospatial attention investigated by unilateral and bilateral TMS over human parietal cortices. *Brain Res.* 1072, 194–199. doi: 10.1016/j.brainres.2005.05.075

de Graaf, T. A., Gross, J., Paterson, G., Rusch, T., Sack, A. T., and Thut, G. (2013). Alpha-band rhythms in visual task performance: phase-locking by rhythmic sensory stimulation. *PLoS ONE* 8, e60035. doi: 10.1371/journal.pone.0060035

Duecker, F., Formisano, E., and Sack, A. T. (2013). Hemispheric differences in the voluntary control of spatial attention: direct evidence for a right-hemispheric dominance within frontal cortex. *J. Cogn. Neurosci.* 25, 1332–1342. doi: 10.1162/jocn_a_00402

Epstein, C. M. (1998). Transcranial magnetic stimulation: language function. *J. Clin. Neurophysiol.* 15, 325–332. doi: 10.1097/00004691-199807000-00004

Farah, M. J., Illes, J., Cook-Deegan, R., Gardner, H., Kandel, E., King, P., et al. (2004). Neurocognitive enhancement: what can we do and what should we do? *Nat. Rev. Neurosci.* 5, 421–425. doi: 10.1038/nrn1390

Hallett, M. (2007). Transcranial magnetic stimulation: a primer. *Neuron* 55, 187–199. doi: 10.1016/j.neuron.2007.06.026

Händel, B. F., Haarmeier, T., and Jensen, O. (2011). Alpha oscillations correlate with the successful inhibition of unattended stimuli. *J. Cogn. Neurosci.* 23, 2494–2502. doi: 10.1162/jocn.2010.21557

Heilman, K. M., and Abell, T. V. D. (1980). Right hemisphere dominance for attention. *Neurology* 30, 327–330. doi: 10.1212/wnl.30.3.327

Hilgetag, C. C., Theoret, H., and Pascual-Leone, A. (2001). Enhanced visual spatial attention ipsilateral to rTMS-induced "virtual lesions" of human parietal cortex. *Nat. Neurosci.* 4, 953–957. doi: 10.1038/nn0901-953

Hummel, F. C., and Cohen, L. G. (2006). Non-invasive brain stimulation: a new strategy to improve neurorehabilitation after stroke? *Lancet Neurol.* 5, 708–712. doi: 10.1016/s1474-4422(06)70525-7

Jensen, O., and Mazaheri, A. (2010). Shaping functional architecture by oscillatory alpha activity: gating by inhibition. *Front. Hum. Neurosci.* 4:186. doi: 10.3389/fnhum.2010.00186

Cohen Kadosh, R., Levy, N., O'Shea, J., Shea, N., and Savulescu, J. (2012). The neuroethics of non-invasive brain stimulation. *Curr. Biol.* 22, R108–R111. doi: 10.1016/j.cub.2012.01.013

Kinsbourne, M. (1977). Hemi-neglect and hemisphere rivalry. *Adv. Neurol.* 18, 41–49.

Klimesch, W. (2012). Alpha-band oscillations, attention, and controlled access to stored information. *Trends Cogn. Sci.* 16, 606–617. doi: 10.1016/j.tics.2012.10.007

Knoch, D., Pascual-Leone, A., Meyer, K., Treyer, V., and Fehr, E. (2006). Diminishing reciprocal fairness by disrupting the right prefrontal cortex. *Science* 314, 829–832. doi: 10.1126/science.1129156

Luber, B., and Lisanby, S. H. (2014). Enhancement of human cognitive performance using transcranial magnetic stimulation (TMS). *Neuroimage* 85(Pt. 3), 961–970. doi: 10.1016/j.neuroimage.2013.06.007

Mesulam, M. M. (1981). A cortical network for directed attention and unilateral neglect. *Ann. Neurol.* 10, 309–325. doi: 10.1002/ana.410100402

Miniussi, C., Cappa, S. F., Cohen, L. G., Floel, A., Fregni, F., Nitsche, M. A., et al. (2008). Efficacy of repetitive transcranial magnetic stimulation/transcranial direct current stimulation in cognitive neurorehabilitation. *Brain Stimul.* 1, 326–336. doi: 10.1016/j.brs.2008.07.002

Mottaghy, F. M., Hungs, M., Brugmann, M., Sparing, R., Boroojerdi, B., Foltys, H., et al. (1999). Facilitation of picture naming after repetitive transcranial magnetic stimulation. *Neurology* 53, 1806–1812. doi: 10.1212/wnl.53.8.1806

Oliviero, A., Mordillo-Mateos, L., Arias, P., Panyavin, I., Foffani, G., and Aguilar, J. (2011). Transcranial static magnetic field stimulation of the human motor cortex. *J. Physiol.* 589, 4949–4958. doi: 10.1113/jphysiol.2011.211953

Paulus, W. (2011a). Transcranial electrical stimulation (tES – tDCS; tRNS, tACS) methods. *Neuropsychol. Rehabil.* 21, 602–617. doi: 10.1080/09602011.2011.557292

Paulus, W. (2011b). Transcranial static magnetic field stimulation in man: making things as simple as possible? *J. Physiol.* 589, 5917–5918. doi: 10.1113/jphysiol.2011.221655

Polanía, R., Nitsche, M. A., Korman, C., Batsikadze, G., and Paulus, W. (2012). The importance of timing in segregated theta phase-coupling for cognitive performance. *Curr. Biol.* 22, 1314–1318. doi: 10.1016/j.cub.2012.05.021

Romei, V., Gross, J., and Thut, G. (2010). On the role of prestimulus alpha rhythms over occipito-parietal areas in visual input regulation: correlation or causation? *J. Neurosci.* 30, 8692–8697. doi: 10.1523/jneurosci.0160-10.2010

Sack, A. T. (2006). Transcranial magnetic stimulation, causal structure-function mapping and networks of functional relevance. *Curr. Opin. Neurobiol.* 16, 593–599. doi: 10.1016/j.conb.2006.06.016

Snowball, A., Tachtsidis, I., Popescu, T., Thompson, J., Delazer, M., Zamarian, L., et al. (2013). Long-term enhancement of brain function and cognition using cognitive training and brain stimulation. *Curr. Biol.* 23, 987–992. doi: 10.1016/j.cub.2013.04.045

Thut, G., Veniero, D., Romei, V., Miniussi, C., Schyns, P., and Gross, J. (2011). Rhythmic TMS causes local entrainment of natural oscillatory signatures. *Curr. Biol.* 21, 1176–1185. doi: 10.1016/j.cub.2011.05.049

van Dijk, H., Schoffelen, J.-M., Oostenveld, R., and Jensen, O. (2008). Prestimulus oscillatory activity in the alpha band predicts visual discrimination ability. *J. Neurosci.* 28, 1816–1823. doi: 10.1523/jneurosci.1853-07.2008

Walsh, V., Ellison, A., Battelli, L., and Cowey, A. (1998). Task-specific impairments and enhancements induced by magnetic stimulation of human visual area V5. *Proc. Biol. Sci.* 265, 537–543. doi: 10.1098/rspb.1998.0328

6

Tapping into rhythm generation circuitry in humans during simulated weightlessness conditions

Irina A. Solopova[1], Victor A. Selionov[1], Francesca Sylos-Labini[2,3], Victor S. Gurfinkel[4], Francesco Lacquaniti[2,3,5] and Yuri P. Ivanenko[2]*

[1] Laboratory of Neurobiology of Motor Control, Institute for Information Transmission Problems, Russian Academy of Science, Moscow, Russia
[2] Laboratory of Neuromotor Physiology, IRCCS Fondazione Santa Lucia, Rome, Italy
[3] Centre of Space Bio-medicine, University of Rome Tor Vergata, Rome, Italy
[4] Biomedical Engineering Department, Oregon Health and Science University, Portland, OR, USA
[5] Department of Systems Medicine, University of Rome Tor Vergata, Rome, Italy

Edited by:
Ioan Opris, Wake Forest University, USA

Reviewed by:
E. Paul Zehr, Centre for Biomedical Research, Canada
Maria Knikou, City University of New York, USA
Elena Yu. Shapkova, State Research Institute for Phthysiopulmonology, Russia

***Correspondence:**
Yuri P. Ivanenko, Laboratory of Neuromotor Physiology, IRCCS Fondazione Santa Lucia, 306 via Ardeatina, 00179 Rome, Italy
e-mail: y.ivanenko@hsantalucia.it

An ability to produce rhythmic activity is ubiquitous for locomotor pattern generation and modulation. The role that the rhythmogenesis capacity of the spinal cord plays in injured populations has become an area of interest and systematic investigation among researchers in recent years, despite its importance being long recognized by neurophysiologists and clinicians. Given that each individual interneuron, as a rule, receives a broad convergence of various supraspinal and sensory inputs and may contribute to a vast repertoire of motor actions, the importance of assessing the functional state of the spinal locomotor circuits becomes increasingly evident. Air-stepping can be used as a unique and important model for investigating human rhythmogenesis since its manifestation is largely facilitated by a reduction of external resistance. This article aims to provide a review on current issues related to the "locomotor" state and interactions between spinal and supraspinal influences on the central pattern generator (CPG) circuitry in humans, which may be important for developing gait rehabilitation strategies in individuals with spinal cord and brain injuries.

Keywords: central pattern generator, sensory input, rhythmogenesis, locomotion, humans

INTRODUCTION

It is now largely accepted that the neural circuitry controlling locomotion involves a central pattern generator (CPG; Grillner, 1981). CPG functioning depends on supraspinal inputs and sensory feedback (Shik, 1997; Orlovsky et al., 1999; Pearson, 2004; Jordan et al., 2008). Most CPGs are quiescent under resting condition and become recruited by supraspinal pathways with command function (Grillner, 2006). Sensory activity establishes the timing of major phase transitions and contributes to the production of motoneuronal drive (Nielsen and Sinkjaer, 2002; Pearson, 2004), and may also trigger a stepping-like output (Sherrington, 1910; Gurfinkel et al., 1998; Gerasimenko et al., 2010).

The capacity of the mammalian lumbosacral spinal cord to generate rhythmic activity in the absence of input from the brain is firmly established in animal models (Sherrington, 1910; Graham Brown, 1912; Grillner, 1981) and there is indirect evidence that CPGs may also be a feature of the human spinal cord (Bussel et al., 1996; Minassian et al., 2004; Shapkova, 2004; Dominici et al., 2011; Hubli and Dietz, 2013; Ivanenko et al., 2013). The available evidence suggests that many locomotor-related movements that humans perform routinely (walking, running, cycling, swimming, crawling, backward walking, etc.) use similar rhythm circuitry but additionally require specialized control circuits (Zehr, 2005; Patrick et al., 2009; Hoogkamer et al., 2014). In fact, the capacity of neural circuits to generate rhythmic activity represents the common core for various locomotor tasks (Zehr, 2005). The aim of this article is to provide a review on current issues related to the excitability of spinal CPG circuitry in humans. Under normal conditions, it is sometimes difficult to investigate impairments in the CPG functioning due to interference with the ongoing task of body weight and balance control (including intense feedback). Therefore, one might examine the rhythmogenesis capacity of spinal circuitry in conditions not-complicated by these two factors.

Body weight support systems coupled with robotic devices or pharmacologic treatments are now often used in the rehabilitation practice to assist locomotor recovery in individuals with neuromotor disorders (Dietz, 2009; Sale et al., 2012; Hubli and Dietz, 2013; Valentin-Gudiol et al., 2013; Meyns et al., 2014; Moraru and Onose, 2014). There is still limited evidence of the efficacy of treadmill interventions with body weight support in some injured populations due to the complex nature of the control of locomotion, compensatory strategies, and plasticity of neuronal networks (Grasso et al., 2004; Picelli et al., 2013; Valentin-Gudiol et al., 2013; Swinnen et al., 2014; Sylos-Labini et al., 2014b). We will not review here any detailed analysis of clinical outcomes for ambulation when using locomotor training with body weight support systems and refer to other reviews (e.g.,

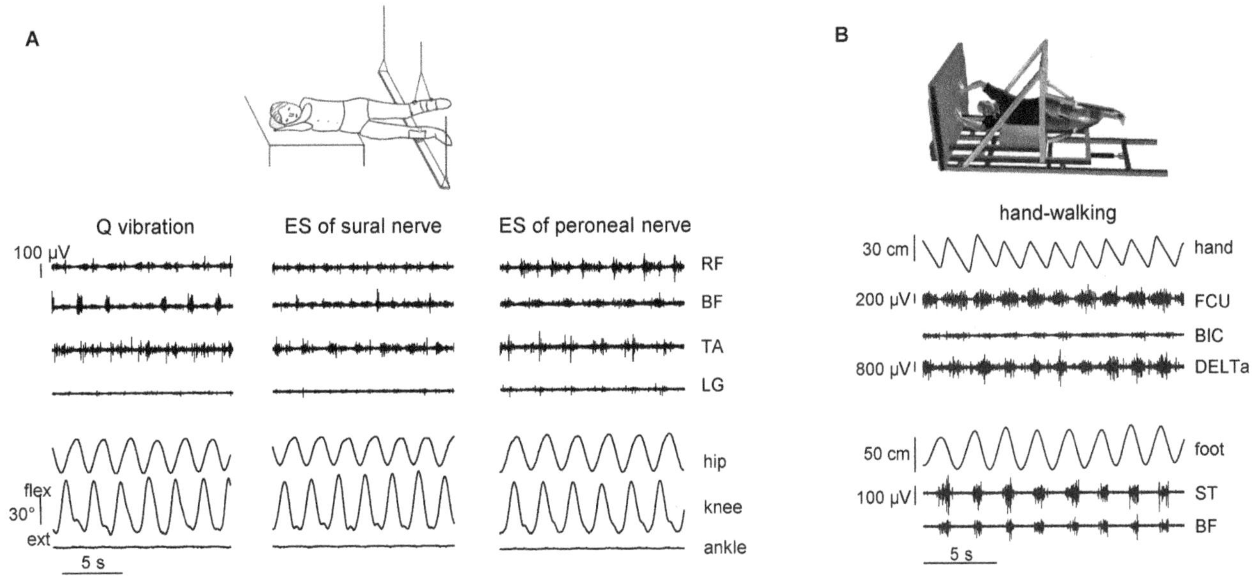

FIGURE 1 | Eliciting non-voluntary limb stepping movements in simulated weightlessness (gravity neutral) conditions. (A) examples of non-voluntary rhythmic movements of the suspended legs induced by quadriceps (Q) muscle vibration and electrical stimulation (ES) of sural and peroneal nerves in one representative subject from the study of Selionov et al. (2009). An upward deflection of traces denotes flexion in the hip and knee joint angles and dorsiflexion in the ankle joint. Note the absence of ankle joint rotations during evoked air-stepping. **(B)** An example of evoked rhythmic leg movements during hand walking in one subject from the study of Sylos-Labini et al. (2014a). RF, rectus femoris, BF, biceps femoris, TA, tibialis anterior, LG, lateral gastrocnemius, FCU, flexor carpi ulnaris, BIC, biceps brachii, DELTa, anterior deltoid, ST, and semitendinosus. Hand and foot denote anterior-posterior displacements of the left hand and foot.

Wirz et al., 2005; Sale et al., 2012; Valentin-Gudiol et al., 2013; Scivoletto et al., 2014). The main focus here is to give emphasis to a facilitatory effect of simulated weightlessness on rhythmogenesis and its potential for assessing the state of the CPG circuits and for gait recovery after spinal cord injury and other neuromotor disorders.

LOCOMOTOR "STATE" OF THE SPINAL CIRCUITY

Historically, Goltz and Freusberg (1874) were the first to report spontaneous air-stepping of the hindlimbs of the spinal dog before voiding the distended bladder, presumably due to some excitatory state of the spinal circuitry. In decerebrated animals exhibiting spontaneous fluctuations in their level of rigidity, rhythmic movements can be evoked by peripheral stimulation, provided there is an appropriate level of background extensor tonus and that the tonus is neither too low nor too high (Beritoff, 1915). In addition, an increase in tonus precedes the initiation of locomotion (Mori et al., 1982). The excitability status or state of the spinal network is thus of particular importance (Edgerton et al., 2008). Air-stepping can be used as a unique and important model for investigating human rhythmogenesis since its manifestation is largely facilitated by a reduction of external resistance, such as that resulting from body weight unloading (Gurfinkel et al., 1998; Selionov et al., 2009). Below we consider various experiments and observations in conditions of reduced gravity effects that help revealing the intrinsic properties of locomotor pattern generators and making evident the facilitation of non-voluntary limb stepping in humans.

The spinal CPG circuitry can be activated in healthy humans by applying tonic central or peripheral sensory inputs. As we previously mentioned, in addition to the control of the timing of major phase transitions and muscle activity production (Nielsen and Sinkjaer, 2002; Pearson, 2004), sensory activity has access to the functional state of CPG and may initiate a stepping-like output (Sherrington, 1910; Gurfinkel et al., 1998; Gerasimenko et al., 2010). **Figure 1A** illustrates different examples of stimulation techniques that were explored for eliciting non-voluntary air-stepping: continuous muscle vibration (40–60 Hz, ~1 mm amplitude), and electrical stimulation of the superficial peroneal or sural nerves (0.3 ms duration pulses, 2–3 mA, 60 Hz) (Selionov et al., 2009). To minimize interference with the ongoing task of body weight and balance control, stepping movements are elicited during air-stepping in the absence of gravity influences and reduced external resistance. The subjects were tested while lying on their side with the legs supported using long ropes attached to the ceiling (**Figure 1A**) or using an exoskeleton (**Figure 1B**) so that they provided low-friction pendulum-like leg motion in the horizontal plane with a limited vertical motion component. The afferent signals due to vibration or electrical stimulation of peripheral nerves may increase the excitability of several segments of the spinal cord, which may facilitate triggering of locomotor-like movements. The latency of the elicited cyclic movements varied significantly across subjects and conditions (range 1–25 s). The delay in the onset of leg movement likely reflects the general property of the pattern generation circuitry and transition from tonic activation to the phasic CPG output. Generally, cyclic movements increased monotonically for 2–10 cycles until they reached a relatively constant amplitude of angular oscillations (Gurfinkel et al., 1998; Selionov et al., 2009; Gerasimenko et al., 2010). The characteristics of non-voluntary air-stepping (amplitude, cycle duration) were similar to the voluntary stepping in the same conditions.

In addition to peripheral sensory stimulation, central tonic facilitatory influences may be used for eliciting rhythmic leg movements, such as the Jendrassik maneuver and the Kohnstamm phenomenon (Gurfinkel et al., 1998; Selionov et al., 2009). An intriguing approach related to the role of tonic influences is the Kohnstamm phenomenon (Kohnstamm, 1915), which consists in the appearance of involuntary tonic activity and a particular sensation of "lightness" after the cessation of a long-lasting (30–40 s) isometric effort. Post-activation phenomena can therefore be used as a tool to study tonic influences. After-effects of a voluntary, long-lasting contraction in the leg muscles featured alternating rhythmic leg movements that lasted for about 20–40 s (Selionov et al., 2009), corresponding roughly to a typical duration of the post-contraction activity (Craske and Craske, 1986; Duclos et al., 2004; Ivanenko et al., 2006b). The difference in the effects of the two techniques (the post-contraction phenomenon and the Jendrassik maneuver) may point to the importance of tonic activation of the lumbosacral enlargement, since voluntary arm contractions (due to the Jendrassik maneuver) are weaker in evoking stepping movements: they act primarily on the cervical spinal cord and are not sufficient to evoke air-stepping unless the experimenter triggers them (Selionov et al., 2009).

Other techniques for triggering stepping movements are based on the more direct stimulation of the spinal cord by electromagnetic (Gerasimenko et al., 2010), transcutaneous or epidural electrical stimulation (Shapkova and Schomburg, 2001; Gorodnichev et al., 2012), which can initiate and sustain movements more robustly than by stimulation of sensory afferent fibers. Transcutaneous electrical spinal cord stimulation (at 5–40 Hz) is applied over T11-T12 vertebrae and presumably activates the locomotor circuitry through the dorsal roots (Gorodnichev et al., 2012; Gerasimenko et al., 2014), while epidural stimulation is based on an implanted array of electrodes directly placed over the back portion of the lower thoracic-upper lumbar spinal cord (**Figure 4A**, upper panel). Rhythmic locomotor-like leg movements in a gravity neutral position can be evoked in ~10–50% of healthy subjects, and the degree of activation may depend on supraspinal influences and the state and the rhythmogenesis capacity of the spinal circuitry (Gurfinkel et al., 1998; Selionov et al., 2009; Gerasimenko et al., 2010). The common feature of all stimulations described above is that they are tonic. In this respect, they corroborate earlier pioneering observations in decerebrate cats that stepping can be induced using a simple tonic stimulation pattern applied to the mesencephalic locomotor region (Shik et al., 1966), but they also show that this type of control can be initiated at the lumbosacral spinal cord level. Overall, the findings suggest that nonspecific tonic excitability may elicit or facilitate CPG activity.

Finally, automatic, alternating movements of the legs can be initiated by upper limb movements by asking participants to move their arms rhythmically, as in hand-walking (**Figure 1B**; Sylos-Labini et al., 2014a). The idea is grounded on the evidence that the coordination between arms and legs during human locomotion shares many features with that in quadrupeds (Falgairolle et al., 2006; Zehr et al., 2007; Patrick et al., 2009; Dietz, 2011; Kuhtz-Buschbeck and Jing, 2012). For instance, inter-limb coupling in humans has previously been demonstrated by evoking reflexes in one limb and observing the extent to which the movement of another limb modulates reflex expression during walking (Haridas and Zehr, 2003; Mezzarane et al., 2011; Massaad et al., 2014). The coupling between the activity of cervical motoneurons underlying hand-walking and the activity of lumbosacral motoneurons underlying leg movements (**Figure 1B**) is presumably indirect, delayed and asynchronous (e.g., leg stepping is often characterized by a non-integer ratio between arm and leg movements frequency). These variable features suggest that signals related to arm movements do not directly entrain the motor commands to leg muscles, but affect the state of the lumbosacral locomotor circuitry, consistent with a facilitatory effect of arm swinging on cyclic leg muscle activity (de Kam et al., 2013). In addition, it has been recently shown that cervical transcutaneous stimulation of the spinal cord significantly facilitates non-voluntary air-stepping leg movements and the lumbosacral locomotor-related neuronal circuitry (Gerasimenko et al., 2014). One possible route for these trigger signals is through the intrinsic spinal pathways (propriospinal interneurons) linking cervical to lumbosacral regions in humans (Nathan et al., 1996). However, considering the latency of the leg responses relative to arm oscillations, supraspinal contributions cannot be excluded. Rhythmic arm movements imitating those during running or walking can also evoke prominent modulation of leg muscle EMGs during standing (Danna-Dos-Santos et al., 2009). Whatever the exact mechanism, these findings (**Figure 1B**) reinforce the idea that there exists a functional coupling between arm and leg CPGs.

INTERACTION BETWEEN RHYTHM-GENERATION ACTIVITY AND SENSORY INPUT

The previous studies, which aimed to activate the CPG circuits using the "air-stepping" paradigm (Gurfinkel et al., 1998; Selionov et al., 2009; Gerasimenko et al., 2010, 2014; Sylos-Labini et al., 2014a), also revealed some essential features of the intrinsic rhythm generation in humans. The evoked cyclic movements share many of their characteristics with animals. For instance, given the extensive evidence for the presence of commissural interneurons driving the contralateral locomotor circuitry (Kiehn, 2011), oscillator mechanisms and tonic influences may not be limb-specific. We found, for example, that treating one limb (e.g., applying electrical stimulation of the peroneal or sural nerves of one leg) can have its output transferred to another limb, even if the treated limb is kept stationary (Selionov et al., 2009). Also, although pattern generators for each limb have the potential to produce relatively autonomous rhythmic patterns (Forssberg et al., 1980; Yang et al., 2005), right

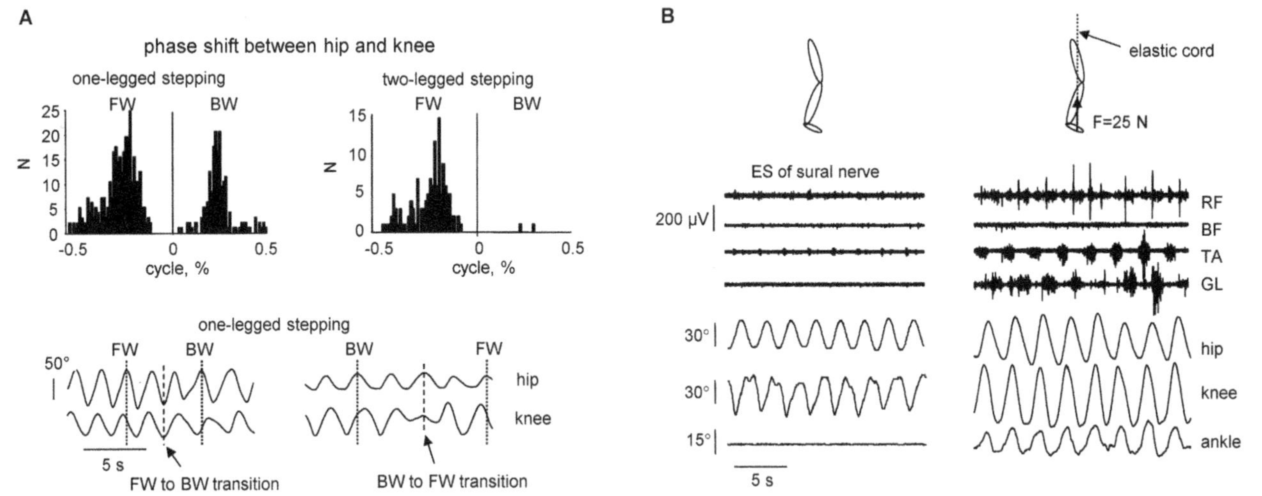

FIGURE 2 | Kinematic features of non-voluntary air-stepping movements. **(A)** one-legged vs. two-legged air-stepping evoked by quadriceps muscle vibration. Upper panels—histogram of the phase shift between hip and knee joints across subjects and probes. Note similar occurrence of forward and backward one-legged air-stepping and predominantly forward 2-legged stepping. Low panels—examples of transitions (in the middle of the record) from FW to BW stepping and vice versa in 2 subjects. **(B)** examples of rhythmic leg movements evoked by continuous electrical stimulation (ES) of the sural nerve in the absence (left) and presence (right) of small (25 N) force applied to the forefoot part of the foot. The force was applied approximately in the direction of the longitudinal axis of the body using a long elastic thread cord. The length of the thread cord was about 5 m so that fluctuations in its force due to the length changes were minimal (<10%) during air-stepping. Eight consecutive cycles are shown for each condition. Note the appearance of noticeable oscillations in the ankle joint angle and activity in the distal muscles in the presence of small load force (adapted from Selionov et al., 2009).

and left sides are strongly coupled under most natural conditions (Orlovsky et al., 1999; Ivanenko et al., 2006a; Maclellan et al., 2014). Further evidence of the importance of bilateral coupling is demonstrated by the finding that two-legged stepping was more stable (and predominantly forward, **Figure 2A**, upper panels), whereas one-legged stepping in some subjects displayed frequent spontaneous transitions from forward to backward direction and vice versa (**Figure 2A**, lower panels).

Air-stepping tends to involve prominent movements in the hip and knee joints, whereas the ankle joint is typically not involved, unless minimal loading forces are applied to the foot (**Figure 2B**). The facilitatory effect of forces is often accompanied by modulation of the EMG activity, consistent with phase-dependent contribution of sensory activity to the pre-programmed motoneuronal drive of the distal muscles during human walking (Duysens et al., 2000; Nielsen and Sinkjaer, 2002). Even individuals with clinically motor complete paralysis demonstrate modulated activity of distal leg muscles during assisted stepping with body weight support (during locomotion with 100% body unloading, no EMG activity was present) (Harkema et al., 1997; Dietz et al., 2002). It can be concluded that afferent input from load-related receptors (including Golgi tendon organs, spindles, cutaneous receptors, and various load mechanoreceptors in the foot arch, Duysens et al., 2000; Pearson, 2004; Gravano et al., 2011) contributes to the generation of locomotor activity in the isolated human spinal cord. Therefore, the sacral pattern generation circuitry (Cazalets and Bertrand, 2000) might be inactivated when the input from the support surface is lacking. The more direct stimulation of the spinal cord locomotor circuitry using repetitive electromagnetic stimuli can evoke ankle joint oscillations (Gerasimenko et al., 2010). However, in this case it likely involves stimulation of the dorsal roots, and thus load-related afferents. Overall, the lack of ankle joint movements during non-voluntary air-stepping (**Figures 1A, 2B**) supports the hypothesis that the upper lumbar pattern generator activity may constitute the major oscillator "pacemaker," whereas the sacral generator could play a subordinator role for adaptation to specific foot-support interactions. Also, minimal contact forces during air-stepping may significantly improve accurate foot trajectory control, suggesting that the support surface represents an importance reference frame and is included in the locomotor body scheme (Ivanenko et al., 2002).

ENGAGEMENT OF SUPRASPINAL MOTOR AREAS

Better understanding of interactions between spinal and supraspinal influences on the state of CPG circuitry may be important for developing gait rehabilitation strategies in individuals with spinal cord and brain injuries. In addition, there is an increasing consensus that motor centers in the brain, and the motor cortex in particular, play an essential and greater role in human walking compared to other mammals (Capaday, 2002; Yang and Gorassini, 2006; Petersen et al., 2012; Beloozerova et al., 2013). For instance, the coherence analysis demonstrated significant coupling between EEG recordings over the leg motor area and EMG from the tibialis anterior muscle prior to heel strike during the swing phase of walking, suggesting that the motor cortex and corticospinal

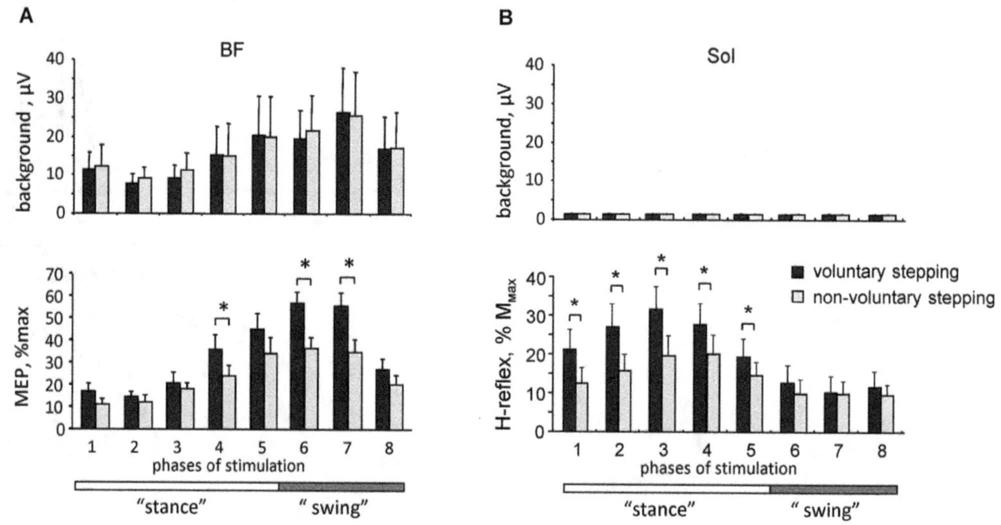

FIGURE 3 | Motor responses during voluntary and non-voluntary air-stepping in healthy subjects. (A) background EMG activity (upper panel) and motor evoked potentials (lower panel) in response to transcranial magnetic stimulation of the motor cortex (MEPs, mean ± SE, $n = 8$ subjects) in the BF muscle during different phases of the step cycle. **(B)** background soleus EMG activity (upper panel) and H-reflex (lower panel) modulation. Asterisks denote significant differences. Note facilitation of motor responses during voluntary stepping. Adapted from Solopova et al. (2014).

tract contribute directly to the muscle activity observed in steady-state human walking (Petersen et al., 2012). Recently, we compared motor evoked potentials (MEP) in response to transcranial magnetic stimulation of the motor cortex and the H-reflex during voluntary and vibration-induced air-stepping movements in healthy humans (Solopova et al., 2014). Both the MEPs and H-reflex were significantly smaller during vibration-induced cyclic leg movements at matched amplitudes of angular motion and muscle activity (**Figure 3**). One may suppose that in both cases the locomotor-like leg movements are evoked via activation of the spinal pattern generation circuitry. The greater responsiveness to central inputs during voluntary CPG activation (**Figure 3**) may be related to facilitation of transcortical reflex pathways (Christensen et al., 1999), increased depolarization of motoneurons, and/or an overall facilitatory effect on spinal motoneurons and interneurons. Interestingly, modulation of the H-reflex was observed in the absence of noticeable background EMG activity of the soleus and tibialis anterior muscles (likely due to the absence of limb loading and ankle joint movements), and occurred during the hypothetical stance phase of the step cycle (**Figure 3**), consistent with a CPG phase-related modulation of spinal reflexes.

These findings highlight differences between voluntary and non-voluntary activation of the spinal pattern generator circuitry, presumably due to an extra facilitatory effect of voluntary control of stepping on spinal motoneurons and interneurons. It has been argued that the engagement of supraspinal motor areas may be beneficial for gait recovery (van den Brand et al., 2012), and there is a link between facilitation of segmental reflexes and the ability to recover gait (Dietz et al., 2009; Thompson and Wolpaw, 2014). Our results (**Figure 3**) support this hypothesis, and show an overall facilitatory effect of supraspinally mediated stepping on reflex responses. Such investigations may contribute to the clinical development of CPG-modulating therapies (Guertin, 2014).

TAPPING INTO RHYTHM GENERATION CIRCUITRY IN NEUROMOTOR DISORDERS

During the last decade, there has been a growing interest in understanding an appropriate state of the spinal circuitry for performing locomotor movements (Hultborn, 2001; Edgerton et al., 2008; van den Brand et al., 2012; Selionov et al., 2013). In particular, to trigger the CPG by neurons with command function (Grillner, 2006), the physiological state of the spinal network needs to be properly prepared (Edgerton et al., 2008) since the same interneurons and motoneurons may contribute to a vast repertoire of motor actions (Hultborn, 2001).

A facilitatory effect of simulated weightlessness can be used for investigating rhythmogenesis of the spinal cord in injured populations and for entraining the spinal locomotor circuitry. Epidural stimulation is a technique that has been used for a number of years to treat individuals with a spinal cord injury, and various experiments emphasized a significant complementary effect of epidural stimulation when combined with pharmacological facilitation, e.g., serotonergic agonists, and step training (Shapkova and Schomburg, 2001; Minassian et al., 2007; Gerasimenko et al., 2008). The existence of a spinal locomotor generator circuitry in humans has been confirmed based on observations in patients with a severe spinal cord injury implanted with an array of electrodes directly placed over the back portion of the lower thoracic-upper lumbar spinal cord (Minassian et al., 2004; Shapkova, 2004). In these experiments, stepping-like movements were produced in patients who were supine with the legs in the resting position (**Figure 4A**) or suspended in the air (**Figure 4B**). Epidural stimulation could

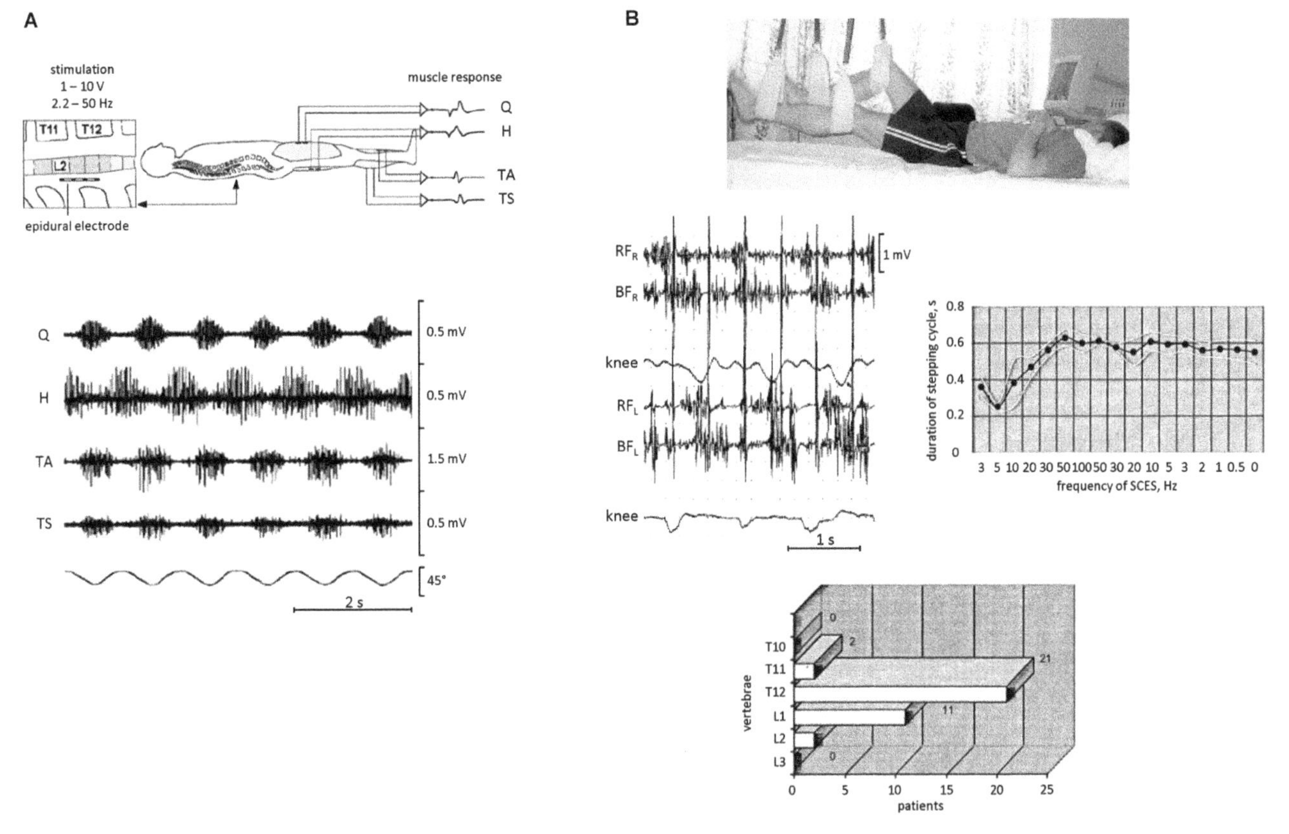

FIGURE 4 | EMG activity and rhythmic leg movements induced by epidural spinal cord electrical stimulation (SCES) in SCI patients in a supine position. **(A)** epidural SCES (upper panel) and an example of EMG recordings (bottom panel) obtained from quadriceps (Q), hamstrings (H), tibialis anterior (TA), and triceps surae (TS) during SCES at 31 Hz. The goniometer traces of the knee joint angle illustrate the corresponding induced rhythmical movements of the lower limbs. Adapted from Minassian et al. (2004). **(B)** SCES-induced rhythmic leg movements in SCI patients. During SCES, the patient was lying supine and the legs were suspended on elastic straps in a position such that the hip and knee joints were in semi-flexion (top panel). Middle panels: an example of stepping-like movements at ~1 Hz evoked with 2 Hz SCES in one SCI patient. On the right—duration of stepping cycle in relationship to the frequency of SCES in this patient. The frequency gradually increased from 3 to 100 Hz and then decreased from 100 to 0.5 Hz. Bottom panel: location of the effective zone for initiating alternating stepping-like movements with SCES in a group of paraplegic patients (n = 29). Adapted from Shapkova (2004).

even produce rhythmic EMG activities without step-related sensory feedback (stationary legs) or with a rhythm frequency independent of that of passive treadmill stepping (Minassian et al., 2013). Nevertheless, leg suspension significantly facilitates the manifestation of rhythmic motion (**Figure 4B**) and permits to reveal its characteristics. For instance, depending on the exact location of the stimulating electrodes, the stimulation could produce different patterns of rhythmic leg movements with different involvements of leg joints (Shapkova, 2004), consistent with the idea that there exist individual CPGs for each limb and/or each segment, and are coordinated during natural locomotion to produce a coherent interlimb pattern (Graham Brown, 1912; Grillner, 1981). Epidural stimulation can also transform the CPG circuitry into the active functional state which persists even after a significant decrease of stimulation frequency (**Figure 4B**, right panel). Interestingly, non-voluntary (evoked by epidural stimulation) air-stepping movements in incomplete spinal cord injury individuals can be sustained for more than 1 h with increasing EMG activity, while voluntarily initiated rhythmic leg movements in these patients demonstrate progressive fatigue after several minutes (Shapkova, 2004). Thus, even though supraspinally mediated activation of stepping has an overall facilitatory effect on reflex responses (**Figure 3**) and pattern generation (Solopova et al., 2014), it may also contribute to the development of "central" fatigue (Taylor et al., 2006). Furthermore, daily sessions with epidural stimulation evoking air-stepping rhythmic movements were effective in restoring the locomotor function in some children with a severe spinal cord injury (Shapkova, 2004).

The residual sensory pathways may be critical in regaining voluntary movement. Moreover, the neuromodulation and activation of the "locomotor state" of the spinal circuitry below the lesion may enable completely paralyzed individuals to process conceptual, auditory and visual inputs, and to regain some voluntary control of paralyzed muscles (Angeli et al., 2014). In this study, a stimulation protocol was developed to allow the individuals to stimulate for ~1 h while practicing intentional movement in the supine position. Four individuals diagnosed with clinically motor complete paralysis (classified as AIS-B and AIS-A before implantation) and implanted with a lumbrosacral spinal cord stimulator at least 2.2 years post injury were able to generate EMG activity and movement during ankle dorsiflexion in the presence of epidural stimulation following a verbal command. No motor activity was present when attempting to move without epidural stimulation. Furthermore, daily training resulted in the generation of voluntary efforts with higher forces and lower stimulation voltages to reach the thresholds that enabled voluntary motor responses that could be modulated by visual and/or auditory input (Angeli et al., 2014). Hence, it is essential to discern how the spinal pattern generation circuitry is controlled by sensory input and supraspinal networks to design new rehabilitation devices that involve modulation of the physiological state of the spinal cord during training. A degradation of spinal neuronal activity takes place following a spinal cord injury, suggesting that a continuous training approach starting early after injury is necessary to maintain neuronal activity below the level of the lesion (Dietz and Müller, 2004). Future studies may focus on the mechanisms underlying the manifestation of early motor symptoms, muscle tone, impaired sensory feedback and their relation to rhythmogenesis investigated under simulated weightlessness conditions. This may also help facilitating the application of neurophysiological analyses as quantification tools for evaluating new medications useful to assess or augment the rhythmogenesis capacity and gait recovery in neurological disorders.

CONCLUDING REMARKS

Novel pharmacological strategies (Roy et al., 2012; Borton et al., 2014; Guertin, 2014) and electromagnetic stimulation techniques (Shapkova and Schomburg, 2001; Minassian et al., 2007; Gerasimenko et al., 2008; Selionov et al., 2009; Angeli et al., 2014) are being developed aimed at modulating spinal activity and restoring the locomotor function. Even though electrochemical or sensory stimulations do not necessarily induce automated stepping by activating CPG networks, they may transform lumbosacral circuits from non-functional to functional states, enabling the information-processing interface in the spinal cord to utilize multifaceted sensory input as a source of control for locomotion (Courtine et al., 2009). Overall, recent findings highlight the importance of investigating the tonic "state" of the spinal circuits. Since the air-stepping is free from many of the mechanical constraints of normal walking, it may provide an effective model for studying how peripheral inputs influence CPG behavior in human adults (Gurfinkel et al., 1998; Shapkova and Schomburg, 2001; Selionov et al., 2009; Gerasimenko et al., 2010; Solopova et al., 2014; Sylos-Labini et al., 2014a). Thus, the beneficial effect of simulated weightlessness on rhythmogenesis may enhance the utility of spinal cord stimulation techniques for developing CPG-modulating therapies and augmentation of function for disabled people.

ACKNOWLEDGMENTS

The work was supported by the Russian Foundation for Basic Research grants #13-04-12076 and #15-04-02825, Italian Health Ministry and Italian Space Agency (COREA Grant).

REFERENCES

Angeli, C. A., Edgerton, V. R., Gerasimenko, Y. P., and Harkema, S. J. (2014). Altering spinal cord excitability enables voluntary movements after chronic complete paralysis in humans. *Brain* 137, 1394–1409. doi: 10.1093/brain/awu038

Beloozerova, I. N., Stout, E. E., and Sirota, M. G. (2013). Distinct Thalamo-cortical controls for shoulder, elbow and wrist during locomotion. *Front. Comput. Neurosci.* 7:62. doi: 10.3389/fncom.2013.00062

Beritoff, J. S. (1915). On the mode of originating of labyrinthine and cervical tonic reflexes and on their part in the reflex reactions of decerebrate preparation. *Q. J. Exp. Physiol.* 6, 199–229. doi: 10.1113/expphysiol.1915.sp000204

Borton, D., Bonizzato, M., Beauparlant, J., DiGiovanna, J., Moraud, E. M., Wenger, N., et al. (2014). Corticospinal neuroprostheses to restore locomotion after spinal cord injury. *Neurosci. Res.* 78, 21–29. doi: 10.1016/j.neures.2013.10.001

Bussel, B., Roby-Brami, A., Néris, O. R., and Yakovleff, A. (1996). Evidence for a spinal stepping generator in man. Electrophysiological study. *Acta Neurobiol. Exp. (Wars)* 56, 465–468.

Capaday, C. (2002). The special nature of human walking and its neural control. *Trends Neurosci.* 25, 370–376. doi: 10.1016/s0166-2236(02)02173-2

Cazalets, J. R., and Bertrand, S. (2000). Coupling between lumbar and sacral motor networks in the neonatal rat spinal cord. *Eur. J. Neurosci.* 12, 2993–3002. doi: 10.1046/j.1460-9568.2000.00169.x

Christensen, L. O., Morita, H., Petersen, N., and Nielsen, J. (1999). Evidence suggesting that a transcortical reflex pathway contributes to cutaneous reflexes in the tibialis anterior muscle during walking in man. *Exp. Brain Res.* 124, 59–68. doi: 10.1007/s002210050600

Courtine, G., Gerasimenko, Y., van den Brand, R., Yew, A., Musienko, P., Zhong, H., et al. (2009). Transformation of nonfunctional spinal circuits into functional states after the loss of brain input. *Nat. Neurosci.* 12, 1333–1342. doi: 10.1038/nn.2401

Craske, B., and Craske, J. D. (1986). Oscillator mechanisms in the human motor system: investigating their properties using the aftercontraction effect. *J. Mot. Behav.* 18, 117–145. doi: 10.1080/00222895.1986.10735374

Danna-Dos-Santos, A., Shapkova, E. Y., Shapkova, A. L., Degani, A. M., and Latash, M. L. (2009). Postural control during upper body locomotor-like movements: similar synergies based on dissimilar muscle modes. *Exp. Brain Res.* 193, 565–579. doi: 10.1007/s00221-008-1659-3

de Kam, D., Rijken, H., Manintveld, T., Nienhuis, B., Dietz, V., and Duysens, J. (2013). Arm movements can increase leg muscle activity during submaximal recumbent stepping in neurologically intact individuals. *J. Appl. Physiol. (1985)* 115, 34 42. doi: 10.1152/japplphysiol.00510.2012

Dietz, V. (2009). Body weight supported gait training: from laboratory to clinical setting. *Brain Res. Bull.* 78, I–VI. doi: 10.1016/s0361-9230(08)00410-3

Dietz, V. (2011). Quadrupedal coordination of bipedal gait: implications for movement disorders. *J. Neurol.* 258, 1406–1412. doi: 10.1007/s00415-011-6063-4

Dietz, V., Grillner, S., Trepp, A., Hubli, M., and Bolliger, M. (2009). Changes in spinal reflex and locomotor activity after a complete spinal cord injury: a common mechanism? *Brain* 132, 2196–2205. doi: 10.1093/brain/awp124

Dietz, V., and Müller, R. (2004). Degradation of neuronal function following a spinal cord injury: mechanisms and countermeasures. *Brain* 127, 2221–2231. doi: 10.1093/brain/awh255

Dietz, V., Müller, R., and Colombo, G. (2002). Locomotor activity in spinal man: significance of afferent input from joint and load receptors. *Brain J. Neurol.* 125, 2626–2634. doi: 10.1093/brain/awf273

Dominici, N., Ivanenko, Y. P., Cappellini, G., d'Avella, A., Mondì, V., Cicchese, M., et al. (2011). Locomotor primitives in newborn babies and their development. *Science* 334, 997–999. doi: 10.1126/science.1210617

Duclos, C., Roll, R., Kavounoudias, A., and Roll, J. P. (2004). Long-lasting body leanings following neck muscle isometric contractions. *Exp. Brain Res.* 158, 58–66. doi: 10.1007/s00221-004-1871-8

Duysens, J., Clarac, F., and Cruse, H. (2000). Load-regulating mechanisms in gait and posture: comparative aspects. *Physiol. Rev.* 80, 83–133.

Edgerton, V. R., Courtine, G., Gerasimenko, Y. P., Lavrov, I., Ichiyama, R. M., Fong, A. J., et al. (2008). Training locomotor networks. *Brain Res. Rev.* 57, 241–254. doi: 10.1016/j.brainresrev.2007.09.002

Falgairolle, M., de Seze, M., Juvin, L., Morin, D., and Cazalets, J.-R. (2006). Coordinated network functioning in the spinal cord: an evolutionary perspective. *J. Physiol. Paris* 100, 304–316. doi: 10.1016/j.jphysparis.2007.05.003

Forssberg, H., Grillner, S., and Halbertsma, J. (1980). The locomotion of the low spinal cat. I. Coordination within a hindlimb. *Acta Physiol. Scand.* 108, 269–281. doi: 10.1111/j.1748-1716.1980.tb06533.x

Gerasimenko, Y., Gorodnichev, R., Machueva, E., Pivovarova, E., Semyenov, D., Savochin, A., et al. (2010). Novel and direct access to the human locomotor spinal circuitry. *J. Neurosci.* 30, 3700–3708. doi: 10.1523/JNEUROSCI.4751-09.2010

Gerasimenko, Y. P., Gorodnichev, R., Puhov, A., Moshonkina, T., Savochin, A., Selionov, V. A., et al. (2014). Initiation and modulation of locomotor circuitry output with multi-site transcutaneous electrical stimulation of the spinal cord in non-injured humans. *J. Neurophysiol.* doi: 10.1152/jn.00609.2014. [Epub ahead of print].

Gerasimenko, Y., Roy, R. R., and Edgerton, V. R. (2008). Epidural stimulation: comparison of the spinal circuits that generate and control locomotion in rats, cats and humans. *Exp. Neurol.* 209, 417–425. doi: 10.1016/j.expneurol.2007.07.015

Goltz, F., and Freusberg, A. (1874). Uber die Funktionen des Lendenmarkes des Hundes. *Pflugers Physiol.* 8, 460–498. doi: 10.1007/BF01612308

Gorodnichev, R. M., Pivovarova, E. A., Pukhov, A., Moiseev, S. A., Savokhin, A. A., Moshonkina, T. R., et al. (2012). Transcutaneous electrical stimulation of the spinal cord: non-invasive tool for activation of locomotor circuitry in human. *Fiziol. Cheloveka* 38, 46–56.

Graham Brown, T. (1912). The factors in rhythmic activity of the nervous system. *Proc. R. Soc. B Biol. Sci.* 85, 278–289. doi: 10.1098/rspb.1912.0051

Grasso, R., Ivanenko, Y. P., Zago, M., Molinari, M., Scivoletto, G., Castellano, V., et al. (2004). Distributed plasticity of locomotor pattern generators in spinal cord injured patients. *Brain* 127, 1019–1034. doi: 10.1093/brain/awh115

Gravano, S., Ivanenko, Y. P., Maccioni, G., Macellari, V., Poppele, R. E., and Lacquaniti, F. (2011). A novel approach to mechanical foot stimulation during human locomotion under body weight support. *Hum. Mov. Sci.* 30, 352–367. doi: 10.1016/j.humov.2010.01.002

Grillner, S. (1981). "Control of locomotion in bipeds, tetrapods and fish," in *Handbook of Physiology: Section 1: The Nervous System, volume II, Part.1 Motor Control*, eds V. B. Brooks, J. M. Brookhart and V. B. Mountcastle (Bethesda, MD: Am. Physiol. Soc.), 1179–1236.

Grillner, S. (2006). Biological pattern generation: the cellular and computational logic of networks in motion. *Neuron* 52, 751–766. doi: 10.1016/j.neuron.2006.11.008

Guertin, P. A. (2014). Preclinical evidence supporting the clinical development of central pattern generator-modulating therapies for chronic spinal cord-injured patients. *Front. Hum. Neurosci.* 8:272. doi: 10.3389/fnhum.2014.00272

Gurfinkel, V. S., Levik, Y. S., Kazennikov, O. V., and Selionov, V. A. (1998). Locomotor-like movements evoked by leg muscle vibration in humans. *Eur. J. Neurosci.* 10, 1608–1612. doi: 10.1046/j.1460-9568.1998.00179.x

Haridas, C., and Zehr, E. P. (2003). Coordinated interlimb compensatory responses to electrical stimulation of cutaneous nerves in the hand and foot during walking. *J. Neurophysiol.* 90, 2850–2861. doi: 10.1152/jn.00531.2003

Harkema, S. J., Hurley, S. L., Patel, U. K., Requejo, P. S., Dobkin, B. H., and Edgerton, V. R. (1997). Human lumbosacral spinal cord interprets loading during stepping. *J. Neurophysiol.* 77, 797–811.

Hoogkamer, W., Meyns, P., and Duysens, J. (2014). Steps forward in understanding backward gait: from basic circuits to rehabilitation. *Exerc. Sport Sci. Rev.* 42, 23–29. doi: 10.1249/JES.0000000000000000

Hubli, M., and Dietz, V. (2013). The physiological basis of neurorehabilitation - locomotor training after spinal cord injury. *J. Neuroeng. Rehabil.* 10:5. doi: 10.1186/1743-0003-10-5

Hultborn, H. (2001). State-dependent modulation of sensory feedback. *J. Physiol.* 533, 5–13. doi: 10.1111/j.1469-7793.2001.0005b.x

Ivanenko, Y. P., Dominici, N., Cappellini, G., Di Paolo, A., Giannini, C., Poppele, R. E., et al. (2013). Changes in the spinal segmental motor output for stepping during development from infant to adult. *J. Neurosci.* 33, 3025a–3036a. doi: 10.1523/JNEUROSCI.2722-12.2013

Ivanenko, Y. P., Grasso, R., Macellari, V., and Lacquaniti, F. (2002). Control of foot trajectory in human locomotion: role of ground contact forces in simulated reduced gravity. *J. Neurophysiol.* 87, 3070–3089.

Ivanenko, Y. P., Poppele, R. E., and Lacquaniti, F. (2006a). Motor control programs and walking. *Neuroscientist* 12, 339–348. doi: 10.1177/1073858406287987

Ivanenko, Y. P., Wright, W. G., Gurfinkel, V. S., Horak, F., and Cordo, P. (2006b). Interaction of involuntary post-contraction activity with locomotor movements. *Exp. Brain Res.* 169, 255–260. doi: 10.1007/s00221-005-0324-3

Jordan, L. M., Liu, J., Hedlund, P. B., Akay, T., and Pearson, K. G. (2008). Descending command systems for the initiation of locomotion in mammals. *Brain Res. Rev.* 57, 183–191. doi: 10.1016/j.brainresrev.2007.07.019

Kiehn, O. (2011). Development and functional organization of spinal locomotor circuits. *Curr. Opin. Neurobiol.* 21, 100–109. doi: 10.1016/j.conb.2010.09.004

Kohnstamm, O. (1915). Demonstration einer katatonieartigen Erscheinung beim Gesunden (Katatonusversuch). *Neurol Zent. Bl* 34S, 290–291.

Kuhtz-Buschbeck, J. P., and Jing, B. (2012). Activity of upper limb muscles during human walking. *J. Electromyogr. Kinesiol.* 22, 199–206. doi: 10.1016/j.jelekin.2011.08.014

Maclellan, M. J., Ivanenko, Y. P., Massaad, F., Bruijn, S. M., Duysens, J., and Lacquaniti, F. (2014). Muscle activation patterns are bilaterally linked during split-belt treadmill walking in humans. *J. Neurophysiol.* 111, 1541–1552. doi: 10.1152/jn.00437.2013

Massaad, F., Levin, O., Meyns, P., Drijkoningen, D., Swinnen, S. P., and Duysens, J. (2014). Arm sway holds sway: locomotor-like modulation of leg reflexes when arms swing in alternation. *Neuroscience* 258, 34–46. doi: 10.1016/j.neuroscience.2013.10.007

Meyns, P., Van de Crommert, H. W. A. A., Rijken, H., van Kuppevelt, D. H. J. M., and Duysens, J. (2014). Locomotor training with body weight support in SCI: EMG improvement is more optimally expressed at a low testing speed. *Spinal Cord* 52, 887–893. doi: 10.1038/sc.2014.172

Mezzarane, R., Klimstra, M., Lewis, A., Hundza, S., and Zehr, E. (2011). Interlimb coupling from the arms to legs is differentially specified for populations of motor units comprising the compound H-reflex during "reduced" human locomotion. *Exp. Brain Res.* 208, 157–168. doi: 10.1007/s00221-010-2467-0

Minassian, K., Hofstoetter, U. S., Danner, S. M., Mayr, W., McKay, W. B., Tansey, K., et al. (2013). Mechanisms of rhythm generation of the human lumbar spinal cord in response to tonic stimulation without and with step-related sensory feedback. *Biomed. Eng. Biomed. Tech.* Available online at: http://www. degruyter. com/ view/j/ bmte.2013.58.issue-s1-A / bmt-2013 –4013/ bmt-2013–4013.xml;jsessionid=AF92C08F8D31046DE80E9B1BB68DC420. Accessed on December 15, 2014.

Minassian, K., Jilge, B., Rattay, F., Pinter, M. M., Binder, H., Gerstenbrand, F., et al. (2004). Stepping-like movements in humans with complete spinal cord injury induced by epidural stimulation of the lumbar cord: electromyographic study of compound muscle action potentials. *Spinal Cord* 42, 401–416. doi: 10.1038/sj.sc.3101615

Minassian, K., Persy, I., Rattay, F., Pinter, M. M., Kern, H., and Dimitrijevic, M. R. (2007). Human lumbar cord circuitries can be activated by extrinsic tonic input to generate locomotor-like activity. *Hum. Mov. Sci.* 26, 275–295. doi: 10.1016/j.humov.2007.01.005

Moraru, E., and Onose, G. (2014). Current issues and considerations about the central role of rehabilitation therapies in the functional recovery of neurological impairments after stroke in adults. *J. Med. Life* 7, 368–372.

Mori, S., Kawahara, K., Sakamoto, T., Aoki, M., and Tomiyama, T. (1982). Setting and resetting of level of postural muscle tone in decerebrate cat by stimulation of brain stem. *J. Neurophysiol.* 48, 737–748.

Nathan, P. W., Smith, M., and Deacon, P. (1996). Vestibulospinal, reticulospinal and descending propriospinal nerve fibres in man. *Brain* 119, 1809–1833. doi: 10.1093/brain/119.6.1809

Nielsen, J. B., and Sinkjaer, T. (2002). Afferent feedback in the control of human gait. *J. Electromyogr. Kinesiol.* 12, 213–217. doi: 10.1016/s1050-6411(02)00023-8

Orlovsky, G. N., Deliagina, T. G., Grillner, S., Orlovskii, G. N., and Grillner, S. (1999). *Neuronal Control of Locomotion: From Mollusc to Man.* Oxford, UK: Oxford University Press.

Patrick, S. K., Noah, J. A., and Yang, J. F. (2009). Interlimb coordination in human crawling reveals similarities in development and neural control with quadrupeds. *J. Neurophysiol.* 101, 603–613. doi: 10.1152/jn.91125.2008

Pearson, K. G. (2004). Generating the walking gait: role of sensory feedback. *Prog. Brain Res.* 143, 123–129. doi: 10.1016/s0079-6123(03)43012-4

Petersen, T. H., Willerslev-Olsen, M., Conway, B. A., and Nielsen, J. B. (2012). The motor cortex drives the muscles during walking in human subjects. *J. Physiol.* 590, 2443–2452. doi: 10.1113/jphysiol.2012.227397

Picelli, A., Melotti, C., Origano, F., Neri, R., Waldner, A., and Smania, N. (2013). Robot-assisted gait training versus equal intensity treadmill training in patients with mild to moderate Parkinson's disease: a randomized controlled trial. *Parkinsonism Relat. Disord.* 19, 605–610. doi: 10.1016/j.parkreldis.2013.02.010

Roy, R. R., Harkema, S. J., and Edgerton, V. R. (2012). Basic concepts of activity-based interventions for improved recovery of motor function after spinal cord injury. *Arch. Phys. Med. Rehabil.* 93, 1487–1497. doi: 10.1016/j.apmr.2012.04.034

Sale, P., Franceschini, M., Waldner, A., and Hesse, S. (2012). Use of the robot assisted gait therapy in rehabilitation of patients with stroke and spinal cord injury. *Eur. J. Phys. Rehabil. Med.* 48, 111–121.

Scivoletto, G., Tamburella, F., Laurenza, L., Torre, M., and Molinari, M. (2014). Who is going to walk? A review of the factors influencing walking recovery after spinal cord injury. *Front. Hum. Neurosci.* 8:141. doi: 10.3389/fnhum.2014.00141

Selionov, V. A., Ivanenko, Y. P., Solopova, I. A., and Gurfinkel, V. S. (2009). Tonic central and sensory stimuli facilitate involuntary air-stepping in humans. *J. Neurophysiol.* 101, 2847–2858. doi: 10.1152/jn.90895.2008

Selionov, V. A., Solopova, I. A., Zhvansky, D. S., Karabanov, A. V., Chernikova, L. A., Gurfinkel, V. S., et al. (2013). Lack of non-voluntary stepping responses in Parkinson's disease. *Neuroscience* 235, 96–108. doi: 10.1016/j.neuroscience.2012.12.064

Shapkova, E. Y. (2004). "Spinal locomotor capabality revealed by electrical stimulation of the lumbar enlargement in paraplegic patients," in *Progress in Motor Control*, eds M. Latash and M. Levin (Champaign, IL: Human Kinetics), 253–289.

Shapkova, E. Y., and Schomburg, E. D. (2001). Two types of motor modulation underlying human stepping evoked by spinal cord electrical stimulation (SCES). *Acta Physiol. Pharmacol. Bulg.* 26, 155–157.

Sherrington, C. S. (1910). Flexion-reflex of the limb, crossed extension-reflex and reflex stepping and standing. *J. Physiol.* 40, 28–121. doi: 10.1113/jphysiol.1910.sp001362

Shik, M. L. (1997). Recognizing propriospinal and reticulospinal systems of initiation of stepping. *Motor Control* 1, 310–313.

Shik, M. L., Severin, F. V., and Orlovskiĭ, G. N. (1966). Control of walking and running by means of electric stimulation of the midbrain. *Biofizika* 11, 659–666.

Solopova, I. A., Selionov, V. A., Kazennikov, O. V., and Ivanenko, Y. P. (2014). Effects of transcranial magnetic stimulation during voluntary and non-voluntary stepping movements in humans. *Neurosci. Lett.* 579, 64–69. doi: 10.1016/j.neulet.2014.07.015

Swinnen, E., Baeyens, J.-P., Pintens, S., Van Nieuwenhoven, J., Ilsbroukx, S., Buyl, R., et al. (2014). Trunk kinematics during walking in persons with multiple sclerosis: the influence of body weight support. *NeuroRehabilitation* 34, 731–740. doi: 10.3233/NRE-141089

Sylos-Labini, F., Ivanenko, Y. P., Maclellan, M. J., Cappellini, G., Poppele, R. E., and Lacquaniti, F. (2014a). Locomotor-like leg movements evoked by rhythmic arm movements in humans. *PloS One* 9:e90775. doi: 10.1371/journal.pone.0090775

Sylos-Labini, F., La Scaleia, V., d' Avella, A., Pisotta, I., Tamburella, F., Scivoletto, G., et al. (2014b). EMG patterns during assisted walking in the exoskeleton. *Front. Hum. Neurosci.* 8:423. doi: 10.3389/fnhum.2014.00423

Taylor, J. L., Todd, G., and Gandevia, S. C. (2006). Evidence for a supraspinal contribution to human muscle fatigue. *Clin. Exp. Pharmacol. Physiol.* 33, 400–405. doi: 10.1111/j.1440-1681.2006.04363.x

Thompson, A. K., and Wolpaw, J. R. (2014). Operant conditioning of spinal reflexes: from basic science to clinical therapy. *Front. Integr. Neurosci.* 8:25. doi: 10.3389/fnint.2014.00025

Valentin-Gudiol, M., Bagur-Calafat, C., Girabent-Farrés, M., Hadders-Algra, M., Mattern-Baxter, K., and Angulo-Barroso, R. (2013). Treadmill interventions with partial body weight support in children under six years of age at risk of neuromotor delay: a report of a Cochrane systematic review and meta-analysis. *Eur. J. Phys. Rehabil. Med.* 49, 67–91.

van den Brand, R., Heutschi, J., Barraud, Q., DiGiovanna, J., Bartholdi, K., Huerlimann, M., et al. (2012). Restoring voluntary control of locomotion after paralyzing spinal cord injury. *Science* 336, 1182–1185. doi: 10.1126/science.1217416

Wirz, M., Zemon, D. H., Rupp, R., Scheel, A., Colombo, G., Dietz, V., et al. (2005). Effectiveness of automated locomotor training in patients with chronic incomplete spinal cord injury: a multicenter trial. *Arch. Phys. Med. Rehabil.* 86, 672–680. doi: 10.1016/j.apmr.2004.08.004

Yang, J. F., and Gorassini, M. (2006). Spinal and brain control of human walking: implications for retraining of walking. *Neuroscientist* 12, 379–389. doi: 10.1177/1073858406292151

Yang, J. F., Lamont, E. V., and Pang, M. Y. C. (2005). Split-belt treadmill stepping in infants suggests autonomous pattern generators for the left and right leg in humans. *J. Neurosci.* 25, 6869–6876. doi: 10.1523/jneurosci.1765-05.2005

Zehr, E. P. (2005). Neural control of rhythmic human movement: the common core hypothesis. *Exerc. Sport Sci. Rev.* 33, 54–60.

Zehr, E. P., Balter, J. E., Ferris, D. P., Hundza, S. R., Loadman, P. M., and Stoloff, R. H. (2007). Neural regulation of rhythmic arm and leg movement is conserved across human locomotor tasks. *J. Physiol.* 582, 209–227. doi: 10.1113/jphysiol.2007.133843

7

How to build better memory training games

Jenni Deveau[1], Susanne M. Jaeggi[2,3], Victor Zordan[4], Calvin Phung[4] and Aaron R. Seitz[1]*

[1] Department of Psychology, University of California, Riverside, Riverside, CA, USA
[2] School of Education, University of California, Irvine, Irvine, CA, USA
[3] Department of Cognitive Sciences, University of California, Irvine, Irvine, CA, USA
[4] Department of Computer Science, University of California, Riverside, Riverside, CA, USA

Edited by:
Mikhail Lebedev, Duke University, USA

Reviewed by:
Jyoti Mishra, University of California San Francisco, USA
Mariano Sigman, Universidad Torcuato Di Tella, Argentina

***Correspondence:**
Aaron R. Seitz, Department of Psychology, University of California, Riverside, 900 University Ave, Riverside, CA 92521, USA
e-mail: aseitz@ucr.edu

Can we create engaging training programs that improve working memory (WM) skills? While there are numerous procedures that attempt to do so, there is a great deal of controversy regarding their efficacy. Nonetheless, recent meta-analytic evidence shows consistent improvements across studies on lab-based tasks generalizing beyond the specific training effects (Au et al., 2014; Karbach and Verhaeghen, 2014), however, there is little research into how WM training aids participants in their daily life. Here we propose that incorporating design principles from the fields of Perceptual Learning (PL) and Computer Science might augment the efficacy of WM training, and ultimately lead to greater learning and transfer. In particular, the field of PL has identified numerous mechanisms (including attention, reinforcement, multisensory facilitation and multi-stimulus training) that promote brain plasticity. Also, computer science has made great progress in the scientific approach to game design that can be used to create engaging environments for learning. We suggest that approaches integrating knowledge across these fields may lead to a more effective WM interventions and better reflect real world conditions.

Keywords: working memory, video games, brain training, perceptual learning, game design

INTRODUCTION

As long as scientists have explored memory, they have strived, and often failed, to improve it. Most approaches to improve memory implement strategies, such as creating mnemonic devices (for example, the method of loci). However, despite evidence these techniques improve memory *performance*, they do not target underlying memory *processes*, and while they do have some influence on memory systems in the brain (Maguire et al., 2003), they typically fail to broadly generalize to untrained activities (Verhaeghen et al., 1992; Maguire et al., 2003; St Clair-Thompson et al., 2010). Recent research on "brain training" renews promise for improving memory and other cognitive skills. Here, we focus on working memory (WM), a limited-capacity system for storing and manipulating information in a given moment. WM underlies performance in virtually all complex cognitive tasks (Shah and Miyake, 1999). Recent approaches targeting skills related to WM (Klingberg et al., 2002, 2005; Jaeggi et al., 2008, 2010; Anguera et al., 2013; Goldin et al., 2014) have shown generalizing benefits to a wide number of non-trained cognitive tasks that are thought to rely on WM, including executive control and fluid reasoning (c.f. Au et al., 2014; Karbach and Verhaeghen, 2014 for recent meta-analyses).

Here we review recent WM training approaches discussing their strengths and limitations and suggest methods that are based on the principles of perceptual learning (PL) and game design to make them more effective. Off-the-shelf computer games and standard cognitive approaches each contain component properties that can benefit WM. We propose that integrating knowledge from psychology and neuroscience along with the science of video game design could critically inform the development of engaging, cognitively immersive challenges that will more optimally train WM memory processes.

SPAN TRAINING

Span training targets WM capacity (Klingberg et al., 2002, 2005) typically relying on two types of tasks, simple and complex. Simple span tasks present sequences of stimuli that vary in set-size with participants typically reporting the items in (reverse) order of presentation. Research has shown that training on simple span tasks results in transfer in a variety of measures, such as non-trained WM tasks, response inhibition, and even fluid reasoning (Klingberg et al., 2002, 2005; Thorell et al., 2009).

In contrast to simple span tasks, which focus predominantly on WM storage, complex span tasks involve a secondary processing task. An example of a complex span task is Reading Span (Daneman and Carpenter, 1980) where participants judge the semantic content of a series of sentences and then later recall the last word of each sentence in order. Simple and complex span tasks used as interventions are typically adaptive, where the number of items to be recalled increases as training progresses. Adaptive complex span training leads to both near and far transfer in a variety of populations. Chein and Morrison (2010) showed that training on verbal and spatial complex span tasks improves verbal and spatial short-term memory, response inhibition, and reading comprehension in young and older adults (Richmond et al., 2011). In another series of studies, typically developing children (Loosli et al., 2012; Karbach et al., 2014) and older adults (Buschkuehl et al., 2008) were trained on complex span (see **Figure 1B**) demonstrating improved reading performance (Loosli et al., 2012; Karbach et al., 2014) and improved visual WM and episodic memory (Buschkuehl et al., 2008). Other groups have found similar effects from complex span training in older adults that were maintained several months after training completion (Borella et al., 2010, 2013, 2014).

N-BACK TRAINING

Among the best known WM tasks used for training is the n-back task (Jaeggi et al., 2008; Smith et al., 2009; Buschkuehl and Jaeggi, 2010). Here, participants memorize and constantly update the serial positions "*n* steps back" in a continuous stimulus stream and report whether or not the current stimulus matches the stimulus *n*-items back in a sequence (**Figure 1A**). Task difficulty (equal to level of *n*) is adaptively adjusted in response to participants' performance. N-back training-related improvements are wide-ranging, including non-trained WM functions (e.g., Lilienthal et al., 2013), executive functioning (e.g., Salminen et al., 2012), episodic memory (e.g., Rudebeck et al., 2012), and even fluid reasoning (Stephenson and Halpern, 2013). Effects are observed across the lifespan ranging from typically developing children (Jaeggi et al., 2011) to older adults (Stepankova et al., 2014). Both the amount of training (Stepankova et al., 2014) and achievement on the training task (Jaeggi et al., 2011) have been related to consequent improvements in the untrained fluid intelligence tasks. However, findings of far transfer (e.g., that WM training leads to improved performance on tasks unrelated to the training), are not ubiquitous in the literature (Shipstead et al., 2012). Some of these inconsistencies across studies may be explained by variations in training schedules, outcome measures, or individual differences (Jaeggi et al., 2012, 2014; Shah et al., 2012).

MECHANISMS THAT PROMOTE LEARNING

While there is growing evidence that WM training impacts performance in a wide variety of tasks, the mechanisms driving plasticity in WM systems remain unclear. However, research of PL has identified numerous mechanisms that promote the magnitude and generalization of learning. PL refers to a long lasting improvement in perceptual abilities as a result of experience. Interestingly, key approaches to working WM training, such as extended practice and adaptive procedures (the latter is to use computer algorithms to customize the challenge to each participant), were originally modeled after successful approaches in PL (Klingberg et al., 2002, 2005). Classically, a translational barrier to PL has been its high degree of specificity to trained stimulus features (Fahle, 2005), such as orientation (Fiorentini and Berardi, 1980), retinal location (Karni and Sagi, 1991) or the eye trained (Poggio et al., 1992; Seitz et al., 2009). This specificity to the training task and stimuli mirrors issues that face modern WM training. However, recent research illustrates how to overcome this "curse of specificity" with approaches that integrate many techniques (Deveau et al., 2014a,b) showing greater generalization of learning.

A key question is what mechanisms gate learning? Seitz and Dinse (2007) proposed a model of PL in which mechanisms including attention, reinforcement, optimal stimulation protocols, and multisensory facilitation interact to boost sensory signals over a learning threshold. This model and a host of empirical research on PL demonstrate that learning generalizes best when: (1) a larger set of stimulus features are trained (Xiao et al., 2008; Hung and Seitz, 2014); (2) using multisensory stimuli (Shams and Seitz, 2008); (3) using motivating tasks (Shibata et al., 2009); (4) participants are confident in their performance (Ahissar and Hochstein, 1997); and (5) consistent reinforcement to the training stimuli is used (Seitz and Watanabe, 2009). Combining these approaches increase the magnitude and generality of learning (Deveau et al., 2014a,b). In the following, we review some of the mechanisms that promote PL and discuss how they could be applied to WM training.

ATTENTION AND REINFORCEMENT

Attention refers to a set of mental processes that selectively modulate the processing of relevant information over irrelevant information; attention influences decisions, guides memory processes and our executive functions to direct resources to act upon the world. Numerous studies show that attention gates learning (Shiu and Pashler, 1992; Ahissar and Hochstein, 1993; Schoups et al., 2001; Leclercq and Seitz, 2012b). For example, Schoups et al. (2001) found neuronal plasticity of V1 cells corresponding to attended stimuli but no plasticity for cells with receptive fields overlapping unattended stimuli, suggesting that attention selects what is learned and what is not. A key aspect of WM capacity entails the ability to avoid distraction and is positively correlated with performance on a variety of attention tasks (Engle, 2002; Hutchison, 2007). Furthermore, WM capacity is highly predictive for scholastic achievement (Gathercole et al., 2003) and it is among the major cognitive deficits of children with attention deficit hyperactivity disorder (ADHD; Klingberg et al., 2002). Using casual games found on the Internet, Baniqued et al. (2013) found that playing games focusing on attention/object tracking improved WM abilities, on the other hand, playing games that focused on WM did not improve measures of attention. These and other findings suggest a key role of attention in WM, and that proper engagement of attention during training may be a key factor in WM training success.

Also, reinforcement processes (rewards, punishments, motivation, etc.) have fundamental importance in guiding learning. For example, Seitz et al. (2009) found improved discrimination of orientation stimuli masked in noise after temporal-pairing between a liquid reward and a subliminal presentation of that orientation stimulus. Seitz and Watanabe (2005) suggested a model where learning is gated by reinforcement signals that trigger learning of aspects of the environment (even those for which the organism is not consciously aware) that are predictive or co-vary with the reinforcing event. They suggested that both attention and reinforcement operate in part through the release of neuromodulatory signals in the brain. For example, the orienting of attention, in the direction of the target-arrow, has been linked with the acetylcholine neuromodulatory system (Davidson and Marrocco, 2000). Of interest, cholinergic enhancement through the use of donepezil improves both the attentional processing

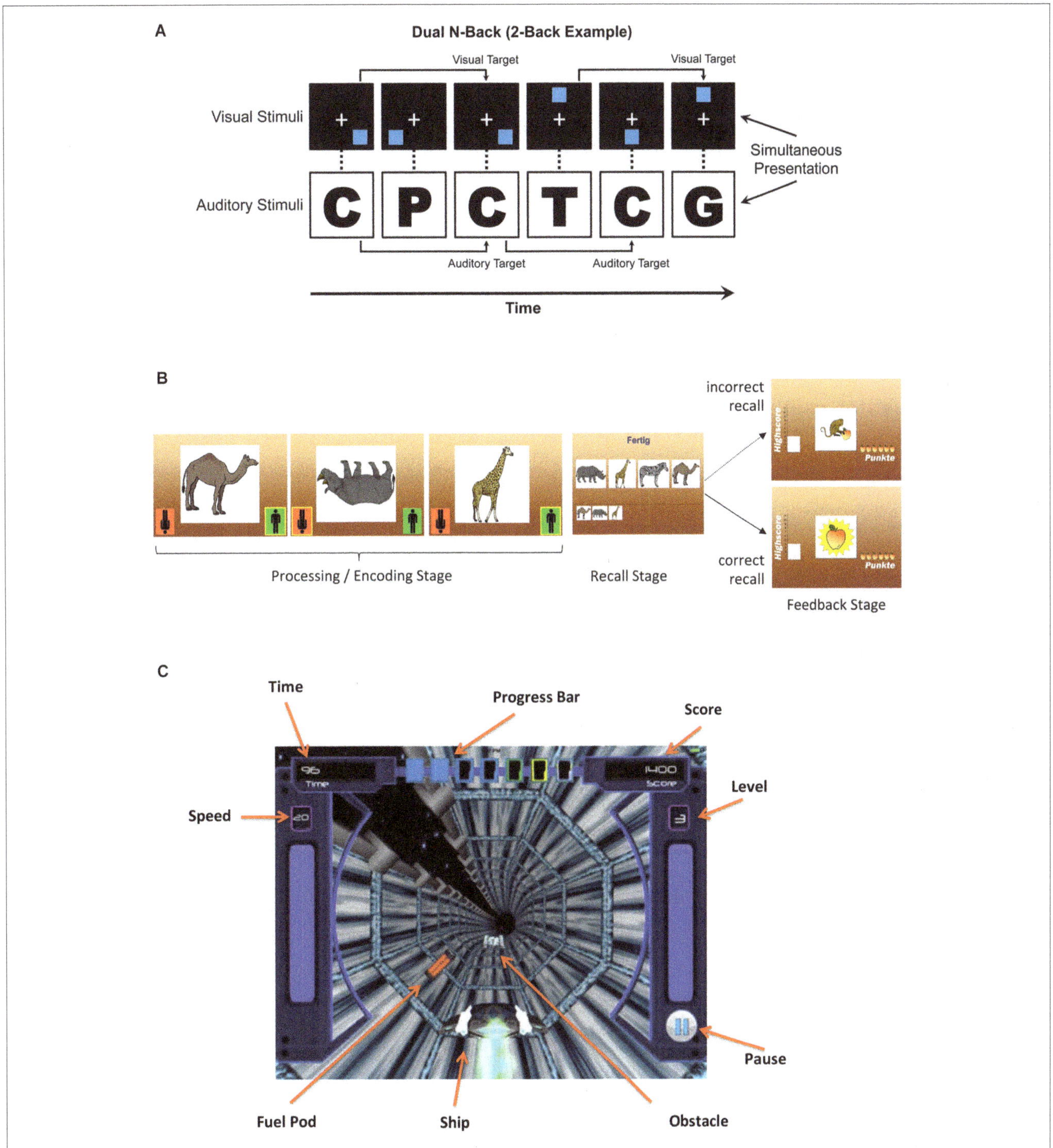

FIGURE 1 | (A) Diagram of an n-back task presented as a 2-back task (Jaeggi et al., 2008, 2010). Here, visual and auditory stimuli are presented simultaneously and participants have to respond to both modality streams independently. **(B)** Diagram of a complex span training task (Buschkuehl et al., 2008; Loosli et al., 2012). Animal pictures are presented sequentially, and participants respond to the orientation of each picture, and then reproduce the sequence in which the animals were presented. **(C)** Schematic of gamified n-back training task.

(Rokem et al., 2010) as well as the magnitude (Rokem and Silver, 2010) and longevity (Rokem and Silver, 2013) of PL. Other neuromodulatory systems, such as dopamine and norepinephrine have also been linked to attention (Posner and Petersen, 1990; Fan et al., 2003), learning (Kilgard and Merzenich, 1998; Bao et al., 2001; Dalley et al., 2001; Blake et al., 2006) and WM (Brehmer et al., 2009; Bellander et al., 2011). These studies suggest that a good training approach should involve the direction of both attention and reinforcement in a coordinated manner to promote learning.

MULTISENSORY FACILITATION

The human brain has evolved to learn and operate optimally in natural environments in which behavior is guided by information integrated across multiple sensory modalities. Crossmodal interactions are ubiquitous in the nervous system and occur even at early stages of perceptual processing (Shimojo and Shams, 2001; Calvert et al., 2004; Schroeder and Foxe, 2005; Ghazanfar and Schroeder, 2006; Driver and Noesselt, 2008). For example, recent research shows that subjects trained with auditory-visual stimuli exhibit a faster rate of learning and a higher degree of improvement than found in subjects trained in silence (Seitz et al., 2006; Kim et al., 2008).

Both memory storage and retrieval involves multiple senses. For example, the smell of a loved one's perfume (olfaction) can invoke memories of their face (vision), and so on. However, existing memory tasks, such as the dual *n*-back, often employ multiple (stimulus) modalities that are not coordinated, which research shows does not promote learning, and may in fact interfere with it (Seitz et al., 2005). Instead, we suggest a different approach where multisensory objects are incorporated into WM training. By defining objects through multi-modal feature sets, each sense can boost learning in the other. For example, an individual with limited visual capabilities will benefit from training utilizing concordant auditory stimuli.

MULTISTIMULUS TRAINING

One way to overcome specificity of learning is by training with multiple stimuli, as demonstrated in PL (Dosher and Lu, 1998; Yu et al., 2004; Xiao et al., 2008; Deveau et al., 2014a,b). For example, the recently developed technique of "double training" found that classically specific learning effects can show broad transfer when more than one stimulus attribute is trained. Xiao et al. (2008) trained participants on a Vernier discrimination task at a specific orientation at a specific location in the visual field, which normally yields location and orientation specific learning (Poggio et al., 1992). However, subsequently training subjects a second orientation at a different spatial location, the training-induced changes for the second orientation transferred to the first location. This data suggests that WM training with a diverse stimulus set might lead to a greater degree of transfer to untrained tasks than training on a narrow set (Estes and Burke, 1953; Schmidt and Bjork, 1992).

Furthermore, PL shows that the arrangement of multiple task elements in space and time can play a pivotal role in determining learning. Poor arrangements, such as when different stimuli are presented in a random order, as opposed to fixed order (Zhang et al., 2008), lead to poor learning (Seitz et al., 2005). Similar rules operate in guiding memory where sudden onsets of task-related stimuli can disrupt memorization of objects paired with those images (Leclercq and Seitz, 2012a). This may explain the recent counter-intuitive finding of WM training where the addition of motivational features in a simple gamification of n-back training led to impaired learning (Katz et al., 2014; see **Figure 2**), by inadvertently leading to greater distraction. We suggest that greater congruence between training stimuli and motivational factors will lead to greater and broader learning from WM training. In the next section we describe how this may be achieved through game design principles.

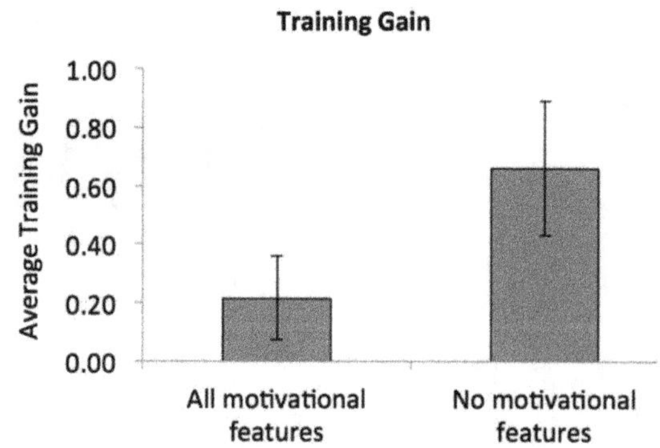

FIGURE 2 | Interference of learning by gamification. Motivational features such as scores, prizes, and scene-changes seem to interfere with learning. Specifically, training with all these features led to a lesser degree of learning compared to training without motivational features over the course of three sessions of *n*-back training (adapted from Katz et al., 2014).

VIDEO GAMES

There are many examples of off-the-shelf video games leading to substantial improvements in a variety of perceptual and cognitive abilities. For example, Green and Bavelier (2003) found that training novices for 10 h on an action video game improved performance on enumeration, useful field of view, and attentional blink tasks when compared to participants trained with a non-action video game. Basak et al. (2008) found that playing a real-time strategy game improved executive control as measured by task switching, visual short-term memory, and reasoning in older adults. Another recent study (Shute et al., 2015) showed that an off-the-shelf video game (Portal 2) led to substantial improvements on measures of problem solving, spatial skills, and persistence (in fact, even more so than training with the popular brain training games of Lumosity). Furthermore, dyslexic children improved reading speed and attentional abilities after playing an action video game (Franceschini et al., 2013). Finally, Goldin et al. (2014) employed several computer games targeting executive control, and found improvements in attention, inhibitory control, and planning, which also translated to school performance (Goldin et al., 2014). Together these studies suggest that video games include important attributes that contribute to learning.

Given the attractive motivational features of video games, recent research in cognitive science is increasingly moving towards adding game-like elements to their assessments. However, without proper design these can impair task performance, and even weaken test quality and learning (Hawkins et al., 2013; Katz et al., 2014). We suggest a better approach is to create training software that will dovetail, and/or implement non-competing concepts from game design that support learning. The video-game field is maturing, proper design rules and constraints are becoming more refined and the practices of coordinated design are becoming better understood and documented (Rabin, 2005). For example, in order to optimally engage players games must establish clear goals and allow players to realize those goals through meaningful actions (Salen and Zimmerman, 2004). Successful game design has critical aspects that make software engaging, including its mechanics, interaction, visual/sensory experience, and progression (Gee, 2007).

Many game design criteria mirror components found to improve learning from the PL literature, and literature on deliberate practice (Ericsson et al., 1993). For example, consistent reinforcement to training stimuli (Seitz and Watanabe, 2009) maps directly to consistent player feedback, a key part of *player-centric interface design* (Adams, 2009). Adams says (of players) "most critically, they need information about whether their efforts are succeeding or failing, taking them closer to victory or closer to defeat". Likewise, motivating tasks (Shibata et al., 2009) and ensuring subjects are confident of their performance (Ahissar and Hochstein, 1997) are consistent with good game-design principles such as establishing clear goals (Salen and Zimmerman, 2004) and balancing games challenges (related to the adaptive approaches used in PL and WM training) to match player performance (Adams, 2009). Applying video-game techniques purposefully into WM training can inject the cognitive benefits found from off-the-shelf video games into principled cognitive training, while also being fun to play.

INTEGRATING LEARNING AND GAMING PRINCIPLES

Two relevant lines of research have made significant breakthroughs in brain training: (1) Studying incidental benefits of off-the-shelf video games; and (2) Transforming standard cognitive tasks into training tasks. We suggest that the most success will come from integrating knowledge of memory systems with that of brain plasticity and modern game-design principles.

As a first attempt to implement this approach, we created a prototype game that incorporates mechanics of the n-back into an engaging 3D space-themed game[1] (see **Figure 1C**). Typically, the n-back task is very basic, e.g., selecting matches from a grid or a picture series. In contrast, our prototype is a space-themed "collection" game with navigation challenges and obstacles, multi-layered progression through levels, and rich, thematic visual and sound effects. The n-back task is integrated into the game mechanics, where players select the "right" fuel cells while avoiding decoys. Levels are designed to get progressively harder through increasing cognitive challenge (n-level) and other game challenges (such as obstacles). While the game is more difficult and attention is spread over more elements than the conventional n-back, participant's control over their environment is anticipated to increase their engagement with the game.

The game also incorporates principles from PL, where participants are trained on multisensory (auditory and visual) features, where sounds and visuals are designed to facilitate each other, and where attention and reinforcement are carefully sculpted to lead to the best learning. While much work is still required to maximize the game's efficacy, e.g., by incorporating a broader stimulus set, adding other memory tasks, and creating an even more compelling game framework, we put it forward as a first example of how to build such an integrative game. Initial piloting with our prototype indicates participants are engaged in the game and improve performance (n-level) across training sessions. However, more research is needed to make firm conclusions regarding its transfer potential.

In summary, we suggest that more integrative approaches will lead to better learning outcomes. We suggest that the general mechanisms that promote PL are shared across brain regions and will also promote WM. Furthermore, there is enough known about the aspects of conventional video games that lead to positive learning outcomes that these principles can be applied to achieve more effective WM training. Additionally, there are other principles, that were beyond the scope of the present review, such as deliberate practice (Ericsson et al., 1993), and many aspects of healthy lifestyles (Walsh, 2011; Sigman et al., 2014) that also promote cognitive fitness. Integrating these approaches with good design could lead to a more comprehensive impact on WM function that might ultimately transfer to real-world conditions.

[1] https://itunes.apple.com/us/app/recall-the-game/id890271623?mt=8

REFERENCES

Adams, E. (2009). *Fundamentals of Game Design (2nd Edn.).* Berkeley, CA: New Riders.

Ahissar, M., and Hochstein, S. (1993). Attentional control of early perceptual learning. *Proc. Natl. Acad. Sci. U S A* 90, 5718–5722. doi: 10.1073/pnas.90.12.5718

Ahissar, M., and Hochstein, S. (1997). Task difficulty and the specificity of perceptual learning. *Nature* 387, 401–406. doi: 10.1038/387401a0

Anguera, J. A., Boccanfuso, J., Rintoul, J. L., Al-Hashimi, O., Faraji, F., Janowich, J., et al. (2013). Video game training enhances cognitive control in older adults. *Nature* 501, 97–101. doi: 10.1038/nature12486

Au, J., Sheehan, E., Tsai, N., Duncan, G. J., Buschkuehl, M., and Jaeggi, S. M. (2014). Improving fluid intelligence with training on working memory: a meta-analysis. *Psychon. Bull. Rev.* doi: 10.3758/s13423-014-0699-x. [Epub ahead of print].

Baniqued, P. L., Lee, H., Voss, M. W., Basak, C., Cosman, J. D., Desouza, S., et al. (2013). Selling points: what cognitive abilities are tapped by casual video games? *Acta Psychol. (Amst)* 142, 74–86. doi: 10.1016/j.actpsy.2012.11.009

Bao, S., Chan, V. T., and Merzenich, M. M. (2001). Cortical remodelling induced by activity of ventral tegmental dopamine neurons. *Nature* 412, 79–83. doi: 10.1038/35083586

Basak, C., Boot, W. R., Voss, M. W., and Kramer, A. F. (2008). Can training in a real-time strategy video game attenuate cognitive decline in older adults? *Psychol. Aging* 23, 765–777. doi: 10.1037/a0013494

Bellander, M., Brehmer, Y., Westerberg, H., Karlsson, S., Furth, D., Bergman, O., et al. (2011). Preliminary evidence that allelic variation in the LMX1A gene influences training-related working memory improvement. *Neuropsychologia* 49, 1938–1942. doi: 10.1016/j.neuropsychologia.2011.03.021

Blake, D. T., Heiser, M. A., Caywood, M., and Merzenich, M. M. (2006). Experience-dependent adult cortical plasticity requires cognitive association between sensation and reward. *Neuron* 52, 371–381. doi: 10.1016/j.neuron.2006.08.009

Borella, E., Carretti, B., Cantarella, A., Riboldi, F., Zavagnin, M., and De Beni, R. (2014). Benefits of training visuospatial working memory in young-old and old-old. *Dev. Psychol.* 50, 714–727. doi: 10.1037/a0034293

Borella, E., Carretti, B., Riboldi, F., and De Beni, R. (2010). Working memory training in older adults: evidence of transfer and maintenance effects. *Psychol. Aging* 25, 767–778. doi: 10.1037/a0020683

Borella, E., Carretti, B., Zanoni, G., Zavagnin, M., and De Beni, R. (2013). Working memory training in old age: an examination of transfer and maintenance effects. *Arch. Clin. Neuropsychol.* 28, 331–347. doi: 10.1093/arclin/act020

Brehmer, Y., Westerberg, H., Bellander, M., Fürth, D., Karlsson, S., and Backman, L. (2009). Working memory plasticity modulated by dopamine transporter genotype. *Neurosci. Lett.* 467, 117–120. doi: 10.1016/j.neulet.2009.10.018

Buschkuehl, M., and Jaeggi, S. M. (2010). Improving intelligence: a literature review. *Swiss Med. Wkly* 140, 266–272. doi: smw-12852

Buschkuehl, M., Jaeggi, S. M., Hutchison, S., Perrig-Chiello, P., Däpp, C., Müller, M., et al. (2008). Impact of working memory training on memory performance in old-old adults. *Psychol. Aging* 23, 743–753. doi: 10.1037/a0014342

Calvert, G., Spence, C., and Stein, B. E. (2004). *The Handbook of Multisensory Processes.* Cambridge, MA: The MIT Press.

Chein, J. M., and Morrison, A. B. (2010). Expanding the mind's workspace: training and transfer effects with a complex working memory span task. *Psychon. Bull. Rev.* 17, 193–199. doi: 10.3758/PBR.17.2.193

Dalley, J. W., McGaughy, J., O'Connell, M. T., Cardinal, R. N., Levita, L., and Robbins, T. W. (2001). Distinct changes in cortical acetylcholine and noradrenaline efflux during contingent and noncontingent performance of a visual attentional task. *J. Neurosci.* 21, 4908–4914.

Daneman, M., and Carpenter, P. A. (1980). Individual differences in working memory and reading. *J. Verbal Learn. Verbal Behav.r* 19, 450–466. doi: 10.1016/s0022-5371(80)90312-6

Davidson, M. C., and Marrocco, R. T. (2000). Local infusion of scopolamine into intraparietal cortex slows covert orienting in rhesus monkeys. *J. Neurophysiol.* 83, 1536–1549.

Deveau, J., Lovcik, G., and Seitz, A. R. (2014a). Broad-based visual benefits from training with an integrated perceptual-learning video game. *Vision Res.* 99, 134–140. doi: 10.1016/j.visres.2013.12.015

Deveau, J., Ozer, D. J., and Seitz, A. R. (2014b). Improved vision and on field performance in baseball through perceptual learning. *Curr. Biol.* 24, R146–R147. doi: 10.1016/j.cub.2014.01.004

Dosher, B. A., and Lu, Z. L. (1998). Perceptual learning reflects external noise filtering and internal noise reduction through channel reweighting. *Proc. Natl. Acad. Sci. U S A* 95, 13988–13993. doi: 10.1073/pnas.95.23.13988

Driver, J., and Noesselt, T. (2008). Multisensory interplay reveals crossmodal influences on 'sensory-specific' brain regions, neural responses and judgments. *Neuron* 57, 11–23. doi: 10.1016/j.neuron.2007.12.013

Engle, R. W. (2002). Working memory capacity as executive attention. *Curr. Dir. sychol. Sci.* 11, 19–23. doi: 10.1111/1467-8721.00160

Ericsson, K. A., Krampe, R. T., and Tesch-Römer, C. (1993). The role of deliberate practice in the acquisition of expert performance. *Psychol. Rev.* 100, 363–406. doi: 10.1037//0033-295x.100.3.363

Estes, W. K., and Burke, C. J. (1953). A theory of stimulus variability in learning. *Psychol. Rev.* 60, 276–286. doi: 10.1037/h0055775

Fahle, M. (2005). Perceptual learning: specificity versus generalization. *Curr. Opin. Neurobiol.* 15, 154–160. doi: 10.1016/j.conb.2005.03.010

Fan, J., Fossella, J., Sommer, T., Wu, Y., and Posner, M. I. (2003). Mapping the genetic variation of executive attention onto brain activity. *Proc. Natl. Acad. Sci. U S A* 100, 7406–7411. doi: 10.1073/pnas.0732088100

Fiorentini, A., and Berardi, N. (1980). Perceptual learning specific for orientation and spatial frequency. *Nature* 287, 43–44. doi: 10.1038/287043a0

Franceschini, S., Gori, S., Ruffino, M., Viola, S., Molteni, M., and Facoetti, A. (2013). Action video games make dyslexic children read better. *Curr. Biol.* 23, 462–466. doi: 10.1016/j.cub.2013.01.044

Gathercole, S. E., Brown, L., and Pickering, S. J. (2003). Working memory assessments at school entry as longitudinal predictors of national curriculum attainment levels. *Educ. Child Psychol.* 20, 109–122.

Gee, J. P. (2007). *What Video Games have to Teach us about Learning and Literacy: Revised and Updated Edition.* New York, NY: Macmillan.

Ghazanfar, A., and Schroeder, C. E. (2006). Is neocortex essentially multisensory? *Trends Cogn. Sci.* 10, 278–285. doi: 10.1016/j.tics.2006.04.008

Goldin, A. P., Hermida, M. J., Shalom, D. E., Elias Costa, M., Lopez-Rosenfeld, M., Segretin, M. S., et al. (2014). Far transfer to language and math of a short software-based gaming intervention. *Proc. Natl. Acad. Sci. U S A* 111, 6443–6448. doi: 10.1073/pnas.1320217111

Green, C. S., and Bavelier, D. (2003). Action video game modifies visual selective attention. *Nature* 423, 534–537. doi: 10.1038/nature01647

Hawkins, G. E., Rae, B., Nesbitt, K. V., and Brown, S. D. (2013). Gamelike features might not improve data. *Behav. Res. Methods* 45, 301–318. doi: 10.3758/s13428-012-0264-3

Hung, S. C., and Seitz, A. R. (2014). Prolonged training at threshold promotes robust retinotopic specificity in perceptual learning. *J. Neurosci.* 34, 8423–8431. doi: 10.1523/jneurosci.0745-14.2014

Hutchison, K. A. (2007). Attentional control and the relatedness proportion effect in semantic priming. *J. Exp. Psychol. Learn. Mem. Cogn.* 33, 645–662. doi: 10.1037/0278-7393.33.4.645

Jaeggi, S. M., Buschkuehl, M., Jonides, J., and Perrig, W. J. (2008). Improving fluid intelligence with training on working memory. *Proc. Natl. Acad. Sci. U S A* 105, 6829–6833. doi: 10.1073/pnas.0801268105

Jaeggi, S. M., Buschkuehl, M., Jonides, J., and Shah, P. (2011). Short- and long-term benefits of cognitive training. *Proc. Natl. Acad. Sci. U S A* 108, 10081–10086. doi: 10.1073/pnas.1103228108

Jaeggi, S. M., Buschkuehl, M., Jonides, J., and Shah, P. (2012). Cogmed and working memory training—current challenges and the search for underlying mechanisms. *J. Appl. Res. Mem. Cogn.* 1, 211–213. doi: 10.1016/j.jarmac.2012.07.002

Jaeggi, S. M., Buschkuehl, M., Shah, P., and Jonides, J. (2014). The role of individual differences in cognitive training and transfer. *Mem. Cognit.* 42, 464–480. doi: 10.3758/s13421-013-0364-z

Jaeggi, S. M., Studer-Luethi, B., Buschkuehl, M., Su, Y. F., Jonides, J., and Perrig, W. J. (2010). The relationship between n-back performance and matrix reasoning—implications for training and transfer. *Intelligence* 38, 625–635. doi: 10.1016/j.intell.2010.09.001

Karbach, J., Strobach, T., and Schubert, T. (2014). Adaptive working-memory training benefits reading, but not mathematics in middle childhood. *Child Neuropsychol.* doi: 10.1080/09297049.2014.899336. [Epub ahead of print]

Karbach, J., and Verhaeghen, P. (2014). Making working memory work: a meta-analysis of executive-control and working memory training in older adults. *Psychol. Sci.* 25, 2027–2037. doi: 10.1177/0956797614548725

Karni, A., and Sagi, D. (1991). Where practice makes perfect in texture discrimination: evidence for primary visual cortex plasticity. *Proc. Natl. Acad. Sci. U S A* 88, 4966–4970. doi: 10.1073/pnas.88.11.4966

Katz, B., Jaeggi, S., Buschkuehl, M., Stegman, A., and Shah, P. (2014). Differential effect of motivational features on training improvements in school-based cognitive training. *Front. Hum. Neurosci.* 8:242. doi: 10.3389/fnhum.2014.00242

Kilgard, M. P., and Merzenich, M. M. (1998). Cortical map reorganization enabled by nucleus basalis activity. *Science* 279, 1714–1718. doi: 10.1126/science.279.5357.1714

Kim, R. S., Seitz, A. R., and Shams, L. (2008). Benefits of stimulus congruency for multisensory facilitation of visual learning. *PLoS One* 3:e1532. doi: 10.1371/journal.pone.0001532

Klingberg, T., Fernell, E., Olesen, P. J., Johnson, M., Gustafsson, P., Dahlström, K., et al. (2005). Computerized training of working memory in children with ADHD—a randomized, controlled trial. *J. Am. Acad. Child Adolesc. Psychiatry* 44, 177–186. doi: 10.1097/00004583-200502000-00010

Klingberg, T., Forssberg, H., and Westerberg, H. (2002). Training of working memory in children with ADHD. *J. Clin. Exp. Neuropsychol.* 24, 781–791. doi: 10.1076/jcen.24.6.781.8395

Leclercq, V., and Seitz, A. R. (2012a). Fast task-irrelevant perceptual learning is disrupted by sudden onset of central task elements. *Vision Res.* 61, 70–76. doi: 10.1016/j.visres.2011.07.017

Leclercq, V., and Seitz, A. R. (2012b). The impact of orienting attention in fast task-irrelevant perceptual learning. *Atten. Percept. Psychophys.* 74, 648–660. doi: 10.3758/s13414-012-0270-7

Lilienthal, L., Tamez, E., Shelton, J. T., Myerson, J., and Hale, S. (2013). Dual n-back training increases the capacity of the focus of attention. *Psychon. Bull. Rev.* 20, 135–141. doi: 10.3758/s13423-012-0335-6

Loosli, S. V., Buschkuehl, M., Perrig, W. J., and Jaeggi, S. M. (2012). Working memory training improves reading processes in typically developing children. *Child Neuropsychol.* 18, 62–78. doi: 10.1080/09297049.2011.575772

Maguire, E. A., Valentine, E. R., Wilding, J. M., and Kapur, N. (2003). Routes to remembering: the brains behind superior memory. *Nat. Neurosci.* 6, 90–95. doi: 10.1038/nn988

Poggio, T., Fahle, M., and Edelman, S. (1992). Fast perceptual learning in visual hyperacuity. *Science* 256, 1018–1021. doi: 10.1126/science.1589770

Posner, M. I., and Petersen, S. E. (1990). The attention system of the human brain. *Annu. Rev. Neurosci.* 13, 25–42. doi: 10.1146/annurev.neuro.13.1.25

Rabin, S. (2005). *Introduction to Game Development.* Rockland, MA: Charles River Media.

Richmond, L. L., Morrison, A. B., Chein, J. M., and Olson, I. R. (2011). Working memory training and transfer in older adults. *Psychol. Aging* 26, 813–822. doi: 10.1037/a0023631

Rokem, A., Landau, A. N., Garg, D., Prinzmetal, W., and Silver, M. A. (2010). Cholinergic enhancement increases the effects of voluntary attention but does not affect involuntary attention. *Neuropsychopharmacology* 35, 2538–2544. doi: 10.1038/npp.2010.118

Rokem, A., and Silver, M. A. (2010). Cholinergic enhancement augments magnitude and specificity of visual perceptual learning in healthy humans. *Curr. Biol.* 20, 1723–1728. doi: 10.1016/j.cub.2010.08.027

Rokem, A., and Silver, M. A. (2013). The benefits of cholinergic enhancement during perceptual learning are long-lasting. *Front. Comput. Neurosci.* 7:66. doi: 10.3389/fncom.2013.00066

Rudebeck, S. R., Bor, D., Ormond, A., O'Reilly, J. X., and Lee, A. C. (2012). A potential spatial working memory training task to improve both episodic memory and fluid intelligence. *PLoS One* 7:e50431. doi: 10.1371/journal.pone.0050431

Salen, K., and Zimmerman, E. (2004). *Rules of Play: Game Design Fundamentals.* (MIT Press).

Salminen, T., Strobach, T., and Schubert, T. (2012). On the impacts of working memory training on executive functioning. *Front. Hum. Neurosci.* 6:166. doi: 10.3389/fnhum.2012.00166

Schmidt, R. A., and Bjork, R. A. (1992). New conceptualizations of practice: common principles in three paradigms suggest new concepts for training. *Psychol. Sci.* 3, 207–217. doi: 10.1111/j.1467-9280.1992.tb00029.x

Schoups, A., Vogels, R., Qian, N., and Orban, G. (2001). Practising orientation identification improves orientation coding in V1 neurons. *Nature* 412, 549–553. doi: 10.1038/35087601

Schroeder, C. E., and Foxe, J. (2005). Multisensory contributions to low-level, 'unisensory' processing. *Curr. Opin. Neurobiol.* 15, 454–458. doi: 10.1016/j.conb.2005.06.008

Seitz, A. R., and Dinse, H. R. (2007). A common framework for perceptual learning. *Curr. Opin. Neurobiol.* 17, 148–153. doi: 10.1016/j.conb.2007.02.004

Seitz, A. R., Kim, R., and Shams, L. (2006). Sound facilitates visual learning. *Curr. Biol.* 16, 1422–1427. doi: 10.1016/j.cub.2006.05.048

Seitz, A. R., Kim, D., and Watanabe, T. (2009). Rewards evoke learning of unconsciously processed visual stimuli in adult humans. *Neuron* 61, 700–707. doi: 10.1016/j.neuron.2009.01.016

Seitz, A., and Watanabe, T. (2005). A unified model for perceptual learning. *Trends Cogn. Sci.* 9, 329–334. doi: 10.1016/j.tics.2005.05.010

Seitz, A. R., and Watanabe, T. (2009). The phenomenon of task-irrelevant perceptual learning. *Vision Res.* 49, 2604–2610. doi: 10.1016/j.visres.2009.08.003

Seitz, A. R., Yamagishi, N., Werner, B., Goda, N., Kawato, M., and Watanabe, T. (2005). Task-specific disruption of perceptual learning. *Proc. Natl. Acad. Sci. U S A* 102, 14895–14900. doi: 10.1073/pnas.0505765102

Shah, P., Buschkuehl, M., Jaeggi, S., and Jonides, J. (2012). Cognitive training for ADHD: the importance of individual differences. *J. Appl. Res. Mem. Cogn.* 1, 204–205. doi: 10.1016/j.jarmac.2012.07.001

Shah, P., and Miyake, A. (1999). "Models of working memory: an introduction," in *Models of Working Memory: Mechanism of Active Maintenance and Executive Control*, eds P. Shah and A. Miyake (New York: Cambridge University Press), 1–26.

Shams, L., and Seitz, A. R. (2008). Benefits of multisensory learning. *Trends Cogn. Sci.* 12, 411–417. doi: 10.1016/j.tics.2008.07.006

Shibata, K., Yamagishi, N., Ishii, S., and Kawato, M. (2009). Boosting perceptual learning by fake feedback. *Vision Res.* 49, 2574–2585. doi: 10.1016/j.visres.2009.06.009

Shimojo, S., and Shams, L. (2001). Sensory modalities are not separate modalities: plasticity and interactions. *Curr. Opin. Neurobiol.* 11, 505–509. doi: 10.1016/s0959-4388(00)00241-5

Shipstead, Z., Hicks, K. L., and Engle, R. W. (2012). Cogmed working memory training: does the evidence support the claims? *J. Appl. Res. Mem. Cogn.* 1, 185–193. doi: 10.1016/j.jarmac.2012.06.003

Shiu, L. P., and Pashler, H. (1992). Improvement in line orientation discrimination is retinally local but dependent on cognitive set. *Percept. Psychophys.* 52, 582–588. doi: 10.3758/bf03206720

Shute, V. J., Ventura, M., and Ke, F. (2015). The power of play: the effects of portal 2 and lumosity on cognitive and noncognitive skills. *Comput. Educ.* 80, 58–67. doi: 10.1016/j.compedu.2014.08.013

Sigman, M., Pñna, M., Goldin, A. P., and Ribeiro, S. (2014). Neuroscience and education: prime time to build the bridge. *Nat. Neurosci.* 17, 497–502. doi: 10.1038/nn.3672

Smith, G. E., Housen, P., Yaffe, K., Ruff, R., Kennison, R. F., Mahncke, H. W., et al. (2009). A cognitive training program based on principles of brain plasticity: results from the Improvement in Memory with Plasticity-based Adaptive Cognitive Training (IMPACT) study. *J. Am. Geriatr. Soc.* 57, 594–603. doi: 10.1111/j.1532-5415.2008.02167.x

St Clair-Thompson, H., Stevens, R., Hunt, A., and Bolder, E. (2010). Improving children's working memory and classroom performance. *Educ. Psychol.* 30, 203–219. doi: 10.1080/01443410903509259

Stepankova, H., Lukavsky, J., Buschkuehl, M., Kopecek, M., Ripova, D., and Jaeggi, S. M. (2014). Dose-response relationship of working memory training and improvements in fluid intelligence: a randomized controlled study in old adults. *Dev. Psychol.* 50, 1049–1059.doi: 10.1037/a0034913

Stephenson, C. L., and Halpern, D. F. (2013). Improved matrix reasoning is limited to training on tasks with a visuospatial component. *Intelligence* 41, 341–357. doi: 10.1016/j.intell.2013.05.006

Thorell, L. B., Lindqvist, S., Bergman Nutley, S., Bohlin, G., and Klingberg, T. (2009). Training and transfer effects of executive functions in preschool children. *Dev. Sci.* 12, 106–113. doi: 10.1111/j.1467-7687.2008.00745.x

Verhaeghen, P., Marcoen, A., and Goossens, L. (1992). Improving memory performance in the aged through mnemonic training: a meta-analytic study. *Psychol. Aging* 7, 242–251. doi: 10.1037//0882-7974.7.2.242

Walsh, R. (2011). Lifestyle and mental health. *Am. Psychol.* 66, 579–592. doi: 10.1037/a0021769

Xiao, L. Q., Zhang, J. Y., Wang, R., Klein, S. A., Levi, D. M., and Yu, C. (2008). Complete transfer of perceptual learning across retinal locations enabled by double training. *Curr. Biol.* 18, 1922–1926. doi: 10.1016/j.cub.2008.10.030

Yu, C., Klein, S. A., and Levi, D. M. (2004). Perceptual learning in contrast discrimination and the (minimal) role of context. *J. Vis.* 4, 169–182. doi: 10.1167/4.3.4

Zhang, J. Y., Kuai, S. G., Xiao, L. Q., Klein, S. A., Levi, D. M., and Yu, C. (2008). Stimulus coding rules for perceptual learning. *PLoS Biol* 6:e197. doi: 10.1371/journal.pbio.0060197

8

Augmentation-related brain plasticity

Giovanni Di Pino[1,2]*, Angelo Maravita[3], Loredana Zollo[2], Eugenio Guglielmelli[2] and Vincenzo Di Lazzaro[1]

[1] Institute of Neurology and Fondazione Alberto Sordi - Research Institute for Ageing, Campus Bio Medico University of Rome, Rome, Italy
[2] Laboratory of Biomedical Robotics and Biomicrosystems CIR - Centre for Integrated Research, Campus Bio Medico University of Rome, Rome, Italy
[3] Department of Psycology, Università di Milano-Bicocca, Milano, Italy

Edited by:
Mikhail Lebedev, Duke University, USA

Reviewed by:
Arvid Guterstam, Karolinska Institutet, Sweden
Bérangère Thirioux, Unité de Recherche Clinique - Centre Hospitalier Henri Laborit, France

***Correspondence:**
Giovanni Di Pino, Institute of Neurology and Fondazione Alberto Sordi - Research Institute for Ageing, Campus Bio Medico University of Rome, Via Alvaro del Portillo 21, Rome 00128, Italy
e-mail: g.dipino@unicampus.it

Today, the anthropomorphism of the tools and the development of neural interfaces require reconsidering the concept of human-tools interaction in the framework of human augmentation. This review analyses the plastic process that the brain undergoes when it comes into contact with augmenting artificial sensors and effectors and, on the other hand, the changes that the use of external augmenting devices produces in the brain. Hitherto, few studies investigated the neural correlates of augmentation, but clues on it can be borrowed from logically-related paradigms: sensorimotor training, cognitive enhancement, cross-modal plasticity, sensorimotor functional substitution, use and embodiment of tools. Augmentation modifies function and structure of a number of areas, i.e., primary sensory cortices shape their receptive fields to become sensitive to novel inputs. Motor areas adapt the neuroprosthesis representation firing-rate to refine kinematics. As for normal motor outputs, the learning process recruits motor and premotor cortices and the acquisition of proficiency decreases attentional recruitment, focuses the activity on sensorimotor areas and increases the basal ganglia drive on the cortex. Augmentation deeply relies on the frontoparietal network. In particular, premotor cortex is involved in learning the control of an external effector and owns the tool motor representation, while the intraparietal sulcus extracts its visual features. In these areas, multisensory integration neurons enlarge their receptive fields to embody supernumerary limbs. For operating an anthropomorphic neuroprosthesis, the mirror system is required to understand the meaning of the action, the cerebellum for the formation of its internal model and the insula for its interoception. In conclusion, anthropomorphic sensorized devices can provide the critical sensory afferences to evolve the exploitation of tools through their embodiment, reshaping the body representation and the sense of the self.

Keywords: supernumerary limbs, sensory substitution, cognitive enhancement, embodiment, brain machine interface (BMI), cross-modal plasticity, hand prostheses, sensorimotor abilities

INTRODUCTION

Humans have always tried to augment their able-body abilities with the help of tools; lenses have been exploited to see further afield or to look at tiny objects, vehicles to travel long distances quicker and pincers and tongs to tightly manipulate objects. Tools use is a unique feature that humans and primates share, whit a loud influence in evolutionary processes, allowing them to push their abilities beyond the boundaries set by evolution and better interact with the environment (Ambrose, 2001).

Today's achievements in biological sciences and engineering might need to reconsider the concept of human-tools interaction in the framework of human augmentation. Human augmentation is a newborn domain of investigation that aims to exploit methodologies proper of medical therapeutic intervention and rehabilitative medicine, such as strategies, drugs and external artificial devices originally designed to compensate for the loss of functions, to increase physical and cognitive ability of able-bodied individuals, beyond the level characteristic of the normal physiological health status. Hence, the health status of the population targeted by the intervention critically sets the difference between rehabilitative functional restoration and human augmentation.

Actually, the idea of augmenting human abilities is not brand new, since, for instance, almost half a century ago, Von Gierke stated that it was among the goals of bionics "to extend man's physical and intellectual capabilities by prosthetic devices in the most general sense" (Von Gierke, 1970). However, more recently, the field of human augmentation started to capture the attention of scientists worldwide and to raise the level of awareness on its ethical and societal implications (for a deep analysis of ethical and societal implications of human augmentation see Clark, 2007; Blanke and Aspell, 2009). Indeed, several features of modern functional prostheses signed a sharp discontinuity with any device previously aimed at enhancing the ability of able-bodied: (i) the achieved high level of anthropomorphism of the tool; (ii) the intimate contact that the tool establishes with the user; and (iii) the absence of bottlenecks in the flow of information from the brain to the environment on which the tool operates. In summary, in recent years we are assisting to the first true attempts to create Hybrid Bionic Systems (HBSs), containing both technical and biological components arranged in a tight complex, where the robotic artifact is directly interfaced with the brain of a human being (Dario et al., 1993). This scenario encompasses, for example, modern cybernetic hand prostheses that exploit neural signals taken by electrodes implanted invasively into the cortex or into peripheral nerves to decode the user's intention of movement (Hochberg et al., 2006; Rossini et al., 2010). This modern approach could eventually lead to an unprecedented degree of man-machine integration.

The development of invasive (Lebedev and Nicolelis, 2006) and non-invasive (Birbaumer and Cohen, 2007) Brain-Machine Interfaces (BMI) and neural interfaces with peripheral nerves (Navarro et al., 2005) allowed to bypass the activity of the muscles and the physical transduction of cutaneous/proprioceptive sensory organs, while directly picking up motor signals from, or delivery sensory inputs to the nervous system. Hitherto, this has been the main determinant of the functional continuity between man and machines and represents the biggest milestone in the enquiry of the human augmentation. Prostheses that the user operates through neural interfaces are often named neuroprostheses. Although this term literally means a prosthesis for replacing a function of the nervous system, as it was originally conceived in the domain of cochlear implant (Terr et al., 1987) and in the stimulation of the sacral roots for bladder control (Brindley, 1974), it was lately used for motor functional electrical stimulation (Popovic et al., 2002) and more recently started to be used also for prostheses interfaced with the nervous system (Lebedev and Nicolelis, 2006). This extended meaning seems to be sufficiently accurate in operational terms and will be use from now on.

The recent advancements in robotics and BMIs are key enabling technologies for the creation of an augmented bionic man. However, can humans adapt themselves to effectively control external additional limbs and other body parts by learning and integrating them into a new sensorimotor representation? In the attempt to answer the question, it might be helpful to make a simple parallelism with the operation of adding a printer or an external hard-drive to our personal computer. The compatibility of the hardware is *conditio sine qua non, moreover* printer and laptop must share, for instance, the same I/O port. However, for a new device to be proficiently controlled the presence of its "representation" in the software that manages external devices is mandatory. In the case the software was not originally designed to allocate that device, it needs to be reprogrammed, often by means of supplemental drivers that plastically adapt it to the new condition. Analogously, human brain can be trained to expand its motor control to a supernumerary, artificial limb or else to receive sensory information from an external accessory sensor and plastically embed them into its representation of the body.

Most of the advancements in the field of human-machine interface have been achieved by pursuing two strategies in parallel: on one hand, the development of devices for restoring sensorimotor functions in disabled and, on the other hand, the development of devices for augmenting sensorimotor capabilities of able-bodied, allowing for instance to operate in impervious environments. However, it is worth considering that a further possible field of application of such technology, located in between rehabilitative functional restoration and human augmentation, is aging. The augmenting technology can be aimed indeed at supporting sensorimotor and cognitive abilities that are lost day-by-day with normal aging. The existence of a net border between therapeutic and augmenting applications seems to be overestimated, since the continuous distribution of individual human performance and its extreme variability could make exploitable for augmentation what has been developed for restoration and vice versa. Along this line, as we will see in the following paragraphs, most brain processes subtending functional restoration match the ones subtending augmentation and can be exploited to understand this phenomenon.

This review is aimed to analyze the neural correlates of human augmentation and, in particular, the plastic process that the brain undergoes when it comes into contact with artificial sensors and effectors meant as external aids and, on the other hand, the changes that the use of external augmenting devices produces in the brain.

BRAIN PLASTICITY: GENERAL CONSIDERATIONS

Brain plasticity is the ability of the brain to adapt its structural and functional connectivity in response to an external condition promoting a novel function, or a new way to perform an old function, or else the suppression of a sensorimotor ability. Plasticity has widely been considered the neural substrate of early development (Hensch, 2005), of the acquisition of new skills (Pascual-Leone et al., 1995) and of the recovery from brain injuries (Chen et al., 2002). It may be intended as an inner property of neural networks that results from the exposure of the system to physiological or pathological conditions (Pascual-Leone et al., 2005).

The Hebb and Paillard's theoretical hypothesis of brain plasticity (Hebb, 1949; Paillard, 1976), postulating that a long lasting strengthening of the connection between two neurons is induced by the simultaneous activation of those cells, has found its neural correlate in the phenomenon of associative learning mediated by long-term potentiation/depression (Bliss and Lomo, 1973; Bailey and Kandel, 2008).

Most of the findings regarding brain plasticity first came from lesion study in animals and, later on, from non-invasive functional imaging in humans. Plastic changes have been widely described in sensorimotor cortices that undergo deep remodeling with an extension of cortical representation of the still functionally active projections (Kaas, 1991). An initial unmasking of already present, but inactive, connections is the effect of increased cortical excitability due to a reduction of GABA-mediated inhibition (Jones, 1993) and an increase of NMDA-mediated activation (Buonomano and Merzenich, 1998). More stable changes often underlie structural modifications, characterized by axonal regeneration and sprouting (Kaas, 1991).

Hitherto, the amount of studies on ability augmentation, nearly all in animals, which investigating the recruited neural networks and/or on the plastic processes involved, are not enough to build a comprehensive body of knowledge on this topic. However, clues about augmentation-related plasticity can be obtained by borrowing insights gained from similar logically-related paradigms, i.e., sensorimotor training, cognitive enhancement, cross-modal plasticity, sensory and motor output functional substitution, use of tools and embodiment.

For instance, sensorimotor abilities can be enhanced by specific training and are boosted in athletes, while cognitive training enhances memory and attentive functions in healthy and brain-damaged, or aged, individuals. Artificial devices for etero-modal sensory substitution are exploited in the deaf and blind and rely on cross-modal plasticity, but the same devices can be exploited for sensory augmentation in sighted and normal hearing people. Motor augmentation, as well as motor functional substitution, involves the use of external effectors, including prostheses. Their optimal functionality relays on their integration in the user body schema, like any other kind of hand-held tool. Starting from those considerations, we will briefly describe the aforementioned paradigms and revise their implications for augmentation-related plasticity.

SENSORIMOTOR TRAINING-INDUCED PLASTICITY

Several effects of sensory motor training have been demonstrated in both the sensory and the motor domains, as well as at cellular level and at the level of whole brain areas or brain networks. Within the sensory domain, the acquisition or improvement of sensory functions is accompanied by plastic changes in the brain. Sensory discrimination training is able to induce changes in primary sensory cortices. Frequency discrimination training in adult owl monkeys results in increased performance and an enlargement of the stimulated skin representation in the primary somatosensory cortex, where the receptive fields of sensory neurons were significantly expanded (Recanzone et al., 1992). For example, monkeys trained in a visual orientation task showed a refined tuning of V1 neurons towards the trained orientation (Schoups et al., 2001).

Within the motor domain, a huge body of literature is devoted to the motor system plasticity induced by training. In rats, practicing a reaching task produced an enlarged representation of the wrist and digit movements in the primary motor cortex (M1) with an increase of the number of synapses per neurons (Kleim et al., 2002). The improvement seen in a reaction task can be well inferred from the activity of the motor neuronal ensemble in charge of the task (Laubach et al., 2000). In awake monkeys, skills acquisition modulates the activity of M1 neurons as assessed through cortical invasive recordings (Germain and Lamarre, 1993). Furthermore, the enlargement of M1 depends more on motor skill acquisition (Nudo et al., 1996) than on the simple repetitive use (Plautz et al., 2000). Long-term training-induced plastic changes in neuronal properties seem to be the substrate for the internal storage of motor skills (Matsuzaka et al., 2007). M1 changes during motor sequence learning, as evidenced by functional magnetic resonance imaging (fMRI), present an initial reduced area of M1 activation, following short-term repetition, but a progressive increased of the extension of M1 activation following motor training. Such a pattern of activation may be the neural substrate underpinning a three-phase motor skill acquisition: initial habituation, consolidation and long-lasting plasticity (Karni et al., 1998). A model that has been largely used to assess sensorimotor plasticity is that of studying the brain of people that hold (or else acquire) peculiar sensorimotor skills, such as sport or music expertise. For example, learning a one-hand piano exercise produces an enlargement of the motor representation of the hand and a facilitation of the corticospinal tract devoted to the muscles of the trained fingers (Pascual-Leone et al., 1995). Expert tennis players have an asymmetry of hand motor cortex with an enlarged representations and increased motor cortex excitability as evaluated by measuring the threshold for motor-evoked potential (MEP) after transcranial brain stimulation, in the cortex controlateral to the hand using the racket (Pearce et al., 2000). Plastic changes take place in the somatosensory system as well. In violin players, the somatosensory cortical representation of the fingers used to play the strings are enlarged and the amount of enlargement correlates with the years of practice (Elbert et al., 1995).

As far as the neurobiological mechanisms of sensorimotor plasticity, evidence from both animal (Rioult-Pedotti et al., 1998, 2000) and human (Ziemann et al., 2004) studies attributes training-induced motor plasticity to long-term potentiation (LTP)-like mechanisms involving the synaptic strength of cortical horizontal connections. However, structural plasticity, in parallel with the modulation of synaptic strength, plays a crucial role even after a few days of training. In humans, learning to juggle induced a bilateral increase in the gray matter of the occipito-temporal cortex, especially in the middle temporal motion-sensitive area (Draganski et al., 2004), after only a week of practice. Such plastic changes were no more present after the training ceased, although the performance did not decrease (Driemeyer et al., 2008). Structural modifications have been reported also for the white matter underlying the intraparietal sulcus (Scholz et al., 2009). Moreover, exercise showed to stimulate neurogenesis in the dentate gyrus of the hippocampus in mice and humans (Pereira et al., 2007).

Sensorimotor plasticity also manifests as a change in the pattern of activation of different brain areas and circuits. Motor skill acquisition recruits brain regions that are not recruited during simple motor task execution (Grafton et al., 1992). Several factors influence which network is recruited by practice, such as the specific task domain and the behavioral and cognitive load required. In general, practice of sensorimotor tasks determines an increased reliance on sensorimotor areas and a decreased recruitment of attentional control exerted by prefrontal, anterior cingulate and posterior parietal cortex (Kelly and Garavan, 2005). Motor practice not only affects the pattern of brain activation involved in the execution of the movement, but also its preparation. It has been shown that during stroke preparation expert golf players, compared to novices, show higher levels of activity in areas involved in visuomotor integration (superior parietal lobule, the dorsal lateral premotor cortex and the occipital area), and decreased activation in attentional/emotional basal ganglia and limbic structures (Milton et al., 2007). In the same paradigm, electroencephalographic (EEG) recordings demonstrated higher frontal theta and parietal alpha power, probably due to attention focusing for sensory processing (Baumeister et al., 2008). Skilled motor performance refines also the activity of the mirror system and goes in parallel with enhanced ability to anticipate the outcome of actions executed by others by resonant motor activation (Aglioti et al., 2008).

In summary, augmentation of sensorimotor skills, and sensorimotor training produce, an enhancement of performance, which is paralleled by specific neurobiological changes in the brain tissue and a change in the pattern of cortical activity, mainly by the focalization of brain activity on sensorimotor cortex both during movement execution and preparation (Yarrow et al., 2009).

COGNITIVE ENHANCEMENT

Cognitive enhancement is the attempt to improve cognitive functions (memory, working memory, attention, fluid intelligence) through training, psychological strategies, drugs or other medical interventions and last, but not least, external technological supports. Today's human augmentation targets cognitive enhancement *per se*, or can affect it as a consequence of sensorimotor augmentation. However, pursuing cognitive enhancement can be considered a foundational goal of humans. For instance, the aim of education always went beyond the mere learning of specific information; even pencil and paper can be regarded as primitive forms of external memory enhancement, while the use of nicotine and caffeine to focus attention, increase alertness and reduce the sense of fatigue can be dated far back in time (Bostrom and Sandberg, 2009).

The amount and quality of the stimuli offered by the environment are main determinants of cognitive development (Taffoni et al., 2014) and can be used to burst cognition. Indeed, in rats, an enriched environment produces an improvement of spatial memory and increases neurogenesis in the dentate gyrus (Nilsson et al., 1999) in a comparable way to chronic cholinergic treatment (Murphy et al., 2006). Also sensorimotor exercise, further than in sensorimotor processes, has a deep impact on cognition and promotes brain plasticity by modulating regional bloody flow and neurotrophic support, especially by releasing brain derived neurotrophic factor (BDNF; Vaynman and Gomez-Pinilla, 2005).

Cognitive enhancement by can be achieved with drugs. These molecules mostly target neurotransmitters of ascending systems from the brainstem nuclei, and have been directed to treat cognitive impairments of attention deficit hyperactivity disorder (ADHD), Parkinson's disease, schizophrenia, while acetylcholinesterase inhibitors are currently used as a the therapy in Alzheimer's disease (Husain and Mehta, 2011). Memory enhancing drugs are of two main classes: (i) LTP inducing drugs, mostly modulating AMPA (α-amino-3-hydroxy-5-methyl-4-isoxazole propionic acid receptors); and (ii) molecules increasing the cAMP response element-binding protein that enhances synapses, stabilizing proteins to allow memory consolidation (Farah et al., 2004). Effects of those drugs can go beyond the cognitive domains and influence non-cognitive symptoms of those clinical conditions. In this line, the acetylcholinesterase inhibitor rivastigmine reversed the abnormality of sensorimotor integration, as evaluated by testing short-latency afferent inhibition, in patients affected by Alzheimer's disease (Di Lazzaro et al., 2005).

It is worth noting that memory enhancement techniques have been developed to counteract memory decline of Alzheimer's and other neurodegenerative disorders, but they are currently extended to the healthy elder population in order to counteract age-related involution. Here again the borders between therapy and augmentation are weak. Similarly, methylphenidate (Ritalin), a catecolamine-like drug that represents the treatment of choice for ADHD and is known to improve cognitive performance also in healthy volunteers, is largely assumed even by children without diagnosed AHDH (Farah et al., 2004). The use of drugs for cognitive enhancement produces structural and functional changes in the brain. In healthy volunteers, the cognitive improvement seen after a single dose of modafinil, a monoamminergic stimulator, goes in parallel with an increased functional connectivity at rest in the anterior cingulate cortex, part of the left fronto-parietal control network and in the bilateral occipito-parietal node of the dorsal attention network (Esposito et al., 2013). Structural changes have been also described following drug treatment. In a rat model of stroke the administration of D-amphetamine induced an amelioration of motor and working memory performance and a significant increase of neurites growth and synaptogenesis in the neocortex (Stroemer et al., 1998).

Does superior memory ability rely on higher Q.I. or particularly developed brain structures or alternatively does it mostly rely on a specific functional engaging strategy? Evidence is in favor of the latter. During memory tasks, people with exceptional memory activate different neural networks involved in spatial learning and navigation, especially the hippocampus. This luckily reflects a "method of loci" memorizing strategy based on the association of each object to memorize with a location in an imagined physical pathway (Maguire et al., 2002). In healthy subjects, spatial memory can be dramatically increased by training, as happens for London taxi drivers that aim to acquire the license. A voxel-based morphometry study documented an increased gray-matter volume of the posterior hippocampus, which correlates with years of works and that can represent the plastic substrate for the allocation of spatial representations (Maguire et al., 2000).

Several attempts to achieve cognitive enhancement target the working memory. Working memory is the ability of retaining information over a brief time. It plays a pivotal role in most cognitive functions and is strictly linked with inhibitory functions, reasoning and intentional allocation of self-attention (Klingberg, 2010). In particular, spatial working memory improvement exerted by methylphenidate has been associated to a task-related activity refinement in the posterior parietal cortex and dorsolateral prefrontal cortex, especially on the left hemisphere, (Mehta et al., 2000); the former locus seems to relate to online organization and storage of information and the latter to their active manipulation and monitoring. Working memory can be enhanced by training. Several training programs have been developed, for instance computerized training devoted to ADHD children (Klingberg et al., 2005), that showed long-term efficacy (Holmes et al., 2009). Training working memory shapes the brain (Klingberg, 2010) by increasing the activity in the middle frontal gyrus, in the superior and inferior parietal cortices (Olesen et al., 2004) and in the caudate nucleus (Dahlin et al., 2008) and decreasing the number of cortical D1 dopamine receptors (McNab et al., 2009). Training affecting the intraparietal-prefrontal network yields effects that are not modality specific and that can be transferred to any different task requiring working memory (Thorell et al., 2009). Indeed, the positive effect in the retention of instrumental activities of daily-living in older adults produced by cognitive training have been documented even after 5 years from the initial intervention (Willis et al., 2006). The extension of performance improvement to untrained domains has a deep impact in the translation to human cognitive augmentation.

Being brain plasticity the base of cognitive enhancement, training programs specifically designed to target its mechanisms gave very promising results. It has been shown in healthy adults over 60, in whom a training program comprising stimulus recognition, discrimination, sequencing, and memory tasks under strict attentional control, high reward, and novelty has been used to target age-related degraded sensory processing and the down-regulation of neuromodulatory control nuclei. The training produced a memory improvement, which generalized to untrained tasks and was maintained over 3 months (Mahncke et al., 2006). Similar findings were demonstrated in children affected by dyslexia. A program composed by auditory and oral language training produced an increased activity during language processing in the right fronto-temporal regions and anterior cingulate cortex and, similarly to unaffected children, in the left inferior frontal gyrus and left temporo-parietal cortex. Activity in the latter area positively correlated with language recovery (Temple et al., 2003).

Currently, the wide diffusion of computer and videogames-based technology for cognitive training gives the opportunity to proficiently self-train cognitive abilities (Jak et al., 2013). Recently, a multitasking performance training videogame has proved effective in restoring, in elder adults, the same brain activity pattern found in younger controls, with an increase in the midline EEG theta band power over the frontal regions and a higher coherence with the posterior regions. EEG changes predicted the improvement of sustained attention and working memory and their maintenance after 6 months (Anguera et al., 2013).

Meditation, in its various forms, is a kind of mental training with a diverse and long-lasting history, that can be exploited as a strategy for cognitive enhancement (So and Orme-Johnson, 2001). It is able to enhance pre-attentive processes, as evidenced by an increase of the amplitude of auditory mismatch negativity waves (Srinivasan and Baijal, 2007) and of the functional activity of anterior cingulate cortex, prefrontal cortex, hippocampus and insula (Lazar et al., 2000; Farb et al., 2007; Hölzel et al., 2008; Lutz et al., 2008). Indeed, meditation induces short and long-term plasticity. High amplitude gamma-band activity has been described during meditation, especially over the lateral fronto-parietal electrodes, and long-distance phase-synchrony, while resting state EEG shows higher gamma/theta+alpha ratio which burst during meditation and persists after it (Lutz et al., 2004). Several studies demonstrated that meditation is able to induce structural changes especially in the prefrontal cortex, hippocampus and the right anterior insula (Lazar et al., 2005; Pagnoni and Cekic, 2007; Hölzel et al., 2008; Luders et al., 2009). Those areas are involved in the regulation of emotions and in their integration with cognition. Changes have been also evidenced in the brainstem (Vestergaard-Poulsen et al., 2009). Recently, a longitudinal follow-up after 8 weeks of meditation documented an increase of gray matter in the left hippocampus, in the posterior cingulate cortex, the temporo-parietal junction, and in the cerebellum (Hölzel et al., 2011).

Brain activity can be voluntarily modulated to pursue cognitive enhancement with the help of neurofeedback, an operant conditioning paradigm, in which participants exploit a feedback of their brain electrical activity to learn to influence it. Several neurofeedback protocols have been attempted so far. For instance, increase of beta/theta+alpha ratio (Rasey et al., 1995) and increase of sensorimotor (12–15 Hz) rhythm to achieve improvement of working memory and attention (Vernon et al., 2003) or perceptual sensitivity and reduced omission errors (Egner and Gruzelier, 2004), beta rhythm to improve reaction time (Egner and Gruzelier, 2004), increase peak of alpha to improve speed of processing and executive function (Angelakis et al., 2007) and frontal-midline theta activity to improve attention and working memory (Wang and Hsieh, 2013). However, changes of EEG rhythm and improvement of cognitive performance have to be taken with caution: in subject exposed to sham neurofeedback the sole attempt to control a bar, that they believed to be driven by EEG rhythm, produced a wide engagement of fronto-parietal and cingulo-opercular network, which are known to be involved in cognitive control (Ninaus et al., 2013).

Further than with the above mentioned drugs, trainings and strategies, cognitive enhancement can be achieved through external technological support and invasive brain stimulation. For instance, computer based memory aids are interactive diaries that can be embedded in portable or wearable devices and that help patients to remind everyday tasks such as calling a relative or taking a medication (Schulze, 2004). As regard as the stimulation, deep brain stimulation of the septal nucleus (Jiang et al., 1997) and high frequency stimulation of caudate and striatum (Williams and Eskandar, 2006) ameliorate learning and memory in humans and rodents, similarly to vagal nerve stimulation (Clark et al., 1999). Coupled cortical stimulating/recordings arrays can be exploited to trigger and support cortical plasticity (Jackson et al., 2006) and to burst inter-regional functional connectivity at the base of cognitive enhancement, or to substitute lost white matter in demyelinating lesions and subcortical atrophies (Serruya and Kahana, 2008). In theory, cognitive enhancement could, one day, completely rely on external modules. Indeed, artificially interfacing a cortical area with a different one is not very dissimilar from interfacing it with external ectopic (namely located in an abnormal position or environment respecting to the one for which they were originally developed) neural modules. Technology could provide surrogates of cortical or basal ganglia circuitries externally grown *in vitro* (Pfister et al., 2007) or hybrid neuron-chips where neurons grow in a silico support (Zeck and Fromherz, 2001; Serruya and Kahana, 2008).

In conclusion, cognitive enhancement can be achieved through appropriate training strategies and drugs and it mostly relies on plastic processes modulating neurotrasmitters ascending systems and involving the frontoparietal network and, in the case of working memory enhancement, the hippocampus.

CROSS-MODAL PLASTICITY AND SENSORY SUBSTITUTION

Literature on plasticity across the systems has been focused on the investigation of the changes that a disrupted sensory modality evokes on different sensorial networks, as occurring in sensory-deprived animals and humans. However, cross-modal plasticity can be considered as an example of the propensity of some brain areas to manage functions that they have not been originally aimed at.

Reading Braille produces an expansion of the S1 representation of the reading fingers in the blind (Pascual-Leone and Torres, 1993), but in parallel, a task-specific activation of V1 (Sadato et al., 1996), which is critically not present if the hand is used for motor tasks others than Braille reading (Gizewski et al., 2003).

Although basic parameters of spared sensory functions, such as visual contrast sensitivity (Finney and Dobkins, 2001), absolute auditory or tactile threshold (Niemeyer and Starlinger, 1981) may not be affected, cross-modal plasticity results in more complex behavioral advantages, as in the case of blind that process sounds faster and better and have enhanced tactile accuracy (Roder and Neville, 2003). This sustains the localization of this plasticity to be primarily in associative cortices. In this line, functional neuroimaging studies documented an increased recruitment of posterior superior temporal sulcus and inferior parietal lobe in the processing of stimuli processed by spared senses in the blind (Büchel et al., 1998) and deaf (Bavelier et al., 2001). However, even primary sensory areas are targets of cross-modal plasticity and in animals the artificial transposition of fibers from the retina to S1 makes S1 responding to light stimulation (Métin and Frost, 1989), while disruptive transcranial magnetic stimulation (TMS) targeting V1 cortex impairs a tactile discrimination task in blind humans (Cohen et al., 1997).

To understand the impact of cross-modal plasticity in augmentation, a first question is whether cross-modal plasticity is active only in response to brain damage or sensory deprivation. Intracortical invasive recordings in animals documented activity in V1 evoked by non-visual stimuli also in non-deprived animals (Murata et al., 1965) and tactile stimulation enhance V1 activity of healthy subjects (Macaluso et al., 2000), thus raising the intriguing possibility that even primary sensory cortices, in physiological conditions, are not completely unimodal. Indeed data support the idea of the existence of heteromodal connection between primary sensory cortices, as found between primary visual and somatosensory cortices in the monkey. Furthermore, connections between primary sensory areas through multisensory cortices may provide feedback projections that may enhance the response to a stimulus presented in one sensory modality when a spatially-temporally congruent stimulus is delivered in a different sensory modality (Macaluso and Maravita, 2010).

The mechanisms at play during cross-modal plasticity are likely the same of intra-modal plasticity and involve changes in local connectivity that warrant for the rearrangements of sensory maps, stabilization of transient long-range connections during development and changes in cortico-cortical feedback (Bavelier and Neville, 2002) and are mostly driven by activity-dependent inputs competition. Those changes are easier during childhood, but still possible along the adult life and may be the consequences of plasticity of subcortical structures, as in the thalamus and/or brainstem nuclei (Jones and Pons, 1998). Cortical feedback exerts also an important role in determining cross-modal changes, involving direct long range connections between primary sensory areas or connections through associative cortices, in line with the finding of enhanced fMRI connectivity between visual and parietal areas in deaf individuals (Bavelier et al., 2000).

Taking together the premises that sensory brain areas that are classically considered unimodal may be not strictly unimodal and that the mechanisms behind cross-modal plasticity are mostly the same at the base of intra-modal plasticity, would raise the hypothesis that the main determinants of plasticity are the features of the experienced stimulus, its timing along the development of the nervous system and the neurobiological features of the targeted system (Bavelier and Neville, 2002). This would happen mostly independently from any a priori restriction related to the modality of the stimulus, allowing therefore to easily conceive, and practically achieve, an artificial heteromodal sensory substitution.

It deserves to be mentioned that cross-modal plasticity could, in some circumstances, be detrimental for sensory-replacement implants, because it sustains a rewiring of the target orphan cortex from areas controlling other modalities, that could compete with inputs coming from the implant (Lee et al., 2001).

Little evidence sustains so far that also the motor system can undergo changes prompted by the incorporation of functions of different modalities: for instance motor cortex representation of the reading fingers is enhanced in Braille-readers far more than the extent only ascribable to its mere increased use (Pascual-Leone et al., 1993). As far as the effect of multi-modal plasticity induced by the introduction of devices offering new motor efferences, it would be extremely interesting to look at widespread brain plastic modifications in primates experiencing the control of a third arm.

Prostheses designed for sensory substitution, rely on cross-modal plasticity where afferences from a sensory modality are employed to guide the accomplishment of tasks that in able-bodied are primarily executed by means of a diverse sense (Bach-y-Rita and W Kercel, 2003). For instance, an electrotactile array laying on the tongue, has been exploited to deliver information coming from two head-mounted accelerometers, in order to stabilize the posture of subjects with bilateral vestibular deficiency (Tyler et al., 2003) or to transfer visual information taken by a camera in blind people (Sampaio et al., 2001).

Direct demonstrations of cross-modal plasticity after training with non-invasive sensory substitution prostheses have been provided. Blind experiencing auditory-to-vision sensory substitution via an ultrasonic echolocation device showed increased occipital cortex activity compared to trained blindfolded sighted control (De Volder et al., 1999), while replacing vision with somesthesis increased the activation of occipital cortex, which correlated with that of posterior parietal cortex (Ptito et al., 2005). Hence, tactile-dependent activation of occipital cortex may occur through feedback projections from multisensory parietal areas.

Heteromodal sensory substitution, relying on cross-modal plasticity, forces the brain towards changes to fulfill the gap between old and new sensory modality. This may involve to fell the replacement as not enough direct and intuitive. An interface able to feedback sensitive information respecting the site and the modality of the cutaneous hand touching and proprioceptive sensations will overcome this issue. We recently demonstrated that the translation of the output of sensors embedded in the prosthesis into patterns of intraneural stimulation allows recognizing shape and stiffness of different objects and consequently choose the appropriate grasp and strength (Raspopovic et al., 2014).

To summarize, cross-modal plasticity has been found to significantly occur in associative areas, such as the parietal cortex, as well as primary sensory areas. Moreover, its occurrence does not only follow compensative mechanisms following brain damage, but may also act as at the basis of sensory substitution.

TOOLS USE INDUCED PLASTICITY

When we think of human augmentation the image that more probably arises is the one of a man, with additional arm-like devices endowed with tools, who operates in hostile or complex environments. Thus, understanding how brain interacts with tools is mandatory to the present paper.

In the late Seventies Gibson defined the concept of affordance of an object or an environment as "a specific combination of the properties of its substance and its surfaces taken with reference to an animal" in Gibson (1977). "It implies the complementarity of the animal and the environment" (Gibson, 1986). The very external appearance of the tool suggest its unique role in enhancing man-environment relationship: one end of the tool is typically, devoted to the interaction with humans and defines their affordance (i.e., the handle of the hammer) and the other is designed for the interaction with the environment (i.e., the weighted head of the hammer).

Critically, the brain encodes different aspects of the tool, from its more perceptual features to its conceptual meaning and its motor feature. Early knowledge on the cognitive representation of the use of tools in the human brain, and on the putative underlying brain areas, comes from reports of patients affected by brain lesions and suffering from apraxia (Goldenberg, 2003), while only more recently functional imaging studies allowed to infer those processes in healthy subjects (Moll et al., 2000). Moreover, much has been inferred capitalizing on findings from non-human primates. However, humans and monkeys exhibit interspecific differences in the way that their brain deals with tools. In monkey, the mirror neuron system, activated when the animal observes an action performed with the hand, is activated very weakly if the same action is performed through a pincer (Gallese et al., 1996). Visuomotor neurons of premotor area F5 are activated by the visual presentation of a specific tool, or by a subclass of objects, and probably code the motor features of the object (Murata et al., 1997). Visual features of the objects are instead coded by the inferior parietal lobe (Shikata et al., 1996) and in the anterior intraparietal area (Murata et al., 2000). Peculiarly in humans, but not in monkey, the inferior parietal lobule, and in particular the anterior supramarginal gyrus, seems to take part in this network by associating the function of the tool with the required action of the hand (Peeters et al., 2009). Human premotor cortex seems instead to host category-specific representation of tools (Perani et al., 1995), probably as a consequence of the precocious exposition to tools during human motor development.

Either observing, performing or only imagining a task recruits different regions when this is done by means of a tool. A task performed with a tool activates the ipsilateral intraparietal sulcus to a greater extent than the same task performed with the hands (Inoue et al., 2001). Furthermore, the imagination of grasping with tools is accompanied by specific activation of premotor and parietal cortices as well as middle temporal and fusiform gyri (Creem-Regehr and Lee, 2005). In humans, observation of tool use produces a suppression of 20 Hz magnetoencephalographic activity, an hallmark of bilateral primary motor cortex function, which is stronger if the tool is involved in goal-directed actions and if the subject is familiar with the use of that specific tool (Järveläinen et al., 2004).

The neural substrates for the representation of the conceptual knowledge of tools, the ones affected in conceptual or ideational apraxia, are different from the ones hosting the representation of dexterous tool use, affected instead in ideomotor apraxia. Both of them are mainly represented in partially dissociable neural networks, primarily of the left hemisphere (Johnson-Frey, 2004), even in left-handed subjects (Lausberg et al., 1999) and converge in the premotor and parietal areas where the conceptual knowledge of the tool is coupled with the motor program to operate it. Key areas of the tool conceptual knowledge network are the fusiform and the middle temporal gyrus, middle and inferior gyrus, and ventral premotor cortex of the frontal lobe, while dorsal premotor cortex, anterior supramarginal gyrus and intraparietal sulcus of the parietal lobe are activated only if conceptual knowledge is mediated by attention. The network dealing with the motor representation of tools comprises the dorsal premotor and middle frontal gyrus plus the posterior parietal cortex and the intraparietal sulcus (Johnson-Frey, 2004).

Cortical structural changes induced by learning to use a tool can take place rapidly. Learning to retrieve food with a rake in a monkey naive for any tool use produced after only 2 weeks a gray matter increase in the superior temporal sulcus, and in the intraparietal sulcus and bilaterally in white matter underlying the cerebellar cortex (Quallo et al., 2009). On a similar token, gene expression was induced while macaque monkeys learned to use a rake. In particular, during the 2 week period necessary for the acquisition of skillful tool use, but not after the learning phase, an increased level of BDNF and its cellular receptors was found in the anterior bank of intraparietal sulcus, witnessing a learning-induced gene expression, which was linked to the reorganization of visuo-tactile integration in parietal cortex following tool use (Ishibashi et al., 2002).

Finally, as in the case of sensory-motor plasticity reviewed above, the pattern of brain recruitment seems to be specific for a given tool and dependent on previous experience. Imagination of tasks performed with a familiar tool, i.e., a tennis racquet in experienced tennis players, produces a facilitation of corticospinal fibers devoted to the muscles needed to operate the tool, which become more excitable. This process does not take place if the subject imagines motor tasks involving similar tools, either a tennis table-paddle or a golf club, or if the subject is an athlete but not an expert tennis player (Fourkas et al., 2008).

Overall, the above reviewed evidence, speaks in favor of a large representation of tool-use in the cortex. Such representation critically depends upon the conceptual categorization of the tool, its motor mechanics and, importantly, the motor goal that it allows to reach. Such a reach coding of tools and tool-mediated actions is particularly important when it comes to include in the brain representation external augmentation devices. The brain is in facts ready to code for the more conceptual, to the more perceptual and motor features of the newly acquired device for optimal performance.

PLASTICITY INDUCED BY ARTIFACT EMBODIMENT

The expansion of the possible interaction between the organism and the environment has been ascribed to the use of tools, while the settlement of the boundary has been ascribed to its practice (Smitsman, 1997). In absence of tools, the part of space where the subject is able to act through his hands and limbs without locomotion, namely the peripersonal space, is coded by dedicated neural structures in the primate brain. A particular relevant role is exerted by visuotactile neurons located in the frontal area 6 and in the inferior parietal lobule (Fogassi et al., 1996). The visual receptive fields of some of those bimodal neurons are arm-centered (Graziano et al., 1994) and surprisingly, following repetitive reaching tasks performed with a rake, increase to cover the expanded range of action of the hand wielding the rake, or increase to encompass the whole length of the tool (Iriki et al., 1996). This seminal finding demonstrated that the human body schema, a mainly unconscious representation of the body arising from the integration of sensory afferences, is not rigid, but maintains a certain plastic flexibility and by integrating sensorimotor inputs (Maravita et al., 2003) can be modulated to embed a tool. Several behavioral data document that how the brain computes tool-use has much more in common with the control of the hands themselves, than that of other objects. Crossing tools affects performance as crossing hands does by producing similar cross-modal interferences and reaching tasks performed with tools are affected in patients with neglect as much as are tasks performed with hands, while, for instance, are spared tasks with pointing devices (Maravita and Iriki, 2004). Moreover a training performed with a grabber extending the range of action, alters the kinematics of subsequent free-hand grasping movements, also reshapes the sensory representation of the arm, inducing subject to localize touch more distally then where it is actually delivered (Cardinali et al., 2009).

Further than body-space interactions, also the sense of ownership towards external objects may be modulated through experience and external interventions (**Figure 1**). The rubber hand illusion is a striking example of how our body image can be tricked to embody a replica of a body segment. The vision of a fake hand stroked with a paintbrush synchronously with the stroking of the hidden real hand induces a sense of ownership of the rubber hand and a proprioceptive drift of the perceived position of the real hand towards the fake one (Botvinick and Cohen, 1998; **Figure 1A**). This process seems to be based on a Bayesian bottom-up integration of convergent multisensory inputs that determines what, within the peripersonal space, belongs to our body (Armel and Ramachandran, 2003) and may involve the activity of multimodal neurons that are activated by proprioceptive, tactile and visual inputs presented in spatial and temporal congruency (Makin et al., 2008). Those neurons have been extensively investigated in non-human primates (Graziano et al., 1994; Fogassi et al., 1996) and their presence has been also documented in humans (Bremmer et al., 2001).

In humans, the rubber hand illusion has been found to activate areas in the premotor cortex (Ehrsson et al., 2004) in the posterior parietal cortex (Ehrsson et al., 2005). Specifically to the mechanisms underlying the illusion, while somatosensory cortex was activated by the rubber-hand situations (comprising asynchronous visuo-tactile stimulation) not inducing embodiment (as assessed by the proprioceptive drift), the occurrence of the RHI was linked to the activation of the posterior insula and frontal operculum (Tsakiris et al., 2007). According to such a different brain substrate, proprioceptive drift and illusory sense of ownership for the rubber hand have been often found to have a low level of correlation (e.g., see Makin et al., 2008; Tsakiris, 2010; Rohde et al., 2011). In particular, the remapping of self body part to the position of an alien hand in external space would include premotor cortex, for the sense of ownership aspect, and the posterior parietal cortex for the monitoring of limb position (Brozzoli et al., 2012). Strikingly, the sense of ownership can be extended even to an empty portion of peripersonal space, thus literally expanding the boundaries of the self, following spatially and temporally congruent visual-proprioceptive signals activating a premotor-intraparietal neural substrate (Guterstam et al., 2013). Finally, brain damage affecting subcortical structures disrupting fronto-parietal connections, may lead to the loss of contralesonal or ipsilesional sensitivity to the RHI (Zeller et al., 2011).

The level of gamma band synchrony over the parietal regions (Kanayama et al., 2009) and a medial shift of the hand representation have also been associated with the strength of the illusion (Schaefer et al., 2009).

When a protocol of repetitive transcranial brain stimulation producing inhibitory effect is delivered over the inferior parietal lobule, it impairs the perceptual component of the illusion, but not the action-oriented component (Kammers et al., 2009), while stroke patients with damage in the white matter connected with prefrontal, premotor and parietal areas have a consistently higher odd to be unable to experience this illusion (Zeller et al., 2011).

However, subjects tested with the rubber hand illusion may experience that the fake hand substitutes their own (Lewis and Lloyd, 2010; Tsakiris et al., 2010) and a sense of disownership toward the real hand (Guterstam et al., 2011). Thus, since the paradigm of augmentation involves the presence of extra-effectors that are controlled in parallel with one's own limbs, an open question is to what extend the brain may show the ability to host a vivid representation of an extra-limb, while preserving that of the physiological ones.

The mirror box illusion was initially developed to give to amputees a normal, though artificial, visual feedback of their lost limb by reflecting the controlateral healthy one in a mirror. This has been shown to readdress amputees' aberrant brain plasticity and improve their phantom limb pain (Ramachandran et al., 1995; Ramachandran and Altschuler, 2009). However, also healthy subjects can be induce to feel the sense of ownership for the reflected image by hiding their intact limb inside the mirror box (**Figure 1B**; Romano et al., 2013).

Reports of humans that, mostly affected by brain lesions located to the right hemisphere, perceive a supernumerary limb in the controlesional side (Halligan and Marshall, 1995) seem to support this possibility. More recently, few modified rubber

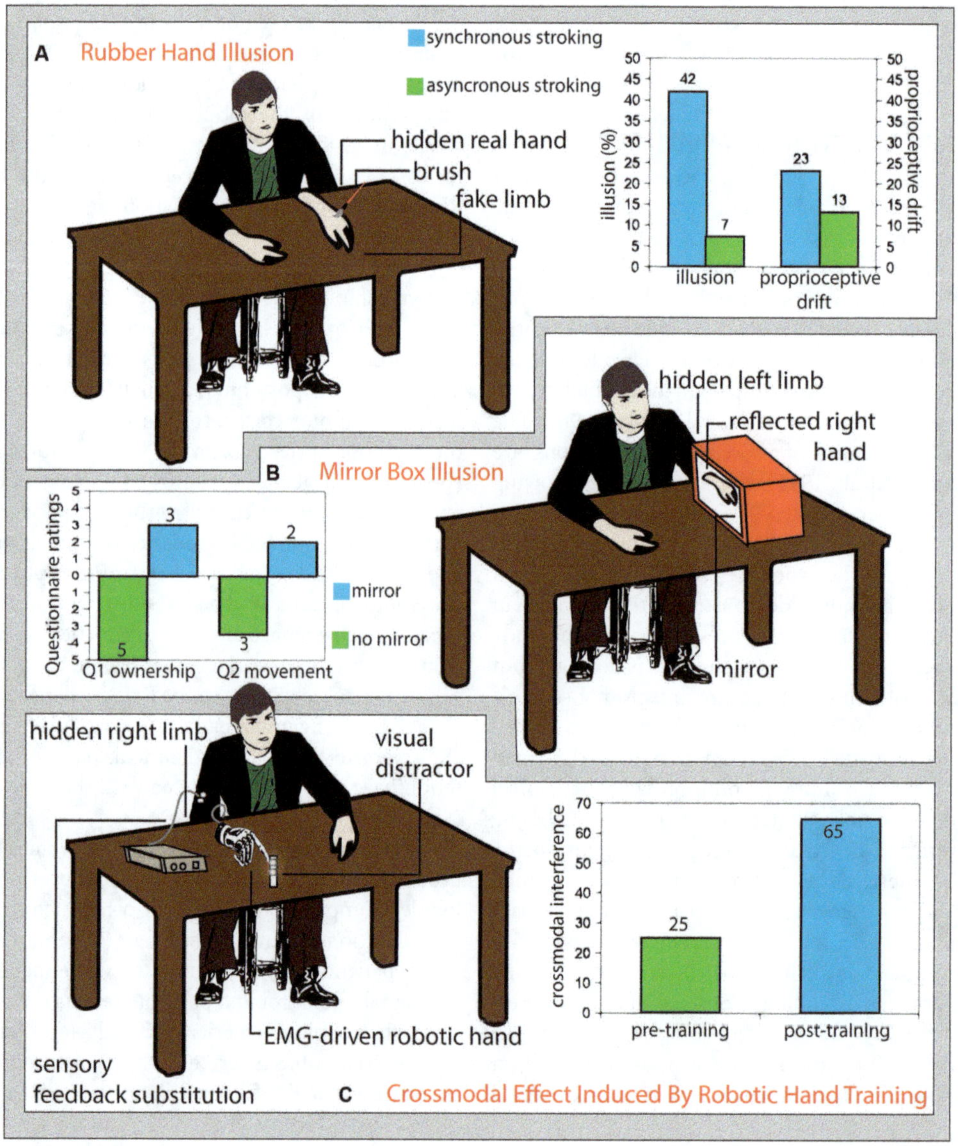

FIGURE 1 | (A) Rubber hand illusion. Participants sit in front of a table with their left hand hidden under the table and a fake limb (white detached arm in figure) placed on the table in front of them. If the fake limb is visibly stroked (schematic red brush in figure) together with the real limb (not visible), participants experience the illusion that the touch is referred to the fake limb (illusion) and that their real limb posture shits toward the fake limb (proprioceptive drift). The size of such effects is greater if the touches on the real and fake limb are delivered synchronously (right panel, light blue columns) than asynchronous (right panel, green columns) (Redrawn from the original data of: Botvinick and Cohen, 1998). **(B)** Mirror box illusion. Participant execute right-hand movements while the left arm is hidden from view and kept still inside a box, the right wall of which is replaced by a mirror (Ramachandran et al., 1995). As compared with a no-mirror condition (left panel, green columns), the mirror reflection of the right hand mimics the movements of the left hand inside the mirror box, biasing the participants feeling (assessed through a questionnaire) of ownership (Question 1: "The reflection in the mirror looks like the hand behind the mirror", left panel, left light blue column) and inducing the illusion of apparent movement (or a true, involuntary, unconscious movement) of the hand inside the box (Question 2: It seems as though the hand behind the mirror is moving; left panel right light blue column) (Romano et al., 2013). **(C)** Crossmodal effects induced by robotic hand training. Prolonged use of an electromyography-driven, detached robot hand (drawn in gray on the right side of the table) providing sensory feedback referred to the participant's arm (white circles), increased the interference from visual distracter leds located near the robot hand fingers (reddish shadowed circles) tested with the crossmodal congruency paradigm (right panel, light blue columns), as compared to the pre-training assessment (right panel, green columns). This pattern of results suggests a training-dependent expansion of crossmodal integration properties, typical of the peripersonal space near the body, to the space surrounding the robot hand (Marini et al., 2014).

hand paradigms documented the embodiment of supernumerary limbs, being them two rubber hands for which the subject proved increased protective autonomic response (Ehrsson, 2009) or two virtual copies of the subject real hand (Newport et al., 2010). In the latter case, subjects integrated the perception of both hands into the body image, but were able to control the movement of only one of them, as if only that limb fully integrated in the body representation for action. Incongruence between efferent and proprioceptive signals and between body image and body schema may sustain the possibility to feel a sense of ownership for both the real and the supernumerary limb (Giummarra et al., 2008). Indeed, aberrant plastic modifications of the hand cortical representation that are common in the amputees' brain (Ramachandran et al., 1992; Flor et al., 1995; Pascual-Leone et al., 1996; Di Pino et al., 2009), not only still allow amputees to experience the rubber hand illusion (Ehrsson et al., 2008), but also to easily embody more than one fake limb at a time (Giummarra et al., 2011). An explanation advanced for this surprising phenomenon is that, in front of multiple, anatomically plausible limbs, the nervous system gradually assigns an equal probability that own limbs may be located at one of the different locations where the fake limbs are, due to multisensory integration (Guterstam et al., 2011).

Which features have to be implemented in the artificial limb to facilitate the process of its embodiment? The level of anthropomorphism of the artifact seems to be a key factor. In front of several objects only realistic prosthetic hands generated strong illusions (Tsakiris et al., 2010), which is prevented by rotating the hand into anatomically implausible postures (Ehrsson et al., 2004). Also proprioceptive afferences play a pivotal role and synchronous active movements of both the real and the fake hand make the embodiment stronger (Tsakiris et al., 2006). Furthermore, the embodiment of virtual hands providing realistic visual input (Slater et al., 2008; Newport et al., 2010).

The embodiment of the supernumerary artificial limb seems like the counterpart of deficit shown by brain-damaged patients who fail to recognize the ownership of their own limbs, attributing them to someone else, and even failing to show anticipatory responses to threatening incoming stimuli (Romano et al., 2014). To the same token, the inclusion of an alien limb in the patient's body representation could provide several advantages that go well beyond the mere improvement of motor control, including an extend sense of protection against forthcoming threats to the artifact. Indeed, it has been shown that, once a rubber hand is embodied, its threatening induces the activation of the insula and the anterior cingulate cortex that is due to interoception and anxiety, together with a motor activation that reflects the replay of the motor properties of the lost limb. Activity in these regions correlates with the level of embodiment (Ehrsson et al., 2007).

Recently, intracortical recordings in primates have revealed that S1 and M1 are involved in the plastic processes responsible for the embodiment of a virtual hand. The time delay of those responses was compatible with an indirect activation of primary sensorimotor areas by visual cortices, probably trough the fronto-parietal cortical circuitry (Shokur et al., 2013).

In order the rubber hand illusion to arise, congruent tactile and visual afferences are needed. Hence, it is plausible to suppose that to enrich the user experience of prosthesis control with a sensory feedback could be a main determinant to prompt the embodiment of prosthetic limbs. Whole nerve electrical stimulation (Mulvey et al., 2012) and vibrotactile stimulation (brushstroke or stick tapping) (D'Alonzo and Cipriani, 2012) of the real hand are able to substitute a real touch in the processes needed to evoke the rubber hand illusion. A pressure stimulator that translated the data acquired by a load cell mounted on a prosthesis into tactile stimulation of the skin reinnervated with nerves originally devoted to the lost hand was able to evoke the rubber hand illusion for a prosthetic device in patients undergoing target muscle reinnervation (Marasco et al., 2011). Moreover, as it happens for the real hands, the embodiment of the prosthesis should produce a cross-modal integration of tactile afferences with visual stimuli coming from the surroundings of the prosthesis, in order to ameliorate manipulation and sensory anticipation of stimuli in its surrounding environment. In healthy participants, long-term use of an electromyographic signal-driven detached robotic hand, able to provide substitutionary sensory feedback from its fingers via vibrotactile stimulation, produces a pattern of visuo-tactile interference from visual stimuli close to the prosthesis fingers, over tactile stimuli referred to the same fingers, in the cross-modal congruency effect, as typically shown when testing the real hand (**Figure 1C**; Marini et al., 2014).

However, a lesson learned from the rubber hand illusion is that, further than its intuitive consequences in a more dexterous control of the prosthesis, the more the afferent feedback from a prosthesis is veridical and close to normal physiology, the more the eventual embodiment of the artifact is likely. This has strong implications for the strategy to adopt for prosthesis-user interfacing.

Finally, the integration of neuroprostheses into the dynamic body image of the users, would likely change the body representation in a proficient, but also unnatural way, giving rise to a potential side effect of the prosthesis (Dobkin, 2007). Indeed, the risk of the arising of perceptual distortions of the body image could produce also detrimental effects due to the possible mismatch between the mental body image and the physical body. For example, psychological/psychiatric symptoms may occur, similar to those suffered by teens affected by body dysmorphic disorders, with consequent severe emotional distress, anxiety and depression or to those reported in the body integrity identity disorders or even somatoparaphrenia, where the subject reports extreme discomfort for a body segment that he feel as not belonging to him (Blom et al., 2012; Romano et al., 2014).

PLASTICITY INDUCED BY THE FUNCTIONAL REPLACEMENT OF MOTOR OUTPUT

Amputation is a straightforward model of deprivation-dependent plasticity and the consequences of the use of prostheses may be taken as a model of brain reorganization following the replacement of sensation and motor output. The interruption of incoming and outgoing flow between the lost segment and the brain triggers, in amputees, a plastic rearrangement of pathways and relays, especially in the cortical sensorimotor representation (Ramachandran et al., 1992; Pascual-Leone et al., 1996). The neural underpinning of phantom limb pain has been primarily ascribed to such an aberrant cortical reorganization (Flor et al., 1995). Long-term use of myoelectric (Lotze et al., 1999) or even body-powered (Weiss et al., 1999) prostheses somehow reduces the maladaptive cortical reorganization and the associated phantom limb pain. The right ventral premotor cortex is strongly activated during the control of an EMG-guided prosthesis, while the right posterior parietal cortex activation may underlie its perceptual assimilation in the body schema (Maruishi et al., 2004).

However, interfacing systems relying on the contraction of far spared muscles transmitted through hidden pulleys and cables or superficial electromyographic sensors, may be inadequate for the control of novel multifingered sensorized prostheses and to effectively readdress the aberrant plasticity. To this aim invasive multicontact electrodes have been developed to be implanted in the peripheral nerves (Navarro et al., 2005) and to reopen a bunch of input/output channels directly toward the nervous system of amputees (Micera et al., 2009, 2010). The surgery needed to implant the electrodes, if performed by experts respecting few restrictions, could be considered a low-risk procedure (Di Pino et al., 2013), that may be eventually available in the near future also for healthy people aiming at augmentation.

In parallel with the anthropomorphism and the manipulative skills own by the prosthesis, a key factor that plays a major role in driving the brain reshaping accompanying the employment of a motor substitution device is the achievement of proper solutions for effective and natural bidirectional human–machine interfacing (Di Pino et al., 2009). Indeed, the training for the control of an anthropomorphic dexterous robotic hand interfaced with intraneural multielectrodes with the forearm nerves of the user, induced consistent reversion of the amputation-induced aberrant cortical plasticity. In particular, it can unmask the motor cortical representation of the lost hand (Rossini et al., 2010) and normalize the EEG activation pattern during movement of the phantom hand (Tombini et al., 2012), the functional interhemispheric interaction (Di Pino et al., 2012c) and the cortico-cortical functional connectivity (Ferreri et al., 2014). Those plastic changes are accompanied by a modulation of patient body image, who referred the reshaping of the perceived phantom of the lost limb, now resembling more closely the healthy real arm, and an improvement of his phantom limb pain (Di Pino et al., 2012a,b).

Also targeted muscle reinnervation, the relocation of sensory and motors nerve fibers once devoted to the missing hand toward spared muscles above the line of amputation, could represent a good solution for human–machine interfacing devoted to prosthesis control (Kuiken et al., 2007). Indeed, in amputees this solution results in the return of motor task execution that reversed the previous shift of lost limb cortical motor representation (Chen et al., 2013).

The readdressing of aberrant cortical changes described so far well matches those produced by the transplantation of biological functional body parts. Recovered intracortical and corticospinal excitability was found in patients undergoing toe-to-thumb transfer for their lost thumb (Ni et al., 2010) or for the correct relocation of the functional sensorimotor representation of the grafted hands in bilateral amputees who underwent transplantation of both hands (Giraux et al., 2001). Reacquiring a lost or a new motor output drives brain plasticity also in case of central nervous system damage. Indeed, stroke patients exploiting a mu rhythm-driven magnetoencephalographic brain computer interface (BCI) to operate an orthesis controlling their paretic hand improved their ability to modulate mu rhythm (Buch et al., 2008).

Therefore, the evidence is in favor of a normalization of the aberrant motor cortical plasticity pushed by the reacquisition of a viable motor efference: The more the regained output resembles the previous physiologic condition, the more the normalization of cortical plasticity.

AUGMENTATION-INDUCED PLASTICITY

Although strictly inherent to human augmentation, the evidence on the evolution of neural plastic processes reviewed so far, is mainly inferred from parallel knowledge acquired from logically related paradigms. From now on, we will focus our discussion on the brain mechanisms that lie behind enhancing able-bodied ability. Augmentation is achieved through BMI, invasive or not, as well as with more traditional devices such as haptic manipulators and vibrotactile stimulators.

Humans have been shown able to acquire new, not-previously experienced, sensory modalities that are instead typical of other animal species. Vibrotactile stimulation can deliver inputs through gyroscopes, accelerometers and magnetometers-embedded in a belt, to be used for space orientation, (Nagel et al., 2005) or for "whisking" through an ad-hoc developed artificial whisker (Saig et al., 2010). Devices for haptic augmented reality are based on the same rationale. Artificial sensors mounted on a fingernail (Ando et al., 2002), on a pen-like tool (Nojima et al., 2002) or directly on an artificial skin layer (Kajimoto et al., 2003) extract from the environment visual information that a tactile display converts mostly into vibrations. A proficient interaction with those devices primarily relies on cross-modal plasticity in the user's brain. They have been designed to touch the untouchable and can find, for instance, in the enhancement of manipulative skills inside particular surgical theaters their operating field. Surgery under microscope and through robotic effectors can be considered a sort of human augmented scenario, as shown by the ability of transfer to the surgical tool, even a virtual one, multisensory integration properties that are proper of the body itself (Sengül et al., 2012). In humans exposed to an augmented task, the features of the tool adopted for functional augmentation influence the activation pattern of the brain. Indeed, surgeons involved in a laparoscopic procedure manifested higher intrahemispheric sensorimotor EEG coherence, probably because operating straight instruments in a bi-dimensional view requests an enhanced activation of primary and high-order areas. Surgeons performing the same task with the da Vinci® robotic surgical system, which offers more dexterous surgical instruments (EndoWrist) articulated like a wrist in a tridimensional view, had instead higher interhemispheric coherence and a more robust alpha and beta activity, perhaps underlying the enhanced exploitation of bimanuality accomplishing robotic-aided surgery (Bocci et al., 2013).

Proves of the acquisition of unnatural new sensory modalities through invasive brain machine interfaces have been documented in rodents. Rats reorganized their foraging behavior in function of infrared cues sensed by an IR detector directly interfaced with their barrel cortex. Here again, cross-modal plasticity demonstrated to be the key of sensory augmentation. Remarkably, as previously described for the artificial transposition of retinal afferences to S1 that makes S1 responding to light (Métin and Frost, 1989), S1 neurons developed bimodal tactile-IR receptive fields. Unfortunately, it is impossible to disentangle if new inputs were perceived by rats as unnatural stimuli coming from the whiskers or as stimuli arising from a brand new sensory modality (Thomson et al., 2013).

Human augmentation realized some of its best potentialities, also starting to attract a wide attention from non-specialists since brain to machine interfaces have been employed to control artificial limbs, assistive grabbers or wheelchairs. Brain-machine (or computer) interfaces are intrinsic promoters of brain plasticity by forcing an unnatural function of cortical neurons that, instead of modulating the inferior spinal motor neuron, start to be the final nervous element of the motor output chain (Wolpaw, 2007). Moreover, brain machine interfaces give to users the opportunity to have a novel feedback of their brain activity, namely neurofeedback, which would be otherwise unavailable. Such a new form of awareness is a further determinant of brain plastic processes (Dobkin, 2007). The more the feedback on the state of the brain is given in an optimal modality and relayed with good accuracy and delay, the more it is able to support the process of reorganization (Grosse-Wentrup et al., 2011).

The execution of actions through brain machine interface is intentional and goal-directed, since those actions are learned worse if the action-reward contingency is altered or the weight of the reward is reduced (Koralek et al., 2012).

Controlling the output of a BCI, although the controlled task has not prevalent motor features, such as in the case of the control of a visual cursor or the modulation of the pitch of an auditory cursor, seems to be resolved by the brain similarly to a motor task. In this line, the achievement of proficiency is not dissimilar to the one involved in motor skills learning with an initial fast improvement of performance and a later phase of slower learning. In epileptic patients undergoing electrocorticography-monitoring, the control of a one degree-of-freedom BCI by volitional modulation of high gamma band produced a diffuse cortical activation, especially sensorimotor and visuomotor areas. The refinement of performance, achieved through the training, corresponded to a focalization of cortical recruitment, akin to what often seen following motor non-BMI training (Kelly and Garavan, 2005), with a decrement of activity in prefrontal, premotor and parietal cortex, probably due to the shift from a fully cognitive towards a more automatic control of the task (Wander et al., 2013). In a similar paradigm, an increase in non REM spindles has been reported, which witness a facilitation of synaptic plasticity (Johnson et al., 2012). Improvement of BMI control is strongly sustained by an increased striatal to M1 functional coupling (enhanced lower band coherence) and increased firing rate of the cortical-striatal projection. It is based on LTP-dependent plasticity, since mice with defective NMDA striatal receptors exhibit impaired ability to refine their performance (Koralek et al., 2012). The finding of a very similar enhancement of cortico-striatal functional coupling in normal subjects who learn to response with the most appropriate motor behavior to given visual stimuli (Toni et al., 2002) strongly supports the neural correlate correspondence of learning tasks executed exploiting physiological motor outputs or BMI.

A key issue explored in the present paper is whether the brain expand its motor control to a supernumerary limb. In monkeys, several studies documented the ability of the brain to control supernumerary, artificial limbs. Monkey implanted in their primary motor cortex were able to control a 5 degrees of freedom actuated arm for self-feeding, while their own real hand was restrained (Velliste et al., 2008). In a previous study, a significant performance decrease took place when the monkey independently used its own hand (Carmena et al., 2003). To the best of the authors' knowledge, so far, these findings have not been replicated in humans.

As far as the independency of real and artificial limb control is concerned, cortical motor neurons with augmented outputs, even if still devoted to the control of the natural arm, are able to arrange their activity in order to create what somehow may be considered as the cortical map of the neuroprosthesis. Indeed, in the presence of a constant transformation function of the recorded activity into movement of the external actuator, the learning process results in the formation of a functional neuronal compound, defined by the refinement of tuning parameters such as, preferred directions, mean firing rates and the depth of modulation (Ganguly and Carmena, 2009). The ensemble of neurons controlling the position of a cursor in a 3D space can also plastically adapt its behavior in front of a modification of the transformation function that produces a visuomotor rotation. Both rotated and especially non-rotated units shift their tuning toward the applied perturbation, but rotated units decrease their modulation depth in order to lower their influence on the preferred direction (Jarosiewicz et al., 2008), showing a relative selectivity of response in different subpopulation of neurons. A similar approach, but scaled at the level of entire brain, has been taken by Imamizu and colleagues, that demonstrated an activation of the posterior superior fissure of the cerebellum in subjects relearning to use a computer mouse that underwent a rotational transformation (Imamizu et al., 2000). Learning the use of two mice with alterations of different parameters (rotation and velocity) of their transformation functions activated contiguous, yet different, cerebellar areas (Imamizu et al., 2003). Authors explain cerebellar activity as the result of the formation of a tool-use internal model, a neural process mimicking the input-output flow of tool motor (and probably cognitive) constraints characterizing the interaction.

Amelioration of the intracortical BMI performance also affects the modulation of neuronal firing rate in motor, premotor supplementary motor and parietal regions to a level not directly correlated with the refinement of cursor kinematic. This firing-rate variance showed an inverse *u*-shape trend, increasing in the initial training and decreasing with the acquisition of proficiency, as if it was driven by a progressive reduction of prediction and execution error due, to a progressive refinement of the internal model of the external controlled device (Zacksenhouse et al., 2007). Such a progressive cortical representation of the neuroprosthesis seems to be stable, and ready to use at each new recording session, critical for task accuracy, (since the removal of neurons from the ensemble deeply impairs performance) and resistant to interference since it keeps working even in parallel with the formation of new maps (Ganguly and Carmena, 2009). This body of evidence has enormous implications in favor of the relative stability of the neurons-behavioral links in neuroprosthetic as well as in natural control.

"To resume the section in a few words, controlling external augmenting devices through neural interfaces is resolved by the brain as it does by controlling normal motor output; in particular by building a cortical map of the motor efferences which change its features to achieve, day after day, a more proficient control".

MODULATING AUGMENTATION RELATED PLASTICITY

Along the present manuscript we showed how the propensity of the brain to be plastic can be considered as the fertile soil needed for a proficient implant of new input/output external aid. This implies that any attempt to increase the efficiency of any plastic brain changes or even to redirect them towards the desired direction could result in a more effective blend between the biological and the artificial component of any hybrid bionic system.

In this view, it is known that brain plasticity can be modulated through drugs. Especially noradrenergic agonists have been exploited to enhance M1 excitability (Ziemann et al., 2002), improve motor skill acquisition (Plewnia et al., 2004), learning language (Breitenstein et al., 2004) and in the motor recovery from stroke and other brain lesions (Gladstone and Black, 2000; Schuster et al., 2011). Recently, it has been hypothesized that motor improvement after the administration of amphetamine-like drugs may be due to a better visuomotor integration, with an increased functional coupling between right intraparietal and superior frontal premotor cortex (Grefkes et al., 2010). We already discussed the primary role that the right fronto-parietal circuit plays in augmentation-related plasticity.

Recently, non-invasive neuromodulatory techniques, mostly based on repetitive transcranial magnetic stimulation and transcranial direct current stimulation, have been introduced and showed to effectively inhibit or facilitate the excitability of the motor cortex, possibly through LTP/LTD-like mechanisms (Ziemann et al., 2008). For instance, in humans, transcranial direct current stimulation showed to be able to enhance not only motor skills (Nitsche et al., 2003) and movement speed accuracy (Reis et al., 2009), but also visuomotor coordination (Antal et al., 2004b), learning (Antal et al., 2004a) and frontal functions (Capone et al., 2014). Stimulation of motor cortex has been also successfully used to control chronic neuropatic pain of different etiology, possibly enhancing descending analgesic effects that limit aberrant afferent noxious signals and overall limiting maladaptive plasticity (Andrade et al., 2013; Bolognini et al., 2013a,b). However not invasive neuromodulation can be used also for modulating plasticity of frontal and associative cortices with the aim of cognitive enhancement in the domain of working memory (Andrews et al., 2011; Cantone et al., 2014), problem solution (Chi and Snyder, 2012) and creative intelligence (Cerruti and Schlaug, 2009). Paired associative stimulation is a neuromodulation paradigm that targets specifically sensorimotor integration process by repeating the coupled electrical stimulus to a peripheral nerve and a time-locked TMS pulse to the contralateral M1 (Stefan et al., 2002). Neither paired associative stimulation nor other non-invasive neuromodulatory techniques, perhaps targeting premotor of posterior parietal cortices have been applied, to our knowledge, to attempt to facilitate the embodiment of tools and prostheses. This should definitely deserve our future efforts.

Also less conventional non-invasive brain stimulation can improve augmentation plasticity, as for alpha frequency visual flickering that improves word recall (Williams, 2001). Sleep is a physiological prolonged activity, taking almost a third of our life, when the brain is extremely prone to undergo plastic remodeling especially linked with consolidation of memories (Diekelmann and Born, 2010). A bad sleep is known to negatively impact plastic processes, such as, for instance, those at the base of the recovery from stroke (Zunzunegui et al., 2011). Therefore its modulation could also enhance learning processes related to augmentation. Indeed, it has been shown how sleep-related plasticity can be modulated with transcranial stimulation (Marshall et al., 2006), or simply by delivering external odors (Rasch et al., 2007), with a significant impact on consolidated memory. The tight relation among BCI-related plasticity and sleep is sustained by the local increase of spindles, signs of a cortical state conductive to synaptic plasticity, in subjects trained to control a computer cursor via an electrocorticographic interface (Johnson et al., 2012).

Furthermore, different genetic substrates could have an impact in the individual propensity to be augmented. This can be inferred from the effect of different haplotypes on plasticity related paradigms. Indeed, The Val66Met polymorphism of the brain derived neurotrophic factor, present in about a third of the Caucasian population, has been associated with reduced sensitivity to plasticity-inducing neuromodulation (Cheeran et al., 2008) and with a worse recovery from stroke (Kim et al., 2012). The response of ADHD children to methylphenidate seems to be affected by the Val158Met polymorphism in the Catechol-O-methyltransferase (Kereszturi et al., 2008) and by the genotype of the dopamine transporter (Winsberg and Comings, 1999), which affects also the outcome of working memory training (Brehmer et al., 2009).

Also age-related effect could be taken into consideration as modulating factors for augmentation-related plasticity. Although the rate of enhancement of motor and cognitive ability is maximal at younger ages, when sensorimotor areas express their critical plastic period (Hensch, 2005), there is also evidence that augmentation-related plasticity can take place throughout the entire life span. Plasticity in primary visual (Kaas et al., 1990), auditory (Recanzone et al., 1993) and somatosensory cortices (Merzenich et al., 1984) has been described at later ages and cats deprived of vision during adulthood showed cross-modal improvement of the ability to localize sound, albeit lower than earlier deprived cats do (Rauschecker and Kniepert, 1994).

Finally, can augmentation-related plasticity always be enhanced or it may suffer from ceiling effects that limit the ability to be further augmented? Overtrained athletes can undergo the burnout syndrome (Winsley and Matos, 2011) and excessive use and training can be responsible of aberrant plasticity in sensorimotor areas and in the basal ganglia at the base of the focal dystonia of expert players and musicians (Defazio et al., 2007). There are also reports of ceiling effect in cognitive enhancement (Kwok et al., 2011) and London taxi drivers, whit exceptional navigation ability, acquired worse new spatial memory as if the hyper-representation of posterior hippocampus may undermined new plasticity in the anterior hippocampus (Maguire et al., 2006). However, sometimes improvement can undergo false ceiling effects due to precocious delegation of not yet consolidated functions to brain networks in charge of automaticity (Ericsson, 2007).

CONCLUSION

SUMMARY OF THE EVIDENCE ON AUGMENTING-RELATED PLASTICITY

From the body of literature reviewed in the present paper, a few conclusions can be drawn.

First, augmentation-related plasticity takes place at the cellular level, likely through synaptic signals, as evidenced by changes of gray matter thickness and even with neurogenesis in the dentate gyrus.

Second, a number of brain areas have been identified as likely actors of augmentation-based plasticity, playing a role at different stage of the process (**Figure 2**). The representation of the external world in primary sensory areas is extremely sensitive to activity that modulates their tuning parameters. These cortices are able to accept afferences from different physiological or artificial sensory modalities by shaping the receptive fields of their neurons to make them sensitive to novel kinds of sensory input.

Also M1 is highly susceptible to modulation of cortical representation and corticospinal excitability. The control of neuroprostheses recruits motor and premotor areas, and the acquisition of the skillful use of them promotes the recovery of the cortical representation of a lost limb and its functional interplay with related regions. Training-based skill acquisition gradually decreases attentional recruitment, focusing the activity on sensorimotor areas and increasing the basal ganglia drive of cortical activity. Indeed, the brain can learn to deal with neuroprostheses as it does with normal motor outputs, producing similar learning curves in both conditions.

The frontoparietal network is another functional actor that plays the key role in augmentation-related plasticity. It is strongly recruited in the initial phase of the acquisition of a new motor ability. Premotor cortex is also activated to learn to control an external effector, controls tool motor representation and together with the intraparietal sulcus, which contributes to extracting the visual features of the tool, is the main substrate for artifact embodiment. In these areas, neurons responsible for multisensory integration can be modified to extend their receptive fields and assimilate a supernumerary limb. An anthropomorphic sensorized prosthesis provides the critical sensory afferences needed for a full, comfortable embodiment, and thus optima efficiency, of the artifact. By operating a neuroprosthesis, the brain builds up a cortical representation of the device. This process selectively involves subgroup of interfaced neurons that plastically adapt their firing rate to refine the kinematic parameters and reduce the execution error.

The mirror system of premotor and parietal areas may exert a role in understanding the meaning of an action performed with anthropomorphic augmentation devices and in learning to operate them. Furthermore, plasticity in posterior parietal cortex is responsible also for the assimilation of artificial sensory modalities and for the complex behavioral advantages that from this derive.

Finally, plasticity in the attentional frontoparietal network is the main target of cognitive enhancement, achieved as a corollary effect of sensorimotor augmentation or, selectively, by modulating the neurochemical signals ascending from the brainstem. The hippocampus contributes by undergoing memory-induced changes. The insula and the cerebellum are involved in augmentation-related plasticity too. The cerebellar cortex is activated during the learning of a tool or a neuroprosthesis, contributing to their embodiment; furthermore its activation is related to the formation of an internal model of the external effector. The insula plays a role in the interoception of the embodied artifact and in the relationship of augmented skills with emotions.

FUTURE PERSPECTIVES

The evidence provided in this review, unmasks the ability of the central nervous system of primates and humans, not only to master the use of external tools, but also to plastically reshape the body representation and the very sense of the self in favor of a more affordable sensing, and operating in the environment (Clark, 2007).

Central to the topic of the present review is the integration of any augmentative device in the global sense of the self of the user. Operatively, the sense that conscious experience is bound to the self has been defined to emerge from a series of elements including the feeling of body ownership, the perception of self-location in space and the observation of our own body and outside world according to a first-person perspective (Blanke, 2012). The sense of self can be notably disrupted in pathological conditions affecting a single body part such as somatoparaphrenia (the denial of ownership of contralesional limbs, following brain damage) (Vallar and Ronchi, 2009) or the whole body, such as in the out-of-the-body experience phenomena (Blanke and Mohr, 2005). An experimental modulation of the sense of the self for the whole body has been famously demonstrated using the "full body illusion" procedures, in which participants receive tactile strokes, while seeing their own body, filmed by a camera, receiving synchronous or asynchronous strokes of homologous body regions (back/chest). Following this procedure, a variety of illusions of self-identification with the virtual body (Lenggenhager et al., 2007), with the camera viewpoint (as if looking to an alien body), as well as modulation of sensory experience (Aspell et al., 2009; Romano et al., 2014) have been obtained. Different aspects of corporeal self consciousness have been linked to the activation of different brain structures, including premotor, parietal (somatosensory and IPS), extrastriate (EBA) and putaminal regions, as well as the temporoparietal junction, as the result of a process of multisensory integration involving visual, somatosensory and vestibular input (see Blanke, 2012 for review).

The knowledge acquired on the mechanisms of body ownership and, in general, self identification, may put the basis for understanding how plasticity-induced brain augmentation may contribute to the recovery or the enhancement of the sense of

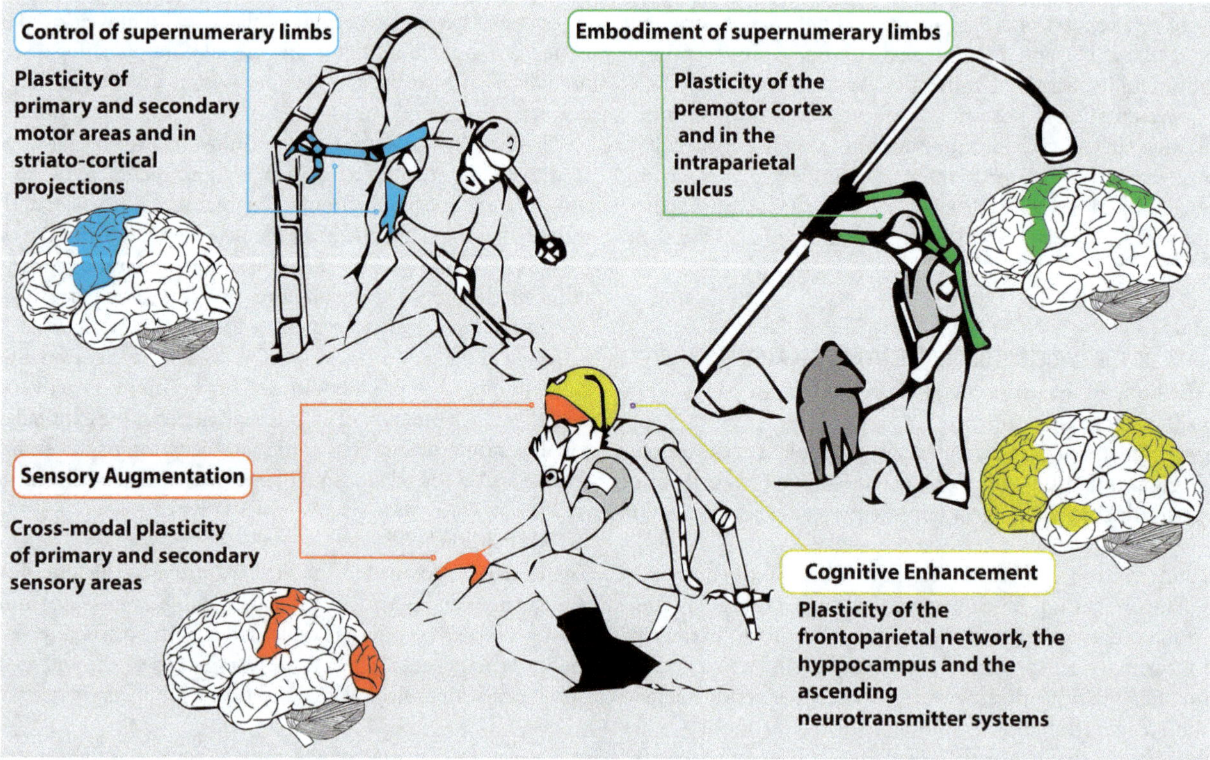

FIGURE 2 | Possible applicative scenario of human augmentation. Rescuers dug through the rubble of collapsed buildings looking for survivors in the wake of an earthquake exploiting artificial supernumerary limbs (light blue and green), artificial organs of sense (red) and cognitive enhancement (yellow). The most relevant areas of the brain recruited by the task are drawn on the side. Control of supernumerary limbs mostly relies on primary and secondary sensorimotor areas and on the facilitation of striato-cortical projection, their embodiment in changes especially taking place in the premotor cortex and in the intraparietal sulcus. Sensory augmentation is enabled by cross-modal plasticity of sensory areas, while cognitive enhancement has in the neural plasticity of the frontoparietal network, of the hippocampus and in the facilitation of the ascending neurotransmitter system its neurobiological substrate.

the self. The more straightforward situation to think about is certainly the case of amputation. As discussed previously, a key role of functional prostheses is to allow the rebuilt of a full sense of ownership and agency of the prosthesis through a process of training-induced, embodiment (Ehrsson et al., 2008; Marasco et al., 2011; D'Alonzo and Cipriani, 2012; Mulvey et al., 2012). In this respect, the plasticity induced by functional prostheses (Di Pino et al., 2009; Rossini et al., 2010; Maruishi et al., 2004), targets similar sensorimotor brain areas as those modulated by paradigms inducing illusory sense of ownership for alien body parts and could constitute the basis of a full inclusion of external devices into the self as well as the extension of visuo-tactile integration properties to an external augmentation device (Marini et al., 2014).

Indeed, the evaluation of whole brain activity, and the monitoring of cortico-cortical connectivity, for instance by means of functional magnetic resonance, in primates undergoing motor output augmentation through BMI, of which literature to the best of authors knowledge is still wanting, would be of utmost value to depict a comprehensive picture of brain processes underlying augmentation. Such studies could be of out-breaking relevance in order to understand the interplay among different brain structures in the buildup of plasticity, as well as for the monitoring of the neural substrates of possible conditions (pain, emotional distress) that may co-occur as severe side effects.

Finally, we saw how the plastic changes resulting from the interaction with external devices are the necessary neural correlates of functional augmentation, of learning new skills and exploiting artificial senses. Plasticity allows evolving the exploitation of tools through their embodiment and it is strongly correlated with how much the interface constituting the hybrid bionic system is direct and intuitive. We thus propose that, in parallel with more classical instruments for performance monitoring, methods for the functional evaluation of the augmentation-related plasticity, can provide reliable and comprehensive measures of the effectiveness achieved by the hybrid bionic system in accomplishing augmentation.

AUTHOR AND CONTRIBUTORS

Giovanni Di Pino chose the topic, conceived the design of the manuscript and wrote the main text. Angelo Maravita was in charge of the sections on tools use and embodiment. Loredana Zollo took care of the section on prostheses. Eugenio Guglielmelli and Vincenzo Di Lazzaro deeply revised the manuscript. All the authors checked and approved the final submitted version of the manuscript.

ACKNOWLEDGMENTS

This work was partially supported by the National Project of the Italian Ministry of Research, PRIN 2010, HANDBOT—Biomechatronic and Prostheses Endowed with Bio-inspired Tactile Perception, Bi-directional Neural Interfaces and Distributed Sensorymotor Control, CUP: B81J12002680008".

REFERENCES

Aglioti, S. M., Cesari, P., Romani, M., and Urgesi, C. (2008). Action anticipation and motor resonance in elite basketball players. *Nat. Neurosci.* 11, 1109–1116. doi: 10.1038/nn.2182

Ambrose, S. H. (2001). Paleolithic technology and human evolution. *Science* 291, 1748–1753. doi: 10.1126/science.1059487

Ando, H., Miki, T., Inami, M., and Maeda, T. (2002). The nail-mounted tactile display for the behavior modeling. Proceedings of the ACM SIGGRAPH 2002. conference abstracts and applications; ACM.

Andrade, D. C., Borges, I., Bravo, G. L., Bolognini, N., and Fregni, F. (2013). Therapeutic time window of noninvasive brain stimulation for pain treatment: inhibition of maladaptive plasticity with early intervention. *Expert Rev. Med. Devices* 10, 339–352. doi: 10.1586/erd.12.90

Andrews, S. C., Hoy, K. E., Enticott, P. G., Daskalakis, Z. J., and Fitzgerald, P. B. (2011). Improving working memory: the effect of combining cognitive activity and anodal transcranial direct current stimulation to the left dorsolateral prefrontal cortex. *Brain Stimul.* 4, 84–89. doi: 10.1016/j.brs.2010.06.004

Angelakis, E., Stathopoulou, S., Frymiare, J. L., Green, D. L., Lubar, J. F., and Kounios, J. (2007). EEG neurofeedback: a brief overview and an example of peak alpha frequency training for cognitive enhancement in the elderly. *Clin. Neuropsychol.* 21, 110–129. doi: 10.1080/13854040600744839

Anguera, J. A., Boccanfuso, J., Rintoul, J. L., Al-Hashimi, O., Faraji, F., Janowich, J., et al. (2013). Video game training enhances cognitive control in older adults. *Nature* 501, 97–101. doi: 10.1038/nature12486

Antal, A., Nitsche, M. A., Kincses, T. Z., Kruse, W., Hoffmann, K. P., and Paulus, W. (2004a). Facilitation of visuo-motor learning by transcranial direct current stimulation of the motor and extrastriate visual areas in humans. *Eur. J. Neurosci.* 19, 2888–2892. doi: 10.1111/j.1460-9568.2004.03367.x

Antal, A., Nitsche, M. A., Kruse, W., Kincses, T. Z., Hoffmann, K.-P., and Paulus, W. (2004b). Direct current stimulation over V5 enhances visuomotor coordination by improving motion perception in humans. *J. Cogn. Neurosci.* 16, 521–527. doi: 10.1162/089892904323057263

Armel, K. C., and Ramachandran, V. S. (2003). Projecting sensations to external objects: evidence from skin conductance response. *Proc. Biol. Sci.* 270, 1499–1506. doi: 10.1098/rspb.2003.2364

Aspell, J. E., Lenggenhager, B., and Blanke, O. (2009). Keeping in touch with one's self: multisensory mechanisms of self-consciousness. *PLoS One* 4:e6488. doi: 10.1371/journal.pone.0006488

Bach-y-Rita, P., and W Kercel, S. (2003). Sensory substitution and the human–machine interface. *Trends Cogn. Sci.* 7, 541–546. doi: 10.1016/j.tics.2003.10.013

Bailey, C. H., and Kandel, E. R. (2008). Synaptic remodeling, synaptic growth and the storage of long-term memory in Aplysia. *Prog. Brain Res.* 169, 179–198. doi: 10.1016/s0079-6123(07)00010-6

Baumeister, J., Reinecke, K., Liesen, H., and Weiss, M. (2008). Cortical activity of skilled performance in a complex sports related motor task. *Eur. J. Appl. Physiol.* 104, 625–631. doi: 10.1007/s00421-008-0811-x

Bavelier, D., Brozinsky, C., Tomann, A., Mitchell, T., Neville, H., and Liu, G. (2001). Impact of early deafness and early exposure to sign language on the cerebral organization for motion processing. *J. Neurosci.* 21, 8931–8942.

Bavelier, D., and Neville, H. J. (2002). Cross-modal plasticity: where and how? *Nat. Rev. Neurosci.* 3, 443–452. doi: 10.1038/nrn848

Bavelier, D., Tomann, A., Hutton, C., Mitchell, T., Corina, D., Liu, G., et al. (2000). Visual attention to the periphery is enhanced in congenitally deaf individuals. *J. Neurosci.* 20, RC93.

Birbaumer, N., and Cohen, L. G. (2007). Brain-computer interfaces: communication and restoration of movement in paralysis. *J. Physiol.* 579, 621–636. doi: 10.1113/jphysiol.2006.125633

Blanke, O. (2012). Multisensory brain mechanisms of bodily self-consciousness. *Nat. Rev. Neurosci.* 13, 556–571. doi: 10.1038/nrn3292

Blanke, O., and Aspell, J. E. (2009). Brain technologies raise unprecedented ethical challenges. *Nature* 458, 703–703. doi: 10.1038/458703b

Blanke, O., and Mohr, C. (2005). Out-of-body experience, heautoscopy, and autoscopic hallucination of neurological origin: implications for neurocognitive mechanisms of corporeal awareness and self-consciousness. *Brain Res. Brain Res. Rev.* 50, 184–199. doi: 10.1016/j.brainresrev.2005.05.008

Bliss, T. V., and Lomo, T. (1973). Long-lasting potentiation of synaptic transmission in the dentate area of the anaesthetized rabbit following stimulation of the perforant path. *J. Physiol.* 232, 331–356.

Blom, R. M., Hennekam, R. C., and Denys, D. (2012). Body integrity identity disorder. *PLoS One* 7:e34702. doi: 10.1371/journal.pone.0034702

Bocci, T., Moretto, C., Tognazzi, S., Briscese, L., Naraci, M., Leocani, L., et al. (2013). How does a surgeon's brain buzz? An EEG coherence study on the interaction between humans and robot. *Behav. Brain Funct.* 9:14. doi: 10.1186/1744-9081-9-14

Bolognini, N., Olgiati, E., Maravita, A., Ferraro, F., and Fregni, F. (2013a). Motor and parietal cortex stimulation for phantom limb pain and sensations. *Pain* 154, 1274–1280. doi: 10.1016/j.pain.2013.03.040

Bolognini, N., Spandri, V., Olgiati, E., Fregni, F., Ferraro, F., and Maravita, A. (2013b). Long-term analgesic effects of transcranial direct current stimulation of the motor cortex on phantom limb and stump pain: a case report. *J. Pain Symptom Manage.* 46, e1–e4. doi: 10.1016/j.jpainsymman.2013.06.014

Bostrom, N., and Sandberg, A. (2009). Cognitive enhancement: methods, ethics, regulatory challenges. *Sci. Eng. Ethics.* 15, 311–341. doi: 10.1007/s11948-009-9142-5

Botvinick, M., and Cohen, J. (1998). Rubber hands "feel" touch that eyes see. *Nature* 391, 756–756. doi: 10.1038/35784

Brehmer, Y., Westerberg, H., Bellander, M., Fürth, D., Karlsson, S., and Bäckman, L. (2009). Working memory plasticity modulated by dopamine transporter genotype. *Neurosci. Lett.* 467, 117–120. doi: 10.1016/j.neulet.2009.10.018

Breitenstein, C., Wailke, S., Bushuven, S., Kamping, S., Zwitserlood, P., Ringelstein, E. B., et al. (2004). D-amphetamine boosts language learning independent of its cardiovascular and motor arousing effects. *Neuropsychopharmacology* 29, 1704–1714. doi: 10.1038/sj.npp.1300464

Bremmer, F., Schlack, A., Shah, N. J., Zafiris, O., Kubischik, M., Hoffmann, K.-P., et al. (2001). Polymodal motion processing in posterior parietal and premotor cortex: a human fMRI study strongly implies equivalencies between humans and monkeys. *Neuron* 29, 287–296. doi: 10.1016/s0896-6273(01)00198-2

Brindley, G. S. (1974). Emptying the bladder by stimulating sacral ventral roots. *J. Physiol.* 237, 15P–16P.

Brozzoli, C., Gentile, G., and Ehrsson, H. H. (2012). That's near my hand! parietal and premotor coding of hand-centered space contributes to localization and self-attribution of the hand. *J. Neurosci.* 32, 14573–14582. doi: 10.1523/jneurosci.2660-12.2012

Buch, E., Weber, C., Cohen, L. G., Braun, C., Dimyan, M. A., Ard, T., et al. (2008). Think to move: a neuromagnetic brain-computer interface (BCI) system for chronic stroke. *Stroke* 39, 910–917. doi: 10.1161/strokeaha.107.505313

Büchel, C., Price, C., Frackowiak, R., and Friston, K. (1998). Different activation patterns in the visual cortex of late and congenitally blind subjects. *Brain* 121, 409–419. doi: 10.1093/brain/121.3.409

Buonomano, D. V., and Merzenich, M. M. (1998). Cortical plasticity: from synapses to maps. *Annu. Rev. Neurosci.* 21, 149–186. doi: 10.1146/annurev.neuro.21.1.149

Cantone, M., Di Pino, G., Capone, F., Piombo, M., Chiarello, D., and Cheeran, B. (2014). The contribution of transcranial magnetic stimulation in the diagnosis and in the management of dementia. *Clin. Neurophysiol.* doi: 10.1016/j.clinph.2014.04.010. [Epub ahead of print].

Capone, F., Capone, G., Ranieri, F., Di Pino, G., Oricchio, G., and Di Lazzaro, V. (2014). The effect of practice on random number generation task: a transcranial direct current stimulation study. *Neurobiol. Learn. Mem.* 114C, 51–57. doi: 10.1016/j.nlm.2014.04.013

Cardinali, L., Frassinetti, F., Brozzoli, C., Urquizar, C., Roy, A. C., and Farnè, A. (2009). Tool-use induces morphological updating of the body schema. *Curr. Biol.* 19, R478–R479. doi: 10.1016/j.cub.2009.05.009

Carmena, J. M., Lebedev, M. A., Crist, R. E., O'Doherty, J. E., Santucci, D. M., Dimitrov, D. F., et al. (2003). Learning to control a brain-machine interface for reaching and grasping by primates. *PLoS Biol.* 1:E42. doi: 10.1371/journal.pbio.0000042

Cerruti, C., and Schlaug, G. (2009). Anodal transcranial direct current stimulation of the prefrontal cortex enhances complex verbal associative thought. *J. Cogn. Neurosci.* 21, 1980–1987. doi: 10.1162/jocn.2008.21143

Cheeran, B., Talelli, P., Mori, F., Koch, G., Suppa, A., Edwards, M., et al. (2008). A common polymorphism in the brain-derived neurotrophic factor gene (BDNF) modulates human cortical plasticity and the response to rTMS. *J. Physiol.* 586, 5717–5725. doi: 10.1113/jphysiol.2008.159905

Chen, A., Yao, J., Kuiken, T., and Dewald, J. P. (2013). Cortical motor activity and reorganization following upper-limb amputation and subsequent targeted reinnervation. *Neuroimage Clin.* 3, 498–506. doi: 10.1016/j.nicl.2013.10.001

Chen, R., Cohen, L. G., and Hallett, M. (2002). Nervous system reorganization following injury. *Neuroscience* 111, 761–773. doi: 10.1016/s0306-4522(02)00025-8

Chi, R. P., and Snyder, A. W. (2012). Brain stimulation enables the solution of an inherently difficult problem. *Neurosci. Lett.* 515, 121–124. doi: 10.1016/j.neulet.2012.03.012

Clark, A. (2007). Re-inventing ourselves: the plasticity of embodiment, sensing and mind. *J. Med. Philos.* 32, 263–282. doi: 10.1080/03605310701397024

Clark, K. B., Naritoku, D. K., Smith, D. C., Browning, R. A., and Jensen, R. A. (1999). Enhanced recognition memory following vagus nerve stimulation in human subjects. *Nat. Neurosci.* 2, 94–98. doi: 10.1038/4600

Cohen, L. G., Celnik, P., Pascual-Leone, A., Corwell, B., Faiz, L., Dambrosia, J., et al. (1997). Functional relevance of cross-modal plasticity in blind humans. *Nature* 389, 180–183. doi: 10.1038/38278

Creem-Regehr, S. H., and Lee, J. N. (2005). Neural representations of graspable objects: are tools special? *Brain Res. Cogn. Brain Res.* 22, 457–469. doi: 10.1016/j.cogbrainres.2004.10.006

D'Alonzo, M., and Cipriani, C. (2012). Vibrotactile sensory substitution elicits feeling of ownership of an alien hand. *PLoS One* 7:e50756. doi: 10.1371/journal.pone.0050756

Dahlin, E., Nyberg, L., Bäckman, L., and Neely, A. S. (2008). Plasticity of executive functioning in young and older adults: immediate training gains, transfer and long-term maintenance. *Psychol. Aging* 23, 720–730. doi: 10.1037/a0014296

Dario, P., Sandini, G., and Aebischer, P. (1993). "Robots and biological systems: towards a new bionics?," in *Proceedings of the NATO Advanced Workshop on Robots and Biological Systems*. Available at http://www.springer.com/computer/ai/book/978-3-540-56158-3

De Volder, A. G., Catalan-Ahumada, M., Robert, A., Bol, A., Labar, D., Coppens, A., et al. (1999). Changes in occipital cortex activity in early blind humans using a sensory substitution device. *Brain Res.* 826, 128–134. doi: 10.1016/s0006-8993(99)01275-5

Defazio, G., Berardelli, A., and Hallett, M. (2007). Do primary adult-onset focal dystonias share aetiological factors? *Brain* 130, 1183–1193. doi: 10.1093/brain/awl355

Di Lazzaro, V., Oliviero, A., Pilato, F., Saturno, E., Dileone, M., Marra, C., et al. (2005). Neurophysiological predictors of long term response to AChE inhibitors in AD patients. *J. Neurol. Neurosurg. Psychiatry* 76, 1064–1069. doi: 10.1136/jnnp.2004.051334

Di Pino, G., Benvenuto, A., Cavallo, G., Denaro, L., Denaro, V., Ferreri, F., et al. (2012a). "In human implant of intraneural multielectrodes for controlling a 5-fingered hand prosthesis and delivering sensorial feedback," in *Grasping the Future: Advances in Powered Upper Limb Prosthetics*, eds V. P. Castelli and M. Troncossi (Beijing, P. R. China: Bentham Science Publishers), 28–38.

Di Pino, G., Benvenuto, A., Tombini, M., Cavallo, G., Denaro, L., Denaro, V., et al. (2012b). Overview of the implant of intraneural multielectrodes in human for controlling a 5-fingered hand prosthesis, delivering sensorial feedback and producing rehabilitative neuroplasticity. Proceedings of the Biomedical Robotics and Biomechatronics (BioRob), 4th IEEE RAS and EMBS International Conference on 2012.

Di Pino, G., Denaro, L., Vadala, G., Marinozzi, A., Tombini, M., Ferreri, F., et al. (2013). Invasive neural interfaces: the perspective of the surgeon. *J. Surg. Res.* 188, 77–87. doi: 10.1016/j.jss.2013.12.014

Di Pino, G., Guglielmelli, E., and Rossini, P. M. (2009). Neuroplasticity in amputees: main implications on bidirectional interfacing of cybernetic hand prostheses. *Prog. Neurobiol.* 88, 114–126. doi: 10.1016/j.pneurobio.2009.03.001

Di Pino, G., Porcaro, C., Tombini, M., Assenza, G., Pellegrino, G., Tecchio, F., et al. (2012c). A neurally-interfaced hand prosthesis tuned inter-hemispheric communication. *Restor. Neurol. Neurosci.* 30, 407–418. doi: 10.3233/RNN-2012-120224

Diekelmann, S., and Born, J. (2010). The memory function of sleep. *Nat. Rev. Neurosci.* 11, 114–126. doi: 10.1038/nrn2762

Dobkin, B. H. (2007). Brain-computer interface technology as a tool to augment plasticity and outcomes for neurological rehabilitation. *J. Physiol.* 579, 637–642. doi: 10.1113/jphysiol.2006.123067

Draganski, B., Gaser, C., Busch, V., Schuierer, G., Bogdahn, U., and May, A. (2004). Neuroplasticity: changes in grey matter induced by training. *Nature* 427, 311–312. doi: 10.1038/427311a

Driemeyer, J., Boyke, J., Gaser, C., Büchel, C., and May, A. (2008). Changes in gray matter induced by learning—revisited. *PLoS One* 3:e2669. doi: 10.1371/journal.pone.0002669

Egner, T., and Gruzelier, J. (2004). EEG biofeedback of low beta band components: frequency-specific effects on variables of attention and event-related brain potentials. *Clin. Neurophysiol.* 115, 131–139. doi: 10.1016/s1388-2457(03)00353-5

Ehrsson, H. H., Holmes, N. P., and Passingham, R. E. (2005). Touching a rubber hand: feeling of body ownership is associated with activity in multisensory brain areas. *J. Neurosci.* 25, 10564–10573. doi: 10.1523/jneurosci.0800-05.2005

Ehrsson, H. H., Rosen, B., Stockselius, A., Ragno, C., Kohler, P., and Lundborg, G. (2008). Upper limb amputees can be induced to experience a rubber hand as their own. *Brain* 131, 3443–3452. doi: 10.1093/brain/awn297

Ehrsson, H. H., Spence, C., and Passingham, R. E. (2004). That's my hand! Activity in premotor cortex reflects feeling of ownership of a limb. *Science* 305, 875–877. doi: 10.1126/science.1097011

Ehrsson, H. H., Wiech, K., Weiskopf, N., Dolan, R. J., and Passingham, R. E. (2007). Threatening a rubber hand that you feel is yours elicits a cortical anxiety response. *Proc. Natl. Acad. Sci. U S A* 104, 9828–9833. doi: 10.1073/pnas.0610011104

Ehrsson, H. H. (2009). How many arms make a pair? Perceptual illusion of having an additional limb. *Perception* 38, 310–312. doi: 10.1068/p6304

Elbert, T., Pantev, C., Wienbruch, C., Rockstroh, B., and Taub, E. (1995). Increased cortical representation of the fingers of the left hand in string players. *Science* 270, 305–307. doi: 10.1126/science.270.5234.305

Ericsson, K. A. (2007). Deliberate practice and the modifiability of body and mind: Toward a science of the structure and acquisition of expert and elite performance. *Int. J. Sport. Psychol.* 38, 4–34.

Esposito, R., Cilli, F., Pieramico, V., Ferretti, A., Macchia, A., Tommasi, M., et al. (2013). Acute effects of modafinil on brain resting state networks in young healthy subjects. *PLoS One* 8:e69224. doi: 10.1371/journal.pone.0069224

Farah, M. J., Illes, J., Cook-Deegan, R., Gardner, H., Kandel, E., King, P., et al. (2004). Neurocognitive enhancement: what can we do and what should we do? *Nat. Rev. Neurosci.* 5, 421–425. doi: 10.1038/nrn1390

Farb, N. A., Segal, Z. V., Mayberg, H., Bean, J., McKeon, D., Fatima, Z., et al. (2007). Attending to the present: mindfulness meditation reveals distinct neural modes of self-reference. *Soc. Cogn. Affect. Neurosci.* 2, 313–322. doi: 10.1093/scan/nsm030

Ferreri, F., Ponzo, D., Vollero, L., Guerra, A., Di Pino, G., Petrichella, S., et al. (2014). Does an intraneural interface short-term implant for robotic hand control modulate sensorimotor cortical integration? An EEG-TMS co-registration study on a human amputee. *Restor. Neurol. Neurosci.* 32, 281–292. doi: 10.3233/RNN-130347

Finney, E. M., and Dobkins, K. R. (2001). Visual contrast sensitivity in deaf versus hearing populations: exploring the perceptual consequences of auditory deprivation and experience with a visual language. *Brain Res. Cogn. Brain Res.* 11, 171–183. doi: 10.1016/s0926-6410(00)00082-3

Flor, H., Elbert, T., Knecht, S., Wienbruch, C., Pantev, C., Birbaumer, N., et al. (1995). Phantom-limb pain as a perceptual correlate of cortical reorganization following arm amputation. *Nature* 375, 482–484. doi: 10.1038/375482a0

Fogassi, L., Gallese, V., Fadiga, L., Luppino, G., Matelli, M., and Rizzolatti, G. (1996). Coding of peripersonal space in inferior premotor cortex (area F4). *J. Neurophysiol.* 76, 141–157.

Fourkas, A. D., Bonavolontà, V., Avenanti, A., and Aglioti, S. M. (2008). Kinesthetic imagery and tool-specific modulation of corticospinal representations in expert tennis players. *Cereb. Cortex* 18, 2382–2390. doi: 10.1093/cercor/bhn005

Gallese, V., Fadiga, L., Fogassi, L., and Rizzolatti, G. (1996). Action recognition in the premotor cortex. *Brain* 119, 593–609. doi: 10.1093/brain/119.2.593

Ganguly, K., and Carmena, J. M. (2009). Emergence of a stable cortical map for neuroprosthetic control. *PLoS Biol.* 7:e1000153. doi: 10.1371/journal.pbio.1000153

Germain, L., and Lamarre, Y. (1993). Neuronal activity in the motor and premotor cortices before and after learning the associations between auditory stimuli and motor responses. *Brain Res.* 611, 175–179. doi: 10.1016/0006-8993(93)91792-q

Gibson, J. J. (1977). "The theory of affordances," in *Perceiving, Acting and Knowing. Towards an Ecological Psychology*, eds R. Shaw and J. Bransford (Hoboken, NJ: John Wiley and Sons Inc.), 67–82.

Gibson, J. J. (1986). *The Ecological Approach to Visual Perception.* Hillsdale, NJ: Psychology Press.

Giraux, P., Sirigu, A., Schneider, F., and Dubernard, J.-M. (2001). Cortical reorganization in motor cortex after graft of both hands. *Nat. Neurosci.* 4, 691–692. doi: 10.1038/89472

Giummarra, M. J., Georgiou-Karistianis, N., Nicholls, M. E., and Bradshaw, J. L. (2011). The third hand: ownership of a rubber hand in addition to the existing (phantom) hand. *Cortex* 47, 998–1000. doi: 10.1016/j.cortex.2011.02.010

Giummarra, M. J., Gibson, S. J., Georgiou-Karistianis, N., and Bradshaw, J. L. (2008). Mechanisms underlying embodiment, disembodiment and loss of embodiment. *Neurosci. Biobehav. Rev.* 32, 143–160. doi: 10.1016/j.neubiorev.2007.07.001

Gizewski, E., Gasser, T., de Greiff, A., Boehm, A., and Forsting, M. (2003). Cross-modal plasticity for sensory and motor activation patterns in blind subjects. *Neuroimage* 19, 968–975. doi: 10.1016/s1053-8119(03)00114-9

Gladstone, D. J., and Black, S. E. (2000). Enhancing recovery after stroke with noradrenergic pharmacotherapy: a new frontier? *Can. J. Neurol. Sci.* 27, 97–105.

Goldenberg, G. (2003). Apraxia and beyond: life and work of Hugo Liepmann. *Cortex* 39, 509–524. doi: 10.1016/s0010-9452(08)70261-2

Grafton, S. T., Mazziotta, J. C., Presty, S., Friston, K. J., Frackowiak, R., and Phelps, M. E. (1992). Functional anatomy of human procedural learning determined with regional cerebral blood flow and PET. *J. Neurosci.* 12, 2542–2548.

Graziano, M. S., Yap, G. S., and Gross, C. G. (1994). Coding of visual space by premotor neurons. *Science* 266, 1054–1057. doi: 10.1126/science.7973661

Grefkes, C., Wang, L. E., Eickhoff, S. B., and Fink, G. R. (2010). Noradrenergic modulation of cortical networks engaged in visuomotor processing. *Cereb. Cortex* 20, 783–797. doi: 10.1093/cercor/bhp144

Grosse-Wentrup, M., Mattia, D., and Oweiss, K. (2011). Using brain-computer interfaces to induce neural plasticity and restore function. *J. Neural Eng.* 8:025004. doi: 10.1088/1741-2560/8/2/025004

Guterstam, A., Gentile, G., and Ehrsson, H. H. (2013). The invisible hand illusion: multisensory integration leads to the embodiment of a discrete volume of empty space. *J. Cogn. Neurosci.* 25, 1078–1099. doi: 10.1162/jocn_a_00393

Guterstam, A., Petkova, V. I., and Ehrsson, H. H. (2011). The illusion of owning a third arm. *PLoS One* 6:e17208. doi: 10.1371/journal.pone.0017208

Halligan, P., and Marshall, J. (1995). Supernumerary phantom limb after right hemispheric stroke. *J. Neurol. Neurosurg. Psychiatry* 59, 341–342. doi: 10.1136/jnnp.59.3.341-a

Hebb, D. O. (1949). *The Organization of Behavior.* New York: Wiley.

Hensch, T. K. (2005). Critical period plasticity in local cortical circuits. *Nat. Rev. Neurosci.* 6, 877–888. doi: 10.1038/nrn1787

Hochberg, L. R., Serruya, M. D., Friehs, G. M., Mukand, J. A., Saleh, M., Caplan, A. H., et al. (2006). Neuronal ensemble control of prosthetic devices by a human with tetraplegia. *Nature* 442, 164–171. doi: 10.1038/nature04970

Holmes, J., Gathercole, S. E., and Dunning, D. L. (2009). Adaptive training leads to sustained enhancement of poor working memory in children. *Dev. Sci.* 12, F9–F15. doi: 10.1111/j.1467-7687.2009.00848.x

Hölzel, B. K., Carmody, J., Vangel, M., Congleton, C., Yerramsetti, S. M., Gard, T., et al. (2011). Mindfulness practice leads to increases in regional brain gray matter density. *Psychiatry Res.* 191, 36–43. doi: 10.1016/j.pscychresns.2010.08.006

Hölzel, B. K., Ott, U., Gard, T., Hempel, H., Weygandt, M., Morgen, K., et al. (2008). Investigation of mindfulness meditation practitioners with voxel-based morphometry. *Soc. Cogn. Affect. Neurosci.* 3, 55–61. doi: 10.1093/scan/nsm038

Husain, M., and Mehta, M. A. (2011). Cognitive enhancement by drugs in health and disease. *Trends Cogn. Sci.* 15, 28–36. doi: 10.1016/j.tics.2010.11.002

Imamizu, H., Kuroda, T., Miyauchi, S., Yoshioka, T., and Kawato, M. (2003). Modular organization of internal models of tools in the human cerebellum. *Proc. Natl. Acad. Sci. U S A* 100, 5461–5466. doi: 10.1073/pnas.0835746100

Imamizu, H., Miyauchi, S., Tamada, T., Sasaki, Y., Takino, R., Pütz, B., et al. (2000). Human cerebellar activity reflecting an acquired internal model of a new tool. *Nature* 403, 192–195. doi: 10.1038/35003194

Inoue, K., Kawashima, R., Sugiura, M., Ogawa, A., Schormann, T., Zilles, K., et al. (2001). Activation in the ipsilateral posterior parietal cortex during tool use: a PET study. *Neuroimage* 14, 1469–1475. doi: 10.1006/nimg.2001.0942

Iriki, A., Tanaka, M., and Iwamura, Y. (1996). Coding of modified body schema during tool use by macaque postcentral neurones. *Neuroreport* 7, 2325–2330. doi: 10.1097/00001756-199610020-00010

Ishibashi, H., Hihara, S., Takahashi, M., Heike, T., Yokota, T., and Iriki, A. (2002). Tool-use learning selectively induces expression of brain-derived neurotrophic factor, its receptor *trk*B and neurotrophin 3 in the intraparietal multisensorycortex of monkeys. *Brain Res. Cogn. Brain Res.* 14, 3–9. doi: 10.1016/s0926-6410(02)00056-3

Jackson, A., Mavoori, J., and Fetz, E. E. (2006). Long-term motor cortex plasticity induced by an electronic neural implant. *Nature* 444, 56–60. doi: 10.1038/nature05226

Jak, A. J., Seelye, A. M., and Jurick, S. M. (2013). Crosswords to computers: a critical review of popular approaches to cognitive enhancement. *Neuropsychol. Rev.* 23, 13–26. doi: 10.1007/s11065-013-9226-5

Jarosiewicz, B., Chase, S. M., Fraser, G. W., Velliste, M., Kass, R. E., and Schwartz, A. B. (2008). Functional network reorganization during learning in a brain-computer interface paradigm. *Proc. Natl. Acad. Sci. U S A* 105, 19486–19491. doi: 10.1073/pnas.0808113105

Järveläinen, J., Schuermann, M., and Hari, R. (2004). Activation of the human primary motor cortex during observation of tool use. *Neuroimage* 23, 187–192. doi: 10.1016/j.neuroimage.2004.06.010

Jiang, F., Racine, R., and Turnbull, J. (1997). Electrical stimulation of the septal region of aged rats improves performance in an open-field maze. *Physiol. Behav.* 62, 1279–1282. doi: 10.1016/s0031-9384(97)00306-5

Johnson, L. A., Blakely, T., Hermes, D., Hakimian, S., Ramsey, N. F., and Ojemann, J. G. (2012). Sleep spindles are locally modulated by training on a brain–computer interface. *Proc. Natl. Acad. Sci. U S A* 109, 18583–18588. doi: 10.1073/pnas.1207532109

Johnson-Frey, S. H. (2004). The neural bases of complex tool use in humans. *Trends Cogn. Sci.* 8, 71–78. doi: 10.1016/j.tics.2003.12.002

Jones, E. G., and Pons, T. P. (1998). Thalamic and brainstem contributions to large-scale plasticity of primate somatosensory cortex. *Science* 282, 1121–1125. doi: 10.1126/science.282.5391.1121

Jones, E. G. (1993). GABAergic neurons and their role in cortical plasticity in primates. *Cereb. Cortex* 3, 361–372. doi: 10.1093/cercor/3.5.361-a

Kaas, J. H., Krubitzer, L. A., Chino, Y. M., Langston, A. L., Polley, E. H., and Blair, N. (1990). Reorganization of retinotopic cortical maps in adult mammals after lesions of the retina. *Science* 248, 229–231. doi: 10.1126/science.2326637

Kaas, J. H. (1991). Plasticity of sensory and motor maps in adult mammals. *Annu. Rev. Neurosci.* 14, 137–167. doi: 10.1146/annurev.neuro.14.1.137

Kajimoto, H., Inami, M., Kawakami, N., and Tachi, S. (2003). Smarttouch-augmentation of skin sensation with electrocutaneous display. Proceedings of the Haptic Interfaces for Virtual Environment and Teleoperator Systems, 2003 HAPTICS 2003 Proceedings 11th Symposium on; IEEE.

Kammers, M. P., Verhagen, L., Dijkerman, H. C., Hogendoorn, H., De Vignemont, F., and Schutter, D. J. (2009). Is this hand for real? Attenuation of the rubber hand illusion by transcranial magnetic stimulation over the inferior parietal lobule. *J. Cogn. Neurosci.* 21, 1311–1320. doi: 10.1162/jocn.2009.21095

Kanayama, N., Sato, A., and Ohira, H. (2009). The role of gamma band oscillations and synchrony on rubber hand illusion and crossmodal integration. *Brain Cogn.* 69, 19–29. doi: 10.1016/j.bandc.2008.05.001

Karni, A., Meyer, G., Rey-Hipolito, C., Jezzard, P., Adams, M. M., Turner, R., et al. (1998). The acquisition of skilled motor performance: fast and slow experience-driven changes in primary motor cortex. *Proc. Natl. Acad. Sci. U S A* 95, 861–868. doi: 10.1073/pnas.95.3.861

Kelly, A. C., and Garavan, H. (2005). Human functional neuroimaging of brain changes associated with practice. *Cereb. Cortex* 15, 1089–1102. doi: 10.1093/cercor/bhi005

Kereszturi, E., Tarnok, Z., Bognar, E., Lakatos, K., Farkas, L., Gadoros, J., et al. (2008). Catechol-O-methyltransferase Val158Met polymorphism is associated with methylphenidate response in ADHD children. *Am. J. Med. Genet. B Neuropsychiatr. Genet.* 147B, 1431–1435. doi: 10.1002/ajmg.b.30704

Kim, J. M., Stewart, R., Park, M. S., Kang, H. J., Kim, S. W., Shin, I. S., et al. (2012). Associations of BDNF genotype and promoter methylation with acute and long-term stroke outcomes in an East Asian cohort. *PLoS One* 7:e51280. doi: 10.1371/journal.pone.0051280

Kleim, J. A., Barbay, S., Cooper, N. R., Hogg, T. M., Reidel, C. N., Remple, M. S., et al. (2002). Motor learning-dependent synaptogenesis is localized to functionally reorganized motor cortex. *Neurobiol. Learn. Mem.* 77, 63–77. doi: 10.1006/nlme.2000.4004

Klingberg, T., Fernell, E., Olesen, P. J., Johnson, M., Gustafsson, P., Dahlström, K., et al. (2005). Computerized training of working memory in children with ADHD–a randomized, controlled trial. *J. Am. Acad. Child Adolesc. Psychiatry* 44, 177–186. doi: 10.1097/00004583-200502000-00010

Klingberg, T. (2010). Training and plasticity of working memory. *Trends Cogn. Sci.* 14, 317–324. doi: 10.1016/j.tics.2010.05.002

Koralek, A. C., Jin, X., Long, J. D. 2nd, Costa, R. M., and Carmena, J. M. (2012). Corticostriatal plasticity is necessary for learning intentional neuroprosthetic skills. *Nature* 483, 331–335. doi: 10.1038/nature10845

Kuiken, T. A., Miller, L. A., Lipschutz, R. D., Lock, B. A., Stubblefield, K., Marasco, P. D., et al. (2007). Targeted reinnervation for enhanced prosthetic arm function in a woman with a proximal amputation: a case study. *Lancet* 369, 371–380. doi: 10.1016/s0140-6736(07)60193-7

Kwok, T. C., Chau, W. W., Yuen, K. S., Wong, A. Y., Li, J. C., Shiu, R. Y., et al. (2011). Who would benefit from memory training? A pilot study examining the ceiling effect of concurrent cognitive stimulation. *Clin. Interv. Aging* 6, 83–88. doi: 10.2147/CIA.S16802

Laubach, M., Wessberg, J., and Nicolelis, M. A. (2000). Cortical ensemble activity increasingly predicts behaviour outcomes during learning of a motor task. *Nature* 405, 567–571. doi: 10.1038/35014604

Lausberg, H., Göttert, R., Müniinger, U., Boegner, F., and Marx, P. (1999). Callosal disconnection syndrome in a left-handed patient due to infarction of the total length of the corpus callosum. *Neuropsychologia* 37, 253–265. doi: 10.1016/s0028-3932(98)00079-7

Lazar, S. W., Bush, G., Gollub, R. L., Fricchione, G. L., Khalsa, G., and Benson, H. (2000). Functional brain mapping of the relaxation response and meditation. *Neuroreport* 11, 1581–1585. doi: 10.1097/00001756-200005150-00041

Lazar, S. W., Kerr, C. E., Wasserman, R. H., Gray, J. R., Greve, D. N., Treadway, M. T., et al. (2005). Meditation experience is associated with increased cortical thickness. *Neuroreport* 16, 1893–1897. doi: 10.1097/01.wnr.0000186598.66243.19

Lebedev, M. A., and Nicolelis, M. A. (2006). Brain-machine interfaces: past, present and future. *Trends Neurosci.* 29, 536–546. doi: 10.1016/j.tins.2006.07.004

Lee, D. S., Lee, J. S., Oh, S. H., Kim, S.-K., Kim, J.-W., Chung, J.-K., et al. (2001). Deafness: cross-modal plasticity and cochlear implants. *Nature* 409, 149–150. doi: 10.1038/35051653

Lenggenhager, B., Tadi, T., Metzinger, T., and Blanke, O. (2007). Video ergo sum: manipulating bodily self-consciousness. *Science* 317, 1096–1099. doi: 10.1126/science.1143439

Lewis, E., and Lloyd, D. M. (2010). Embodied experience: a first-person investigation of the rubber hand illusion. *Phenomenology Cogn. Sci.* 9, 317–339. doi: 10.1007/s11097-010-9154-2

Lotze, M., Grodd, W., Birbaumer, N., Erb, M., Huse, E., and Flor, H. (1999). Does use of a myoelectric prosthesis prevent cortical reorganization and phantom limb pain? *Nat. Neurosci.* 2, 501–502. doi: 10.1038/9145

Luders, E., Toga, A. W., Lepore, N., and Gaser, C. (2009). The underlying anatomical correlates of long-term meditation: larger hippocampal and frontal volumes of gray matter. *Neuroimage* 45, 672–678. doi: 10.1016/j.neuroimage.2008.12.061

Lutz, A., Brefczynski-Lewis, J., Johnstone, T., and Davidson, R. J. (2008). Regulation of the neural circuitry of emotion by compassion meditation: effects of meditative expertise. *PLoS One* 3:e1897. doi: 10.1371/journal.pone.0001897

Lutz, A., Greischar, L. L., Rawlings, N. B., Ricard, M., and Davidson, R. J. (2004). Long-term meditators self-induce high-amplitude gamma synchrony during mental practice. *Proc. Natl. Acad. Sci. U S A* 101, 16369–16373. doi: 10.1073/pnas.0407401101

Macaluso, E., Frith, C. D., and Driver, J. (2000). Modulation of human visual cortex by crossmodal spatial attention. *Science* 289, 1206–1208. doi: 10.1126/science.289.5482.1206

Macaluso, E., and Maravita, A. (2010). The representation of space near the body through touch and vision. *Neuropsychologia* 48, 782–795. doi: 10.1016/j.neuropsychologia.2009.10.010

Maguire, E. A., Gadian, D. G., Johnsrude, I. S., Good, C. D., Ashburner, J., Frackowiak, R. S., et al. (2000). Navigation-related structural change in the hippocampi of taxi drivers. *Proc. Natl. Acad. Sci. U S A* 97, 4398–4403. doi: 10.1073/pnas.070039597

Maguire, E. A., Valentine, E. R., Wilding, J. M., and Kapur, N. (2002). Routes to remembering: the brains behind superior memory. *Nat. Neurosci.* 6, 90–95. doi: 10.1038/nn988

Maguire, E. A., Woollett, K., and Spiers, H. J. (2006). London taxi drivers and bus drivers: a structural MRI and neuropsychological analysis. *Hippocampus* 16, 1091–1101. doi: 10.1002/hipo.20233

Mahncke, H. W., Connor, B. B., Appelman, J., Ahsanuddin, O. N., Hardy, J. L., Wood, R. A., et al. (2006). Memory enhancement in healthy older adults using a brain plasticity-based training program: a randomized, controlled study. *Proc. Natl. Acad. Sci. U S A* 103, 12523–12528. doi: 10.1073/pnas.0605194103

Makin, T. R., Holmes, N. P., and Ehrsson, H. H. (2008). On the other hand: dummy hands and peripersonal space. *Behav. Brain Res.* 191, 1–10. doi: 10.1016/j.bbr.2008.02.041

Marasco, P. D., Kim, K., Colgate, J. E., Peshkin, M. A., and Kuiken, T. A. (2011). Robotic touch shifts perception of embodiment to a prosthesis in targeted reinnervation amputees. *Brain* 134, 747–758. doi: 10.1093/brain/awq361

Maravita, A., and Iriki, A. (2004). Tools for the body (schema). *Trends Cogn. Sci.* 8, 79–86. doi: 10.1016/j.tics.2003.12.008

Maravita, A., Spence, C., and Driver, J. (2003). Multisensory integration and the body schema: close to hand and within reach. *Curr. Biol.* 13, R531–R539. doi: 10.1016/s0960-9822(03)00449-4

Marini, F., Tagliabue, C. F., Sposito, A. V., Hernandez-Arieta, A., Brugger, P., Estevez, N., et al. (2014). Crossmodal representation of a functional robotic hand arises after extensive training in healthy participants. *Neuropsychologia* 53, 178–186. doi: 10.1016/j.neuropsychologia.2013.11.017

Marshall, L., Helgadóttir, H., Mölle, M., and Born, J. (2006). Boosting slow oscillations during sleep potentiates memory. *Nature* 444, 610–613. doi: 10.1038/nature05278

Maruishi, M., Tanaka, Y., Muranaka, H., Tsuji, T., Ozawa, Y., Imaizumi, S., et al. (2004). Brain activation during manipulation of the myoelectric prosthetic hand: a functional magnetic resonance imaging study. *Neuroimage* 21, 1604–1611. doi: 10.1016/j.neuroimage.2003.12.001

Matsuzaka, Y., Picard, N., and Strick, P. L. (2007). Skill representation in the primary motor cortex after long-term practice. *J. Neurophysiol.* 97, 1819–1832. doi: 10.1152/jn.00784.2006

McNab, F., Varrone, A., Farde, L., Jucaite, A., Bystritsky, P., Forssberg, H., et al. (2009). Changes in cortical dopamine D1 receptor binding associated with cognitive training. *Science* 323, 800–802. doi: 10.1126/science.1166102

Mehta, M. A., Owen, A. M., Sahakian, B. J., Mavaddat, N., Pickard, J. D., and Robbins, T. W. (2000). Methylphenidate enhances working memory by modulating discrete frontal and parietal lobe regions in the human brain. *J. Neurosci.* 20, RC65, 1–6.

Merzenich, M. M., Nelson, R. J., Stryker, M. P., Cynader, M. S., Schoppmann, A., and Zook, J. M. (1984). Somatosensory cortical map changes following digit amputation in adult monkeys. *J. Comp. Neurol.* 224, 591–605. doi: 10.1002/cne.902240408

Métin, C., and Frost, D. O. (1989). Visual responses of neurons in somatosensory cortex of hamsters with experimentally induced retinal projections to somatosensory thalamus. *Proc. Natl. Acad. Sci. U S A* 86, 357–361. doi: 10.1073/pnas.86.1.357

Micera, S., Citi, L., Rigosa, J., Carpaneto, J., Raspopovic, S., Di Pino, G., et al. (2010). Decoding information from neural signals recorded using intraneural electrodes: towards the development of a neurocontrolled hand prosthesis. *Proceedings of the IEEE* 98, 407–417. doi: 10.1109/jproc.2009.2038726

Micera, S., Rigosa, J., Carpaneto, J., Citi, L., Raspopovic, S., Guglielmelli, E., et al. (2009). On the control of a robot hand by extracting neural signals from the PNS: Preliminary results from a human implantation. *Conf. Proc. IEEE Eng. Med. Biol. Soc.* 2009, 4586–4589. doi: 10.1109/IEMBS.2009.5332764

Milton, J., Solodkin, A., Hluštík, P., and Small, S. L. (2007). The mind of expert motor performance is cool and focused. *Neuroimage* 35, 804–813. doi: 10.1016/j.neuroimage.2007.01.003

Moll, J., de Oliveira-Souza, R., Passman, L., Cunha, F. C., Souza-Lima, F., and Andreiuolo, P. (2000). Functional MRI correlates of real and imagined tool-use pantomimes. *Neurology* 54, 1331–1336. doi: 10.1212/wnl.54.6.1331

Mulvey, M. R., Fawkner, H. J., Radford, H. E., and Johnson, M. I. (2012). Perceptual embodiment of prosthetic limbs by transcutaneous electrical nerve stimulation. *Neuromodulation* 15, 42–46; discussion 47. doi: 10.1111/j.1525-1403.2011.00408.x

Murata, A., Fadiga, L., Fogassi, L., Gallese, V., Raos, V., and Rizzolatti, G. (1997). Object representation in the ventral premotor cortex (area F5) of the monkey. *J. Neurophysiol.* 78, 2226–2230.

Murata, A., Gallese, V., Luppino, G., Kaseda, M., and Sakata, H. (2000). Selectivity for the shape, size and orientation of objects for grasping in neurons of monkey parietal area AIP. *J. Neurophysiol.* 83, 2580–2601.

Murata, K., Cramer, H., and Bach-y-Rita, P. (1965). Neuronal convergence of noxious, acoustic and visual stimuli in the visual cortex of the cat. *J. Neurophysiol.* 28, 1223–1239.

Murphy, K. J., Foley, A. G., O'Connell, A. W., and Regan, C. M. (2006). Chronic exposure of rats to cognition enhancing drugs produces a neuroplastic response identical to that obtained by complex environment rearing. *Neuropsychopharmacology* 31, 90–100. doi: 10.1038/sj.npp.1300810

Nagel, S. K., Carl, C., Kringe, T., Martin, R., and Konig, P. (2005). Beyond sensory substitution—learning the sixth sense. *J. Neural. Eng.* 2, R13–R26. doi: 10.1088/1741-2560/2/4/r02

Navarro, X., Krueger, T. B., Lago, N., Micera, S., Stieglitz, T., and Dario, P. (2005). A critical review of interfaces with the peripheral nervous system for the control of neuroprostheses and hybrid bionic systems. *J. Peripher. Nerv. Syst.* 10, 229–258. doi: 10.1111/j.1085-9489.2005.10303.x

Newport, R., Pearce, R., and Preston, C. (2010). Fake hands in action: embodiment and control of supernumerary limbs. *Exp. Brain Res.* 204, 385–395. doi: 10.1007/s00221-009-2104-y

Ni, Z., Anastakis, D. J., Gunraj, C., and Chen, R. (2010). Reversal of cortical reorganization in human primary motor cortex following thumb reconstruction. *J. Neurophysiol.* 103, 65–73. doi: 10.1152/jn.00732.2009

Niemeyer, W., and Starlinger, I. (1981). Do the blind hear better? Investigations on auditory processing in congenital or early acquired blindness II. central functions. *Int. J. Audiol.* 20, 510–515. doi: 10.3109/00206098109072719

Nilsson, M., Perfilieva, E., Johansson, U., Orwar, O., and Eriksson, P. S. (1999). Enriched environment increases neurogenesis in the adult rat dentate gyrus and improves spatial memory. *J. Neurobiol.* 39, 569–578. doi: 10.1002/(sici)1097-4695(19990615)39:4<569::aid-neu10>3.0.co;2-f

Ninaus, M., Kober, S. E., Witte, M., Koschutnig, K., Stangl, M., Neuper, C., et al. (2013). Neural substrates of cognitive control under the belief of getting neurofeedback training. *Front. Hum. Neurosci.* 7:914. doi: 10.3389/fnhum.2013.00914

Nitsche, M. A., Schauenburg, A., Lang, N., Liebetanz, D., Exner, C., Paulus, W., et al. (2003). Facilitation of implicit motor learning by weak transcranial direct current stimulation of the primary motor cortex in the human. *J. Cogn. Neurosci.* 15, 619–626. doi: 10.1162/089892903321662994

Nojima, T., Sekiguchi, D., Inami, M., and Tachi, S. (2002). The smarttool: a system for augmented reality of haptics. Proceedings of the Virtual Reality, 2002 Proceedings IEEE.

Nudo, R., Milliken, G., Jenkins, W. M., and Merzenich, M. (1996). Use-dependent alterations of movement representations in primary motor cortex of adult squirrel monkeys. *J. Neurosci.* 16, 785–807.

Olesen, P. J., Westerberg, H., and Klingberg, T. (2004). Increased prefrontal and parietal activity after training of working memory. *Nat. Neurosci.* 7, 75–79. doi: 10.1038/nn1165

Pagnoni, G., and Cekic, M. (2007). Age effects on gray matter volume and attentional performance in Zen meditation. *Neurobiol. Aging* 28, 1623–1627. doi: 10.1016/j.neurobiolaging.2007.06.008

Paillard, J. (1976). [Neural coding of motor commands]. *Rev. Electroencephalogr. Neurophysiol. Clin.* 6, 453–472. doi: 10.1016/s0370-4475(76)80006-8

Pascual-Leone, A., Amedi, A., Fregni, F., and Merabet, L. B. (2005). The plastic human brain cortex. *Annu. Rev. Neurosci.* 28, 377–401. doi: 10.1146/annurev.neuro.27.070203.144216

Pascual-Leone, A., Cammarota, A., Wassermann, E. M., Brasil-Neto, J. P., Cohen, L. G., and Hallett, M. (1993). Modulation of motor cortical outputs to the reading hand of braille readers. *Ann. Neurol.* 34, 33–37. doi: 10.1002/ana.410340108

Pascual-Leone, A., Nguyet, D., Cohen, L. G., Brasil-Neto, J. P., Cammarota, A., and Hallett, M. (1995). Modulation of muscle responses evoked by transcranial magnetic stimulation during the acquisition of new fine motor skills. *J. Neurophysiol.* 74, 1037–1045.

Pascual-Leone, A., Peris, M., Tormos, J. M., Pascual, A. P., and Catala, M. D. (1996). Reorganization of human cortical motor output maps following traumatic forearm amputation. *Neuroreport* 7, 2068–2070. doi: 10.1097/00001756-199609020-00002

Pascual-Leone, A., and Torres, F. (1993). Plasticity of the sensorimotor cortex representation of the reading finger in Braille readers. *Brain* 116, 39–52. doi: 10.1093/brain/116.1.39

Pearce, A. J., Thickbroom, G. W., Byrnes, M. L., and Mastaglia, F. L. (2000). Functional reorganisation of the corticomotor projection to the hand in skilled racquet players. *Exp. Brain Res.* 130, 238–243. doi: 10.1007/s002219900236

Peeters, R., Simone, L., Nelissen, K., Fabbri-Destro, M., Vanduffel, W., Rizzolatti, G., et al. (2009). The representation of tool use in humans and monkeys: common and uniquely human features. *J. Neurosci.* 29, 11523–11539. doi: 10.1523/JNEUROSCI.2040-09.2009

Perani, D., Cappa, S., Bettinardi, V., Bressi, S., Gorno-Tempini, M., Matarrese, M., et al. (1995). Different neural systems for the recognition of animals and man-made tools. *Neuroreport* 6, 1637–1641. doi: 10.1097/00001756-199508000-00012

Pereira, A. C., Huddleston, D. E., Brickman, A. M., Sosunov, A. A., Hen, R., McKhann, G. M., et al. (2007). An in vivo correlate of exercise-induced neurogenesis in the adult dentate gyrus. *Proc. Natl. Acad. Sci. U S A* 104, 5638–5643. doi: 10.1073/pnas.0611721104

Pfister, B. J., Huang, J. H., Kameswaran, N., Zager, E. L., and Smith, D. H. (2007). Neural engineering to produce in vitro nerve constructs and neurointerface. *Neurosurgery* 60, 137–141; discussion 141–142. doi: 10.1227/01.neu.0000249197.61280.1d

Plautz, E. J., Milliken, G. W., and Nudo, R. J. (2000). Effects of repetitive motor training on movement representations in adult squirrel monkeys: role of use versus learning. *Neurobiol. Learn. Mem.* 74, 27–55. doi: 10.1006/nlme.1999.3934

Plewnia, C., Hoppe, J., Cohen, L. G., and Gerloff, C. (2004). Improved motor skill acquisition after selective stimulation of central norepinephrine. *Neurology* 62, 2124–2126. doi: 10.1212/01.wnl.0000128041.92710.17

Popovic, M. R., Popovic, D. B., and Keller, T. (2002). Neuroprostheses for grasping. *Neurol. Res.* 24, 443–452. doi: 10.1179/016164102101200311

Ptito, M., Moesgaard, S. M., Gjedde, A., and Kupers, R. (2005). Cross-modal plasticity revealed by electrotactile stimulation of the tongue in the congenitally blind. *Brain* 128, 606–614. doi: 10.1093/brain/awh380

Quallo, M., Price, C., Ueno, K., Asamizuya, T., Cheng, K., Lemon, R., et al. (2009). Gray and white matter changes associated with tool-use learning in macaque monkeys. *Proc. Natl. Acad. Sci. U S A* 106, 18379–18384. doi: 10.1073/pnas.0909751106

Ramachandran, V. S., and Altschuler, E. L. (2009). The use of visual feedback, in particular mirror visual feedback, in restoring brain function. *Brain* 132, 1693–1710. doi: 10.1093/brain/awp135

Ramachandran, V. S., Rogers-Ramachandran, D., and Cobb, S. (1995). Touching the phantom limb. *Nature* 377, 489–490. doi: 10.1038/377489a0

Ramachandran, V. S., Rogers-Ramachandran, D., and Stewart, M. (1992). Perceptual correlates of massive cortical reorganization. *Science* 258, 1159–1160. doi: 10.1126/science.1439826

Rasch, B., Büchel, C., Gais, S., and Born, J. (2007). Odor cues during slow-wave sleep prompt declarative memory consolidation. *Science* 315, 1426–1429. doi: 10.1126/science.1138581

Rasey, H. W., Lubar, J. F., McIntyre, A., Zoffuto, A. C., and Abbott, P. L. (1995). EEG biofeedback for the enhancement of attentional processing in normal college students. *J. Neurother.* 1, 15–21. doi: 10.1300/j184v01n03_03

Raspopovic, S., Capogrosso, M., Petrini, F. M., Bonizzato, M., Rigosa, J., Di Pino, G., et al. (2014). Restoring natural sensory feedback in real-time bidirectional hand prostheses. *Sci. Transl. Med.* 6:222ra219. doi: 10.1126/scitranslmed.3006820

Rauschecker, J. P., and Kniepert, U. (1994). Auditory localization behaviour in visually deprived cats. *Eur. J. Neurosci.* 6, 149–160. doi: 10.1111/j.1460-9568.1994.tb00256.x

Recanzone, G. A., Schreiner, C., and Merzenich, M. M. (1993). Plasticity in the frequency representation of primary auditory cortex following discrimination training in adult owl monkeys. *J. Neurosci.* 13, 87–103.

Recanzone, G. H., Merzenich, M. M., Jenkins, W. M., Grajski, K. A., and Dinse, H. R. (1992). Topographic reorganization of the hand representation in cortical area 3b owl monkeys trained in a frequency-discrimination task. *J. Neurophysiol.* 67, 1031–1056.

Reis, J., Schambra, H. M., Cohen, L. G., Buch, E. R., Fritsch, B., Zarahn, E., et al. (2009). Noninvasive cortical stimulation enhances motor skill acquisition over multiple days through an effect on consolidation. *Proc. Natl. Acad. Sci. U S A* 106, 1590–1595. doi: 10.1073/pnas.0805413106

Rioult-Pedotti, M.-S., Friedman, D., and Donoghue, J. P. (2000). Learning-induced LTP in neocortex. *Science* 290, 533–536. doi: 10.1126/science.290.5491.533

Rioult-Pedotti, M.-S., Friedman, D., Hess, G., and Donoghue, J. P. (1998). Strengthening of horizontal cortical connections following skill learning. *Nat. Neurosci.* 1, 230–234. doi: 10.1038/678

Roder, B., and Neville, H. (2003). Developmental functional plasticity. *Handbook of Neuropsychology* 9, 231–270.

Rohde, M., Di Luca, M., and Ernst, M. O. (2011). The rubber hand illusion: feeling of ownership and proprioceptive drift do not go hand in hand. *PLoS One* 6:e21659. doi: 10.1371/journal.pone.0021659

Romano, D., Bottini, G., and Maravita, A. (2013). Perceptual effects of the mirror box training in normal subjects. *Restor. Neurol. Neurosci.* 31, 373–386. doi: 10.3233/RNN-120273

Romano, D., Gandola, M., Bottini, G., and Maravita, A. (2014). Arousal responses to noxious stimuli in somatoparaphrenia and anosognosia: clues to body awareness. *Brain* 137, 1213–1223. doi: 10.1093/brain/awu009

Rossini, P. M., Micera, S., Benvenuto, A., Carpaneto, J., Cavallo, G., Citi, L., et al. (2010). Double nerve intraneural interface implant on a human amputee for robotic hand control. *Clin. Neurophysiol.* 121, 777–783. doi: 10.1016/j.clinph.2010.01.001

Sadato, N., Pascual-Leone, A., Grafman, J., Ibanez, V., Deiber, M.-P., Dold, G., et al. (1996). Activation of the primary visual cortex by Braille reading in blind subjects. *Nature* 380, 526–528. doi: 10.1038/380526a0

Saig, A., Arieli, A., and Ahissar, E. (2010). "What is it like to be a rat? sensory augmentation study," in *Haptics: Generating and Perceiving Tangible Sensations*, eds A. M. L. Kappers, J. B. F. van Erp, W. M. Bergmann Tiest and F. C. T. van der Helm (Berlin Heidelberg: Springer), 298–305.

Sampaio, E., Maris, S., and Bach-y-Rita, P. (2001). Brain plasticity: 'visual' acuity of blind persons via the tongue. *Brain Res.* 908, 204–207. doi: 10.1016/S0006-8993(01)02667-1

Schaefer, M., Heinze, H. J., and Rotte, M. (2009). My third arm: shifts in topography of the somatosensory homunculus predict feeling of an artificial supernumerary arm. *Hum. Brain Mapp.* 30, 1413–1420. doi: 10.1002/hbm.20609

Scholz, J., Klein, M. C., Behrens, T. E. J., and Johansen-Berg, H. (2009). Training induces changes in white-matter architecture. *Nat. Neurosci.* 12, 1370–1371. doi: 10.1038/nn.2412

Schoups, A., Vogels, R., Qian, N., and Orban, G. (2001). Practising orientation identification improves orientation coding in V1 neurons. *Nature* 412, 549–553. doi: 10.1038/35087601

Schulze, H. (2004). MEMOS: a mobile extensible memory aid system. *Telemed. J. E Health* 10, 233–242. doi: 10.1089/1530562041641228

Schuster, C., Maunz, G., Lutz, K., Kischka, U., Sturzenegger, R., and Ettlin, T. (2011). Dexamphetamine improves upper extremity outcome during rehabilitation after stroke: a pilot randomized controlled trial. *Neurorehabil. Neural Repair* 25, 749–755. doi: 10.1177/1545968311405674

Sengül, A., van Elk, M., Rognini, G., Aspell, J. E., Bleuler, H., and Blanke, O. (2012). Extending the body to virtual tools using a robotic surgical interface: evidence from the crossmodal congruency task. *PLoS One* 7:e49473. doi: 10.1371/journal.pone.0049473

Serruya, M. D., and Kahana, M. J. (2008). Techniques and devices to restore cognition. *Behav. Brain Res.* 192, 149–165. doi: 10.1016/j.bbr.2008.04.007

Shikata, E., Tanaka, Y., Nakamura, H., Taira, M., and Sakata, H. (1996). Selectivity of the parietal visual neurones in 3D orientation of surface of stereoscopic stimuli. *Neuroreport* 7, 2389–2394. doi: 10.1097/00001756-199610020-00022

Shokur, S., O'Doherty, J. E., Winans, J. A., Bleuler, H., Lebedev, M. A., and Nicolelis, M. A. (2013). Expanding the primate body schema in sensorimotor cortex by virtual touches of an avatar. *Proc. Natl. Acad. Sci. U S A* 110, 15121–15126. doi: 10.1073/pnas.1308459110

Slater, M., Perez-Marcos, D., Ehrsson, H. H., and Sanchez-Vives, M. V. (2008). Towards a digital body: the virtual arm illusion. *Front. Hum. Neurosci.* 2:6. doi: 10.3389/neuro.09.006.2008

Smitsman, A. W. (1997). "The development of tool use: changing boundaries between organism and environment," in *Evolving Explanations of Development: Ecological Approaches to Organism-Environment Systems*, eds C. Dent-Read and P. Zukow-Goldring (Washington DC: American Psychological Association).

So, K.-T., and Orme-Johnson, D. W. (2001). Three randomized experiments on the longitudinal effects of the Transcendental Meditation technique on cognition. *Intelligence* 29, 419–440. doi: 10.1016/s0160-2896(01)00070-8

Srinivasan, N., and Baijal, S. (2007). Concentrative meditation enhances preattentive processing: a mismatch negativity study. *Neuroreport* 18, 1709–1712. doi: 10.1097/wnr.0b013e3282f0d2d8

Stefan, K., Kunesch, E., Benecke, R., Cohen, L. G., and Classen, J. (2002). Mechanisms of enhancement of human motor cortex excitability induced by interventional paired associative stimulation. *J. Physiol.* 543, 699–708. doi: 10.1113/jphysiol.2002.023317

Stroemer, R. P., Kent, T. A., Hulsebosch, C. E., and Feeney, D. M. (1998). Enhanced neocortical neural sprouting, synaptogenesis and behavioral recovery with d-amphetamine therapy after neocortical infarction in rats editorial comment. *Stroke* 29, 2381–2395. doi: 10.1161/01.str.29.11.2381

Taffoni, F., Tamilia, E., Focaroli, V., Formica, D., Ricci, L., Di Pino, G., et al. (2014). Development of goal-directed action selection guided by intrinsic motivations: an experiment with children. *Exp. Brain Res.* doi: 10.1007/s00221-014-3907-z. [Epub ahead of print].

Temple, E., Deutsch, G. K., Poldrack, R. A., Miller, S. L., Tallal, P., Merzenich, M. M., et al. (2003). Neural deficits in children with dyslexia ameliorated by behavioral remediation: evidence from functional MRI. *Proc. Natl. Acad. Sci. U S A* 100, 2860–2865. doi: 10.1073/pnas.0030098100

Terr, L. I., Sinha, U. K., and House, W. F. (1987). Anatomical relationships of the cochlear nuclei and the pontobulbar body: possible significance for neuroprosthesis placement. *Laryngoscope* 97, 1009–1011. doi: 10.1288/00005537-198709000-00001

Thomson, E. E., Carra, R., and Nicolelis, M. A. (2013). Perceiving invisible light through a somatosensory cortical prosthesis. *Nat. Commun.* 4:1482. doi: 10.1038/ncomms2497

Thorell, L. B., Lindqvist, S., Bergman Nutley, S., Bohlin, G., and Klingberg, T. (2009). Training and transfer effects of executive functions in preschool children. *Dev. Sci.* 12, 106–113. doi: 10.1111/j.1467-7687.2008.00745.x

Tombini, M., Rigosa, J., Zappasodi, F., Porcaro, C., Citi, L., Carpaneto, J., et al. (2012). Combined analysis of cortical (EEG) and nerve stump signals improves robotic hand control. *Neurorehabil. Neural Repair* 26, 275–281. doi: 10.1177/1545968311408919

Toni, I., Rowe, J., Stephan, K. E., and Passingham, R. E. (2002). Changes of cortico-striatal effective connectivity during visuomotor learning. *Cereb. Cortex* 12, 1040–1047. doi: 10.1093/cercor/12.10.1040

Tsakiris, M., Carpenter, L., James, D., and Fotopoulou, A. (2010). Hands only illusion: multisensory integration elicits sense of ownership for body parts but not for non-corporeal objects. *Exp. Brain Res.* 204, 343–352. doi: 10.1007/s00221-009-2039-3

Tsakiris, M., Hesse, M. D., Boy, C., Haggard, P., and Fink, G. R. (2007). Neural signatures of body ownership: a sensory network for bodily self-consciousness. *Cereb. Cortex* 17, 2235–2244. doi: 10.1093/cercor/bhl131

Tsakiris, M., Prabhu, G., and Haggard, P. (2006). Having a body *versus* moving your body: How agency structures body-ownership. *Conscious. Cogn.* 15, 423–432. doi: 10.1016/j.concog.2005.09.004

Tsakiris, M. (2010). *My* body in the brain: a neurocognitive model of body-ownership. *Neuropsychologia* 48, 703–712. doi: 10.1016/j.neuropsychologia.2009.09.034

Tyler, M., Danilov, Y., and Bach-y-Rita, P. (2003). Closing an open-loop control system: vestibular substitution through the tongue. *J. Integr. Neurosci.* 2, 159–164. doi: 10.1142/s0219635203000263

Vallar, G., and Ronchi, R. (2009). Somatoparaphrenia: a body delusion. A review of the neuropsychological literature. *Exp. Brain Res.* 192, 533–551. doi: 10.1007/s00221-008-1562-y

Vaynman, S., and Gomez-Pinilla, F. (2005). License to run: exercise impacts functional plasticity in the intact and injured central nervous system by using neurotrophins. *Neurorehabil. Neural Repair* 19, 283–295. doi: 10.1177/1545968305280753

Velliste, M., Perel, S., Spalding, M. C., Whitford, A. S., and Schwartz, A. B. (2008). Cortical control of a prosthetic arm for self-feeding. *Nature* 453, 1098–1101. doi: 10.1038/nature06996

Vernon, D., Egner, T., Cooper, N., Compton, T., Neilands, C., Sheri, A., et al. (2003). The effect of training distinct neurofeedback protocols on aspects of cognitive performance. *Int. J. Psychophysiol.* 47, 75–85. doi: 10.1016/s0167-8760(02)00091-0

Vestergaard-Poulsen, P., van Beek, M., Skewes, J., Bjarkam, C. R., Stubberup, M., Bertelsen, J., et al. (2009). Long-term meditation is associated with increased gray matter density in the brain stem. *Neuroreport* 20, 170–174. doi: 10.1097/wnr.0b013e328320012a

Von Gierke, H. (1970). Principles and Practice of Bionics. Proceedings of the Proc 44th AGARD—Conference Brüssel.

Wander, J. D., Blakely, T., Miller, K. J., Weaver, K. E., Johnson, L. A., Olson, J. D., et al. (2013). Distributed cortical adaptation during learning of a brain-computer interface task. *Proc. Natl. Acad. Sci. U S A* 110, 10818–10823. doi: 10.1073/pnas.1221127110

Wang, J. R., and Hsieh, S. (2013). Neurofeedback training improves attention and working memory performance. *Clin. Neurophysiol.* 124, 2406–2420. doi: 10.1016/j.clinph.2013.05.020

Weiss, T., Miltner, W. H., Adler, T., Bruckner, L., and Taub, E. (1999). Decrease in phantom limb pain associated with prosthesis-induced increased use of an amputation stump in humans. *Neurosci. Lett.* 272, 131–134. doi: 10.1016/s0304-3940(99)00595-9

Williams, J. H. (2001). Frequency-specific effects of flicker on recognition memory. *Neuroscience* 104, 283–286. doi: 10.1016/s0306-4522(00)00579-0

Williams, Z. M., and Eskandar, E. N. (2006). Selective enhancement of associative learning by microstimulation of the anterior caudate. *Nat. Neurosci.* 9, 562–568. doi: 10.1038/nn1662

Willis, S. L., Tennstedt, S. L., Marsiske, M., Ball, K., Elias, J., Koepke, K. M., et al. (2006). Long-term effects of cognitive training on everyday functional outcomes in older adults. *JAMA* 296, 2805–2814. doi: 10.1001/jama.296.23.2805

Winsberg, B. G., and Comings, D. E. (1999). Association of the dopamine transporter gene (*DAT1*) with poor methylphenidate response. *J. Am. Acad. Child Adolesc. Psychiatry* 38, 1474–1477. doi: 10.1097/00004583-199912000-00006

Winsley, R., and Matos, N. (2011). Overtraining and elite young athletes. *Med. Sport Sci.* 56, 97–105. doi: 10.1159/000320636

Wolpaw, J. R. (2007). Brain-computer interfaces as new brain output pathways. *J. Physiol.* 579, 613–619. doi: 10.1113/jphysiol.2006.125948

Yarrow, K., Brown, P., and Krakauer, J. W. (2009). Inside the brain of an elite athlete: the neural processes that support high achievement in sports. *Nat. Rev. Neurosci.* 10, 585–596. doi: 10.1038/nrn2672

Zacksenhouse, M., Lebedev, M. A., Carmena, J. M., O'Doherty, J. E., Henriquez, C., and Nicolelis, M. A. (2007). Cortical modulations increase in early sessions with brain-machine interface. *PLoS One* 2:e619. doi: 10.1371/journal.pone.0000619

Zeck, G., and Fromherz, P. (2001). Noninvasive neuroelectronic interfacing with synaptically connected snail neurons immobilized on a semiconductor chip. *Proc. Natl. Acad. Sci. U S A* 98, 10457–10462. doi: 10.1073/pnas.181348698

Zeller, D., Gross, C., Bartsch, A., Johansen-Berg, H., and Classen, J. (2011). Ventral premotor cortex may be required for dynamic changes in the feeling of limb ownership: a lesion study. *J. Neurosci.* 31, 4852–4857. doi: 10.1523/jneurosci.5154-10.2011

Ziemann, U., Iliać, T. V., Pauli, C., Meintzschel, F., and Ruge, D. (2004). Learning modifies subsequent induction of long-term potentiation-like and long-term depression-like plasticity in human motor cortex. *J. Neurosci.* 24, 1666–1672. doi: 10.1523/JNEUROSCI.5016-03.2004

Ziemann, U., Paulus, W., Nitsche, M. A., Pascual-Leone, A., Byblow, W. D., Berardelli, A., et al. (2008). Consensus: motor cortex plasticity protocols. *Brain Stimul.* 1, 164–182. doi: 10.1016/j.brs.2008.06.006

Ziemann, U., Tam, A., Butefisch, C., and Cohen, L. G. (2002). Dual modulating effects of amphetamine on neuronal excitability and stimulation-induced plasticity in human motor cortex. *Clin. Neurophysiol.* 113, 1308–1315. doi: 10.1016/s1388-2457(02)00171-2

Zunzunegui, C., Gao, B., Cam, E., Hodor, A., and Bassetti, C. L. (2011). Sleep disturbance impairs stroke recovery in the rat. *Sleep* 34, 1261–1269. doi: 10.5665/sleep.1252

9

Enhancement of cognitive and neural functions through complex reasoning training: evidence from normal and clinical populations

Sandra B. Chapman[1]* and Raksha A. Mudar[2]

[1] Center for BrainHealth®, The University of Texas at Dallas, Dallas, TX, USA
[2] Department of Speech and Hearing Science, University of Illinois at Urbana-Champaign, Champaign, IL, USA

Edited by:
Mikhail Lebedev, Duke University, USA

Reviewed by:
Jitendra Sharma, Massachusetts Institute of Technology, USA
Aaron P. Blaisdell, University of California, Los Angeles, USA

***Correspondence:**
Sandra B. Chapman, Center for BrainHealth®, The University of Texas at Dallas, 2200 W Mockingbird Ln, Dallas, TX, 75235, USA
e-mail: schapman@utdallas.edu

Public awareness of cognitive health is fairly recent compared to physical health. Growing evidence suggests that cognitive training offers promise in augmenting cognitive brain performance in normal and clinical populations. Targeting higher-order cognitive functions, such as reasoning in particular, may promote generalized cognitive changes necessary for supporting the complexities of daily life. This data-driven perspective highlights cognitive and brain changes measured in randomized clinical trials that trained gist reasoning strategies in populations ranging from teenagers to healthy older adults, individuals with brain injury to those at-risk for Alzheimer's disease. The evidence presented across studies support the potential for Gist reasoning training to strengthen cognitive performance in trained and untrained domains and to engage more efficient communication across widespread neural networks that support higher-order cognition. The meaningful benefits of Gist training provide compelling motivation to examine optimal dose for sustained benefits as well as to explore additive benefits of meditation, physical exercise, and/or improved sleep in future studies.

Keywords: cognitive training, gist reasoning, cognition, neural, brain plasticity

INTRODUCTION

Five decades of research have shown that the brain is modifiable in the context of stimulating cognitive experiences and in response to cognitive training (e.g., Bennett et al., 1964; Schooler, 1984; Schooler et al., 1999). Cognitive training involves guided practice on tasks targeting specific cognitive functions (e.g., working memory, attention) or specific cognitive strategies (Clare and Woods, 2004; Martin et al., 2011). In general, evidence from most cognitive training studies reveal improvements in performance, especially in cognitive functions directly targeted by training (Nyberg et al., 2003; Dahlin et al., 2008; Jaeggi et al., 2008; Valenzuela et al., 2008; Carlson et al., 2009; Zelinski, 2009; Anguera et al., 2013; Chapman et al., 2013). However, much remains to be learned about the kinds of training programs that provide meaningful changes beyond the specific skills trained. From a public health perspective, cognitive training will be deemed useful if the training has generalized benefits and builds cognitive capacities to support performance in day-to-day tasks (Anand et al., 2011).

Concerted efforts are being directed toward exploring the realities of augmenting cognitive performance. Memory training has been a key focus of cognitive training programs motivated by extant evidence that declines in memory commonly occur with normal aging and brain diseases/injuries (e.g., Papp et al., 2009; Gates et al., 2011). Memory training mostly yields short-term improvements in memory; however, benefits do not generalize/transfer to other cognitive functions (Papp et al., 2009; Valenzuela and Sachdev, 2009; Martin et al., 2011; Tardif and Simard, 2011; Reijnders et al., 2012; Teixeira et al., 2012; Thompson et al., 2013), nor do they produce long-term benefits (Rebok et al., 2014). Emerging evidence suggests that reasoning training has widespread and lasting benefits that may guard against and restore cognitive losses in aging and/or disease (Willis et al., 2006; Anand et al., 2011; Chapman et al., 2013; Rebok et al., 2014). For instance, in one of the largest randomized cognitive training trials to date, i.e., the Advanced Cognitive Training for Independent and Vital Elderly (ACTIVE) trial, participants who underwent reasoning training (i.e., focused on solving problems related to serial patterns and sequences) showed less decline in self-reported Independent Activities of Daily Living over a 10-year period compared to the memory training group (i.e., strategies to improve verbal episodic memory) (Rebok et al., 2014).

A growing body of evidence suggests that advanced reasoning engages gist-based processing (Reyna and Brainerd, 1995, 2011; Reyna and Lloyd, 2006). In the current paper, we present a perspective on a particular type of reasoning training that targets *gist-based reasoning* abilities. Gist reasoning is defined as the ability to synthesize and create abstract meanings from the literal content/information, a skill essential for academic, occupational, and functional competence. The primary objective of strategy-driven Gist reasoning training is to improve the ability to abstract generalized meanings from complex information and to incorporate these strategies into everyday tasks. Gist training is informed by cognitive theories of discourse meaning structure (Van Dijk et al., 1983) and information processing (Reyna and Brainerd,

1995), specifically van Dijk and Kintsch's macrostructure/global meanings and Reyna and Brainerd's gist representation. In this perspective paper, we provide a general framework of Gist reasoning training and highlight converging findings from Gist reasoning training studies across adolescent and adult populations. This novel strategy-based approach to cognitive training may provide insights and future directions to guide testing and development of training protocols that have ecological validity/real life application.

GENERAL OVERVIEW OF COGNITIVE TRAINING PROTOCOLS

In the distinct studies summarized below, we examined the potential for Gist reasoning training to improve cognitive performance as compared to control protocol/s (active control/wait-list control) (see **Table 1**) using a pseudo-randomized control design. We present data from studies on two groups of adolescents [i.e., typically developing eighth graders; youth with traumatic brain injury (TBI)] and three adult populations (i.e., adults with TBI, adults with early mild cognitive impairment, and cognitive healthy adults). Overall, the length of the training period across studies was short-term, ranging from 8 to 12 sessions delivered over one to two months in 45 to 60 min. duration, with each study protocol being identical for all participants within the trial. When an active control protocol was used (Memory strategy or New learning), it was comparable to the Gist reasoning training in length, complexity, and active group discussion/engagement.

Table 1 | Brief description of experimental and control training protocols.

Training	Description
EXPERIMENTAL TRAINING	
Gist Reasoning Training (Gamino et al., 2010; Anand et al., 2011; Vas et al., 2011; Chapman et al., 2013; Mudar et al., 2013; Motes et al., 2014; Cook et al., under review)	Hierarchical Strategies Strategic Attention: Consciously blocking/inhibiting distractions and irrelevant/less relevant information Integrated Reasoning: Binding explicit facts with world knowledge to construct generalized/abstracted meanings Innovation: Deriving multiple interpretations and generalized applications beyond the concrete content reflecting fluency and fluidity of thinking
CONTROL TRAINING	
Memory Strategy Training (Gamino et al., 2010; Cook et al., under review)	Training of bottom-up memory strategies: focus on encoding, rehearsal, retrieval practice, cross modality associations and developing mnemonics
New Learning Training (Vas et al., 2011; Mudar et al., 2013) (Gamino et al., 2010)	New Learning about brain functions and influences on cognition Example topics covered: Brain Structures and Functions; The Neuron; Neuroplasticity and Neurogenesis; Memory and the Brain; Executive Functions of the Brain; Effects of Sleep and Stress on the Brain; Diet and Exercise and the Brain; Social Bonds and the Brain. This program was originally developed at the Rotman Institute, Canada and is referred to as Brain health workshop (Binder et al., 2008).
Wait-list controls (Chapman et al., 2013; Motes et al., 2014)	No contact group

GIST REASONING TRAINING

The Gist reasoning training (also referred to as gist training) is a strategy- rather than content-based program. The protocol entails three core strategies: *strategic attention, integrated reasoning*, and *innovation* summarized in **Table 1**, delineated in a training manual, and defined in more detail elsewhere (e.g., Gamino et al., 2010; Vas et al., 2011; Chapman et al., 2012; Chapman and Mudar, 2013). The strategies facilitate cognitive control and depth of encoding to facilitate knowledge acquisition and creation. The strategy instruction is hierarchical and dynamically interdependent, with each strategy building on previous strategies, and involves practice that encourages integrating all steps when tackling mental activities both inside and outside of training.

EVIDENCE OF GAINS FROM GIST TRAINING vs. CONTROL CONDITIONS

COGNITIVE TRAINING IN YOUTH (GAMINO ET AL., 2010; MOTES ET AL., 2014; COOK ET AL., UNDER REVIEW)

Typically developing adolescents

In this study, middle-school students (8th graders) were randomly assigned to one of three training protocols, either the Gist reasoning, or one of two control groups, i.e., the Memory training or the New learning (Gamino et al., 2010). The trainings were delivered over 9 class periods lasting 45 min over four weeks. These students were from lower SES backgrounds (92% living in poverty). The three groups were comparable in age, gender, memory, and cognitive abilities at baseline. Outcomes comparing pre- to post- training performances were scored by researchers blinded to individuals and group identity.

Results revealed that gist-trained students improved ability to abstract novel meanings from lengthy classroom-type texts. Additionally, these gist-trained students showed significant improvement in memory for facts, a skill not targeted in training. We found a significant relation between gains in ability to abstract meanings and a real life school measure, the Texas Assessment of Knowledge and Skills (TAKS) reading testing "Applying Critical Thinking Skills." In contrast, students in the Memory training showed improvements only in memory for isolated facts with no gains in abstracting meanings. The New learning group did not show any significant gains. These findings suggest that gist reasoning strategies may have a broader impact on learning that improves deeper understanding of information encountered beyond shallow learning of isolated facts.

In a subsequent study Motes et al. (2014) examined the effects of Gist training on neural mechanisms related to inhibitory control using electroencephalograph (EEG). Participants in the Gist training group vs. a Wait-list control group completed three visual go/no-go tasks that involved varying levels of semantic categorization (basic to more abstract superordinate categorization) both before and after training or a comparable duration in the case of the controls. The findings revealed that participants in the Gist group showed significant improvement in inhibition (i.e., ability to withhold behavioral responses on no-go trials) following training unlike the control group across basic and superordinate categorization tasks. Furthermore, those in the Gist trained group showed EEG changes suggestive of improved processing efficiency, as reflected by significant reduction in P3 no-go amplitude post-training compared to pre-training. No such differences were observed in the Wait-list controls. Overall, both the behavioral findings and the electrophysiological data across these two studies suggest that Gist training appears to enhance inhibitory responses both at the behavioral and neural level in typically developing middle school children. However, these findings have to be further validated using additional procedures (e.g., positive and negative patterning) in future studies.

Adolescents with TBI

The benefits of Gist training vs. Memory training in adolescents with TBI (ages 12–20 years) at chronic stages post injury (>6 months) was evaluated in a recent study (Cook et al., under review). Participants received one-on-one training delivered in eight sessions of 45 min duration over a four week period. The text materials for the Memory training were largely the same content as used in the Gist protocol. The findings revealed that the Gist-trained group significantly improved in their ability to abstract/synthesize meanings as compared to the Memory-trained group. The Gist-trained group also showed enhanced performance on cognitive measures for memory for facts, working memory (Digit Span backwards and Letter-Number Sequencing—WAIS III or WISC IV), and inhibition (Color Word Interference—D-KEFS). None of these latter cognitive skills were specifically targeted during training, suggesting spill-over effects of the Gist training to untrained cognitive domains. The Memory trained group's performance on memory for facts approached significance; however, results failed to show significant gains in domains of abstracting meaning, working memory, inhibition, or other cognitive areas.

Taken together, evidence from these three studies implicates the potential to enhance cognitive performance in areas of cognitive control in typically developing teens and teens with TBI, beyond the traditional treatment phase of 3 months post injury. Augmenting cognitive performance in normally developing populations and individuals at chronic stages post brain injury represents newer and promising areas of investigation.

ADULT COGNITIVE TRAINING TRIALS (ANAND ET AL., 2011; VAS ET AL., 2011; CHAPMAN ET AL., 2013)

Adults with TBI

In a randomized trial, the effects of Gist-reasoning training were compared to an active control training involving New learning in adults with TBI (ages 29–65 years) in chronic stages post-injury (>one year) (Vas et al., 2011). The Gist-trained group exhibited significant gains in abstracting meanings from complex information as compared to the New learning training group. Moreover, the Gist-trained group showed significant enhancement on measures of immediate memory (Digit Span Forward—WAIS-III), executive functions of working memory (Letter Number-Sequence—WAIS III and Daneman and Carpenter listening span) and cognitive switching (Color-Word Interference task—D-KEFS), and non-verbal reasoning (Matrix Reasoning—WAIS III). None of these latter cognitive processes were specifically targeted during training, adding further evidence of generalized benefits from Gist training. Furthermore, this group reported significant improvement in daily life skills (GOS-E, Functional Status Examination, Community Integration Questionnaire), such as increased socialization (e.g., initiating and planning activities with family and friends), higher levels of life productivity (e.g., active job seeking, setting up interviews, improved work efficiency and output), improved personal management (e.g., completing household responsibilities and house upkeep) and better sense of overall well-being. These reported real life gains from Gist training are not likely due to placebo effects since both groups believed they were receiving the experimental training. These training-related gains were maintained at 6-month follow-up. Despite comparable levels of active and engaged learning, the New Learning group failed to show significant gains on any of the performance measures.

Adults with pre-clinical Alzheimer's (Mild Cognitive Impairment)

This study compared immediate benefits of Gist training vs. New learning on cognition in individuals with Mild Cognitive Impairment (MCI) in a random assignment design (Mudar et al., 2013). Groups were comparable in age, Mini-Mental State Examination (MMSE) and episodic memory scores at baseline. Both groups received 8 h of training over a period of 4 weeks. We found differential cognitive gains between the two groups. Significant improvement was observed in the Gist-trained group on measures of abstract meaning, strategic attention, memory (immediate and delayed recall Logical Memory subtest-WMS III) and abstract verbal reasoning (Similarities-WAIS III). In contrast, participants in the New learning group showed significant improvements in remembering facts on an experimental text memory measure and on the Sorting test (D-KEFS). These findings suggest that both trainings offered some benefit for those with a progressive neurologic disease; however, Gist training offered broader benefits. Given the lack of pharmacological treatment options in slowing cognitive deterioration in pre-clinical stages of dementia, one current focus is on identifying non-pharmacological options (e.g., cognitive training) that can slow the rate of cognitive deterioration. Although maintenance of gains from Gist training needs to be studied in larger trials, even short-term increases in cognitive performance offer a glimmer of hope. Different doses and more frequent time intervals of cognitive training needs to be examined to harness optimal benefits in terms of maintaining cognitive capacity and slowing decline.

Cognitively healthy adults

The short-term effects of (i.e., 12 weeks of 1-h in-person training/week + 2 h/week homework) Gist training on cognitive and neural plasticity was examined in cognitively healthy

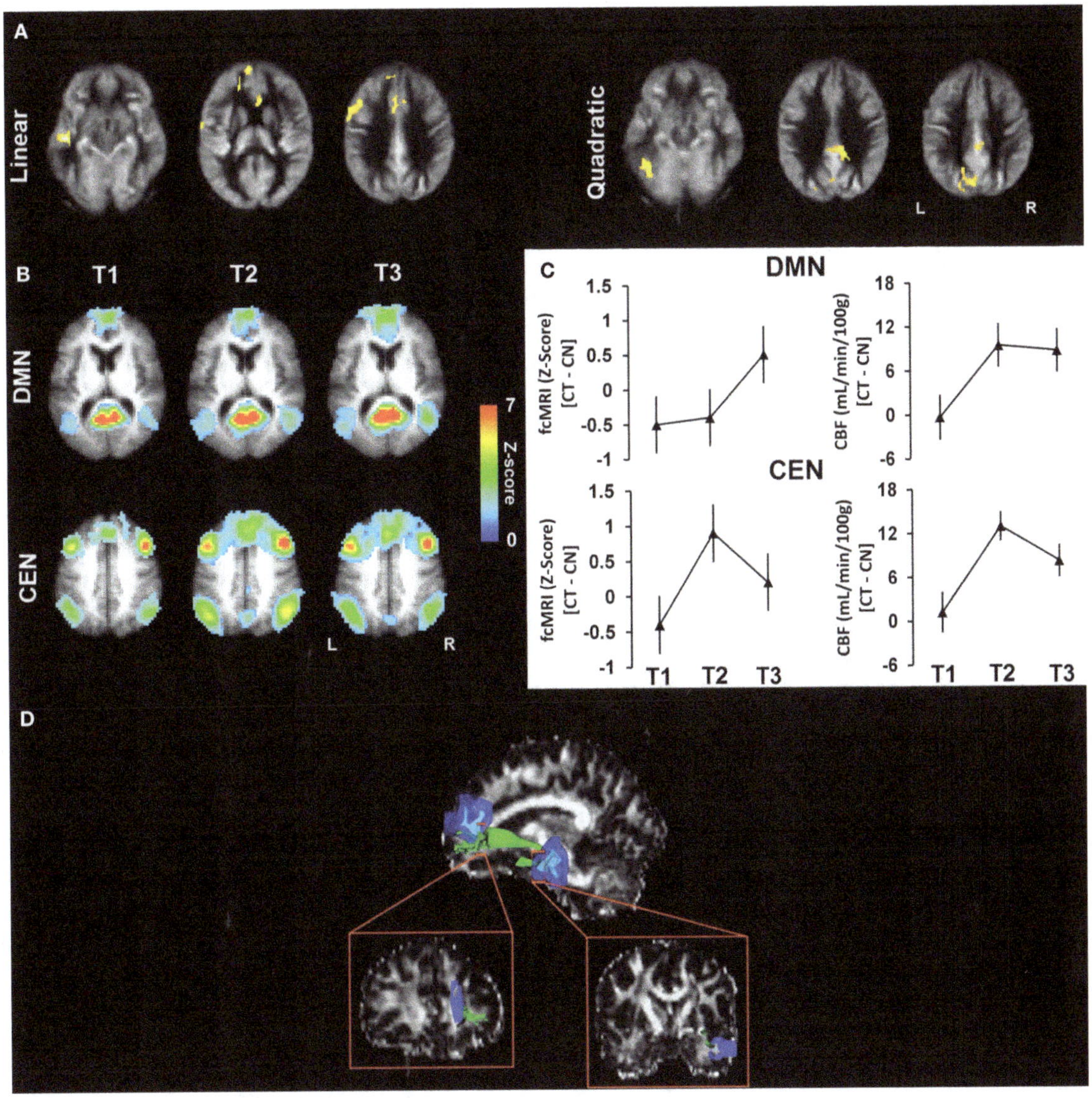

FIGURE 1 | This figure illustrates the convergence of neural plasticity findings in the cognitive training vs. control group across cerebral blood flow, functional connectivity, and structural DTI changes implicating functional brain changes more frequent and rapid than structural plasticity comparing changes at T2 and T3 to baseline T1 measures. (A) Results of CBF voxel-based comparison superimposed on an average CBF map of all participants for linear and quadratic interaction contrasts. **(B)** The average functional connectivity maps (i.e., DMN and CEN) of the cognitive training group are overlaid on their average T1-weighted image. **(C)** Mean increase in fcMRI z-scores (left column) and mean change in absolute CBF (right column) are shown for DMN and CEN across time periods. **(D)** A representative participant's uncinate fasciculus (green) is overlaid on his fractional anisotropy map from DTI (Chapman et al., 2013).

adults (55—75 years of age), well-screened to rule out early dementia, as compared to a Wait-list control group (Chapman et al., 2013). Individuals were assessed at baseline, at mid-point and immediately post-training. The Gist-trained group showed generalized cognitive gains consistent with an earlier pilot study in healthy older adults in which participants improved in cognitive switching (Trail Making Test Part B), concept abstraction (Similarities-WAIS III), and fluency (COWAT letter fluency) (Anand et al., 2011). We examined changes in large-scale brain networks in terms of brain blood flow (CBF) and functional and structural connectivity, in addition to the relationship between improved cognitive performance and brain changes. Results revealed significant increases in global CBF (total brain) as well as increased regional CBF measures as measured with Arterial Spin Labeling in two distinct and major brain networks tied to higher-order cognition, namely the Default Mode Network (DMN) and the Central Executive Network (CEN). Specifically, the DMN and CEN have been associated with top-down, cognitive control processes (Bressler and Menon, 2010). We also found corroborating patterns of increased functional connectivity in these very same major brain networks as the increased CBF (**Figure 1**). Additionally, we found significantly increased structural connectivity as measured with diffusion tensor imaging (DTI) in the left uncinate fasciculus—the white matter tract that connects the middle temporal lobe to the superior medial frontal gyri after 12 weeks of training. The finding of increased white matter integrity in this select brain region perhaps suggests that some degree of atrophy at the level of white matter tracts in healthy aging may be reversible through Gist training. The expansion of the uncinate is intriguing and perhaps suggests that this pathway plays a role in synthesizing new learning—linking the memory center (left middle temporal region) to a brain region that is implicated in abstraction skills (e.g., the left superior medial frontal gyrus).

Whereas a handful of studies have reported cognitive gains and brain changes in response to cognitive training (Nyberg et al., 2003; Boyke et al., 2008; Belleville et al., 2011; Rosen et al., 2011), this study provided some of the first convergent findings across multiple brain imaging platforms (CBF, connectivity, white matter) and cognition supporting the promise of strategy-based top-down cognitive training to enhance brain integrity (Chapman et al., 2013). We acknowledge these findings are preliminary and should be interpreted with caution since the gist training group was compared to a wait-list control group. Nonetheless, the significant relation between brain changes and cognitive improvement provides impetus that the brain gains from gist-training may be possible and warrant further study with active controls.

CONCLUSIONS AND FUTURE OPPORTUNITIES

This synopsis of key findings across studies in normal and clinical populations indicates Gist reasoning training has the potential to improve cognitive performance beyond skills trained with the likelihood of enhancing underlying neural systems, as well as real life functional abilities. The significant improvements were achieved after relatively short-term training periods. The gains were documented in pseudo-randomly assigned trials comparing the experimental Gist reasoning training to control groups using objective measures.

We postulate that top-down strategy-based cognitive training may yield efficient and easily adoptable methods of mental practice to achieve broad-based benefits. To guide future cognitive training trials, we offer several explanations why Gist reasoning training may augment higher-order executive functions. First, gist reasoning takes advantage of the human brain's preferential bias toward understanding generalized/gist meanings (Bartlett, 1932; Reyna, 1996; Gabrieli, 2004). Extant evidence has demonstrated that while memory for details is lost fairly quickly, memory for global/gist meanings is preserved when delayed recall is examined, whether tested 30 min, one day or even a week later (Bransford and Franks, 1971; Bransford et al., 1972; Mandler and Rabinowitz, 1981; Reyna, 1996; Norman and Schacter, 1997; Kahana and Wingfield, 2000; Gabrieli, 2004). Second, gist reasoning requires an active process of meaning-abstraction where the incoming details are integrated within one's repository of world knowledge by a conscious, controlled manipulation of input into précised ideas (Johnson-Laird, 1983; Van Dijk et al., 1983; Frederksen and Donin, 1991; Zwaan and Radvansky, 1998; Chapman and Mudar, 2013). This integration of incoming data with prior knowledge necessitates activation of top-down processing with enhanced depth of encoding compared to simple representation of literal input. Third, gist reasoning is a practical skill that the majority of people from adolescence to old age can implement and practice throughout their daily normal mental activities (Lloyd and Reyna, 2009; Gamino et al., 2010; Vas et al., 2011; Motes et al., 2014). Examples of gist reasoning are meaning-creations illustrated by generating interpretations, themes, take-home messages, synopses, or generalized statements, to mention a few forms. Fourth, accruing evidence suggests that such a top-down approach to processing engages broad-based brain networks (Gazzaley et al., 2005; Chen et al., 2006, 2011; Chapman et al., 2013). We propose that when the neural activity of major brain networks is increased through complex and meaningful cognitive activities involving gist reasoning, the outcomes may be manifested at multiple levels of cognitive performance and neural health.

Immense potential exists to augment cognitive performance and enhance neural systems through top-down cognitive activity, such as gist reasoning. Future research opportunities should combine multiple approaches simultaneously from the growing armamentaria shown to enhance cognitive performance and brain functions to examine additive benefits. The current reported benefits from Gist reasoning training motivate future trials where the gist training protocol is combined with methods such as short-term meditation (Tang et al., 2007), sensory processing training (Mahncke et al., 2006), aerobic exercise (Kramer and Erickson, 2007; Chapman et al., 2013), or protocols to improve sleep (Nedergaard, 2013). Also critical is examining subjects' motivational level as a factor. Expanded efforts to identify combinatorial protocols that strengthen cognitive performance and recoup losses will be of major public health significance, with the ultimate goal to more fully harness the brain's capacity to be strengthened in health, disease, and injury.

FUNDING

This work was supported by grant from the National Institute of Health (RC1-AG035954, R01-NS067015, R01-AG033106, NICHD R21-HD062835), Department of Defense (W81XWH-11-2-0194) and by grants from the T. Boone Pickens Foundation, the RGK foundation, the Lyda Hill Foundation, Dallas Foundation, and Dee Wyly Distinguished University Endowment.

ACKNOWLEDGMENTS

The authors thank Jacquelyn Gamino, Lori Cook, Asha Vas, Mike Motes, Molly Keebler, Audette Rackley, Jennifer Zientz, Erin Venza, Hsueh-Sheng Chiang, Justin Eroh, Ali Perez, and the rest of the cognitive training team for their contribution to the research discussed in this perspective.

REFERENCES

Anand, R., Chapman, S. B., Rackley, A., Keebler, M., Zientz, J., and Hart, J. (2011). Gist reasoning training in cognitively normal seniors. *Int. J. Geriatr. Psychiatry* 26, 961–968. doi: 10.1002/gps.2633

Anguera, J. A., Boccanfuso, J., Rintoul, J. L., Al-Hashimi, O., Faraji, F., Janowich, J., et al. (2013). Video game training enhances cognitive control in older adults. *Nature* 501, 97–101. doi: 10.1038/nature12486

Bartlett, F. C. (1932). *Remembering: An Experimental and Social Study.* Cambridge: Cambridge University.

Belleville, S., Clément, F., Mellah, S., Gilbert, B., Fontaine, F., and Gauthier, S. (2011). Training-related brain plasticity in subjects at risk of developing Alzheimer's disease. *Brain* 134, 1623–1634. doi: 10.1093/brain/awr037

Bennett, E. L., Diamond, M. C., Krech, D., and Rosenzweig, M. R. (1964). Chemical and Anatomical Plasticity of the Brain. *Science* 610–619. doi: 10.1126/science.146.3644.610

Binder, D. T. G., O'Connor, C., Levine, B. (2008). *Brain HealthWorkshop*. Rotman Research Institute, Baycrest, Toronto: ON; University of California, Berkeley: CA.

Boyke, J., Driemeyer, J., Gaser, C., Büchel, C., and May, A. (2008). Training-induced brain structure changes in the elderly. *J. Neurosci.* 28, 7031–7035. doi: 10.1523/JNEUROSCI.0742-08.2008

Bransford, J. D., Barclay, J. R., and Franks, J. J. (1972). Sentence memory: a constructive versus interpretive approach. *Cogn. Psychol.* 3, 193–209. doi: 10.1016/0010-0285(72)90003-5

Bransford, J. D., and Franks, J. J. (1971). The abstraction of linguistic ideas. *Cogn. Psychol.* 2, 331–350. doi: 10.1016/0010-0285(71)90019-3

Bressler, S. L., and Menon, V. (2010). Large-scale brain networks in cognition: emerging methods and principles. *Trends Cogn. Sci.* 14, 277–290. doi: 10.1016/j.tics.2010.04.004

Carlson, M. C., Erickson, K. I., Kramer, A. F., Voss, M. W., Bolea, N., Mielke, M., et al. (2009). Evidence for neurocognitive plasticity in at-risk older adults: the experience corps program. *J. Gerontol. A Biol. Sci. Med. Sci.* 64, 1275–1282. doi: 10.1093/gerona/glp117

Chapman, S. B., Aslan, S., Spence, J. S., Hart, J. J., Bartz, E. K., Didehbani, N., et al. (2013). Neural mechanisms of brain plasticity with complex cognitive training in healthy seniors. *Cereb. Cortex*. doi: 10.1093/cercor/bht234. [Epub ahead of print].

Chapman, S. B., Gamino, J. F., and Mudar, R. A. (2012). "Higher-order strategic gist reasoning in adolescence," in *The Adolescent Brain: Learning, Reasoning, and Decison Making*, eds V. Reyna, S. B. Chapman, M. R. Dougherty, and J. Confrey, 123–151. doi: 10.1037/13493-005

Chapman, S. B., and Mudar, R. A. (2013). Discourse gist: a window into the brain's complex cognitive capacity. *Discourse Stud.* 15, 519–533. doi: 10.1177/1461445613501444

Chen, A. J., Nycum, T. J., Novakovic-Agopian, T., Song, S., Gary, T., Rome, S., et al. (2011). Training of goal-directed attention regulation enhances control over neural processing for individuals with brain injury. *Brain* 134, 1541–1554. doi: 10.1093/brain/awr067

Chen, A. J.-W., Abrams, G. M., and D'Esposito, M. (2006). Functional reintegration of prefrontal neural networks for enhancing recovery after brain injury. *J. Head Trauma Rehabil.* 21, 107–118. doi: 10.1097/00001199-200603000-00004

Clare, L., and Woods, R. T. (2004). Cognitive training and cognitive rehabilitation for people with early-stage Alzheimer's disease: a review. *Neuropsychol. Rehabil.* 14, 385–401. doi: 10.1080/09602010443000074

Dahlin, E., Neely, A. S., Larsson, A., Bäckman, L., and Nyberg, L. (2008). Transfer of learning after updating training mediated by the striatum. *Science* 320, 1510–1512. doi: 10.1126/science.1155466

Frederksen, C. H., and Donin, J. (1991). Constructing multiple semantic representations in comprehending and producing discourse. *Adv. Psychol.* 79, 19–44. doi: 10.1016/S0166-4115(08)61547-2

Gabrieli, J. (2004). Memory: pandora's hippocampus? *Cerebrum* 6, 39–48.

Gamino, J. F., Chapman, S. B., Hull, E. L., and Lyon, G. R. (2010). Effects of higher-order cognitive strategy training on gist-reasoning and fact-learning in adolescents. *Front. Psychol.* 1:188. doi: 10.3389/fpsyg.2010.00188

Gates, N. J., Sachdev, P. S., Fiatarone Singh, M. A., and Valenzuela, M. (2011). Cognitive and memory training in adults at risk of dementia: a systematic review. *BMC Geriatr.* 11:55. doi: 10.1186/1471-2318-11-55

Gazzaley, A., Cooney, J. W., McEvoy, K., Knight, R. T., and D'Esposito, M. (2005). Top-down enhancement and suppression of the magnitude and speed of neural activity. *J. Cogn. Neurosci.* 17, 507–517. doi: 10.1162/0898929053279522

Jaeggi, S. M., Buschkuehl, M., Jonides, J., and Perrig, W. J. (2008). Improving fluid intelligence with training on working memory. *Proc. Natl. Acad. Sci. U.S.A.* 105, 6829–6833. doi: 10.1073/pnas.0801268105

Johnson-Laird, P. N. (1983). *Mental Models: Towards a Cognitive Science of Language, Inference, and Consciousness.* Cambridge, MA: Harvard University Press.

Kahana, M. J., and Wingfield, A. (2000). A functional relation between learning and organization in free recall. *Psychon. Bull. Rev.* 7, 516–521. doi: 10.3758/BF03214365

Kramer, A. F., and Erickson, K. I. (2007). Capitalizing on cortical plasticity: influence of physical activity on cognition and brain function. *Trends Cogn. Sci.* 11, 342–348. doi: 10.1016/j.tics.2007.06.009

Lloyd, F. J., and Reyna, V. F. (2009). Clinical gist and medical education. *JAMA* 302, 1332–1333. doi: 10.1001/jama.2009.1383

Mahncke, H. W., Connor, B. B., Appelman, J., Ahsanuddin, O. N., Hardy, J. L., Wood, R. A., et al. (2006). Memory enhancement in healthy older adults using a brain plasticity-based training program: a randomized, controlled study. *Proc. Natl. Acad. Sci. U.S.A.* 103, 12523–12528. doi: 10.1073/pnas.0605194103

Mandler, G., and Rabinowitz, J. C. (1981). Appearance and reality: does a recognition test really improve subsequent recall and recognition? *J. Exp. Psychol. Hum. Learn. Mem.* 7, 79. doi: 10.1037/0278-7393.7.2.79

Martin, M., Clare, L., Altgassen, A. M., Cameron, M. H., and Zehnder, F. (2011). Cognition-based interventions for healthy older people and people with mild cognitive impairment. *Cochrane Database Syst. Rev.* CD006220. doi: 10.1002/14651858.CD006220.pub2

Motes, M. A., Gamino, J. F., Chapman, S. B., Rao, N. K., Maguire, M. J., Brier, M. R., et al. (2014). Inhibitory control gains from higher-order cognitive strategy training. *Brain Cogn.* 84, 44–62. doi: 10.1016/j.bandc.2013.10.007

Mudar, R. A., Chiang, H., Eroh, J. T., Rackley, A., Venza, E., Martin-Cook, K., et al. (2013). "Benefits of cognitive training in individuals with mild cognitive impairment," in *Poster Presentation - Cognitive Neuroscience Society Annual Meeting*, April 2013 (San Francisco, CA).

Nedergaard, M. (2013). Garbage truck of the brain. *Science* 340, 1529–1530. doi: 10.1126/science.1240514

Norman, K. A., and Schacter, D. L. (1997). False recognition in younger and older adults: exploring the characteristics of illusory memories. *Mem. Cognit.* 25, 838–848. doi: 10.3758/BF03211328

Nyberg, L., Sandblom, J., Jones, S., Neely, A. S., Petersson, K. M., Ingvar, M., et al. (2003). Neural correlates of training-related memory improvement in adulthood and aging. *Proc. Natl. Acad. Sci. U.S.A.* 100, 13728–13733. doi: 10.1073/pnas.1735487100

Papp, K. V., Walsh, S. J., and Snyder, P. J. (2009). Immediate and delayed effects of cognitive interventions in healthy elderly: a review of current literature and future directions. *Alzheimers Dement.* 5, 50–60. doi: 10.1016/j.jalz.2008.10.008

Rebok, G. W., Ball, K., Guey, L. T., Jones, R. N., Kim, H. Y., King, J. W., et al. (2014). Ten year effects of the advanced cognitive training for independent and vital elderly cognitive training trial on cognition and everyday functioning in older adults. *J. Am. Geriatr. Soc.* 62, 16–24. doi: 10.1111/jgs.12607

Reijnders, J., Van Heugten, C., and Van Boxtel, M. (2012). Cognitive interventions in healthy older adults and people with mild cognitive impairment; a systematic review. *Ageing Res. Rev.* 12, 263–275. doi: 10.1016/j.arr.2012.07.003

Reyna, V. F. (1996). Conceptions of memory development with implications for reasoning and decision making. *Ann. Child Dev.* 12, 87–118.

Reyna, V. F., and Brainerd, C. J. (1995). Fuzzy-trace theory: an interim synthesis. *Learn. Individ. Differ.* 7, 1–75. doi: 10.1016/1041-6080(95)90031-4

Reyna, V. F., and Brainerd, C. J. (2011). Dual processes in decision making and developmental neuroscience: a Fuzzy-Trace model. *Dev. Rev.* 31, 180–206. doi: 10.1016/j.dr.2011.07.004

Reyna, V. F., and Lloyd, F. J. (2006). Physician decision making and cardiac risk: effects of knowledge, risk perception, risk tolerance, and fuzzy processing. *J. Exp. Psychol. Appl.* 12, 179–195. doi: 10.1037/1076-898X.12.3.179

Rosen, A. C., Sugiura, L., Kramer, J. H., Whitfield-Gabrieli, S., and Gabrieli, J. D. (2011). Cognitive training changes hippocampal function in mild cognitive impairment: a pilot study. *J. Alzheimers Dis.* 26, 349–357. doi: 10.3233/JAD-2011-0009

Schooler, C. (1984). Psychological effects of complex environments during the life span: a review and theory. *Intelligence* 8, 259–281. doi: 10.1016/0160-2896(84)90011-4

Schooler, C., Mulatu, M. S., and Oates, G. (1999). The continuing effects of substantively complex work on the intellectual functioning of older workers. *Psychol. Aging* 14, 483. doi: 10.1037/0882-7974.14.3.483

Tang, Y.-Y., Ma, Y., Wang, J., Fan, Y., Feng, S., Lu, Q., et al. (2007). Short-term meditation training improves attention and self-regulation. *Proc. Natl. Acad. Sci. U.S.A.* 104, 17152–17156. doi: 10.1073/pnas.0707678104

Tardif, S., and Simard, M. (2011). Cognitive stimulation programs in healthy elderly: a review. *Int. J. Alzheimers Dis.* 2011:378934. doi: 10.4061/2011/378934

Teixeira, C. V. L., Gobbi, L. T. B., Corazza, D. I., Stella, F., Costa, J. L. R., and Gobbi, S. (2012). Non-pharmacological interventions on cognitive functions in older people with mild cognitive impairment (MCI). *Arch. Gerontol. Geriatr.* 54, 175–180. doi: 10.1016/j.archger.2011.02.014

Thompson, T. W., Waskom, M. L., Garel, K.-L. A., Cardenas-Iniguez, C., Reynolds, G. O., Winter, R., et al. (2013). Failure of working memory training to enhance cognition or intelligence. *PLoS ONE* 8:e63614. doi: 10.1371/journal.pone.0063614

Valenzuela, M. J., Sachdev, P., Wen, W., Chen, X., and Brodaty, H. (2008). Lifespan mental activity predicts diminished rate of hippocampal atrophy. *PLoS ONE* 3:e2598. doi: 10.1371/journal.pone.0002598

Valenzuela, M., and Sachdev, P. (2009). Can cognitive exercise prevent the onset of dementia? Systematic review of randomized clinical trials with longitudinal follow-up. *Am. J. Geriatr. Psych.* 17, 179–187. doi: 10.1097/JGP.0b013e3181953b57

Van Dijk, T. A., Kintsch, W., and Van Dijk, T. A. (1983). *Strategies of Discourse Comprehension.* New York, NY: Academic Press.

Vas, A. K., Chapman, S. B., Cook, L. G., Elliott, A. C., and Keebler, M. (2011). Higher-order reasoning training years after traumatic brain injury in adults. *J. Head Trauma Rehabil.* 26, 224–239. doi: 10.1097/HTR.0b013e318218dd3d

Willis, S. L., Tennstedt, S. L., Marsiske, M., Ball, K., Elias, J., Koepke, K. M., et al. (2006). Long-term effects of cognitive training on everyday functional outcomes in older adults. *JAMA* 296, 2805–2814. doi: 10.1001/jama.296.23.2805

Zelinski, E. M. (2009). Far transfer in cognitive training of older adults. *Restor. Neurol. Neurosci.* 27, 455–471. doi: 10.3233/RNN-2009-0495

Zwaan, R. A., and Radvansky, G. A. (1998). Situation models in language comprehension and memory. *Psychol. Bull.* 123:162. doi: 10.1037/0033-2909.123.2.162

10

"Messing with the mind": evolutionary challenges to human brain augmentation

Arthur Saniotis[1,2]*, Maciej Henneberg[1,2], Jaliya Kumaratilake[1] and James P. Grantham[1]

[1] Biological Anthropology and Comparative Anatomy Unit, School of Medical Sciences, The University of Adelaide, Adelaide, SA, Australia
[2] Centre for Evolutionary Medicine, University of Zürich, Zürich, Switzerland

Edited by:
Ioan Opris, Wake Forest University, USA

Reviewed by:
Victor Manuel Pulgar, Wake Forest University, USA
Daniel James Miller, Vanderbilt University, USA

****Correspondence:***
Arthur Saniotis, Biological Anthropology and Comparative Anatomy Unit, School of Medical Sciences, The University of Adelaide, North Terrace, Adelaide, SA 5005, Australia
e-mail: arthur.saniotis@adelaide.edu.au

The issue of brain augmentation has received considerable scientific attention over the last two decades. A key factor to brain augmentation that has been widely overlooked are the complex evolutionary processes which have taken place in evolving the human brain to its current state of functioning. Like other bodily organs, the human brain has been subject to the forces of biological adaptation. The structure and function of the brain, is very complex and only now we are beginning to understand some of the basic concepts of cognition. Therefore, this article proposes that brain-machine interfacing and nootropics are not going to produce "augmented" brains because we do not understand enough about how evolutionary pressures have informed the neural networks which support human cognitive faculties.

Keywords: brain size, hominin brain, memory formation, brain-machine interfaces, nootropic agents

INTRODUCTION

The issue of brain augmentation has received considerable scientific attention over the last two decades. Much of this focus has been prompted by the increase in human aging population and the concomitant rise in dementiae and neuro-degenerative disease. Moreover, brain augmentation has become a central theme for transhumanists who argue for the creation of various biotechnologies in order to transcend the limitations of the biological body (Drexler, 1992; Roco and Bainbridge, 2002; Bostrom, 2003; Ramez, 2005). Kurzweil (2000) has suggested that development of brain-machine interfaces will be necessary to cope with the informational demands of future high tech societies. He even proposes the supplanting of a "cognitively superior" nanotech brain to supplement the biological human brain (Kurzweil, 2000). Transhumanists have overlooked the complex and plural selective pressures which have led to the human brain's current functioning. Like other bodily organs, the human brain has been subject to the forces of biological adaptation (Hawks et al., 2007; Henneberg and Saniotis, 2009), thus it is continuously changing. The challenges that humans are faced with are the continuously changing living environment and to a very much lesser extent the "technological advancement". Being a result of the trial-and-error processes of biological adaptation the structure and function of the human brain are very complex and only now we are beginning to understand some of the basic concepts of cognition (i.e., in relation to memory, memory consolidation and retrieval). Therefore, this article proposes that brain-machine interfacing is not going to produce "augmented" brains because we do not understand enough about how evolutionary pressures have informed the neural networks which support human cognitive faculties.

EVOLUTION OF HUMAN BRAIN SIZE AND INTELLIGENCE

There is no doubt that humans display behavioral complexity greater than other mammals, and there is ample archeological evidence for the historical development of human mind that is a system of informational processes manifesting itself in symbolic communication transmissible from one individual to others (Bednarik, 1997; Butler, 2005; Bar-Yosef, 2007; Burke, 2010; Lycett and Chauhan, 2010). However, it is still difficult to pinpoint and identify what is special about a biological substrate that led to the evolution of human complex behaviors.

Human brain is a mammalian organ that in no single particular way is exceptional. Its anatomy is very similar to that of other primate brains (Radinsky, 1979). For the long time it has been widely accepted that during several million years of hominin evolution the human brain became especially large, thus indicating anatomical basis for our unusual abilities. This, however, turns out not to be true at closer scrutiny of the fossil record of hominin evolution. True enough, the volume of hominin braincase tripled in the last, approximately, 3 million years (from about 450 ml to current 1350 ml, De Miguel and Henneberg, 2001). During that time, however, hominin body size increased, too. Body size is measured either as the linear height, or weight, that in humans scales approximately to the second power of height (Henneberg et al., 1989), a fact generally recognized by the construction of the Body Mass index as a ratio of weight to height squared. When the size of human brain is expressed as a linear dimension (a cube root of volume), its increases over the last 3 million years are comparable to those of height (Henneberg and Saniotis, 2009) and weight (**Figure 1**). The size of the human brain is proportional to the size of musculoskeletal system mass (Rogers, 1992); scaling of

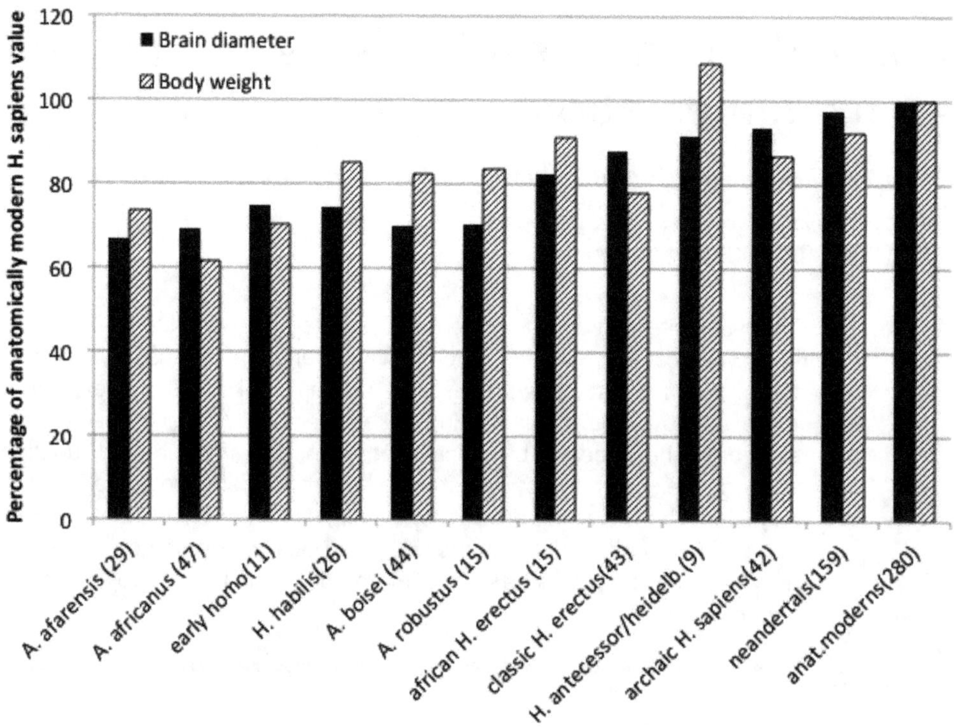

FIGURE 1 | Average brain diameters (a cubic root of endocranial capacity) and estimated body weights of hominids expressed as percentages of anatomically modern human averages. Data from De Miguel and Henneberg (2001) and Mathers and Henneberg supplemented with newer finds. Numbers in brackets are numbers of individual estimates taken into account.

human brain size to body size, in contrast to other vertebrates and mammals, where brain size increases allometrically at a fraction of body size (Jerison, 1973; Martin, 1990) is isometric, due to changes of body structure related to erect bipedalism, high quality diet and extraoral food processing together reducing body size (Henneberg, 1998). Physiological regulation of the human brain by endocrine exchanges follows the same principles as that of all other mammals, but the quantities of specific active substances may differ (Previc, 1999, 2009).

The size of the human brain does not correlate meaningfully with the mental abilities (Henneberg et al., 1985; McDaniel, 2005); the size explains at best about 10% of the variation in "intelligence" and even this number is debatable. Higher intellectual functions are difficult to localize precisely to specific regions of the brain compared to processing of sensory inputs and motor outputs (Power et al., 2011), while many tasks controlled by brains are processed in complex networks widely distributed across the cortex (Bullmore and Sporns, 2009). Researchers have tried to justify human uniqueness, since the rise of modern scientism by quoting various "exceptional" human brain characteristics. These were mostly associated with anatomical character due to the slow progress in physiological research on the human brain (because of ethical constraints), especially those related to neurotransmitter and hormone regulation of the central nervous system functions (i.e., primarily, synaptic function). The most common among the indices defining the uniqueness of the human brain are variously constructed "encephalization" indices. They combine in various forms information on brain size and body size, with the assumption that mammalian brains need to have a certain number of neurons to receive sensory information and process it to control functions of the body. The prevailing hypothesis states that the larger the brain in relation to body size, the greater the ability to process information. Averages of encephalization indices calculated in various ways (**Table 1**) place humans clearly above other mammals and human ancestors. However, when the range of variability in human brain size and the body size is taken into account differences between individual humans may be greater than those between Australopithecines and modern *Homo sapiens*. South African *Australopithecus robustus* had 4.3×10^9 extraneurons, while modern *Homo sapiens* have 8.2×10^9 extraneurons (McHenry, 1976, extra-neuron numbers were calculated using Jerison, 1973 formula). The large difference of 3.9×10^9, however, is smaller than the differences between some modern humans (see range in **Table 1**). When normal intraspecies variation is taken into account, it follows that individual members of our species, *H. sapiens*, do not differ from some individuals of *H. erectus* since the ranges of encephalization indices of these two species overlap widely.

Brains of different species have different neuronal densities and different levels of myelination in various regions (Haug, 1987; Glasser et al., 2014), which means that bigger brain does not necessarily contain more neurons. Usually neuronal density decreases with increasing brain size (Haug, 1987).

Table 1 | Ranges of various indices of encephalization in modern humans expressed as the lower and upper limits of 99% confidence intervals and their midpoints compared with *Homo erectus* midpoints (data from Henneberg, 1990) supplemented by *H. erectus* ranges calculated in a similar way using data from Henneberg and Thackeray, 1995.

Index (Author)	*H. erectus* lower limit	*H. erectus* midpoint	*H. erectus* upper limit	*H. sapiens* lower limit	*H. sapiens* midpoint	*H. sapiens* upper limit
Extraneurons (Jerison, 1973)	5.96×10^9	7.02×10^9	8.38×10^9	6.94×10^9	9.17×10^9	11.39×10^9
Encephalization Quotient (Jerison, 1973)	3.70	5.51	8.11	5.64	8.51	11.38
Index of Progression (Stephan, 1972)	18.59	23.0	32.33	23.6	35.0	46.4

Note that H. erctus midpoints are close to H. sapiens lower limits while H. sapiens midpoints are close to H. erectus upper limits. There is an obvious overlap between ranges of the two taxa.

BRAIN-MACHINE INTERFACES: EVOLUTIONARY CHALLENGES

Animal research in brain-machine interfaces has led to an improved understanding of memory and sensory processes and neural firing patterns, leading to possible prosthetic therapies for the restoration of motor function (Nicolelis, 2003; Nicolelis and Srinivasan, 2003; Sanchez et al., 2003; Lebedev and Nicolelis, 2006; Moritz et al., 2008; Ethier et al., 2012). These developments have prompted some thinkers to suggest that humans are on the verge of a "technological cognitive revolution" (Nicolelis and Srinivasan, 2003). Current research is focusing on the use of computers to ascertain information on a user's cognitive state by observing their physiology (Tan and Nijholt, 2010), thus therapeutically directed brain-machine interfaces appear to be promising (Collinger et al., 2012; Shih et al., 2012; Borton et al., 2013; Ifft et al., 2013; Thakor, 2013; Raspopovic et al., 2014). Recent developments have focussed on stimulation of ulner and median nerve fascicles using transversal multichannel intrafascicular electrodes, which enables an amputee to adapt their grasping force (Raspopovic et al., 2014). In another recent study a bimanual BMI has been developed that enables rhesus monkeys to simultaneously control two avatar arms. The bimanual BMI is based on extracellular activity of 374 to 497 neurons monitored from various parietal and cortical areas (Ifft et al., 2013). These developments should assist in the design of BMIs which enable human patients better manual control.

While neuroscience research is advancing BMI therapeutic capabilities, there is yet no existing brain-machine interface based on exchange of electrical (electromagnetic) signals that would improve human cognitive abilities above and beyond what a natural brain can do. We do not have yet a theory correctly approximating physical substrate of higher cognitive processes. Brain did not evolve by adding defined units for more complex functions, it improved its performance by physiological modulation enabled by biochemical alterations of neuroactive substances.

Therefore, the belief that brain-machine interfaces offer a viable method for augmenting cognitive processes lacks scientific credibility (Kurzweil, 2000). The mainstay of this rhetoric has come via futurists who have generally ignored evolutionary processes, which have produced the current structure and functions of the human brain. What we have to remember is that our advanced technology that is in use in society is not the product of the brain of one person, who generated it in a short time. Rather it is the combined effect of multitudinous brains over a long historical period (i.e., learning, processing of learned information, researching and planning) together or separately over a long period of time. The brain is a unique organ that "changes" with learning and processing of the learned material to generate novel ideas that could be researched or tested. In short, the brain is continuously changing to generate the complex technological advances of the modern world. Therefore, a normal brain does not need a brain-machine interface to cope with the ever increasing technology or new information; what the brain needs is continuous input of the new information (i.e., learning). Furthermore, when an individual executes an action (mental or physical), it results from the complex interactions of information inputs and outputs from many regions of the brain (e.g., a muscular action—sensory cortex, motor cortex, basal nuclei, cerebellum, etc.) and the level and type of interaction from each region vary (Blumenfeld, 2010; Michael-Titus et al., 2010). Therefore, proper understanding of all these process is critical, before manufacturing "brain-machine" interfaces to augment brain functions. If this path is not taken, brain-machine interfaces could cause more harm than benefits.

We may infer from this that any attempts to augment human intelligence via brain-machine interfaces will be problematic due to evolutionary dynamics underpinning the human brain. Furthermore, the incredibly complex nature of neural networks, chemical complexity of nerve signals conduction and individual anatomical and physiological variation pose enormous challenges for interaction of engineered devices with association networks in the human brain. However, in the current environment, brain-machine interfaces may have some therapeutic benefits in individuals developing dementiae, neuro-degenerative diseases and sensory input inadequacies (blindness, deafness). For example, neuromodulation using deep brain stimulation (DBS) is currently being used to reduce Parkinsonian symptoms in selected patients. A goal of DBS is not merely to slow down cognitive decline, but also to lead to a restoration of function, thereby increasing life quality (Zibly et al., 2014). Advantages of DBS surgery are its low complication rates and comparatively higher safety levels when performed by expert neurosurgeons (Zibly et al., 2014).

Since complex cognitive tasks rely on widely dispersed intersecting neural networks involving various parts of the brain, it is thought to be difficult to connect to the brain an engineered device that would assist or augment complex thoughts. Since transmission of signal from one neuron to other neurons is mediated chemically, it may be more feasible to introduce into brains substances that alter the efficiency of neurotransmission. Chemical engineering may be more efficient than electronic engineering.

NOOTROPIC AGENTS AND EVOLUTION

There are a number of chemically based methods of augmenting the human brain, forming an important element of cosmetic neurology (Dees, 2004). The field of cosmetic neurology is increasingly dependent on the development and application of nootropic agents (Cakic, 2009). A nootropic agent is a substance that may alter, nourish or augment cognitive performance, predominantly through the stimulation or inhibition of certain neurotransmitters (Nishizaki et al., 1999). These agents may occur in nature or be synthetically derived (Dielenberg, 2013). These substances have been proven to increase concentration, harness memory potential and expedite cognitive functioning (Turner et al., 2003, 2004). Many of these agents act under the premise of manipulating neurochemistry in a targeted fashion and are predominantly stimulatory in nature (Copani et al., 1992). Most traditional and modern nootropics activate an excitatory neurotransmitter or suppress the action of its inhibitory counterpart (Ito et al., 1990; Nicoletti et al., 1991; Staubli et al., 1994; Lynch and Gall, 2006; Huff, 2012).

Many authors support the co-evolution of early hominins with the use of nootropic substances and the attainment of altered states of consciousness (Winkelman, 2000, 2001; Sullivan and Hagen, 2002; Saniotis, 2010). Indeed, the desire to augment cognitive performance through the consumption of particular substances predates antiquity.

There is evidence to support the long-standing and widespread use of nootropic agents on every inhabited continent. For example Aboriginal Australians have used the stimulatory effects of *Nicotiani gossei* for millennia (Watson, 1983; Sullivan and Hagen, 2002). The use of tobacco throughout North and Central America has been well established and coca, the pre-cursor of cocaine, was cultivated along the western coast of South America as long as 7,000 years ago (Balick and Cox, 1996; Sullivan and Hagen, 2002). This cultivation ran contemporaneously with the use of cannabis in Europe (Schultes and Hofmann, 1979). The modest potency of organically derived substances and the long-standing, stable use of the aforementioned products in these ancient cultures proved to be beneficial (Saniotis and Henneberg, 2011). The strongest evidence to support this development is the presence of encoding DNA specific for the metabolization of these substances, such as the cytochrome P450 2D6 (CYP2D6) gene (Saniotis and Henneberg, 2011). These examples illustrate the inextricable involvement of environmental substances in altering or augmenting cognitive performance.

The affiliation with biological neuro-stimulants has continued through to recent history. The industrial revolution permitted the production of mind-altering substances on an unprecedented scale. Throughout the 20th century, there was a proliferation of synthetically derived substances applicable to cosmetic neurology. Today, nootropic agents are used to intentionally augment cognitive performance. University students appear to be amongst major perpetrators as they complete assignments and prepare for examinations (Greely et al., 2008). Prescription medications such as methylphenidate (Ritalin) and dextroamphetamine (Adderall) are being increasingly used and modafinil, an analeptic prescription medication has been used as a study aid by one-fifth of UK university students (Ghahremani et al., 2011; Fitzsimons and McDonald, 2014). Modafinil is believed to increase concentrations of glutamate and decrease GABA within the posterior hypothalamus, producing an overall neuro-excitatory effect (Ferraro et al., 1999). The drug has been shown to improve attention and working memory in medical practitioners and aviators and may be used in other challenging professions (Turner et al., 2003; Chatterjee, 2004; Müller et al., 2004; Walsh et al., 2004; Czeisler et al., 2005; Warren et al., 2009; Garcia et al., 2013).

However, the over-application of modern cosmetic neurology is fraught with danger and has been proven deleterious in many instances. In the short term, modafinil is known to produce nausea, vomiting, diarrhea, dyspepsia, headache, insomnia and anxiety with its long-term complications remaining largely unknown (Ballon and Feifel, 2006; Sahakian and Morein-Zamir, 2007). More alarmingly, the consumption of commonly used psycho-stimulants, including Ritalin and Adderall, has been linked to the precipitation or exacerbation of underlying mental illness, sleep disturbances and cerebrovascular disease (Cakic, 2009). This is likely due to the modern human brain being maladaptive to the exaggerated pharmacological alteration of neurochemistry (Sullivan and Hagen, 2002). Increased drug potency associated with synthetic production has outpaced the brain's capacity to metabolize and clear toxic substances, leading to prolonged exposure to these potentially harmful products (Sullivan and Hagen, 2002). This may be an example of evolutionary mismatch (Sullivan and Hagen, 2002). Whatever the mechanism, it appears these ill-adapted responses to modern nootropic agents may account for the bulk of the observed negative outcomes.

The potential scope of application for nootropic agents is vast. Mind-altering substances have the capacity to optimize cognitive performance and maximize human achievement. However, the limits of pharmacologically aided human cognition should not exceed the capacities of the brain. The human brain is a complex organ, thus pushing its performance beyond its adaptive capacity using pharmacological products could lead to failure. Therefore, caution must be taken when approaching the inherent risks of exacerbating the existing evolutionary mismatch in order to avoid deleterious outcomes. The majority of these outcomes are likely to relate to unbalancing salubrious and delicate neurochemical concentrations. Many psychiatric conditions, including schizophrenia, bipolar disorder and major depression, have illustrated neurochemical etiologies (Knable and Weinberger, 1997; Hirschfeld, 2000; López-Figueroa et al., 2004; Berk et al., 2007). Evolutionary challenges aside, there are also unresolved ethical and practical issues related to the intentional consumption of nootropic agents, not the least of which being whether it is fair, ethical and sensible to do so.

CONCLUSION

Many believe it to be evident that the human brain has a tremendous propensity for technologically driven augmentation. Several authors have discussed the potential for anatomical and physiological enhancement via brain-machine interfaces and cosmetic neurology. Despite the hypothetical applications of cognitive improvement, this article has argued that human brain augmentation possesses a number of inherent challenges, many of which are informed during prehistory. The daunting complexity of neurological processes which inform cognitive abilities, combined with a current lack of understanding will likely confound any attempts in creating "smarter" minds. In fact, any attempt to circumvent the archaic substructures of the human brain may only serve to exacerbate the already existing maladaptive responses. For this reason, great caution must be adopted in approaching further attempts to go "messing with the mind".

REFERENCES

Balick, M. J., and Cox, P. A. (1996). *Plants, People and Culture: The Science of Ethnobotany.* New York: Scientific American Library.

Ballon, J. S., and Feifel, D. (2006). A systematic review of modafinil: potential clinical uses and mechanisms of action. *J. Clin. Psychiatry* 67, 554–566. doi: 10.4088/jcp.v67n0406

Bar-Yosef, O. (2007). The archaeological framework of the upper paleolithic revolution. *Diogenes* 54, 3–18. doi: 10.1177/0392192107076869

Bednarik, R. G. (1997). The global evidence of early human symboling behaviour. *Hum. Evol.* 12, 147–168. doi: 10.1007/bf02438065

Berk, M., Dodd, S., Kauer-Sant Anna, M., Malhi, G. S., Bourin, M., Kapczinski, F., et al. (2007). Dopamine dysregulation syndrome: implications for a dopamine hypothesis of bipolar disorder. *Acta Psychiatr. Scand. Suppl.* 116, 41–49. doi: 10.1111/j.1600-0447.2007.01058.x

Blumenfeld, H. (2010). *Neuroanatomy Through Clinical Cases.* 2nd Edn. Sunderland, Massachusetts: Sinauer Associates, Inc.

Borton, D., Silvestro Micera, S., Millán, J. R., and Courtine, G. (2013). Robotics and neuroprosthetics: personalizsed neuroprosthetics. *Sci. Transl. Med.* 5:210rv2. doi: 10.1126/scitranslmed.3005968

Bostrom, N. (2003). Are you living in a computer simulation?. *Philos. Q.* 53, 243–255. doi: 10.1111/1467-9213.00309

Bullmore, E., and Sporns, O. (2009). Complex brain networks: graph theoretical analysis of structural and functional systems. *Nat. Rev. Neurosci.* 10, 186–198. doi: 10.1038/nrn2575

Burke, A. (2010). Spatial abilities, cognition and the pattern of Neanderthal and modern human dispersals. *Quat. Int.* 247, 230–235. doi: 10.1016/j.quaint.2010.10.029

Butler, C. (2005). *Prehistoric Flintwork.* Tempus: Stroud.

Cakic, V. (2009). Smart drugs for cognitive enhancement: ethical and pragmatic considerations in the era of cosmetic neurology. *J. Med. Ethics* 35, 611–615. doi: 10.1136/jme.2009.030882

Chatterjee, A. (2004). Cosmetic neurology: the controversy over enhancing movement, mentation and mood. *Neurology* 63, 968–974. doi: 10.1212/01.wnl.0000138438.88589.7c

Collinger, J. L., Wodlinger, B., Downey, J. E., Wang, W., Tyler-Kabara, E. C., Weber, D. J., et al. (2012). High-performance neuroprosthetic control by an individual with tetraplegia. *Lancet* 381, 557–564. doi: 10.1016/S0140-6736(12)61816-9

Copani, A., Genazzani, A. A., Aleppo, G., Casabona, G., Canonico, P. L., Scapagnini, U., et al. (1992). Nootropic drugs positively modulate α-amino-3-hydroxy-5-methyl-4-isoxazolepropionic acid-sensitive glutamate receptors in neuronal cultures. *J. Neurochem.* 58, 1199–1204. doi: 10.1111/j.1471-4159.1992.tb11329.x

Czeisler, C. A., Walsh, J. K., Roth, T., Hughes, R. J., Wright, K. P., Kingsbury, L., et al. (2005). Modafinil for excessive sleepiness associated with shift-work sleep disorder. *N. Engl. J. Med.* 353, 476–486. doi: 10.1056/nejm200509083531028

Dees, R. H. (2004). Slippery slopes, wonder drugs and cosmetic neurology the neuroethics of enhancement. *Neurology* 63, 951–952. doi: 10.1212/01.wnl.0000140733.62305.af

De Miguel, C., and Henneberg, M. (2001). Variation in hominid brain size: how much is due to method? *Homo* 52, 3–58. doi: 10.1078/0018-442x-00019

Dielenberg, R. A. (2013). The speculative neuroscience of the future human brain. *Humanities* 2, 209–252. doi: 10.3390/h2020209

Drexler, K. E. (1992). *Nanosystems: Molecular Machinery, Manufacturing and Computation.* New York: John Wiley and Sons, Inc.

Ethier, C., Oby, E. R., Bauman, M. J., and Miller, L. E. (2012). Restoration of grasp following paralysis through brain-controlled stimulation of muscles. *Nature* 485, 368–371. doi: 10.1038/nature10987

Ferraro, L., Antonelli, T., Tanganelli, S., O'Connor, W. T., Perez de la Mora, M., Mendez-Franco, J., et al. (1999). The vigilance promoting drug modafinil increases extracellular glutamate levels in the medial preoptic area and the posterior hypothalamus of the conscious rat: prevention by local GABAA receptor blockade. *Neuropsychopharmacology* 20, 346–356. doi: 10.1016/s0893-133x(98)00085-2

Fitzsimons, S., and McDonald, M. (2014). *One in Five Students have Used Modafinil: Study Drug Survey Results.* Cambrige: The Tab.com (Online).

Garcia, V. A., Hirotsu, C., Matos, G., Alvarenga, T., Pires, G. N., Kapczinski, F., et al. (2013). Modafinil ameliorates cognitive deficits induced by maternal separation and sleep deprivation. *Behav. Brain Res.* 253, 274–279. doi: 10.1016/j.bbr.2013.07.029

Ghahremani, D. G., Tabibnia, G., Monterosso, J., Hellemann, G., Poldrack, R. A., and London, E. D. (2011). Effect of modafinil on learning and task-related brain activity in methamphetamine-dependent and healthy individuals. *Neuropsychopharmacology* 36, 950–959. doi: 10.1038/npp.2010.233

Glasser, M. F., Goyal, M. S., Preuss, T. M., Raichle, M. E., and Van Essen, D. C. (2014). Trends and properties of human cerebral cortex: correlations with cortical myelin content. *Neuroimage* 93, 165–175. doi: 10.1016/j.neuroimage.2013.03.060

Greely, H., Sahakian, B., Harris, J., Kessler, R. C., Gazzaniga, M., Campbell, P., et al. (2008). Towards responsible use of cognitive-enhancing drugs by the healthy. *Nature* 456, 702–705. doi: 10.1038/456702a

Haug, H. (1987). Brain sizes, surfaces and neuronal sizes of the cortex cerebri: a stereological investigation of man and his variability and a comparison with some mammals (primates, whales, marsupials, insectivores and one elephant). *Am. J. Anat.* 180, 126–142. doi: 10.1002/aja.1001800203

Hawks, J., Wang, E. T., Cochran, G. M., Harpending, H. C., and Moyzis, R. K. (2007). Recent acceleration of human adaptive evolution. *Proc. Natl. Acad. Sci. U S A* 104, 20753–20758. doi: 10.1073/pnas.0707650104

Henneberg, M. (1990). Brain size/body weight variability in Homo sapiens: consequences for interpreting hominid evolution. *Homo* 39, 121–130.

Henneberg, M. (1998). Evolution of the human brain: is bigger better? *Clin. Exp. Pharmacol. Physiol.* 25, 745–749. doi: 10.1111/j.1440-1681.1998.tb02289.x

Henneberg, M., Budnik, A., Pezacka, M., and Puch, A. E. (1985). Head size body size and intelligence intraspecific correlation in Homo sapiens species. *Homo* 36, 207–218.

Henneberg, M., Hugg, J., and Townsend, E. J. (1989). Body weight/height relationship an exponential solution. *Am. J. Hum. Biol.* 1, 483–491. doi: 10.1002/ajhb.1310010412

Henneberg, M., and Saniotis, A. (2009). Evolutionary origins of human brain and spirituality. *Anthropol. Anz.* 67, 427–438. doi: 10.1127/0003-5548/2009/0032

Henneberg, M., and Thackeray, J. F. (1995). A single-lineage hypothesis of hominid evolution. *Evol. Theory* 13, 31–38.

Hirschfeld, R. M. A. (2000). History and evolution of the monoamine hypothesis of depression. *J. Clin. Psychiatry* 61, 4–6.

Huff, M. M. (2012). *Cosmetic Neurology: Enhancement of the Mind and Attention Deficit Hyperactive Disorder Medication Abuse among College Students.* Lynchburg: Liberty University.

Ifft, P. J., Shokur, S., Li, Z., Lebedev, M. A., and Nicolelis, M. A. L. (2013). A brain-machine interface enables bimanual arm movements in monkeys. *Sci. Transl. Med.* 5:210ra154. doi: 10.1126/scitranslmed.3006159

Ito, I., Tanabe, S., Kohda, A., and Sugiyama, H. (1990). Allosteric potentiation of receptors by a nootropic drug aniracetam. *J. Physiol.* 424, 533–543.

Jerison, H. J. (1973). *Evolution of the Brain and Intelligence.* New York: Academic Press.

Knable, M. B., and Weinberger, D. R. (1997). Dopamine, the pre-frontal cortex and schizophrenia. *J. Psychopharmacol.* 11, 123–131. doi: 10.1177/026988119701100205

Kurzweil, R. (2000). *The Age of Spiritual Machines: When Computers Exceed Human Intelligence.* New York: Penguin Books.

Lebedev, M., and Nicolelis, M. A. L. (2006). Brain-machine interfaces: past, present and future. *Trends Neurosci.* 29, 536–546. doi: 10.1016/j.tins.2006.07.004

López-Figueroa, A. L., Norton, C. S., Lopez-Figueroa, M. O., Armellini-Dodel, D., Burke, S., Akil, H., et al. (2004). Serotonin 5-HT1A, 5-HT1B and 5-HT2A receptor mRNA expression in subjects with major depression, bipolar disorder and schizophrenia. *Biol. Psychiatry* 55, 225–233. doi: 10.1016/j.biopsych.2003.09.017

Lycett, S. P., and Chauhan, P. eds. (2010). *Newperspectives on Old Stones: Analytical Approaches to Palaeolithic Techniques.* New York: Springer.

Lynch, G., and Gall, C. M. (2006). Ampakines and the threefold path to cognitive enhancement. *Trends Neurosci.* 29, 554–562. doi: 10.1016/j.tins.2006.07.007

Martin, R. D. (1990). *Primate Origins and Evolution.* New Jersey: Princeton University Press.

McDaniel, M. A. (2005). Big-brained people are smarter: a meta-analysis of the relationship between in vivo brain volume and intelligence. *Intelligence* 33, 337–346. doi: 10.1016/j.intell.2004.11.005

McHenry, H. M. (1976). Early hominid body weight and encephalisation. *Am. J. Phys. Anthropol.* 45, 77–83. doi: 10.1002/ajpa.1330450110

Michael-Titus, A., Revest, P., and Shortland, P. (2010). *Systems of the Body: The Nervous System—Basic Science and Clinical Conditions.* 2nd Edn. New York, Oxford: Elsevier.

Moritz, C. T., Perlmutter, S. I., and Fetz, E. E. (2008). Direct control of paralysed muscles by cortical neurons. *Nature* 456, 639–642. doi: 10.1038/nature07418

Müller, U., Steffenhagen, N., Regenthal, R., and Bublak, P. (2004). Effects of modafinil on working memory processes in humans. *Psychopharmacology (Berl)* 177, 161–169. doi: 10.1007/s00213-004-1926-3

Nicolelis, M. A. L. (2003). Brain-machine interfaces to restore motor function and probe neural circuits. *Nat. Rev. Neurosci.* 4, 417–422. doi: 10.1038/nrn1105

Nicolelis, M. A. L., and Srinivasan, M. (2003). "Human-machine interactions: potential impact of nanotechnology in the design of neuroprosthetic devices aimed at restoring or augmenting human performance," in *Converging Technologies for Improving Human Performance: Nanotechnology, Biotechnology, Information Technology and Cognitive Science*, eds M. C. Roco and W. S. Bainbridge (Dordrecht, The Netherlands: Kluwer Academic Press), 251–255.

Nicoletti, F., Casabona, G., Genazzani, A. A., Copani, A., Aleppo, G., Canonico, P. L., et al. (1991). Excitatory amino acids and neuronal plasticity: modulation of AMPA receptors as a novel substrate for the action of nootropic drugs. *Funct. Neurol.* 7, 413–422.

Nishizaki, T., Matsuoka, T., Nomura, T., Matsuyama, S., Watabe, S., Shiotani, T., et al. (1999). A 'long-term-potentiation-like' facilitation of hippocampal synaptic transmission induced by the nootropic nefiracetam. *Brain Res.* 826, 281–288. doi: 10.1016/s0006-8993(99)01312-8

Power, J. D., Alexander, J., Cohen, L., Nelson, S. M., Wig, G. S., Barnes, K. A., et al. (2011). Functional network organization of the human brain. *Neuron* 72, 665–678. doi: 10.1016/j.neuron.2011.09.006

Previc, F. (1999). Dopamine and the origins of human intelligence. *Brain Cogn.* 41, 299–350. doi: 10.1006/brcg.1999.1129

Previc, F. (2009). *The Dopaminergic Mind in Human Evolution and History.* New York: Cambridge University Press.

Radinsky, L. B. (1979). *The Fossil Record of Primate Brain Evolution. 49th James Arthur Lecture, 1979.* New York: American Museum of Natural History.

Ramez, N. (2005). *More Than Human: Enhancing the Promise of Biological Enhancement.* New York: Broadway Books.

Raspopovic, S., Capogrosso, M., Petrini, F. M., Bonizzato, M., Rigosa, J., Di Pino, G., et al. (2014). Restoring natural sensory feedback in real-time bidirectional hand prostheses. *Sci. Transl. Med.* 6:222ra19. doi: 10.1126/scitranslmed.3006820

Roco, M. C., and Bainbridge, W. S. (2002). *Nanotechnology, Biotechnology, Information Technology and Cognitive Science.* Washington, DC: National Science Foundation.

Rogers, A. W. (1992). *A Textbook of Anatomy.* Edinburgh: Churchill Livingstone.

Sahakian, B., and Morein-Zamir, S. (2007). Professor's little helper. *Nature* 450, 1157–1159. doi: 10.1038/4501157a

Sanchez, J. C., Erdogmus, D., Rao, Y. N., Principe, J. C., Nicolelis, M., and Wessberg, J. (2003). "Learning the contributions of the motor, premotor and posterior parietal cortices for hand trajectory reconstruction in a brain machine interface," in Presented at the *IEEE EMBS Neural Engineering Conference.* Capri, Italy.

Saniotis, A. (2010). Evolutionary and anthropological approaches towards understanding human need for psychotropic and mood altering substances. *J. Psychoactive Drugs* 42, 477–484. doi: 10.1080/02791072.2010.10400710

Saniotis, A., and Henneberg, M. (2011). An evolutionary approach to exploring altered states of consciousness, mind-body techniques and non-local mind. *World Futures* 67, 182–200. doi: 10.1080/02604027.2011.555250

Schultes, R., and Hofmann, A. (1979). "An overview of hallucinogens in the western hemisphere," in *Flesh of the Gods*, ed P. Furst (New York: Praeger), 3–54.

Shih, J. J., Krusienski, D. J., and Wolpaw, J. R. (2012). Brain-computer interfaces in medicine. *Mayo Clin. Proc.* 87, 268–279. doi: 10.1016/j.mayocp.2011.12.008

Staubli, U., Rogers, G., and Lynch, G. (1994). Facilitation of glutamate receptors enhances memory. *Proc. Natl. Acad. Sci. U S A* 91, 777–781. doi: 10.1073/pnas.91.2.777

Stephan, H. (1972). "Evolution of primate brains: a comparative anatomical invesitigation," in *Functional and Evolutionary Biology of Primates*, ed R. Tuttle (Chicago: Aldine Atherton), 155–174.

Sullivan, R. J., and Hagen, E. H. (2002). Psychotropic substance-seeking: evolutionary pathology or adaptation?. *Addiction* 97, 389–400. doi: 10.1046/j.1360-0443.2002.00024.x

Tan, D. S., and Nijholt, A. (2010). "Brain-computer interfaces and human-computer interaction," in *Brain-Computer Interfaces*, eds D. S. Tan and A. Nijholt (London: Springer-Verlag Limited), 3–19.

Thakor, N. V. (2013). Translating the brain-machine interface. *Sci. Transl. Med.* 5:210ps17. doi: 10.1126/scitranslmed.3007303

Turner, D. C., Clark, L., Dowson, J., Robbins, J., and Sahakian, B. J. (2004). Modafinil improves cognition and response inhibition in adult attention-deficit/hyperactivity disorder. *Biol. Psychiatry* 55, 1031–1040. doi: 10.1016/j.biopsych.2004.02.008

Turner, D. C., Robbins, T. W., Clark, L., Aron, A. R., Dowson, J., and Sahakian, B. J. (2003). Cognitive enhancing effects of modafinil in healthy volunteers. *Psychopharmacology (Berl)* 165, 260–269.

Walsh, J. K., Randazzo, A. C., Stone, K. L., and Schweitzer, P. K. (2004). Modafinil improves alertness, vigilance and executive function during simulated night shifts. *Sleep* 27, 434–439.

Warren, O. J., Leff, D. R., Athanasiou, T., Kennard, C., and Darzi, A. (2009). The neurocognitive enhancement of surgeons: an ethical perspective. *J. Surg. Res.* 152, 167–172. doi: 10.1016/j.jss.2007.12.761

Watson, P. L. (1983). *This Precious Foliage: A Study of the Aboriginal Psycho-Active Drug Pituri.* Sydney: University of Sydney.

Winkelman, M. (2000). *The Neural Ecology of Consciousness and Healing.* Westport, Conneticut, London: Bergin and Garvey.

Winkelman, M. (2001). Alternative and traditional medicine approaches for substance abuse programs: a shamanic approach. *Int. J. Drug Policy* 12, 337–351. doi: 10.1016/s0955-3959(01)00100-1

Zibly, Z., Shawa, A., Harnof, S., Sharma, M., Graves, C., and Deogaonkar, M. (2014). Modulation of mind: therapeutic neuromodulation for cognitive disability. *J. Clin. Neurosci.* doi: 10.1016/j.jocn.2013.11.040. [Epub ahead of print].

11

A survey of substance use for cognitive enhancement by university students in the Netherlands

Kimberly J. Schelle[1,2]*, Bas M. J. Olthof[1,3], Wesley Reintjes[1,4], Carsten Bundt[1,5], Joyce Gusman-Vermeer[1] and Anke C. C. M. van Mil[1,6]

[1] Radboud Honours Academy, Radboud University, Nijmegen, Netherlands
[2] Department of Industrial Design, Eindhoven University of Technology, Eindhoven, Netherlands
[3] Faculty of Medical Sciences, Institute of Neuroscience, Newcastle University, Newcastle upon Tyne, UK
[4] Department of Neurology, Isala Clinics, Zwolle, Netherlands
[5] Department of Experimental Psychology, Ghent University, Ghent, Belgium
[6] Department of Physiology, Radboud Institute for Health Sciences, Radboud University Medical Center, Nijmegen, Netherlands

Edited by:
Mikhail Lebedev, Duke University, USA

Reviewed by:
Wanja Wolff, University of Potsdam, Germany
Eshetu Haileselassie Engeda, University of Gondar, Ethiopia

****Correspondence:***
Kimberly J. Schelle, Radboud Honours Academy, Radboud University, Comeniuslaan 4, 6525 HP Nijmegen, Netherlands
e-mail: kimberlyschelle@gmail.com

Background: Pharmacological cognitive enhancement, using chemicals to change cellular processes in the brain in order to enhance one's cognitive capacities, is an often discussed phenomenon. The prevalence among Dutch university students is unknown.

Methods: The study set out to achieve the following goals: (1) give an overview of different methods in order to assess the prevalence of use of prescription, illicit and lifestyle drugs for cognitive enhancement (2) investigate whether polydrug use and stress have a relationship with cognitive enhancement substance use (3) assessing opinions about cognitive enhancement prescription drug use. A nationwide survey was conducted among 1572 student respondents of all government supported Dutch universities.

Results: The most detailed level of analysis—use of specific substances without a prescription and with the intention of cognitive enhancement—shows that prescription drugs, illicit drugs and lifestyle drugs are respectively used by 1.7, 1.3, and 45.6% of the sample. The use of prescription drugs and illicit drugs is low compared to other countries. We have found evidence of polydrug use in relation to cognitive enhancement. A relation between stress and the use of lifestyle drugs for cognitive enhancement was observed. We report the findings of several operationalizations of cognitive enhancement drug use to enable comparison with a wider variety of previous and upcoming research.

Conclusions: Results of this first study among university students in the Netherlands revealed a low prevalence of cognitive enhancement drug use compared to other countries. Multiple explanations, such as a difference in awareness of pharmacological cognitive enhancement among students, accessibility of drugs in the student population and inclusion criteria of enhancement substances are discussed. We urge enhancement researchers to take the different operationalizations and their effects on the prevalence numbers into account.

Keywords: cognitive enhancement, neuroenhancement, smart drugs, prescription stimulants, non-medical use, illicit drugs, lifestyle drugs, self-report

INTRODUCTION

Recently the topic of cognitive enhancement has received much attention, both in popular media (e.g., Schwarz, 2012; Sharrett, 2012; Shiner, 2013; Monks, 2014) and academic literature (e.g., a special issue on cognitive enhancers by Neuropharmacology Lynch et al., 2013). Cognitive enhancement can be accomplished in a variety of ways. Some methods use advanced technology to modulate brain activity, e.g., deep brain stimulation, whilst other methods are based on chemicals that are aimed at changing the cellular processes in the brain, also named pharmacological cognitive enhancement. Pharmacological cognitive enhancement refers to boosting cognitive capacities by using substances, with the aim to enhance one's performance above baseline levels (e.g., Bostrom and Sandberg, 2009). Most substances regularly referred to in the discussion about pharmacological cognitive enhancement were originally developed to treat neuropsychiatric disorders that are often accompanied by cognitive deficits. A drug widely reported to be used with the purpose of pharmacological cognitive enhancement is methylphenidate (e.g., Ritalin, Concerta), which was developed as a treatment for attention deficit hyperactivity disorder (ADHD). Other drugs often used to boost cognitive capacities include modafinil and amphetamines (Ragan et al., 2013). However, recently also other substances, such as caffeine and nicotine as well as several illicit drugs, are included in the discussion of the cognitive enhancement literature (e.g., Franke et al., 2011b, 2012; Wolff et al., 2014).

The expectations of the effect prescription drugs for cognitive enhancement exert in healthy individuals often exceed their real effect (Repantis et al., 2010). Whether effective or not, the prevalence studies have shown that some people do experiment with drugs to boost their (cognitive) performance (Smith and Farah, 2011).

Herman-Stahl et al. (2007) suggested that the use of prescription drugs to improve one's cognitive performance is especially common among individuals in cognitively demanding environments, such as schools and universities. The authors showed that college students are more likely to use prescription stimulants for nonmedical purposes than young adults who are not enrolled in college, although no intentions of use (e.g., recreational, or to enhance performance) were examined in this study. In addition, most of the prevalence studies conducted so far have focused on the university student population. Smith and Farah (2011) give an overview of 28 epidemiological studies on the prevalence of nonmedical prescription drug use that were conducted among secondary and post-secondary students in the US and Canada before July 2010. The prevalence numbers of lifetime nonmedical stimulant use among university students ranged from 5.3% in an online study reaching over 2000 respondents (DuPont et al., 2008) to 55% in a study among 307 fraternity members (DeSantis et al., 2009). Smith and Farah (2011) conclude that it is hard to draw quantitative conclusions from the list of studies, as they differ in many ways. For example, there are marked differences in the way the prevalence numbers are calculated, where some studies include all nonmedical use, others only include nonmedical use with the intention to enhance ones cognitive performance. This means that in the latter condition users with solely recreational or experimental intentions are excluded from the prevalence numbers that are presented. Moreover, some studies focus solely on the intention, meaning that also individuals with a prescription are counted as a cognitive enhancement drug user when they report to use these drugs for nonmedical reasons, while others exclude all users with a prescription regardless of their intention of use. Smith and Farah (2011) also describe a large variation between studies in sampling method and demographic characteristics, ranging from studies examining a single department at a single institution to nationwide epidemiological surveys on nonmedical drug use. These differences have a major influence on the outcome of the studies because of several factors that can vary between institutions or regions. In a national cross-section study of over 10,000 students enrolled at 4-year colleges McCabe et al. (2005) demonstrated, that the nonmedical use of prescription stimulants was higher in the North-Eastern region of the US, compared to other regions, and higher for institutions with more competitive admission criteria compared to less competitive admission criteria. Finally, a difference can be found in the way that cognitive enhancement drugs are addressed in the questionnaire, for example by either questioning general drug use for the purpose of enhancement or questioning the use of specific types of stimulants (e.g., Ritalin) and/or active ingredient (e.g., methylphenidate) for this purpose. The latter limits the number of stimulants and/or active ingredients that are taken into account in the survey, but leads to more specific questions for the respondent.

Recently more and more studies have been conducted on the university student population in (mostly Western) Europe. The aforementioned variety in definitions and demographic characteristics cause difficulty in comparing the prevalence numbers of these studies as well. For example, Holloway and Bennett (2012) are sometimes mentioned in the discussion on cognitive enhancement drugs, while they focus on general nonmedical use and only briefly mention the intention of cognitive enhancement. From the sample of 1614 students 33% reported to use prescription drugs nonmedical, but only three students reported the reason "to study." Castaldi et al. (2012) on the other hand, focus solely on the intention, and thus include two students who have a prescription in their prevalence number of 16% of students who use cognitive enhancement drugs in a sample of 77 Italian medical students. Also Pustovrh and Mali (2014) did a (pilot) study in only a single institution, in Slovenia, resulting in a prevalence of 11 out of 211 students (5.21%) who had ever used prescription drugs for cognitive enhancement.

In contrast to the aforementioned studies, the focus of studies seems to shift from prevalence of substance use for cognitive enhancement toward broader topics, such as the motives behind the use, differences between users and non-users, or theoretically grounded accounts of why certain students choose to use drugs for cognitive enhancement while others do not (Eickenhorst et al., 2012; Sattler and Wiegel, 2013; Wolff and Brand, 2013; Wolff et al., 2013, 2014; Ott and Biller-Andorno, 2014). However, prevalence numbers are usually presented as well and will be reviewed here even though they are not always the primary aim of study. Larger studies in Germany and Switzerland demonstrate differences in targeting specific substances or a more general group of pharmacological cognitive enhancers. Sattler and Wiegel (2013), for example, examined prior use by asking whether respondents had ever used a prescription medicine without medical necessity to enhance cognitive efficiency, resulting in a lifetime prevalence of 4.56%. Ott and Biller-Andorno (2014) examined the particular use of Ritalin, Adderall or Modasomil among 1765 students at one Swiss university, and found a prevalence of 6.2% of 1765 students who use prescription drugs without a prescription to increase concentration or alertness, of which 4.7% more specifically reported study purposes. However, they claim the questionnaire is not designed to be representative for their population. Maier et al. (2013) examined the use of 17 specific substances with the intention to enhance cognitive performance, categorized as prescription drugs (e.g., methylphenidate), drugs of abuse (e.g., alcohol) and other substances (e.g., caffeine). They found a prevalence of 7.6% for nonmedical prescription drug use for cognitive enhancement and 7.8% for drugs of abuse for cognitive enhancement among their sample of 6275 students from three Swiss universities. This points to a more widespread phenomenon among several surveys in Germany, to not only include prescription drugs as potential enhancers, but also illicit drugs and/or more commonly available substances (also: lifestyle drugs) such as coffee and energy drinks. Most studies clearly separate them, such as Wolff et al. (2014), who demonstrated the use of lifestyle, prescription and illicit drugs for cognitive enhancement among approximately 1000 students all over Germany, and found a lifetime prevalence of respectively, 83.2, 5.8, and 3.5%.

Franke et al. (2011a,b) surveyed the use of coffee, caffeinated drinks, caffeine tablets, prescription drugs, and illicit drugs for cognitive enhancement among high school and undergraduate students and found a prevalence of respectively, 53.2, 39, 10.5, 1.3, and 2.6%. However, other researchers in Germany diverge from this distinction between lifestyle, prescription and illicit drugs, and group them in one general class of cognitive enhancers. Dietz et al. (2013), for instance, report a 12-month prevalence of use of cognitive-enhancing drugs of 20%. In this number the authors include the use of prescription drugs, illicit drugs and caffeine tablets. Eickenhorst et al. (2012) grouped prescription drug use and illicit drug use to improve cognitive performance or mood, and found a prevalence of 7% among 1324 students and graduates.

The current study does not aim to solve the problems that arise due to different definitions, sampling methods or questions, nor do we aim to provide a theoretical framework for pharmacological cognitive enhancement drug use. We aim to contribute to the discussion by examining different study methods in the same sample. This creates the possibility to directly compare the influence of certain questions and inclusion criteria on the resulting prevalence number. Furthermore, the present study sets out to assess the prevalence of pharmacological cognitive enhancement by means of a web-based survey administered to university students in the Netherlands, a sample that to our knowledge has not been examined before. There are only a few studies investigating the use of cognitive enhancers in the Dutch population. Ganpat et al. (2009) surveyed the illicit use of prescription drugs with the intention to improve performance in sport and study among adolescents between 14 and 17 years old and found an overall prevalence rate of 1.7%. A second study assessed the quantity of psychopharmacological enhancement among Dutch psychiatrists and other physicians working in psychiatry (Timmer and Glas, 2012). The results demonstrated a lifetime prevalence of 11%. This latter number is comparable to recent results of a survey among German surgeons (Franke et al., 2013).

In an attempt to reach a representative sample our survey has been advertised online and offline among students of all 14 government supported universities in the Netherlands. The survey examines the prevalence of general nonmedical use of prescription drugs, and the use of particular prescription drugs (methylphenidate, modafinil, beta blockers, and rivastigmine) with the specific purpose of cognitive enhancement with and without a prescription. Furthermore, we will assess the use of prescription drugs for cognitive enhancement with a question not targeted at particular drugs, but at the general group of prescription drugs. Furthermore, we will describe the use of lifestyle and illicit drugs with the purpose of cognitive enhancement. It is impossible to make a comparison of all definitions and study methods in previous studies, but in this way many differences of prior studies are addressed, which makes it possible to directly compare prevalence numbers by different methods within this study and to studies with similar methods abroad.

In addition of giving an overview of different prevalence numbers of the use of substances for cognitive enhancement in the student population in the Netherlands, we also examine two topics that have been found to relate to pharmacological cognitive enhancement, being polydrug use and the relationship between using cognitive enhancement substances and stress. Polydrug use considers the finding that there is a positive relationship between the use of prescription drugs for cognitive enhancement and the use of other substances in general (Barret et al., 2005; McCabe et al., 2005; Eickenhorst et al., 2012; Mazanov et al., 2013). Furthermore, it regards a positive relationship between the use of prescription drugs for cognitive enhancement, the use of illicit drugs for cognitive enhancement and the use of lifestyle drugs for cognitive enhancement, meaning that if somebody uses one of these for cognitive enhancement, there is a higher chance of using substances from the other groups with the purpose of cognitive enhancement as well (Maier et al., 2013; Wolff and Brand, 2013; Ott and Biller-Andorno, 2014). We hypothesize that university students in the Netherlands will also display polydrug use, meaning that (1) users of prescription drugs for the purpose of cognitive enhancement are more likely to use other substances than non-users and (2) there is a correlation between the use of prescription, illicit and lifestyle drugs for cognitive enhancement.

Second, Maier et al. (2013) demonstrated that prescription and illicit drug use for cognitive enhancement is related to perceived pressure to perform. Wolff et al. (2014) found a similar relation for the use of prescription and lifestyle drug use for cognitive enhancement and self-reported strain. Wolff and Brand (2013) demonstrated that overwhelming demands in school could predict the use of prescription drugs and lifestyle drugs for cognitive enhancement. With a longitudinal design Sattler and Wiegel (2013) demonstrated that increased cognitive test anxiety increased the prevalence of nonmedical prescription drug use for cognitive enhancement over time. We hypothesize that a similar relation between the use of cognitive enhancement substances and stress will be prevalent among students in the Netherlands; and thus that students who use substances for the purpose of cognitive enhancement will report more stress than students who do not use substances for the purpose of cognitive enhancement.

Finally, several surveys have examined attitudes toward the use of prescription drugs for cognitive enhancement. In general, the public displays similar concerns as described in the academic literature on the topic, concerning topics such as the safety of using prescription drugs by healthy people, the possibility of being coerced in using a drug for cognitive enhancement and the fairness of using drugs to enhance ones cognitive performance (Schelle et al., 2014). To add to this discussion we assessed opinions in the current sample toward several statements regarding the safety and policy surrounding the use of prescription drugs for cognitive enhancement.

To sum up, the survey aimed at (1) giving an overview of different methods to assess the prevalence of use of substances for cognitive enhancement and apply these methods to a new sample of university students in the Netherlands (2) investigating whether findings of polydrug use and the relationship between cognitive enhancement substance use and stress can also be applied to this population and (3) assessing opinions about the use of prescription drugs for cognitive enhancement.

METHODS

RESPONDENTS

In the current study, 1572 respondents of a total population of approximately 245,000 students registered at Dutch universities, replied to a nationwide poster spread, social media advertisements and a letter to student organizations. Prior to analysis 69 respondents were excluded [exclusion criteria were not being a student at a Dutch university, technical difficulties with the online questionnaire and an affirmative answer on a control question (see below)], resulting in a final sample of 1503 respondents with a mean age of 21.8 years (± sd 2.8 years; 70% women). The sample included students of all 14 government supported Dutch universities, although the relative distribution of respondents was not equal for different universities. Respondents were stimulated to complete the questionnaire by raffling one tablet PC, 30 shopping vouchers (€15,-) and 20 cinema vouchers (€7, 50).

PROCEDURE

The questionnaire was an anonymous online survey in Dutch, which could only be accessed after signing a digital informed consent form. This form was followed by the questionnaire as described in a next section. After submission of the questionnaire a new non-related website opened where the respondent was offered the opportunity to enter in the lottery for the tablet PC and vouchers. Data were stored in an offline database for later analysis. Care was taken not to store IP addresses from the respondents in the dataset. Contact information needed for distribution of the prizes was stored in a separate data file. The procedure and questionnaire are approved by the Ethics Committee Faculty of Social Sciences (ECSS) of the Radboud University, Nijmegen, the Netherlands.

QUESTIONNAIRE

The first section of our questionnaire assessed demographics and background characteristics. Furthermore, we assessed study behavior (e.g., time spent studying) and study outcome to be able to further characterize the cognitive enhancement substance user. After that, we translated and adapted the "Perceived Stress Scale" (Cohen et al., 1983) to a version assessing "Perceived Study Stress" by inserting the word "study" in front of the word "stress" each time this was mentioned in the original scale. The remainder of the survey focused on the use of and the opinion about several substances, the main outcome measures of this study.

The length of the survey depended on the amount of substances used, because respondents were routed toward more specific questions about substances. All questions had a forced response format, meaning that respondents could not skip the question. For most respondents the survey was about 80 questions long. On average, respondents took approximately 18 min to complete the survey.

MAIN OUTCOME MEASURES

Type of substances

The main outcome measures concern the use of prescription drugs, illicit drugs (stimulants, soft drugs and hard drugs) and lifestyle drugs (alcohol, nicotine, and caffeine). We asked respondents to indicate their use of prescription drugs in two different ways, namely with questions about four prescription drugs in particular (methylphenidate, modafinil, beta blockers, and rivastigmine) and questions about the use of prescription drugs in general.

The use of specific prescription drugs was part of a single question in which we asked respondents to indicate whether they had used one or more of the following substances since the start of their university studies, followed by examples as shown in the following overview: alcohol (e.g., in beer, wine, liquor), nicotine (e.g., in cigarettes, roll-ups), caffeine (e.g., in coffee, energy drinks), pharmacy products (such as painkillers, nutritional supplements), soft drugs (such as marihuana), smart shop products (such as memory boosters, herb pills), stimulants (such as amphetamine, cocaine), hard drugs (such as lysergic acid diethylamide (LSD), heroine), methylphenidate (e.g., in Ritalin), modafinil (e.g., in Provigil), beta blockers (e.g., in Propanolol) and rivastigmine (e.g., in Exelon). We added a non-existent drug to the list of possible substances respondents could indicate to have used. This drug was named "Hoxazine (e.g., in Hypersotaline)" and was placed there to detect untrustworthy results. Respondents who admitted to have used this non-existent drug were excluded from further analysis.

Because we only included four often discussed prescription drugs that could potentially be used for cognitive enhancement we also asked a question regarding general prescription drug use. Respondents were asked to indicate whether they had ever used a prescription drug without having a prescription themselves. If they confirmed this question they were routed toward a question about their reasons for using prescription drugs.

Use of substances

If respondents indicated to have been in contact with a substance they were routed toward questions about the specific substance(s) to indicate amount, times and reasons of usage. In the case of prescription drugs they were also asked to indicate whether they had a prescription or not. The answer options for amount, times and reasons of usage were based on questions that have previously been developed for the questionnaire "Family and Health 2003/2004" of the project "Family and Health" of the Radboud University Nijmegen (Heatherton et al., 1991; Engels et al., 1999; Engels and Knibbe, 2000; Harakeh et al., 2005). Specific categories and answer options for amount and times of usage were different for certain substance categories. Therefore, they will be discussed in the following sections regarding the specific substances. Answer options for amounts and times of usage of substances which were not present in the "Family and Health 2003/2004" were created based on questions asked on a similar substance in the questionnaire.

The "Family and Health 2003/2004" questionnaire discusses four general reasons for substance usage: coping with stress, conformity to peers, enhancement (feeling good) and social substance use, related to the four-factor model of alcohol use (Cooper, 1994). We added four answer options in the question about reasons for usage for each substance: (1) "to enhance study performance" as this was our main target of interest, (2) "medical reasons" and (3) "to lose weight" as it applied to some of the

Box 1 | Description of the term "smart pills" (translated from Dutch).

Some students use drugs which are only available with a prescription, without having a prescription themselves. Some other students do have a prescription, but they use a higher dose than prescribed. When they use those drugs to improve their study results, these drugs are called smart pills. The statements below are all about smart pills. Please fill in to what extent you agree with these statements.

Table 1 | The number of respondents using specific routes of obtainment for prescription drugs with the purpose of cognitive enhancement from the group of respondents who indicated to "less than often" have a prescription for the drug themselves.

Ways of obtainment	Friends, free	Friends, paid	Online	Stolen	Work/School	Other
Methylphenidate ($N = 21$)	17	8	5	2	0	0
Beta blocker ($N = 7$)	2	2	2	0	0	2

substances different than alcohol on which the four-factor model was based, and (4) "other" to provide respondents with an answer option in case their answer was not in the list.

From these questions specific measures per substance (category) were derived. The amount of nonmedical users was calculated by including all users of the substance (category) who reported to at least sometimes (on a four-point scale of seldom; sometimes; regularly; often) use the substance for any other than "medical reasons" (exception: general prescription drug use, for which this measure could only be calculated for users who do not have a prescription themselves). The amount of users using a substance (category) without a prescription was calculated by including all users of the substance (category) minus the users who reported to use the substance without "regularly" or "often" (similar four-point scale of seldom; sometimes; regularly; often) to have a prescription. The amount of users using the substance (category) with the purpose of cognitive enhancement was calculated by including all users of the substance who reported to use the substance at least sometimes "to enhance study performance" (similar four-point scale).

Opinions: prescription drug use for cognitive enhancement

Further, we were interested in the attitude of our respondents toward the use of prescription drugs for the purpose of cognitive enhancement. Respondents were presented with 17 statements and consequently asked to provide a response on a five-point Likert scale, indicating their (dis) agreement with the statement at hand (see **Table 2** for the list of statements). Before reading these statements we presented a short description of the term "smart pills" to the respondents (see **Box 1** for a translated version of the Dutch text).

DATA ANALYSIS

The first hypothesis, regarding polydrug use, has two components. Chi-square analyses were conducted to examine whether users of prescription drugs are more or less likely to use other substances than non-users. Secondly, Chi-square analyses were conducted to examine the association between the use of prescription drugs, illicit drugs, and lifestyle drugs for the purpose of cognitive enhancement. The second hypothesis, regarding the relationship between substance use for cognitive enhancement and stress, was examined with One-Way ANOVA's for the differences in perceived study stress scores between users and non-users according to our different operationalizations. *P*-values <0.05 (two-tailed) were considered statistically significant. The analyses were conducted with IBM SPSS Statistics version 22.0.

RESULTS

PRESCRIPTION DRUG USE

Use of specific prescription drugs

None of the respondents reported to use rivastigmine or modafinil. In our sample, 52 students indicated to have used methylphenidate, while 36 students indicated to have used beta blockers. Nonmedical use (at least "sometimes" use for any other reason than medical) of methylphenidate was self-reported by 80.8% of methylphenidate users (2.8% of the total sample of respondents) and 61.1% of beta blockers users (1.5% of the total sample of respondents). Total nonmedical use of specific prescription drugs in the sample is 4.0% (due to four users using both beta blockers and methylphenidate at least sometimes for nonmedical purposes). Excluding the respondents who indicated to "regularly" or "often have a prescription" results in 2.4% of respondents reporting to use prescription drugs at least sometimes for a nonmedical purpose without having prescription.

From the methylphenidate users 73.1% (2.5% of the total sample of respondents) reported to use methylphenidate at least sometimes for the specific purposes of improving ones study results (cognitive enhancement). From the beta blocker users 38.9% (0.9% of the total sample of respondents) reported to use beta blockers at least sometimes for the specific purpose of improving ones study results. Total specific prescription drug use with the intention of cognitive enhancement in the sample is 3.2%.

Furthermore, to examine the prevalence of the use of prescription drugs for the purpose of cognitive enhancement without having a prescription, we excluded respondents who indicated to use prescription drugs regularly or often with a prescription. A group of 40.4% of the methylphenidate users reported to use methylphenidate less than often with a prescription, and at least sometimes for the purpose of cognitive enhancement (1.4% of the total sample of respondents). For beta blockers this prevalence was 19.4% (0.5% of the total sample of respondents). Total use of specific prescription drugs with (at least sometimes) the intention of cognitive enhancement without (regularly or often) having a prescription is 1.7%. **Table 1** shows via which other methods these respondents obtained their prescription drug. Most users without a prescription acquire the drugs via people they know.

Use of a general group of prescription drugs

Sixty respondents (4.0% of the total sample of respondents) admitted to use a prescription drug without having a prescription for the drug. Forty-six respondents (3.1% of the total sample of respondents) reported nonmedical use without a prescription (at least "sometimes" use for any other reason than medical). From the 60 respondents, 40% used these prescription drugs at least sometimes to improve their study results (2.7% of the total sample of respondents).

Opinions about prescriptions drug use for cognitive enhancement

The percentage of respondents that (dis)agreed with 17 statements about the use of "smart pills" are presented in **Table 2.** Most respondents disagree with statements regarding the respondent being aware of the use of smart pills. There is less agreement about statements regarding the risks related to the use of smart pills, the fairness of the use of smart pills, and the regulation of the use of smart pills.

ILLICIT DRUG USE

Soft drugs, hard drugs and stimulants are considered illicit drugs. **Table 3** displays the prevalence of the use of the three categories of illicit drugs, the use of illicit drugs for nonmedical reasons (at least "sometimes" use for any other reason than medical) and the use of illicit drugs with the specific purpose of cognitive enhancement. Total use of illicit drugs is 20.5%. The use of illicit drugs for nonmedical reasons is 20.4% and with the specific purpose of cognitive enhancement (CE) 1.3%.

LIFESTYLE DRUG USE

Alcohol, nicotine, caffeine, over the counter pharmacy products, and (legal) smart shop products are considered lifestyle drugs. **Table 4** displays the prevalence of the use of the categories of lifestyle drugs, the use of lifestyle drugs for nonmedical reasons (at least "sometimes" use for any other reason than medical) and the use of lifestyle drugs with the specific purpose of cognitive enhancement. Total use of lifestyle drugs is 92.8%. The use of lifestyle drugs for nonmedical reasons is 90.5% and with the specific purpose of cognitive enhancement 45.6%.

Table 5 provides an overview of the prevalence of the use of certain drugs according to the above described definitions.

POLYDRUG USE

Users of specific prescription drugs with/without a prescription reported more often the use of soft drugs, stimulants, nicotine and over the counter pharmacy products. Users of prescription drugs without a prescription were more likely than non-users to report use of soft drugs, nicotine, caffeine and over the counter pharmacy drugs. **Table 6** provides the test statistics for these tests. For most substances the data confirm the hypothesis that users of prescription drugs for the purpose of cognitive enhancement are more likely to use other substances than non-users of prescription drugs for the purpose of cognitive enhancement.

Furthermore, Chi square tests of the association between prescription drugs, illicit drugs, and lifestyle drugs for the

Table 3 | Prevalence of the use of soft drugs, hard drugs and stimulants, calculated from the total sample.

	Soft drugs (%)	Hard drugs (%)	Stimulants (%)
Use	19.1	1.9	4.9
Nonmedical use	19.0	1.9	4.8
Use for CE	0.7	0.1	0.6

Table 2 | Percentages of agreement toward statements about smart pills (N = 1503).

Options	Strongly disagree	Disagree	Neutral	Agree	Strongly Agree
1. I am aware of students using "smart pills" regularly.	85.5	4.6	2.9	5.1	1.9
2. I am aware of students using "smart pills" during finals week.	83.3	4.8	2.5	6.9	2.5
3. I have spoken about "smart pills" with other students.	78.2	5.1	3.0	9.0	4.7
4. I have been offered stimulant drugs by another student.	92.6	1.7	1.3	2.8	1.6
5. I know students that I can get "smart pills" from.	84.1	3.2	2.8	5.9	4.1
6. "Smart pills" are easily accessible on this campus.	70.1	4.9	22.2	1.8	1.0
7. "Smart pills" should be freely accessible.	73.6	11.0	11.9	2.6	0.9
8. I think that it is harmless to use "smart pills."	57.6	16.8	19.9	4.0	1.7
9. I think students consider the risks of using "smart pills" before taking them.	36.5	25.1	33.9	3.9	0.5
10. I know enough about "smart pills" to safely use them.	67.7	13.0	11.4	4.7	3.3
11. Students should be informed about the risks and possibilities of "smart pills."	12.3	8.0	20.4	35.0	24.3
12. I think that "smart pills" provide an unfair advantage for students compared to those that don't take the drugs.	32.5	19.4	27.1	15.0	5.9
13. I think that the university board on the campus are aware of the use of "smart pills,"	16.2	14.0	64.7	3.8	1.3
14. I am aware of a policy on campus that bans the use of "smart pills."	67.4	15.9	13.2	2.1	1.4
15. The use of "smart pills" should be prohibited on this campus.	10.6	11.2	38.9	21.0	18.3
16. A policy surrounding "smart pills" would allow a fair academic standard for students.	23.8	15.4	36.3	14.9	9.6
17. I think that it is illegal to take "smart pills."	11.2	10.6	51.8	15.1	11.2

Table 4 | Prevalence of the use of alcohol, nicotine, caffeine, over the counter pharmacy products and (legal) smart shop products, calculated from the total sample.

	Alcohol (%)	Nicotine (%)	Caffeine (%)	Pharmacy (%)	Smart shop (%)
Use	84.3	20.3	69.1	59.6	3.7
Nonmedical use	83.2	19.8	66.2	36.8	3.2
Use for CE	1.8	3.0	41.7	9.0	0.5

Table 5 | An overview of the prevalence of the use of drugs for CE.

Nonmedical use of specific prescription drugs with/without prescription	4.0%
Nonmedical use of specific prescription drugs without a prescription	2.4%
Use of specific prescription drugs with/without prescription with the intention of CE	3.2%
Use of specific prescription drugs without a prescription with the intention of CE	1.7%
Nonmedical use of general group of prescription drugs without a prescription	3.1%
Use of general group of prescription drugs without a prescription with the intention of CE	1.6%
Nonmedical use of illicit drug	20.4%
Use of illicit drugs with the intention of CE	1.3%
Nonmedical use of lifestyle drugs	90.5%
Use of lifestyle drugs with the intention of CE	45.6%

Table 6 | Results of the Chi square comparisons of substance use between users and nonusers of prescription drugs, with/without and only without a prescription.

	With and without a prescription ($N = 48$)		Without a prescription ($N = 25$)	
	χ^2	Odds ratio	χ^2	Odds ratio
Alcohol	2.03		2.36	
Nicotine	30.98**	4.56	35.77**	8.78
Caffeine	3.41		4.24*	3.32
Pharmacy	7.87**	2.64	6.28*	3.62
Soft drugs	13.47**	2.90	22.41**	5.62
Smart shop products	X		X	
Stimulant drugs	20.71**	5.02	X	
Hard drugs	X		X	

*Significance levels are indicated with *$P < 0.05$ and **$P < 0.01$. X is used to indicate that a statistical test was not performed as small cell sizes precluded significance testing.*

purpose of cognitive enhancement demonstrate that users of lifestyle drugs for the purpose of cognitive enhancement are more likely to use prescription drugs and illicit drugs for the purpose of cognitive enhancement. This partly confirms the hypothesis that there is an association between the use of prescription, illicit, and lifestyle drugs for cognitive enhancement. **Table 7** provides the test statistics for these tests. Similar tests for the relation between the use of illicit drugs for the purpose of cognitive enhancement and prescription drugs for the purpose of cognitive enhancement could not be performed because small cell sizes precluded significance testing.

COGNITIVE ENHANCEMENT AND STRESS

Users of specific prescription drugs with/without a prescription for the purpose of cognitive enhancement and users of lifestyle drugs for the purpose of cognitive enhancement report more study related stress than their respective non-user groups. This means that our hypothesis that students who use substances for the purpose of cognitive enhancement will report more stress than students who do not use substances for the purpose of cognitive enhancement is only confirmed for certain definitions of cognitive enhancement drug use. **Table 8** provides the according test statistics.

DISCUSSION

The present study demonstrates the prevalence of the nonmedical use and the use with the specific purpose of cognitive enhancement of prescription drugs, illicit drugs, and lifestyle drugs among university students in the Netherlands. General use and nonmedical use is larger for lifestyle drugs than illicit drugs, and larger for illicit drugs than prescription drugs. Even though prevalence numbers differ for general and nonmedical use, the use of prescription drugs and illicit drugs with the purpose of cognitive enhancement is rather similar and low in occurrence in the current sample. However, almost half of the respondents use lifestyle drugs with the intention to cognitively enhance themselves. Users of prescription drugs for the purpose of cognitive enhancement are more likely to use other substances than non-users. There is a relation between the use of prescription drugs and the use of illicit drugs, but not with the use of lifestyle drugs when it comes to using these substances to cognitively enhance oneself. The hypothesis, that respondents who use substances for cognitive enhancement experience more stress than non-users, is confirmed for the group of users of specific prescription drugs that include both users with and without a prescription and for users of lifestyle drugs.

The use of substances for cognitive enhancement has not previously been examined in the university student population in the Netherlands. However, the prevalence of the use of prescription drugs without a prescription for the purpose of cognitive enhancement, is in line with a study within a younger Dutch population (14–17 year) in which 1.7% reported to use prescription drugs—which were not prescribed to themselves or in a different way than prescribed to them—with the intention the

Table 7 | Results of the Chi square association between the use of prescription drugs (specific prescription drugs with/without a prescription; specific prescription drugs without a prescription; general prescription drugs without a prescription), illicit and lifestyle drugs for cognitive enhancement.

	Specific with/without		Specific without		General without		Illicit	
	χ^2	OR	χ^2	OR	χ^2	OR	χ^2	OR
Lifestyle	22.56**	4.75	12.15**	4.89	8.51**	3.65	9.68**	4.87

*Significance levels are indicated with *P < 0.05 and **P < 0.01. The odds ratio (OR) is calculated as a measure of the effect size.*

Table 8 | Results of One-Way ANOVAs for the relation between the use of prescription drugs (specific prescription drugs with/without a prescription; specific prescription drugs without a prescription; general prescription drugs without a prescription), illicit and lifestyle drugs for cognitive enhancement and study related stress.

	Users M (sd)	Nonusers M (sd)	F (df 1,1501)	r
Specific w/wo	39.29 (7.74)	36.67 (6.81)	35.75*	0.067
Specific wo	38.68 (8.61)	36.72 (6.82)	2.02	
General wo	38.25 (8.56)	36.73 (6.82)	1.17	
Illicit	38.00 (6.61)	36.73 (6.86)	0.67	
Lifestyle	37.89 (6.99)	35.79 (6.59)	35.75**	0.153

*Significance levels are indicated with *P < 0.05 and **P < 0.01.*

enhance performance (Ganpat et al., 2009). Compared to the nonmedical use of prescription drugs in Wales, our result of non-medical use is far lower (Holloway and Bennett, 2012). The same trend is observed for the use of substances for the specific purpose of cognitive enhancement. The use of specific prescription drugs and general prescription drugs with this intention (1.7 and 1.6%) is lower than most lifetime prevalence numbers in Europe (ranging from 4.6 to 16%) (Castaldi et al., 2012; Maier et al., 2013; Sattler and Wiegel, 2013; Ott and Biller-Andorno, 2014; Pustovrh and Mali, 2014; Wolff et al., 2014). It might be suggested that our numbers are lower due to their timeframe being based on "during respondent's university studies" instead of lifetime prevalence. However, Eickenhorst et al. (2012) also examined use "during studies" and found a prevalence of 7%, similar to other lifetime reports. Furthermore, the only two studies with a low prevalence more similar to our prevalence are conducted in Germany by Franke et al. (2011a) with a lifetime prevalence of 0.8% and by Mache et al. (2012) with a lifetime prevalence up to 2%.

The use of illicit drugs to enhance cognitive performance in our sample (1.3%) is a little lower than previous prevalence numbers of 2.9% (Franke et al., 2011a) and 3.5% in Germany (Wolff et al., 2014; however, a smaller difference is found when comparing to their finding of the point prevalence of 1.7%). When we combine our prevalence of the use of illicit drugs and alcohol for cognitive enhancement and compare it with the category of drugs of abuse (7.8%) by Maier et al. (2013), the resulting prevalence of our study is clearly lower. The use of lifestyle drugs to enhance cognitive performance (45.6%) is lower than found by Wolff et al. (2014; 83.2%), but more in line with the prevalence of the use of coffee for this purpose by 53% respondents of Franke et al. (2011a) and what the authors report as soft enhancers (e.g., coffee) by about half of the respondents of Maier et al. (2013). Again, when looking at the point prevalence instead of lifetime prevalence of the use of lifestyle drugs for cognitive enhancement (52.3%) by Wolff et al. (2014), the difference is smaller. In general our prevalence numbers of prescription drugs and illicit drugs appear to be low compared to research in other European countries, whilst our results for lifestyle drugs are more in line.

One potential reason that explains the low prevalence of the use of substances for cognitive enhancement among university students in the Netherlands can be found by taking a closer look at responses to statements regarding the awareness about the use of prescription drugs for cognitive enhancement purposes. Whereas in a Swiss sample 93.7% of the respondents and in a German sample almost 60% knew that substances could and are being used for the purpose of cognitive enhancement, only 13.7% of our current sample has ever spoken about the use of prescription drugs for cognitive enhancement (Franke et al., 2011a; Maier et al., 2013). Lesser awareness of the possibility to use substances for the purpose of cognitive enhancement among peers can have an impact on the prevalence, in particular for prescription drugs which, when not obtained by a prescription, are often obtained via peers. This is in line with previous research (McCabe and Boyd, 2005; Maier et al., 2013; Ott and Biller-Andorno, 2014).

Although awareness of the use of cognitive enhancement drugs by others is rather low (10%), it is still considerably higher than the actual prevalence of the use of prescription drugs for cognitive enhancement (1.6–3.2%). It remains unclear whether this difference is based on the fact that respondents know the same users, whether students overestimate the use of prescription drugs for cognitive enhancement by other students, whether there is a bias in sampling toward more non-users, or whether they did not report their own use truthfully. Recent research suggests that prevalence rates vary depending on the type of questions. Previous research by Franke et al. (2011a) showed a prevalence in Germany of below 1% while a more recent study, using an altered version of the Randomized Response Technique estimated a prevalence of 20% prescription drugs use for cognitive enhancement in the German student population (Dietz et al., 2013). Dietz et al. (2013) relates this difference to the stigmatized nature of the topic of enhancement drug use, which would indicate that our results demonstrate an underestimated prevalence rate due to non-truthful answers. However, other researchers emphasize the overestimation of the use of cognitive enhancement drugs by peers, which would suggest that the number of 9%, of students who know other students to be users, is unreliable, while our actual prevalence rate is more reliable (Lucke et al., 2011).

In spite of the low prevalence numbers, the majority of the students believe they ought to be receiving adequate information about the risks and opportunities of using prescription drugs for cognitive enhancement. This is in line with findings from previous studies on the opinions about pharmacological cognitive enhancement in which people argued that it was important to be able to make autonomous decisions about the use of such substances (Schelle et al., 2014). However, deciding whether or not to give students or the general population more information about the use of substances for cognitive enhancement is a difficult task. Sandberg (2013) argues that on the one hand the lack of information can create irrational demand and employer coercion when hype will dominate, but at the same time there is not enough information yet—especially on the long term effects—to create a proper risk/benefit analysis.

Modafinil and rivastigmine were not reported as being used by the students in our sample, while being proposed as two of four specific prescription drugs that could be used for cognitive enhancement. One explanation for this discrepancy could be that these two drugs are not as often prescribed in the Netherlands to students compared to methylphenidate and beta blockers. For example, while modafinil is only 10,500 times provided by the public pharmacies in the Netherlands in 2009, the amount of times methylphenidate was provided was already rising to a million prescriptions per year, which it passed in 2011 (Stichting Farmaceutische Kengetallen, 2010, 2012). In contrast, rivastigmine is often prescribed to older people, which may lead to its accessibility being scarce in the student population, especially when compared to the amount of methylphenidate prescriptions in the population. This explanation based on the amount of prescriptions in the corresponding age population is supported by the fact that most prescription drugs which are not obtained by a prescription are obtained via peers, either freely or paid. This corroborates previous studies in other countries (McCabe and Boyd, 2005). It would be interesting to further examine whether different populations in the Netherlands do use prescription drugs like rivastigmine and modafinil for the purpose of cognitive enhancement, especially focusing on those populations for whom the specific effect of the substance is more desirable, or the substance is more accessible. Examples of specific target populations are academics, pilots and surgeons (see e.g., Franke et al., 2013).

As hypothesized, users of prescription drugs for cognitive enhancement reported more often the use of other substances such as soft drugs, nicotine and stimulants than non-users. This polydrug use is consistent with previous studies (Barret et al., 2005; McCabe et al., 2005; Teter et al., 2006; Eickenhorst et al., 2012; Mazanov et al., 2013). Polydrug use is also found in other domains, such as doping in sport (Dunn et al., 2009; Backhouse et al., 2013). Based on their co-occurrence Backhouse et al. (2013) suggest that athletes who engage in legal performance enhancement are an "at-risk" group for transition toward doping, the gateway hypothesis. Our findings display that users of lifestyle drugs for the purpose of cognitive enhancement are more likely to use illicit drugs and prescription drugs for the purpose of cognitive enhancement and thus support previous findings in suggesting that this hypothesis not only plays a role in physical performance enhancement but also for cognitive performance enhancement.

Furthermore, in accordance with previous studies there is an association between the use of prescription drugs and illicit drugs for cognitive enhancement purposes. In contrast to previous findings, no such relation was found between the use of prescription drugs and lifestyle drugs for cognitive enhancement purposes (Maier et al., 2013; Wolff and Brand, 2013; Ott and Biller-Andorno, 2014). An explanation of this discrepancy can be found in the way that the category of lifestyle drugs is approached and measured. Ott and Biller-Andorno (2014) found that use of cigarettes could explain variance in their logistic regression model about cognitive enhancement drug use, while coffee did not. Another explanation might be found in the low awareness about the use of prescription drugs for cognitive enhancement in the current sample. There might be a higher discrepancy between the awareness of the use of prescription drugs for cognitive enhancement and the use of lifestyle drugs for cognitive enhancement than in other countries, resulting in less association between the two types of cognitive enhancement drug use.

Finally, it was proposed that students who use substances for the purpose of cognitive enhancement report more stress than non-users. This hypothesis is confirmed for the group of users of specific prescription drugs that include users with and without a prescription, and for the group of users of lifestyle drugs for cognitive enhancement. Lifestyle drugs are most commonly used for cognitive enhancement in our sample, by almost half of all respondents. Our findings suggest that stress might be a predicting factor for using lifestyle drugs for cognitive enhancement. A similar longitudinal study as Sattler and Wiegel (2013) conducted on the relation between cognitive test anxiety and the use of prescription drugs for cognitive enhancement would inform whether the use of lifestyle drug use is a coping mechanism for (study related) stress or a potential cause of stress. The finding that there is no relation between the use of illicit drugs for cognitive enhancement and stress is supported by previous findings of Wolff et al. (2014) and Wolff and Brand (2013) but not Maier et al. (2013). More research is needed to explore these contrasting findings. Furthermore, future research can also give more insight in why students in the Netherlands who indicate to use a general group of prescription drugs for cognitive enhancement, or specific prescription drugs without having a prescription, do not confirm the previous associations between prescription drugs use for cognitive enhancement and stress (Maier et al., 2013; Sattler and Wiegel, 2013; Wolff et al., 2014).

In this study, a differentiation between different operationalizations of cognitive enhancement substance use is presented. By displaying results based on different operationalizations we aim to create the possibility to compare our results with as many studies as possible and inform the debate about differences in the result due to different research methods. As several of the prevalence numbers of the use of substances for cognitive enhancement in our sample are rather low, large differences between the operationalizations have not arisen. However, our findings suggest that there is less influence of asking about specific prescription drugs vs. a general kind of prescription drugs than there is influence of including or not including users with a prescription for a prescription drug. Furthermore, our findings demonstrate a large difference between asking nonmedical use of any substance or asking about use for the specific purpose of cognitive enhancement. This supports the importance of a means-to-end relation as proposed by Wolff and Brand (2013) and Wolff et al. (2014).

In addition to the different operationalizations that were proposed in an attempt to tackle most differences between studies on the prevalence of the use of substances for cognitive enhancement, a further topic of interest is found. Recently, more and more researchers start including not only the use of prescription drugs, but also the use of illicit and lifestyle drugs in the debate about cognitive enhancement. It was hard to define which substances belong to which overarching categories, as several frameworks can be chosen to underlie these categories (e.g., legal; normative acceptance; accessibility). Therefore, different categories are used, such as lifestyle drugs vs. soft enhancers (Maier et al., 2013; Wolff et al., 2014) and illicit drugs vs. drugs of abuse (Franke et al., 2011a; Maier et al., 2013; Wolff et al., 2014). When one wants to relate the use of a certain category of substances to for example stress, it is clear that these relations depend on the type of substances included in a certain category. We aimed to create transparency about this topic by providing the prevalence number for each specific substance within each category separately.

LIMITATIONS

A limitation to this study is the sample which, due to convenience sampling, constituted only an approximate representation of the student population in the Netherlands. Women, for example, were oversampled. In addition, the sample was not equally distributed for different universities, as well as not distributed in line with the absolute difference in amount of students of the 14 Dutch government supported universities. However, the percentages of recreational substance use obtained in our sample are lower, but within normal limits, than numbers specified in the National Drug Monitor in the Netherlands (Van Laar et al., 2012). This indicates that, regarding our main topic of drug use, our sample is representative for the population. Therefore, no weighting strategies are applied.

Furthermore, it is clear that although the use of substances for cognitive enhancement is mostly examined in student populations, it is probably not possible to generalize this to other populations. This is supported by the prevalence rate of prescription drug use for cognitive enhancement of 11% among Dutch psychiatrists, which is rather high compared to the prevalence in the current sample (Timmer and Glas, 2012). Even similar aged non-student populations may demonstrate a different pattern of use (Herman-Stahl et al., 2007). Future studies will need to give more insight in the use of substances for cognitive enhancement in other target groups such as in specific occupations, or specific age groups, both within the Netherlands as abroad.

A final limitation regards the study methods. The research is conducted by an online large-scale self-report questionnaire with many questions which might have given rise to a decrease of the feeling of anonymity, a burden in the time that was needed to complete the questionnaire, or for example a lack of memory about certain situations and feelings during the use of certain substances. It is possible that the use of certain substances is stigmatized (Dietz et al., 2013), which may lead to a different reported prevalence rate compared to the actual prevalence rates.

CONCLUSION

To sum up, the present study indicates that the use of prescription drugs and illicit drugs to increase cognitive performance among students in Dutch universities is rather low compared to other European countries, while the use of lifestyle drugs for cognitive enhancement fits the European context better. We have found further evidence of polydrug use in relation to cognitive enhancement, while previous findings of the relation between cognitive enhancement drug use and stress have not been confirmed consistently. We have decided to report the findings of several operationalizations of cognitive enhancement drug use to enable comparison with a wider variety of previous and upcoming research. We urge future researchers to take the discussion about these different operationalizations and the effects that they have on the prevalence numbers into account in designing and reporting future experiments on the use of substances for cognitive enhancement.

ACKNOWLEDGMENTS

We thank prof. dr. H. Zwart and prof. dr. R. Cools for their feedback on previous versions of this article.

REFERENCES

Backhouse, S. H., Whitaker, L., and Petróczi, A. (2013). Gateway to doping? Supplement use in the context of preferred competitive situations, doping attitude, beliefs, and norms. *Scand. J. Med. Sci. Sports* 23, 244–252. doi: 10.1111/j.1600-0838.2011.01374.x

Barret, S. P., Darredeau, C., and Bordy, L. E. (2005). Characteristics of methylphenidate misuse in a university sample. *Can. J. Psychiatry* 50, 457–461.

Bostrom, N., and Sandberg, A. (2009). Cognitive enhancement: methods, ethics, regulatory challenges. *Sci. Eng. Ethics* 15, 311–341. doi: 10.1007/s11948-009-9142-5

Castaldi, S., Gelatti, U., Orizio, G., Hartung, U., Moreno-Londono, A. M., Schulz M., et al. (2012). Use of cognitive enhancement medication among Northern Italian university students. *J. Addict. Med.* 6, 112–117. doi: 10.1097/ADM.0b013e3182479584

Cohen, S., Kamarck, T., and Mermelstein, R. (1983). A global measure of perceived stress. *J. Health Soc. Behav.* 24, 4, 385–396. doi: 10.2307/2136404

Cooper, M. L. (1994). Motivations for alcohol use among adolescents: development and validation of a four-factor model. *Pscyhol. Assess.* 6, 117–128.

DeSantis, A., Noar S. M., and, Webb, E. M. (2009). Nonmedical ADHD stimulant use in fraternities. *J. Stud. Alcohol Drugs* 70, 952–954. doi: 10.3200/JACH.57.3.315-324

Dietz, P., Striegel, H., Franke, A. G., Lieb, K., Simon, P., and Ulrich, R. (2013). Randomized response estimates for the 12-month prevalence of cognitive-enhancing drug use in university students. *Pharmacotherapy* 33, 44–50. doi: 10.1002/phar.1166

Dunn, M., Mazanov, J., and Sitharthan, G. (2009). Predicting future anabolic-androgenic steroid use intentions with current substance use: findings from an internet-based suvery. *Clin. J. Sport Med.* 19, 222–227. doi: 10.1097/JSM.0b013e31819d65ad.

DuPont, R. L., Coleman, J. J., Bucher, R. H., and Wilford, B. B. (2008). Characteristics and motives of college students who engage in nonmedical use of methylphenidate. *Am. J. Addict.* 17, 167–171. doi: 10.1080/10550490802019642

Eickenhorst, P., Vitzthum, K., Klapp, B. F., Groneberg, D., and Mache, S. (2012). Neuroenhancement among German University students: motives, expectations, and relationship with psychoactive lifestyle drugs. *J. Psychoactive Drugs* 44, 418–427. doi: 10.1080/02791072.2012.736845

Engels, R. C. M. E., and Knibbe, R. A. (2000). Alcohol use and intimate relationships in adolescence: when love comes to town. *Addict. Behav.* 25, 435–439. doi: 10.1016/S0306-4603(98)00123-3

Engels, R. C. M. E., Knibbe, R. A., and Drop, M. J. (1999). Why do late adolescents drink at home? A study on psychological well-being, social integration and drinking context. *Addict Res.* 7, 31–46. doi: 10.3109/16066359909004373

Franke, A. G., Bagusat, C., Dietz, P., Hoffmann, I., Simon, P., Ulrich, R., et al. (2013). Use of illicit and prescription drugs for cognitive or mood enhancement among surgeons. *BMC Med.* 11:102. doi: 10.1186/1741-7015-11-102

Franke, A. G., Bonertz, C., Christmann, M., Huss, M., Fellgiebel, A., Hildt, E., et al. (2011a). Non-medical use of prescription stimulants and illicit use of stimulants for cognitive enhancement in pupils and students in Germany. *Pharmacopsychiatry* 44, 60–66. doi: 10.1055/s-0030-1268417

Franke, A. G., Christmann, M., Bonertz, C., Fellgiebel, A., Huss, M., and Lieb, K. (2011b). Use of coffee, caffeinated drinks and caffeine tablets for cognitive enhancement in pupils and students in Germany. *Pharmacopsychiatry* 44, 331–338. doi: 10.1055/s-0031-1286347

Franke, A. G., Lieb, K., and Hildt, E. (2012). What users think about the differences between caffeine and illicit/prescription stimulants for cognitive enhancement. *PLoS ONE* 7:e40047. doi: 10.1371/journal.pone.0040047

Ganpat, S., Kleinjan, M., and Van de Mheen, D. (2009). *Oneigenlijk Medicijngebruik Onder Nederlandse Jongeren: Aard en Omvang.* Rotterdam: Instituut voor Verslavingsonderzoek (IVO).

Harakeh, Z., Scholte, R. H., De Vries, H., and Engels, R. C. (2005). Parental rules and communication: their association with adolescent smoking. *Addiction* 100, 862–870. doi: 10.1111/j.1360-0443.2005.01067.x

Heatherton, T. F., Kozlowski, L. T., Frecker, R. C., and Fagerström, K. O. (1991). The Fagerström test for nicotine dependence: a revision of the Fagerström Tolerance Questionnaire. *Br. J. Addict.* 86, 1119–1127. doi: 10.1111/j.1360-0443.1991.tb01879.x

Herman-Stahl, M. A., Krebs, C. P., Kroutil, L. A., and Heller, D. C. (2007). Risk and protective factors for methamphetamine use and nonmedical use of prescription stimulants among young adults aged 18 to 25. *Addict. Behav.* 32, 1003–1015. doi: 10.1016/j.addbeh.2006.07.010

Holloway, K., and Bennett, T. (2012). Prescription drug misuse among university staff and students: a survey of motives, nature and extent. *Drug Educ. Prev. Policy* 19, 137–144. doi: 10.3109/09687637.2011.594114

Lucke, J. C., Bell, S., Partridge, B., and Hall, W. D. (2011). Deflating the neuroenhancement bubble. *AJOB Neurosci.* 2, 38–43. doi: 10.1080/21507740.2011.611122

Lynch, G., Sahakian, B., Collingridge, G. L., Crawley, J. N., Nye, J. S., and Frenguelli, B. G. (2013). Cognitive enhancers: molecules, mechanisms and minds, 22nd neuropharmacology conference: cognitive enhancers [special issue]. *Neuropharmacology* 64, 1–596. doi: 10.1016/j.neuropharm.2012.08.005

Mache, S., Eickenhorst, P., Vitzthum, K., Klapp, B. F., and Groneberg, D. A. (2012). Cognitive-enhancing substance use at German universities: frequency, reasons and gender differences. *Wien. Med. Wochenschr.* 162, 262–271. doi: 10.1007/s10354-012-0115-y

Maier, L. J., Liechti, M. E., Herzig, F., and Schaub, M. P. (2013). To dope or not to dope: neuroenhancement with prescription drugs and drugs of abuse among Swiss university students. *PLoS ONE* 8:e77967. doi: 10.1371/journal.pone.0077967

Mazanov, J., Dunn, M., Connor, J., and Fielding, M. L. (2013). Substance use to enhance academic performance among Australian university students. *Perform. Enhanc. Health* 2, 110–118. doi: 10.1016/j.peh.2013.08.017

McCabe, S. E., and Boyd, C. J. (2005). Sources of prescription drugs for illicit use. *Addict. Behav.* 30, 1342–1350. doi: 10.1016/j.addbeh.2005.01.012

McCabe, S. E., Knight, J. R., Teter, C. J., and Wechsler, H. (2005). Non-medical use of prescription stimulants among US college students: prevalence and correlates from a national survey. *Addiction* 99, 96–106. doi: 10.1111/j.1360-0443.2005.00944.x

Monks, K. (2014). *Pimp My Brain: A Week on Smart Drugs. Metro World News.* Available online at: http://www.metro.us/newyork/news/national/2014/02/12/pimp-my-brain-a-week-on-smart-drugs/ (June 1, 2014).

Ott, R., and Biller-Andorno, N. (2014). Neuroenhancement among swiss students - A comparison of users and non-users. *Pharmacopsychiatry* 47, 22–28. doi: 10.1055/s-0033-1358682

Pustovrh, T., and Mali, F. (2014). Exploring some challenges of the pharmaceutical cognitive enhancement discourse: users and policy recommendations. *Neuroethics* 7, 137–158. doi: 10.1007/s12152-013-9192-x

Ragan, C. I., Bard, I., and Singh, I. (2013). What should we do about student use of cognitive enhancers? An analysis of current evidence. *Neuropharmacology* 64, 588–595. doi: 10.1016/j.neuropharm.2012.06.016

Repantis, D., Schlattmann, P., Laisney, O., and Heuser, I. (2010). Modafinil and methylphenidate for neuroenhancement in healthy individuals: a systematic review. *Pharmacol. Res.* 62, 187–206. doi: 10.1016/j.phrs.2010.04.002

Sandberg, A. (2013). Enhancement policy and the value of information. *Am. J. Bioeth.* 13, 34–55. doi: 10.1080/15265161.2013.795826

Sattler, S., and Wiegel, C. (2013). Cognitive test anxiety and cognitive enhancement: the influence of students' worries on their use of performance-enhancing drugs. *Subst. Use Misuse* 48, 220–232. doi: 10.3109/10826084.2012.751426

Schelle, K. J., Faulmüller, N., Caviola, L., and Hewstone, M. (2014). Attitudes toward pharmacological cognitive enhancement - a review. *Front. Syst. Neurosci.* 8:53. doi: 10.3389/fnsys.2014.00053

Schwarz, A. (2012). *Risky Rise of the Good-Grade Pill.* The New York Times. Available online at: http://www.nytimes.com/ (Accessed July 23, 2013).

Sharrett, L. (2012). *In Their Own Words: Study Drugs.* The New York Times. Available online at: http://www.nytimes.com/ (Accessed July 23, 2013).

Shiner, F. (2013). *Drug test Students, Says Scientist Barbara Sahakian, But is it Right? The Huffington Post UK.* Available online at: http://www.huffingtonpost.co.uk/2013/07/02/drug-testing-students-barbara-sahakiann3533065.html (Accessed June 1, 2014).

Smith, M. E., and Farah, M. J. (2011). Are prescription stimulants smart pills? The epidemiology and cognitive neuroscience of prescription stimulant use by normal healthy individuals. *Psychol. Bull.* 137, 717–741. doi: 10.1037/a0023825

Stichting Farmaceutische Kengetallen. (2010). Nog geen rem op ADHD. *Pharmaceutisch Weekblad.* 145, 16–17.

Stichting Farmaceutische Kengetallen. (2012). Gebruik ADHD-middelen niet in te tomen. *Pharmaceutisch Weekblad.* 147, 30–31.

Teter, C. J., McCabe, S. E., LaGrange, M. S. W. K., Cranford, J. A., and Boyd, C. J. (2006). Illicit use of specific prescription stimulants among college students: prevalence, motives, and routes of administration. *Pharmacotherapy* 26, 1501–1510. doi: 10.1592/phco.26.10.1501

Timmer, S. J., and Glas, G. (2012). Pillen voor de psych(e); een exploratief onderzoek naar neuro-enhancement onder Nederlandse psychiaters en artsen. *Tijdschr Psychiatry* 54, 371–376.

Van Laar, M. W., Cruts, A. A. N., van Ooyen-Houben, M. M. J., Meijer, R. F., Croes, E. A., Ketelaars, A. P. M., et al. (eds) (2012). *Nationale Drug Monitor, Jaarbericht.* Den Haag: Trimbos Instituut, 2013.

Wolff, W., Baumgarten, F., and Brand, R. (2013). Reduced self-control leads to disregard of an unfamiliar behavioral option: an experimental approach to the study of neuroenhancement. *Subst. Abuse Treat. Prev. Policy* 8:41. doi: 10.1186/1747-597X-8-41

Wolff, W., and Brand, R. (2013). Subjective stressors in school and their relation to neuroenhancement: a behavioral perspective on students' everyday life "doping." *Subst. Abuse Treat. Prev. Policy* 8:23. doi: 10.1186/1747-597X-8-23

Wolff, W., Brand, R., Baumgarten, F., Lösel, J., and Ziegler, M. (2014). Modeling students instrumental (mis-) use of substances to enhance cognitive performance: neuroenhancement in the light of job demands-resources theory. *Biopsychosoc. Med.* 8:12. doi: 10.1186/1751-0759-8-12

12

The reactivation of somatosensory cortex and behavioral recovery after sensory loss in mature primates

Hui-Xin Qi *, Jon H. Kaas and Jamie L. Reed

Department of Psychology, Vanderbilt University, Nashville, TN, USA

Edited by:
Mikhail Lebedev, Duke University, USA

Reviewed by:
Preston E. Garraghty, Indiana University, USA
Ioan Opris, Wake Forest University, USA

****Correspondence:***
Hui-Xin Qi, Department of Psychology, Vanderbilt University, 111 21st Ave. S., Nashville, TN 37240, USA
e-mail: huixin.qi@vanderbilt.edu

In our experiments, we removed a major source of activation of somatosensory cortex in mature monkeys by unilaterally sectioning the sensory afferents in the dorsal columns of the spinal cord at a high cervical level. At this level, the ascending branches of tactile afferents from the hand are cut, while other branches of these afferents remain intact to terminate on neurons in the dorsal horn of the spinal cord. Immediately after such a lesion, the monkeys seem relatively unimpaired in locomotion and often use the forelimb, but further inspection reveals that they prefer to use the unaffected hand in reaching for food. In addition, systematic testing indicates that they make more errors in retrieving pieces of food, and start using visual inspection of the rotated hand to confirm the success of the grasping of the food. Such difficulties are not surprising as a complete dorsal column lesion totally deactivates the contralateral hand representation in primary somatosensory cortex (area 3b). However, hand use rapidly improves over the first post-lesion weeks, and much of the hand representational territory in contralateral area 3b is reactivated by inputs from the hand in roughly a normal somatotopic pattern. Quantitative measures of single neuron response properties reveal that reactivated neurons respond to tactile stimulation on the hand with high firing rates and only slightly longer latencies. We conclude that preserved dorsal column afferents after nearly complete lesions contribute to the reactivation of cortex and the recovery of the behavior, but second-order sensory pathways in the spinal cord may also play an important role. Our microelectrode recordings indicate that these preserved first-order, and second-order pathways are initially weak and largely ineffective in activating cortex, but they are potentiated during the recovery process. Therapies that would promote this potentiation could usefully enhance recovery after spinal cord injury.

Keywords: area 3b, cuneate nucleus, monkey, plasticity, spinal cord, ventroposterior nucleus, somatosensory system

INTRODUCTION

The last 30 years of intensive research has led to a greatly improved understanding of how the somatosensory system of mature primates and other mammals responds to sensory loss, as reviewed by others (Buonomano and Merzenich, 1998; Jones, 2000; Wall et al., 2002; Kaas et al., 2008; Darian-Smith, 2009; Xerri, 2012). The types of sensory loss that have been experimentally studied have varied, ranging from the loss of peripheral nerves, especially the median nerve to the glabrous skin of the hand (Merzenich et al., 1983a,b; Silva et al., 1996; Florence et al., 1998; Xu and Wall, 1999), the sectioning of dorsal roots of peripheral nerve afferents as they enter the spinal cord (Pons et al., 1991; Jones and Pons, 1998; Darian-Smith and Brown, 2000; Darian-Smith, 2004; Darian-Smith and Ciferri, 2005, 2006), the loss of a digit or part of forelimb (Kelahan and Doetsch, 1984; Crockett et al., 1993; Florence and Kaas, 1995; Sengelaub et al., 1997; Florence et al., 1998; Li et al., 2013), the section of peripheral nerve afferents as they travel in the dorsal columns of spinal cord (Jain et al., 1997, 1998, 2000, 2008; Weng et al., 2003; Graziano and Jones, 2009; Qi et al., 2011a), or spinal cord injury in rodents (Ghosh et al., 2009; Aguilar et al., 2010; Humanes-Valera et al., 2013). All these types of sensory loss deactivate topographically matched parts of the somatosensory system, including parts of the ipsilateral dorsal column-trigeminal complex in lower brainstem and the contralateral ventroposterior nucleus (VP) of the thalamus, and the primary (area 3b) and other areas (1 and 2) of contralateral somatosensory cortex. These extensive deactivations were expected from the somatotopic organization and hierarchical arrangement of these processing stations.

What was not expected, at least by most investigators, was that over various amounts of time, the deactivated parts of the somatosensory system became responsive to tactile stimulation again, based on the somatosensory inputs that remained. Some changes in the receptive fields of neurons in the somatosensory system were apparent as soon as they could be measured after sensory loss (Wall, 1977; Calford and Tweedale, 1988; Faggin et al., 1997; Xu and Wall, 1997, 1999; Krupa et al., 1999), and these immediate changes could be attributed to the removal of the excitatory drive on central inhibitory neurons that normally constrain the receptive fields of relay neurons by keeping some of the excitatory inputs subthreshold. Other reactivations with greater changes in the receptive field locations of central neurons occurred over hours to weeks, such as the reactivation of cortical neurons previously activated from the glabrous skin of the hand by touch on the back of the hand after sectioning of the median nerve to the glabrous skin of digits 1–3 (Merzenich et al., 1983a,b). Such rapid reactivations may largely result from the potentiation of previously existing subthreshold inputs, especially in the cuneate nucleus representing the hand in the lower brainstem, by homeostatic mechanisms (Garraghty et al., 1991; Turrigiano, 1999; Wellman et al., 2002), and possibly by new axon growth over short distances (Darian-Smith and Gilbert, 1994; Jain et al., 2000; Darian-Smith, 2004; Hickmott and Steen, 2005; Cheetham et al., 2008; Yamahachi et al., 2009; Marik et al., 2010, 2014). Other reactivations that follow the loss or denervation of the forelimb, including invasion by inputs from the face (Pons et al., 1991; Jain et al., 1997, 2000; Wu and Kaas, 1999; Florence et al., 2000), may take many months to emerge (Jain et al., 1997), and depend on longer distances of new axon growth at subcortical and cortical levels (Florence et al., 1998; Jain et al., 2000). Cortical reorganization after limb amputations in humans can be found in several studies (Flor et al., 1995, 1998; Elbert et al., 1997; Davis et al., 1998; Lotze et al., 1999; Brugger et al., 2000; Moore et al., 2000; Curt et al., 2002). Thus, reactivations commonly occur in humans and other primates after a total loss of a subset of peripheral nerve inputs. In part, the reactivations after injury involve activity-dependent homeostatic cellular mechanisms, but also require the growth of new connections for greater changes in somatotopy. Because of the need for longer axon growth, greater changes in somatotopy take a longer time to emerge. Finally, somatotopic reorganization in cortex may usefully compensate for some of the sensory loss, but extensive reorganizations appear to lead to persisting mislocalization of sensory stimuli, such that the activation of hand cortex by inputs from the face leads to sensation felt on a phantom hand (Ramachandran, 1993; Davis et al., 1998; Ramachandran and Rogers-Ramachandran, 2000). Hence, somatosensory reactivations that restore much of normal somatotopy may be the most useful in restoring lost functions after sensory system damage. For example, highly somatotopic reactivations may occur when a loss of peripheral nerve afferents from any given region of skin is incomplete, as the subsequent potentiation of remaining weak or subthreshold inputs allows aspects of normal somatotopic order in central representations to be restored, at least partially. This may happen after selective sections of the dorsal roots of peripheral nerves as they enter the spinal cord (Darian-Smith and Brown, 2000; Darian-Smith and Ciferri, 2005, 2006), as similar inputs from a region of skin may enter over several dorsal roots (Welker, 1973), including roots left intact. In a similar manner, sectioning of peripheral nerve afferents as they ascend in the dorsal column of the spinal cord may leave a scattering of afferents that can restore some of the normal somatotopy of the deactivated somatosensory cortex (Jain et al., 1997). Alternatively, the information provided by cutting dorsal column afferents may not be totally lost, because these afferents branch as they enter the spinal cord. One branch ascends in the dorsal columns and the other terminates on the dorsal horn neurons in the spinal cord. As this sensory information is preserved, a more useful somatotopic reactivation of cortex may emerge based on the connections of the spinal cord neurons. The remainder of this review mainly focuses on the consequences of dorsal column lesions of the spinal cord in primates, including characteristics of natural recoveries and potential for augmented recoveries, but it is not intended to be a comprehensive literature review of other types of injuries and recovery mechanisms.

DORSAL COLUMN LESIONS IN PRIMATES

Dorsal column lesions in monkeys and other primates provide a number of advantages in studies of central nervous system reorganization after sensory loss. Most importantly, the loss is selective for the afferents that convey low-threshold, rapidly conducting tactile inputs from the slowly adapting and rapidly adapting receptors in the skin, while less rapidly conducting afferents for pain, temperature, and crude touch are left intact, as these afferents bypass the dorsal columns (Kaas, 2012). In addition, proprioceptive information from receptors located in muscles and joints travels in peripheral nerve afferents that ascend lateral to the dorsal column afferents in the spinal cord, where they are damaged only if the dorsal column lesion includes the fibers of the lateral spinal cord. Furthermore, the peripheral nerve afferents that contribute to the dorsal columns branch, such that one branch terminates in the dorsal horn of the spinal cord while another branch ascends in the dorsal columns to terminate in the brainstem. Although one branch is cut by the dorsal column lesion, the other branch may still function in the dorsal horn, where the afferents continue to contribute to spinal cord reflexes and other spinal cord functions, and possibly to ascending sensory pathways that compensate for dorsal column lesions. Studies of the effects of dorsal column lesions in rats have produced useful information (for reviews, see Kaas et al., 2008; Onifer et al., 2011); however, unlike the separation between the sensory and motor pathways in primates, corticospinal (motor) projections course in the dorsal columns in rodents (Hicks and D'Amato, 1975; D'Amato and Hicks, 1978; Vahlsing and Feringa, 1980; Paxino and Watson, 2007). Therefore, dorsal column lesions in rodents involve a direct motor loss in addition to the sensory loss. Thus, the use of dorsal column lesions in primates has the advantages of producing a rather specific loss of tactile capacities, while leaving other functions intact. Importantly, these specific lesions in primates are followed by unexpected levels of behavioral recovery (see below). While the lesions do not mimic the typical types of injury that occur in most cases of spinal cord injury in humans, where damage may be extensive and somewhat non-specific, the lesions can be made with precision and consistency so that useful results can be obtained from a few subjects. Consistent results from similar lesions allow therapeutic procedures to be evaluated. Thus, experimental results from monkeys have the potential of providing information that can usefully guide the interpretations and predictions of consequences of spinal cord damage in humans, and hopefully guide the development of therapeutic procedures.

Our experiments typically involve a unilateral lesion of the dorsal columns at a C4–C5 level of the spinal cord (**Figure 1**). This removes the primary afferent tactile inputs to the cuneate nucleus from one hand, while leaving the inputs from the other hand intact. All inputs to the dorsal horn neurons of the spinal cord are preserved, as are the primary proprioceptive afferents in the lateral spinal cord pathway. Neurons in the elongated cuneate nucleus project to the hand and forelimb subnucleus of

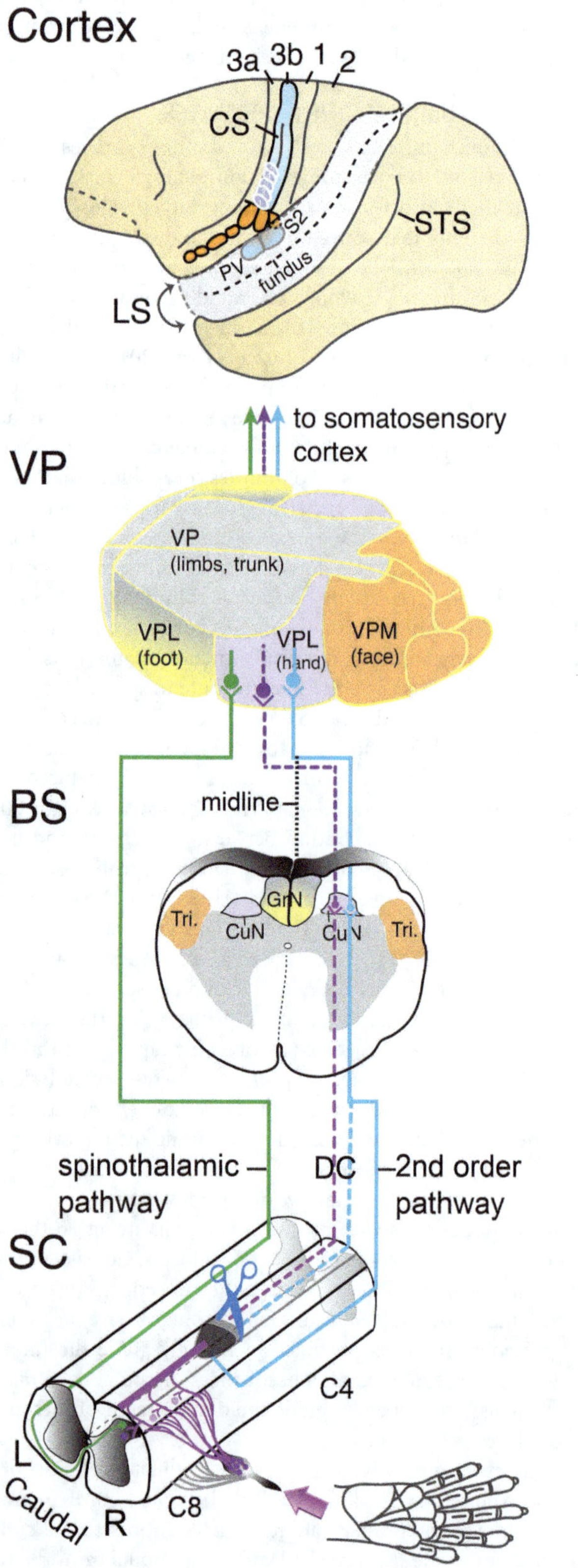

FIGURE 1 | Somatosensory pathways from the spinal cord to cortex of a squirrel monkey. Cutaneous afferents from the hand that enter the cervical spinal cord between C4 and C8 levels via the dorsal roots are *(Continued)*

FIGURE 1 | Continued
shown in the lower panel. In the spinal cord (SC), one branch of the afferents enters the ascending dorsal column pathway to terminate in the ipsilateral cuneate nucleus (violet line). The other branch terminates in the dorsal horn of the spinal cord. Second-order neurons activated in the dorsal horn by cutaneous primary afferents project to the ipsilateral cuneate nucleus via dorsal column, the dorsolateral pathway, or other pathways (blue line). Other dorsal horn neurons send axons to the contralateral spinal cord and form the spinothalamic pathway (green line). Cutting (scissors) the dorsal column pathway at a C4–C5 level deactivates the cuneate nucleus by removing the direct primary afferent inputs from the hand. The dashed lines mark the partially deafferented pathways from spinal cord to cortex after the spinal cord lesion. Most of the afferents of second-order tactile neurons in the dorsal horn that course in the dorsal columns may be preserved as well, but others may join the dorsal columns above the lesions, or travel outside the lesion in the dorsal lateral fiber tracts. The spinothalamic afferents may contribute to the reactivation of the ventroposterior nucleus and somatosensory cortex. The location of the elongated cuneate nucleus at the junction of the upper spinal cord with the lower brainstem (BS) is shown to represent how the pathways for touch on the hand travel. CuN, cuneate nucleus; Tri, trigeminal nucleus; ECN, external cuneate nucleus of the contralateral (left) somatosensory thalamus. In the somatosensory thalamus (VP), the larger ventroposterior lateral division, VPL, contains subnuclei for the hand and foot, which is capped by a region for the upper (proximal) portions of the limbs and trunk. The medial division, VPM, separates the face. Inputs from the hand are relayed to the hand subnucleus of VPL. The spinothalamic pathway terminates in the ventroposterior inferior nucleus (not shown) as well as VP. In cortex, somatosensory areas of the left cerebral hemisphere are shown. Squirrel monkeys have a short, shallow central sulcus, CS, so that the primary cortical area for touch, area 3b of Brodmann, is largely exposed on the brain surface. The region of the hand representation is indicated below the central tip of the central sulcus. Area 3b receives tactile information from VP. Area 1 contains a higher-order representation of touch just caudal to area 3b. Area 3a receives proprioceptive information from the ventroposterior superior nucleus of the thalamus (not shown). Area 2 is a higher-order somatosensory area just caudal to area 1. The second somatosensory area, S2, and the posterior ventral area, PV, are located on the upper bank of the lateral sulcus, LS. The superior temporal sulcus, STS, is shown for reference.

the ventroposterior nucleus (VP) of the contralateral thalamus. VP is commonly divided into a lateral "nucleus" (VPL) representing the contralateral upper and lower body, and a medial "nucleus" (VPM) representing the contralateral face and both the contralateral and ipsilateral tongue and teeth (Kaas et al., 2006). VP projects to primary somatosensory cortex, area 3b, in a somatotopic pattern, so that the hand subnucleus projects to the hand representation in area 3b just medial to that of the face and lateral to that of the arm and trunk. The VP inputs activate area 3b neurons, while VP provides subthreshold projections to area 1 (e.g., Nelson and Kaas, 1981; Garraghty et al., 1990a), which has a somatotopic organization that parallels and mirrors that in area 3b (Kaas et al., 1979).

In our experiments, we typically determine the effects of dorsal column lesions by recording from the hand subdivision of contralateral area 3b in squirrel monkeys or owl monkeys with microelectrodes. Squirrel monkeys have only a short, shallow central sulcus, and owl monkeys have only a short central dimple. For both of these primates, the representations of the hand in area 3b and in adjoining areas 3a and 1 are exposed on the surface of the brain. This exposure of the cortical areas allows activity patterns to be mapped in detail with densely spaced microelectrode penetrations. Microelectrode mapping can also be done at thalamic and brainstem levels, but not under visual guidance. Therefore, the somatotopy of these subcortical representations is both harder to determine in detail, and harder to illustrate compared to the two-dimensional cortical maps. In addition, reorganized area 3b maps reflect both subcortical alterations and those that originate in area 3b. Thus, area 3b is a key location for investigation in most experiments. We and others have also studied area 3b reorganization in macaque monkey (Pons et al., 1991; Florence and Kaas, 1995; Florence et al., 1998; Darian-Smith and Brown, 2000; Jain et al., 2008), where area 3b is hidden on the caudal bank of a deep central fissure, as in humans. These more difficult studies are important because macaques are used as a more common model for human brain organization, as macaque brains have some features of the somatosensory system that more closely resemble those of humans.

Neurons in the hand portion of area 3b typically have small excitatory receptive fields, mostly located on the glabrous skin of the hand, especially on the distal phalanges of digits, and they are often confined to part of a single phalange of a digit or pad of the palm. Nearby neurons have similar receptive fields, and a systematic partial map of the hand representation in area 3b can be reconstructed from a dense array of microelectrode recordings across the hand region by outlining all electrode penetration sites with receptive fields centered on any digit phalanges or pad of the palm, or part of the body (Merzenich et al., 1978; Nelson et al., 1980; Sur et al., 1982; Krubitzer and Kaas, 1990). Such maps are extremely consistent in somatotopy across individuals, and they conform to the orderly arrangement of projections from VP to area 3b (Jones et al., 1982; Kaas et al., 1984; Cusick and Gould, 1990; Qi et al., 2011b; Liao et al., 2013). In addition, narrow cell-poor septa separate the representations of digits in area 3b so that digit territories are histologically visible (Qi and Kaas, 2004). The most apparent of these cortical septa separates the representation of digit 1, the thumb, from that of the face; and this septum serves as a highly useful landmark when recording sites are related to cortical histology (Jain et al., 1998, 2001).

THE REACTIVATION AND REORGANIZATION OF SOMATOSENSORY CORTEX AFTER DORSAL COLUMN LESIONS

As the primary somatosensory cortical area for tactile stimuli, area 3b has been the most studied area after dorsal column injury. Most of the results have been obtained from multiple microelectrode recordings where receptive fields for cortical neurons have been defined by stimulating the skin with hand-held probes. Traditionally, near-threshold skin indentations are used to define the "minimal excitatory receptive field" (Merzenich et al., 1983a). In reactivated regions of cortex deprived of their normal sources of activation, neuron responses are subjectively classified as good or excellent, meaning that the neuron responses to light touch closely resemble those in normal cortex, or as poor, or non-responsive. Recordings in deprived cortex immediately after a dorsal column lesion reveal that this cortex is totally unresponsive to light tactile stimuli. Thus, no neuronal spikes are evoked in deprived cortex, while neurons in un-deprived cortex, such as face cortex, respond normally. After a dorsal column lesion at a high cervical level above C4, the hand cortex in area 3b is completely deprived and unresponsive. Over a period of 3–4 weeks, much of the deprived hand cortex starts to respond to touch on the hand, with a distorted but crudely normal somatotopy. Thus, neurons responsive to touch on digit 1 (thumb) are in cortex lateral to those for digit 2, and digits 1–5 are represented in a lateral to medial order. However, this pattern is often disrupted by displaced islands of neurons that represent the same digit, patches of cortex that remain unresponsive, and neurons with discontinuous receptive fields that represent more than one location on the hand. Such results have been reported in a number of studies, including those from owl monkeys, squirrel monkeys, marmosets, and macaque monkeys (Jain et al., 1997, 1998, 2008; Qi et al., 2011a; Bowes et al., 2012, 2013).

Studies of the reactivation process in monkeys with dorsal column lesion using imaging methods, such as fMRI, optical imaging, and radiographic imaging, have been limited but informative (Tommerdahl et al., 1996; Chen et al., 2012; Dutta et al., 2013; Yang et al., under revision). As an example, results from one squirrel monkey from Chen et al. (2012) are shown in **Figure 2**. Before a dorsal column lesion, tactile stimulation of each of the five digits resulted in a focus of activity in the hand region of area 3b, with foci for digits 1–5 in the expected lateral to medial order (**Figure 2A**. In this anesthetized monkey, responses in area 1 were not reliably obtained. Four weeks after a dorsal column lesion at the C4–C5 level, area 3b was responsive to touch on the digits, and the somatotopic order of foci activated from each digit was roughly in the normal order, but distorted from the normal pattern (**Figure 2B**). After 8 weeks, the cortex was more responsive, and the somatotopic pattern appeared more normal (**Figure 2C**). When the final somatotopic pattern from fMRI was compared to an optical imaging pattern and a microelectrode map in the same monkey, there was good agreement between the activation patterns from the three methods, but optical imaging produced a more detailed map than the fMRI imaging, and greatest detail was provided by the microelectrode maps. Although the fMRI mapping provides less sensitive somatotopic detail than the microelectrode recordings or the optical imaging, fMRI allows the same cortex to be imaged multiple times non-invasively. Over an eight-week or even longer period of recovery, there was no evidence that the deprived hand cortex was reactivated by any other part of the body, including the face. However, after longer periods of 6–8 months to years, face inputs from the region of the chin often activate parts of the hand cortex (Jain et al., 1997).

When the dorsal column lesion is incomplete, perhaps as an unintended result, or because the lesion was intentionally placed at a lower C5–C6 level in order to preserve some inputs from digit 1 and a few from digit 2, then these preserved inputs come to represent larger than normal territories in area 3b after 5–8 weeks of recovery with sensorimotor training and testing. However, much of the activation is in the normal territories for those digits. Somatotopic organization of reactivated cortex after recovery is likely dependent on the level and extent of the lesion, as indicated by studies using single microelectrodes to map the cortex (Qi et al., 2011a; Chen et al., 2012) and using multi-electrode arrays implanted in cortex (Qi et al., 2014). For example, receptive field mapping of neurons recorded with a 100-electrode array

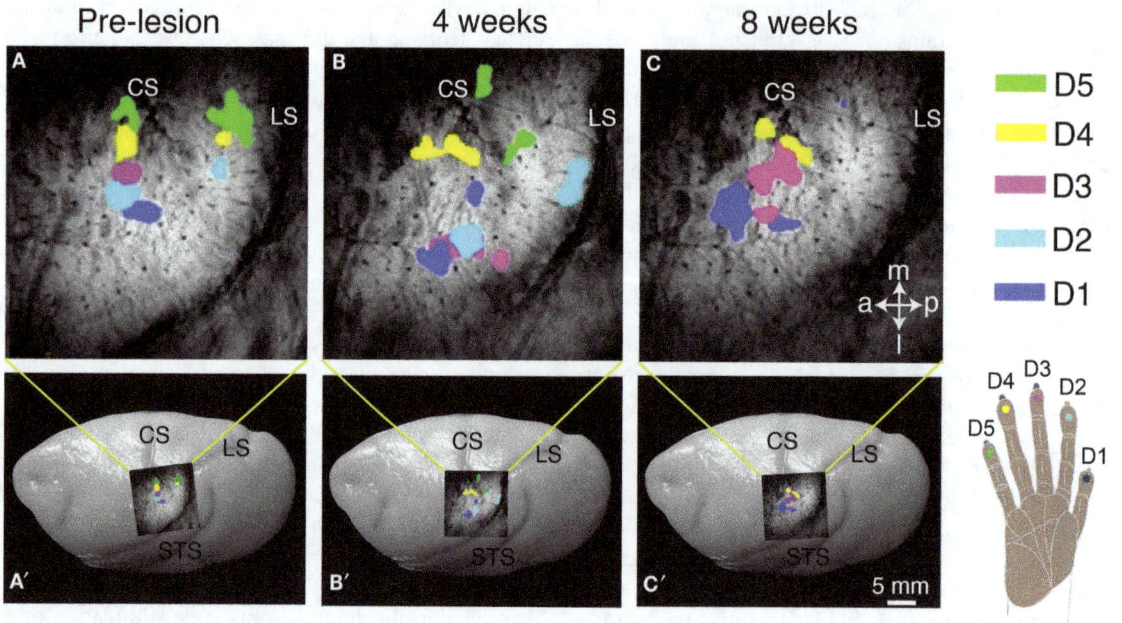

FIGURE 2 | Longitudinal mapping of fMRI activation to vibrotactile stimulation on digits 1–5 pre-lesion (A) and after 4-weeks (B) and 8-weeks (C) post-lesion following unilateral dorsal column section in a squirrel monkey (SM-O). Activation foci from trial blocks of stimulation on individual digits were superimposed for the composite images **(A–C)**. The location of the top panel on the brain is shown for each panel below. Dots on the hand schematic (lower right) are color-coded to represent the activation in cortex when that digit location was stimulated **(A–C)**. Superimposed images of the fMRI activation on photograph of a squirrel monkey brain indicates the approximate location of the region of interest **(A′–C′)**. Abbreviations: a, anterior; CS, central sulcus; D1–5, digits 1–5; l, lateral; LS, lateral sulcus; m, medial; p, posterior; STS, superior temporal sulcus. Adapted from Chen et al. (2012).

in area 3b in a squirrel monkey showed that somatotopic organization in reactivated cortex was largely normal after behavioral recovery from a dorsal column lesion at the C6 level (compare **Figures 3B,C**). However, the cortical territories occupied by spared inputs for digits 1 and 2 encroached into regions deprived of input by the C6 lesion (digits 3–5). This monkey received sensorimotor training and testing for use of the impaired hand over the course of 6 weeks prior to recording with the array, and it is unknown what effect this behavioral intervention may have had on the cortical reactivation beyond what would have occurred spontaneously. In this case, preserved inputs activated their normal locations in cortex, but also came to activate larger than normal territories.

Finally, the reactivation of area 3b hand cortex should result in the reactivation of the hand territories of other cortical areas that depend on area 3b for activation, such as areas 1, S2, and PV, as reported previously (Pons et al., 1987; Burton et al., 1990; Garraghty et al., 1990b). Indeed, the area 1 representation of touch is restored in a somatotopic pattern that generally parallels that in area 3b, but it is less precise in detailed somatotopy, and the neuronal responses tend to be weaker in the reactivated regions (Merzenich et al., 1983a; Jain et al., 2008; Qi et al., 2011a). Responses to tactile stimuli also return to areas 3a and 2 (Garraghty et al., 1990a; Bowes et al., 2013) and the hand region of areas S2 and PV (Pons et al., 1987, 1992; Burton et al., 1990; Garraghty et al., 1990b; Tandon et al., 2009; Wang et al., 2013; Yang et al., under revision). Areas 3a and 2 receive proprioceptive input from the ventroposterior superior nucleus of the thalamus (Kaas, 2012), so neurons in these areas may remain responsive to hand manipulation after dorsal column lesions that spare the proprioceptive axons in the lateral spinal cord. As all these areas recover responsiveness to tactile stimuli and provide direct and indirect inputs to motor and premotor cortex (Krubitzer and Kaas, 1990; Stepniewska et al., 1993; Disbrow et al., 2003; Fang et al., 2005; Qi et al., 2010; Kambi et al., 2011; see Wise et al., 1997 for review), considerable sensory guidance of motor behavior is restored.

THE RESPONSE PROPERTIES OF REACTIVATED NEURONS IN AREA 3b

Reactivated cortical neurons may have disorganized excitatory receptive fields, or larger than normal receptive fields, but these responses to light touch on the hand appear to range from subjectively normal amplitude to weak responses (Qi et al., 2014). Over recovery periods longer than 4–8 weeks, more neurons likely become capable of stronger responses. Quantifying response properties beyond receptive field organization is a growing focus of study in the somatosensory system (Doetsch et al., 1996; Wang et al., 2013; Qi et al., 2014), but some support for these studies comes from studies of reactivated neurons in primary visual cortex after retinal lesions (Chino et al., 1995, 2001; Darian-Smith and Gilbert, 1995). Our quantitative studies of the response properties of reactivated cortical neurons after dorsal column lesions have been limited (Wang et al., 2013; Qi et al., 2014), but there is already evidence that reactivated neurons have responses to tactile stimuli (indentation of the skin with an electromechanical

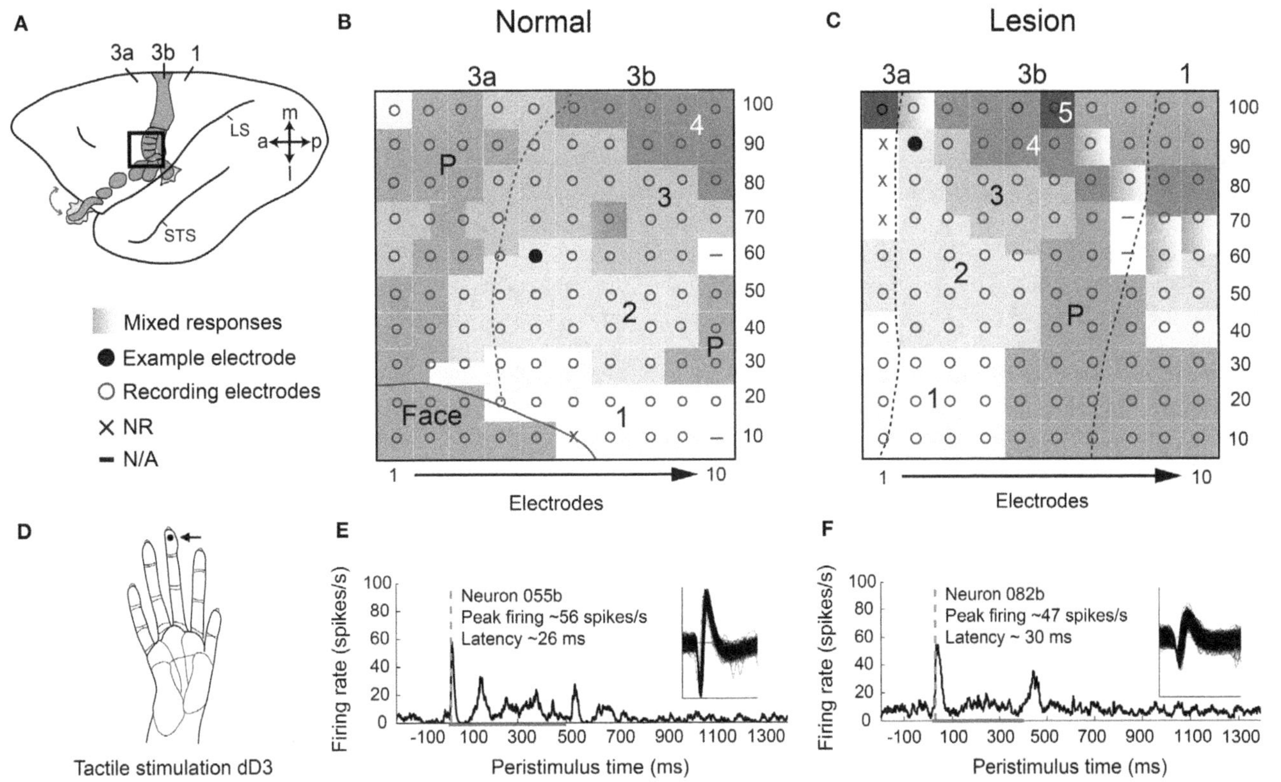

FIGURE 3 | Response properties of area 3b neurons after behavioral recovery from dorsal column lesion are similar to those in a monkey with no lesion. (A) A schematic of the left hemisphere of an owl monkey brain with area 3b shaded shows the approximate placement of a 100-electrode array for monkey OM-A with no lesion (see **B**). The array placement for a monkey SM-G with a dorsal column lesion was similar, but slightly more medial and posterior (see **C**). Note the key for the somatotopic mapping of the array applies to **(B)** and **(C)**. **(B)** Representation of coverage of 100-electrode array in cortex for a normal monkey with somatotopic map reconstructed from locations of receptive fields for neurons at each electrode. Coverage included part of the area 3b hand and face representation as well as area 3a, with somatotopy consistent with previous reports from normal monkeys. The electrode location from which the example neuron for the lower panel **(E)** was recorded is indicated by the filled circle. **(C)** Representation of coverage of 100-electrode array in cortex for monkey SM-G after behavioral recovery from partial DC lesion at the C6 spinal cord level. This lesion preserved many of the dorsal column afferents from digits 1 and 2. SM-G experienced sensorimotor training and testing using the impaired hand for 6 weeks following DC lesion prior to recording with the multi-electrode array. All digits are represented within expected somatotopic locations, but D1 and D2 appear to be represented in more territory than D3–D5. Electrode location for the example neuron in the lower panel **(F)** is indicated by the filled circle. **(D)** Activities of neurons from monkeys with and without a lesion in **(B–C)** are shown in **(E–F)** during tactile stimulation on right distal digit 3 (dD3). The stimulation site is indicated by a dot (see arrow) on drawing of a monkey hand. **(E)** Example of a single unit 055b shows typical peak firing rates and latencies for an example normal case, monkey OM-A. Spikes during 100 trials of tactile stimulation on dD3 are averaged in the peristimulus-time histogram (PSTH). Waveforms of the recorded unit are shown (inset). **(F)** Example of a single unit 082b shows typical responses for a case with a dorsal column lesion, monkey SM-G, following recovery of reaching behavior with the impaired hand. Activity during 150 trials of tactile stimulation on dD3 is shown in the PSTH. In **(B–C)**, dashed lines indicate area 3b borders based on receptive field topography and myelin architecture. In **(E–F)**, dashed gray line indicates the latency of the peak firing response that exceeds 2 times the standard deviation of the average baseline firing. Peak firing value listed is baseline-subtracted. Horizontal gray line indicates stimulus duration in each trial (500 ms in OM-A, 400 ms in SM-G). Abbreviations: 1–5, digits 1–5; 3a, 3b, 1, area 3a, area 3b, area 1; a, anterior; dD3, distal digit 3; l, lateral; LS, lateral sulcus; m, medial; p, posterior; STS, superior temporal sulcus. Modified from Reed et al. (2010) and Qi et al. (2014).

probe) that are in the normal or near-normal range, as indicated by examples of cortical activity (**Figure 3**) from an intact monkey (Reed et al., 2010) and a monkey 6 weeks after mid-cervical dorsal column lesion (Qi et al., 2014).

Qi et al. (2014) found that fewer neurons in area 3b responded to tactile stimulation on the hand in monkeys after sensory loss followed by behavioral training compared to normal monkeys. However, peak firing rates of responsive neurons were similar in monkeys with and without lesions. An example neuron from a normal monkey (**Figure 3E**) maintained low levels of spontaneous firing and increased firing to about 56 spikes/s in response to the onset of a 500 ms depression of the skin on distal digit 3. This example showed some increased firing during the sustained indentation of the stimulus and a response to the removal of the stimulus from the skin. Such "off responses" are common in normal animals (Sur et al., 1984; Pei et al., 2009). The neuron's response with some maintained discharge during the duration of skin indentation is common in area 3b neurons, as these neurons can show mixtures of properties reflecting both rapidly-adapting and slowly-adapting afferents (Sur et al., 1984; Pei et al., 2009). The example neuron in the reactivated cortex after nearly complete dorsal column lesion (**Figure 3F**) responded to both stimulus onset and removal, while maintaining some firing during the sustained skin indentation on distal digit 3. Notably, the neuron in reactivated cortex had somewhat lower peak firing rates during tactile stimulation at about 47 spikes/s, but still greater than the median response rates reported previously (about 18 spikes/s) and seemingly close to rates expected normally (Reed et al., 2010; Qi et al., 2014). In 3 monkeys with dorsal column lesions and after hand use in a reaching task recovered to normal levels, response latencies of neurons in reactivated area 3b to skin indentation were similar to normal or slightly longer than normal, averaging about 31 ms [Reed et al., 2012 (abstract)]. Using similar recording methods and data analysis, Reed et al. (2010) found that response latencies of area 3b neurons in normal monkeys averaged about 21 ms. The example of neuronal activity in **Figure 3** shows a neuron in a lesioned monkey with a response latency to skin indentation that was slightly longer than the latency of a normal neuron (compare **Figure 3E** to **Figure 3F**). Similar response rates with slightly longer latencies than normal may suggest that some sensory input reaches area 3b after dorsal column lesions through alternative pathways that require additional synapses to reach the target. More study is needed, but the reactivated neurons clearly have response properties that could usefully guide behavior.

THE EFFECTS OF DORSAL COLUMN LESION ON BEHAVIOR

There is no doubt that spinal cord injuries often have devastating consequences for functional outcomes. A large number of studies in rodents (e.g., Anderson et al., 2005; Courtine et al., 2008; Zorner et al., 2010) and monkeys (e.g., Schmidlin et al., 2011; Nout et al., 2012a,b) have investigated the behavioral deficits that occur after spinal cord injury. Other studies have focused on the effects of a restricted interruption of the ascending dorsal column somatosensory pathway on the dexterity of the forepaws in rodents (e.g., McKenna and Whishaw, 1999; Ballermann et al., 2001) and monkeys (e.g., Beck, 1976; Glendinning et al., 1992; Leonard et al., 1992; Cooper et al., 1993; Vierck, 1998; Vierck and Cooper, 1998; Qi et al., 2013). In humans and monkeys, the effects of dorsal column lesions on sensory behavior have been interpreted in two quite different ways in early reports. Thus, Rose and Mountcastle (1959) concluded that the "destruction of the posterior columns in man leads to a loss of the capacity to appreciate the position and movement of the limbs," and "severe"—"disturbance in tactile sensations." Later, Mountcastle further stated, "What remains in the mechanoreceptive sphere after... dorsal column lesion is the capacity to recognize that a mechanical stimulus has occurred; it is no longer possible to specify it exactly as to location, intensity or shape" (Mountcastle and Darian-Smith, 1968). These pronouncements clearly reflect what would be expected after damage of such a major sensory pathway. However, Wall (1970) quite differently concluded that "no sensory defect has been shown to follow isolated dorsal column lesion" in human, and "animals with complete dorsal column section can carry out discriminations of weight, texture, vibration, two points and position." Later, Azulay and Schwartz (1975) summarized the effects of dorsal column lesion in monkeys by stating that "surprisingly little, if any, tactile functions are impaired after extensive damage to the dorsal funiculus." Subsequent to these early reports, several studies have reported impairments of hand use after lesion of the dorsal columns in macaque monkeys (Glendinning et al., 1992; Leonard et al., 1992), and sensory alterations have been described in macaques (Vierck, 1973, 1974) and humans (Nathan et al., 1986).

How can we explain these great differences in conclusions about the effects of dorsal column lesion in primates? There are several possible reasons for differences in findings and conclusions. (1) One possibility is that different lesions produce different results. For performance with the hand, the dorsal column lesion should be at the C4–C5 level or higher to remove all afferents from the hand, the lower lesions at C5–C6 of the cervical spinal cord spare some afferents from digit 1 and 2, and still lower lesions would spare inputs from most of the hand. Even with C4–C5 lesions or higher, various afferents in the dorsal columns could be spared. (2) Compensations likely occur. As described below for our study of the effects of dorsal column lesions on behavior, vision appears to supplement tactile feedback in food retrieval tasks after dorsal column lesions. Other compensations for sensory impairments are likely to be rapidly acquired as well. (3) Plasticity of the somatosensory system, even in mature primates appears to be a major source of recovery after dorsal column lesions. Recoveries of activation within the system and use of the hand may result from the potentiation of the activating effects of preserved dorsal columns afferents, even when they are very few. This possibility is well demonstrated by the effects of cutting most of the dorsal sensory roots of nerves of the forearm in monkeys, while leaving a few inputs from that hand that initially fail to activate cortex. However, several months later cortex responded to cutaneous stimulation of the largely deafferented digits. **Figure 4** illustrates such an example reprinted from Figure 10 of Darian-Smith (2004; see also, Darian-Smith and Brown, 2000; Darian-Smith and Ciferri, 2005, 2006; Darian-Smith, 2009). This reactivation of cortex is due in part to the potentiation of preserved afferents likely through axon growth and the formation of new synaptic contacts on deactivated neurons occurring at brainstem, thalamic, and cortical levels (Darian-Smith and Gilbert, 1994, 1995; Florence et al., 1998; Jain et al., 2000; Darian-Smith et al., 2010). A related possibility is that after dorsal column lesion second-order spinal cord neuron inputs to the cuneate nucleus are also potentiated and thereby come to reactivate that nucleus by touch on the hand, effectively replacing some of the lost direct dorsal column inputs to the cuneate nucleus. We return to this possibility in the last section of this review. (4) Finally, some of the effects attributed to damage to the dorsal columns in previous studies may reflect damage to other afferents, as motor impairments may occur when the lesions extend into the lateral spinal cord where the dorsal lateral funiculus with proprioceptive afferents and the lateral corticospinal motor tract are located.

The results of our recent study of hand use in squirrel monkeys after a unilateral dorsal column lesion provide evidence that the sensory loss produced by lesions confined to the dorsal columns do produce impairments in a food retrieval task (Qi et al., 2013). Monkeys were trained to reach for and retrieve small sugar pellets from wells that ranged from easy (shallow) to difficult (deep). Several results are presented in **Figure 5**. Before the spinal cord

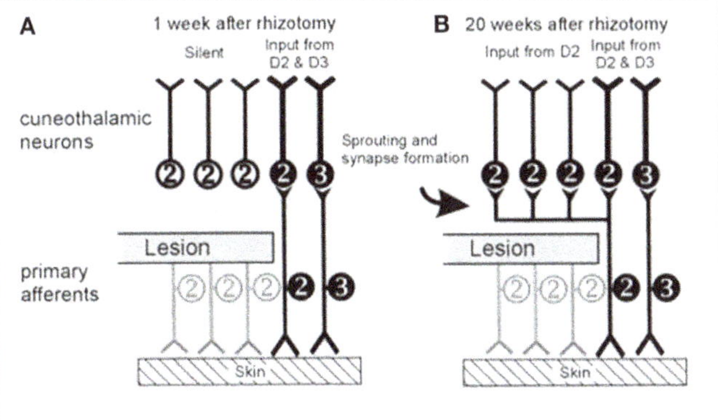

FIGURE 4 | Schematics represent hypothesized effects of a dorsal rootlet section that blocks sensory input from digit 1 (thumb) and digit 2 (index finger) in a macaque monkey after 1 week (A) and after 20 weeks (B). Inputs from digits 1 and 2 are labeled together as 2. After cutting the dorsal rootlet, some fraction of neurons innervating digits 1 and 2 may be spared, but a population of cuneate (and dorsal horn) neurons will be left without peripheral input. By 20 weeks after the dorsal rootlet section, terminals of the spared neurons innervating digits 1 and 2 have sprouted collaterals to innervate the previously deafferented target neurons in the cuneate nucleus. Similar mechanisms are hypothesized to occur at all levels of processing hierarchy from the brainstem to cortex.

lesion, monkeys were very good at the task, even for the most difficult well. They quickly reached to grasp the pellet after briefly visualizing it, and retrieved it with one or sometimes 2 flexes of the digits to bring the pellet from the well to the mouth. When behavioral testing was continued two weeks after a complete or nearly complete lesion of the dorsal columns, the behavior was clearly impaired in that it took more than one attempt to successfully grasp objects from the difficult wells, and more flexes of the digits were needed. The video recordings of the task performance revealed another change in the behavior. Before the dorsal column lesion, the monkey looked at the pellet in the well only briefly as the monkey started the reach, and instead watched the investigator during the grasp and retrieval. This may seem strange, but extensive visual guidance was unnecessary, and the monkey may regard the investigator as a potential competitor for the food, as it would another monkey, or as potentially dangerous and in need of watching. In contrast, after the lesion, the monkey acted as if it could not sense by touch if the pellet was in the hand, and always looked to see if the pellet was there. During the retrieval, the palm was turned up so the presence of the pellet could be visually confirmed. Overall, we think that the deficits in the retrieval behavior were due to the sensory loss, as they occurred when the lesions did not include motor axons lateral to the dorsal columns. Early successes likely related to behavioral compensations, especially the visual assurance that the pellet had been grasped. In addition, sensory perception likely improved as early as 3–4 weeks after the lesion, as cortex became progressively more responsive to touch on the hand due to cortical reactivation.

MECHANISMS OF CORTICAL REACTIVATION AND THE POTENTIAL FOR THERAPEUTIC TREATMENTS

The reactivation of deprived hand cortex weeks to months after high cervical dorsal column lesion depends on the potentiation

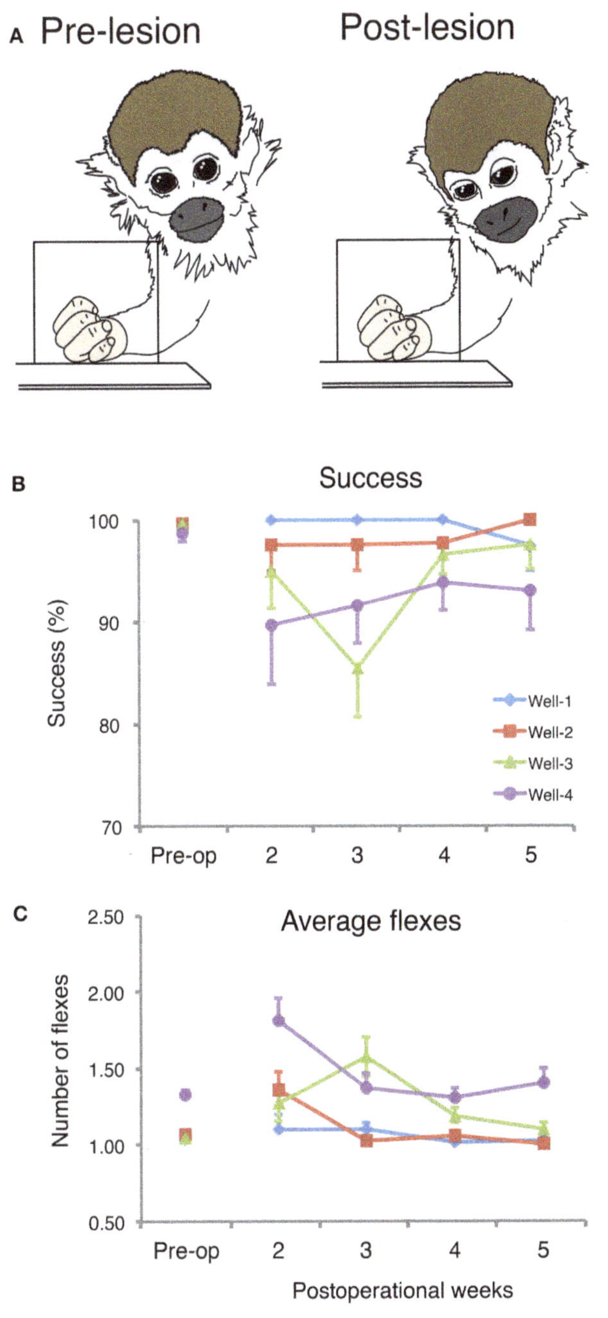

FIGURE 5 | Spontaneous recoveries after dorsal column injury can be incomplete or incorporate various compensations. (A) Drawings from the captured photo-frames taken from a squirrel monkey (SM-O) during the reach-to-grasp task pre-lesion (left) and on post-op Day 15 (right). The schematic summarizes observations that after the spinal cord lesion, monkeys compensate for reduced tactile sensation by relying more often on vision. **(B)** Post-operational changes in the percentage of successful retrievals (mean, ± *SD*) in the reach-to-grasp task. Success scores in percent of the retrieval success for summed trials from each of the 4 testing wells per post-op week for monkey SM-O. Pre-op final week trials were summed. **(C)** Post-operational changes in mean number of flexes (mean, ± *SD*) for monkey SM-O. Each data point within each panel is the averaged number of flexes from the sum of the trials from each of the 4 wells over each testing week. Adapted from Qi et al. (2013).

of preserved sensory pathways through axon growth and the formation of new synapses. We have previously suggested that dorsal column lesions are often incomplete, and that preserved but subthreshold dorsal column inputs to the cuneate nucleus gain strength by forming more synapses on more neurons as the result of reduced competition for synaptic space (Rasmusson and Northgrave, 1997; Xu and Wall, 1997; Darian-Smith, 2004; Darian-Smith and Ciferri, 2006). Similar changes likely occur at the levels of the ventroposterior nucleus and somatosensory cortex (Garraghty et al., 1991, 2006; Rasmusson, 1996; Wellman et al., 2002). Under conditions of extreme loss of afferents to the cuneate nucleus, we had evidence that even afferents from the adjacent trigeminal complex for the face could sprout and grow to innervate the cuneate nucleus (Jain et al., 2000), providing relays to the hand subnucleus of the contralateral ventroposterior nucleus and then to the hand territory of primary somatosensory cortex. While such reactivations of the cuneate nucleus by inputs from the hand that were preserved after the dorsal column lesion, as well as those that grow into the cuneate nucleus from the face, do occur, we have observed reactivations of hand cortex after lesions of the dorsal columns that were 95–100% complete (Qi et al., 2011a). Although it can be difficult to accurately determine the completeness of a lesion of the dorsal columns from histological sections through the lesion site, we feel confident about the completeness of experimental lesions because we injected tracers into the fingers of both hands in monkeys with unilateral lesions to demonstrate the loss of labeled axon terminations in the cuneate nucleus on the lesioned compared to the non-lesioned side (Qi et al., 2011a). Thus, we have strong evidence that there are reactivations that do not depend on preserved dorsal column first-order afferents, and thus depend mostly on other afferents from the hand.

The most likely alternative pathway is from neurons in the dorsal horn of the spinal cord that project to the dorsal column nuclei (Perl et al., 1962; Rustioni et al., 1979; Bennett et al., 1983). These neurons are directly activated by one of the bifurcated branches of peripheral nerve axons that terminates in the dorsal horn, while the other branch ascends in the dorsal columns and terminates in the dorsal column nuclei (Wall, 1970; Willis and Coggeshall, 2004). These dorsal column neurons would receive the same information for the skin of the hand that the cuneate nucleus directly receives, although there may be differences in the amounts of convergence of inputs and inhibitory mechanisms so that receptive field sizes may differ for neurons in the dorsal horn or cuneate nucleus (Dykes and Craig, 1998; Witham and Baker, 2011). However, the normal role of second-order spinal cord inputs to the cuneate nucleus most likely would be to provide subthreshold activation, because cortical reactivation after a loss of the primary inputs to the cuneate nucleus takes weeks to emerge.

In order to be effective, the projections to the cuneate nucleus by second-order dorsal horn neurons must survive the dorsal column lesion. Some axons from second-order neurons might enter the dorsal columns below the lesion and be lost. Others might enter above the lesion, or travel in some other pathway, such as the lateral funiculus, which is dominated by proprioceptive afferents (Rustioni et al., 1979). This possibility seems likely in that larger

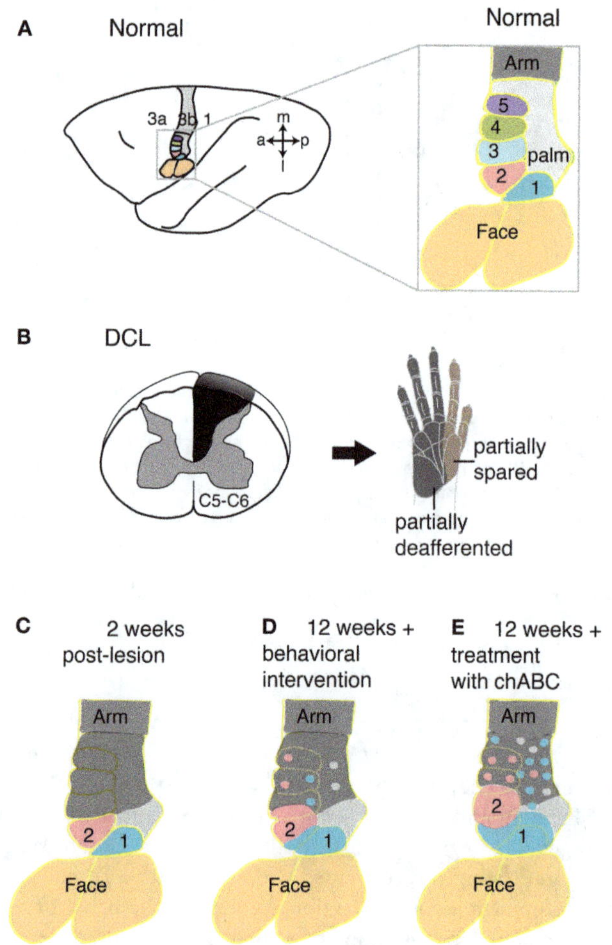

FIGURE 6 | Spontaneous and augmented recoveries from sensory loss in monkey cortex. (A) Schematic view of the left hemisphere of an owl monkey brain with area 3b highlighted in color and expanded (right) to focus on the hand representation. **(B)** When afferents devoted to the hand are cut in the cervical spinal cord at the C5 or C6 level in squirrel monkeys and owl monkeys (left), inputs from much of digit 1 and digit 2 are spared, while inputs from most of the rest of the hand are disrupted, as indicated by the hand schematic (right). **(C)** After such a lesion **(B)**, the hand representation in primary somatosensory cortex is immediately rendered largely unresponsive to tactile stimuli (gray shading), with the exception of much of the digit 1 and digit 2 representations (blue and pink shading, respectively), for which the majority of axons enter the spinal cord above the level of the lesion. Over weeks of spontaneous post-lesion recovery without augmentation, the deactivated cortex becomes partly reactivated by inputs from the hand with activation from the spared dorsal column inputs (digits 1 and 2), and possibly other pathways (not shown). **(D)** This schematic summarizes expected results in monkeys with dorsal column lesions that received behavioral intervention when the cortex is studied 12 weeks after the lesion. Sensorimotor training and testing for use of the impaired hand appears to promote reactivation of cortex, but further study is needed to determine how effective behavioral intervention is beyond spontaneous recoveries and in comparison with other types of treatments. Based on previous findings and ongoing research, we expect that the representations of spared digits will expand their territories and islands of responsiveness will emerge in previously unresponsive zones. **(E)** The effectiveness of a few preserved dorsal column afferents for activating cortex can be enhanced by treatment of the target site in the cuneate nucleus with the enzyme chondroitinase ABC shortly after the spinal cord injury. Digestion of

(Continued)

FIGURE 6 | Continued
components of the extracellular matrix in the cuneate that inhibit axon sprouting allows axons spared from the lesion to sprout collaterals and innervate additional territory, which is reflected at the cortical level (examined 12 weeks after lesion and enzyme treatment). Thus, augmentation in this way produces expanded representations of the spared inputs from digits 1 and 2 in cortex, and possibly enhances ability of axons of second-order spinal cord neurons to sprout and innervate islands of the deprived cuneate nucleus. Abbreviations: 1–5, digits 1–5; 1, 3a and 3b, areas 1, 3a and 3b; a, anterior; C5–6, cervical spinal cord segments 5–6; chABC, chondroitinase ABC; DCL, dorsal column lesion; l, lateral; m, medial; p, posterior. Based on Jain et al. (1997), Bowes et al. (2012), and Qi et al. (2014).

lesions of the dorsal column that extend into the lateral fiber tracts appear to reduce the extent of the reactivation of the hand cortex from inputs from the hand.

Given the evidence that the reactivation of the cortex by inputs from the hand is important for the recovery of manual dexterity, what can be done to promote these reactivations? Recently, we have investigated two interventions for promoting reactivations. First, we found promising evidence that behavioral training after sensory loss improved the recovery of hand use in a retrieval task and correlated with cortical reorganization [Qi et al., 2010, 2012 (abstracts)]. Second, we found that an injection of an enzyme, chondroitinase ABC, into the cuneate nucleus after the lesion of the dorsal columns promotes the reactivation of hand cortex by preserved dorsal column afferents (Bowes et al., 2012). This enzyme digests chondroitin sulphate proteoglycans, which make up the extracellular matrix around neurons and glia. Treatment with chondroitinase ABC was first shown to promote recovery after spinal cord injury in rats by Bradbury et al. (2002). The extracellular matrix around neurons in the cuneate nucleus provide a chemical and physiological barrier that appears to inhibit new axon growth into and within the nucleus, thereby limiting the reactivation of deprived neurons in the nucleus, and the relay of driven activity to higher levels of the somatosensory system. By intentionally sparing dorsal column afferents from the thumb (digit 1) in squirrel monkeys by placing the dorsal column lesion at a lower cervical level (C6), and using the chondroitinase ABC enzyme injections near the targets for new growth from the spinal cord into the brainstem, more of the hand representation in contralateral somatosensory cortex was activated than in monkeys without this injection (**Figure 6**). Chondroitinase ABC has been used by others in a number of different experiments to increase axon sprouting, including the growth of dorsal column axons past a lesion site in rats (Massey et al., 2006, see reviews by Onifer et al., 2011; Garcia-Alias and Fawcett, 2012). Other promising treatments for recovery after sensory loss or spinal cord injury include the use of antibodies to a major myelin-associated neurite growth inhibitor, named Nogo-A (see Fawcett et al., 2012). The local placement of factors that promote growth and provide attraction to a target may also be useful (Schnell et al., 1994). Additional treatments for spinal cord injury have been reviewed by others (He and Koprivica, 2004; Buchli and Schwab, 2005; Bradbury and McMahon, 2006; Cafferty et al., 2008; Giger et al., 2010; Cregg et al., 2014; Silva et al., 2014). Sensorimotor training and testing for use of the impaired hand in monkeys (Qi et al., 2013, 2014) or impaired limbs in rodent (Kao et al., 2009; Krajacic et al., 2010; Graziano et al., 2013), appears to promote functional recovery and reactivation of cortex, but further study is needed to determine how effective behavioral intervention is beyond spontaneous recoveries or in relation to pharmacological treatments such as chondroitinase ABC. Combining pharmacological and behavioral interventions may promote even more useful recoveries in primates, as promising results have been reported in rodent models (Tetzlaff et al., 2009; Garcia-Alias and Fawcett, 2012; Zhao et al., 2013). In conclusion, we stress that much progress has been made over the last several years in understanding the recovery process that occurs after sensory loss following dorsal column injury. Much of this plasticity was unexpected, but the spontaneous recovery accounts for the early misinterpretations that the dorsal column pathway has little sensory significance. In addition to the unexpected spontaneous recovery, there are also hopeful signs that various therapeutic treatments have the potential of greatly improving the course of recovery.

AUTHOR CONTRIBUTIONS

All authors contributed to the writing of the manuscript. The findings reviewed are those of the authors, as well as those of other investigators.

ACKNOWLEDGMENTS

Our research was supported by NIH grants NS057399 and NS067017 to Hui-Xin Qi; NIH grant NS16446 to Jon H. Kaas, and awards from the Christopher and Dana Reeve Foundation to Jamie L. Reed and to Jon H. Kaas.

REFERENCES

Aguilar, J., Humanes-Valera, D., Alonso-Calvino, E., Yague, J. G., Moxon, K. A., Oliviero, A., et al. (2010). Spinal cord injury immediately changes the state of the brain. *J. Neurosci.* 30, 7528–7537. doi: 10.1523/JNEUROSCI.0379-10.2010

Anderson, K. D., Gunawan, A., and Steward, O. (2005). Quantitative assessment of forelimb motor function after cervical spinal cord injury in rats: relationship to the corticospinal tract. *Exp. Neurol.* 194, 161–174. doi: 10.1016/j.expneurol.2005.02.006

Azulay, A., and Schwartz, A. S. (1975). The role of the dorsal funiculus of the primate in tactile discrimination. *Exp. Neurol.* 46, 315–332. doi: 10.1016/0014-4886(75)90138-7

Ballermann, M., McKenna, J., and Whishaw, I. Q. (2001). A grasp-related deficit in tactile discrimination following dorsal column lesion in the rat. *Brain Res. Bull.* 54, 237–242. doi: 10.1016/S0361-9230(01)00431-2

Beck, C. (1976). Forelimb performance by squirrel monkeys (Saimiri sciureus) before and after dorsal column lesions. *J. Comp. Physiol. Psychol.* 90, 353–362. doi: 10.1037/h0077206

Bennett, G. J., Seltzer, Z., Lu, G. W., Nishikawa, N., and Dubner, R. (1983). The cells of origin of the dorsal column postsynaptic projection in the lumbosacral enlargements of cats and monkeys. *Somatosens Res.* 1, 131–149. doi: 10.3109/07367228309144545

Bowes, C., Burish, M., Cerkevich, C., and Kaas, J. (2013). Patterns of cortical reorganization in the adult marmoset after a cervical spinal cord injury. *J. Comp. Neurol.* 521, 3451–3463. doi: 10.1002/cne.23360

Bowes, C., Massey, J. M., Burish, M., Cerkevich, C. M., and Kaas, J. H. (2012). Chondroitinase ABC promotes selective reactivation of somatosensory cortex in squirrel monkeys after a cervical dorsal column lesion. *Proc. Natl. Acad. Sci. U.S.A.* 109, 2595–2600. doi: 10.1073/pnas.1121604109

Bradbury, E. J., and McMahon, S. B. (2006). Spinal cord repair strategies: why do they work? *Nat. Rev. Neurosci.* 7, 644–653. doi: 10.1038/nrn1964

Bradbury, E. J., Moon, L. D., Popat, R. J., King, V. R., Bennett, G. S., Patel, P. N., et al. (2002). Chondroitinase ABC promotes functional recovery after spinal cord injury. *Nature* 416, 636–640. doi: 10.1038/416636a

Brugger, P., Kollias, S. S., Muri, R. M., Crelier, G., Hepp-Reymond, M. C., and Regard, M. (2000). Beyond re-membering: phantom sensations of congenitally absent limbs. *Proc. Natl. Acad. Sci. U.S.A.* 97, 6167–6172. doi: 10.1073/pnas.100510697

Buchli, A. D., and Schwab, M. E. (2005). Inhibition of Nogo: a key strategy to increase regeneration, plasticity and functional recovery of the lesioned central nervous system. *Ann. Med.* 37, 556–567. doi: 10.1080/07853890500407520

Buonomano, D. V., and Merzenich, M. M. (1998). Cortical plasticity: from synapses to maps. *Annu. Rev. Neurosci.* 21, 149–186. doi: 10.1146/annurev.neuro.21.1.149

Burton, H., Sathian, K., and Shao, D. H. (1990). Altered responses to cutaneous stimuli in the second somatosensory cortex following lesions of the postcentral gyrus in infant and juvenile macaques. *J. Comp. Neurol.* 291, 395–414. doi: 10.1002/cne.902910307

Cafferty, W. B., McGee, A. W., and Strittmatter, S. M. (2008). Axonal growth therapeutics: regeneration or sprouting or plasticity? *Trends Neurosci.* 31, 215–220. doi: 10.1016/j.tins.2008.02.004

Calford, M. B., and Tweedale, R. (1988). Immediate and chronic changes in responses of somatosensory cortex in adult flying-fox after digit amputation. *Nature* 332, 446–448. doi: 10.1038/332446a0

Cheetham, C. E., Hammond, M. S., McFarlane, R., and Finnerty, G. T. (2008). Altered sensory experience induces targeted rewiring of local excitatory connections in mature neocortex. *J. Neurosci.* 28, 9249–9260. doi: 10.1523/JNEUROSCI.2974-08.2008

Chen, L. M., Qi, H. X., and Kaas, J. H. (2012). Dynamic reorganization of digit representations in somatosensory cortex of nonhuman primates after spinal cord injury. *J. Neurosci.* 32, 14649–14663. doi: 10.1523/JNEUROSCI.1841-12.2012

Chino, Y., Smith, E. L. 3rd., Zhang, B., Matsuura, K., Mori, T., and Kaas, J. H. (2001). Recovery of binocular responses by cortical neurons after early monocular lesions. *Nat. Neurosci.* 4, 689–690. doi: 10.1038/89469

Chino, Y. M., Smith, E. L. 3rd., Kaas, J. H., Sasaki, Y., and Cheng, H. (1995). Receptive-field properties of deafferentated visual cortical neurons after topographic map reorganization in adult cats. *J. Neurosci.* 15, 2417–2433.

Cooper, B. Y., Glendinning, D. S., and Vierck, C. J. Jr. (1993). Finger movement deficits in the stumptail macaque following lesions of the fasciculus cuneatus. *Somatosens Mot. Res.* 10, 17–29. doi: 10.3109/08990229309028820

Courtine, G., Song, B., Roy, R. R., Zhong, H., Herrmann, J. E., Ao, Y., et al. (2008). Recovery of supraspinal control of stepping via indirect propriospinal relay connections after spinal cord injury. *Nat. Med.* 14, 69–74. doi: 10.1038/nm1682

Cregg, J. M., Depaul, M. A., Filous, A. R., Lang, B. T., Tran, A., and Silver, J. (2014). Functional regeneration beyond the glial scar. *Exp. Neurol.* 253C, 197–207. doi: 10.1016/j.expneurol.2013.12.024

Crockett, D. P., Maslany, S., Harris, S. L., and Egger, M. D. (1993). Enhanced cytochrome-oxidase staining of the cuneate nucleus in the rat reveals a modifiable somatotopic map. *Brain Res.* 612, 41–55. doi: 10.1016/0006-8993(93)91642-6

Curt, A., Alkadhi, H., Crelier, G. R., Boendermaker, S. H., Hepp-Reymond, M. C., and Kollias, S. S. (2002). Changes of non-affected upper limb cortical representation in paraplegic patients as assessed by fMRI. *Brain* 125, 2567–2578. doi: 10.1093/brain/awf250

Cusick, C. G., and Gould, H. J. 3rd. (1990). Connections between area 3b of the somatosensory cortex and subdivisions of the ventroposterior nuclear complex and the anterior pulvinar nucleus in squirrel monkeys. *J. Comp. Neurol.* 292, 83–102. doi: 10.1002/cne.902920106

D'Amato, C. J., and Hicks, S. P. (1978). Normal development and post-traumatic plasticity of corticospinal neurons in rats. *Exp. Neurol.* 60, 557–569. doi: 10.1016/0014-4886(78)90010-9

Darian-Smith, C. (2004). Primary afferent terminal sprouting after a cervical dorsal rootlet section in the macaque monkey. *J. Comp. Neurol.* 470, 134–150. doi: 10.1002/cne.11030

Darian-Smith, C. (2009). Synaptic plasticity, neurogenesis, and functional recovery after spinal cord injury. *Neuroscientist* 15, 149–165. doi: 10.1177/1073858408331372

Darian-Smith, C., and Brown, S. (2000). Functional changes at periphery and cortex following dorsal root lesions in adult monkeys. *Nat. Neurosci.* 3, 476–481. doi: 10.1038/74852

Darian-Smith, C., and Ciferri, M. (2006). Cuneate nucleus reorganization following cervical dorsal rhizotomy in the macaque monkey: its role in the recovery of manual dexterity. *J. Comp. Neurol.* 498, 552–565. doi: 10.1002/cne.21088

Darian-Smith, C., and Ciferri, M. M. (2005). Loss and recovery of voluntary hand movements in the macaque following a cervical dorsal rhizotomy. *J. Comp. Neurol.* 491, 27–45. doi: 10.1002/cne.20686

Darian-Smith, C., and Gilbert, C. D. (1994). Axonal sprouting accompanies functional reorganization in adult cat striate cortex. *Nature* 368, 737–740. doi: 10.1038/368737a0

Darian-Smith, C., and Gilbert, C. D. (1995). Topographic reorganization in the striate cortex of the adult cat and monkey is cortically mediated. *J. Neurosci.* 15, 1631–1647.

Darian-Smith, C., Hopkins, S., and Ralston, H. J. 3rd. (2010). Changes in synaptic populations in the spinal dorsal horn following a dorsal rhizotomy in the monkey. *J. Comp. Neurol.* 518, 103–117. doi: 10.1002/cne.22216

Davis, K. D., Kiss, Z. H., Luo, L., Tasker, R. R., Lozano, A. M., and Dostrovsky, J. O. (1998). Phantom sensations generated by thalamic microstimulation. *Nature* 391, 385–387. doi: 10.1038/34905

Disbrow, E., Litinas, E., Recanzone, G. H., Padberg, J., and Krubitzer, L. (2003). Cortical connections of the second somatosensory area and the parietal ventral area in macaque monkeys. *J. Comp. Neurol.* 462, 382–399. doi: 10.1002/cne.10731

Doetsch, G. S., Harrison, T. A., Macdonald, A. C., and Litaker, M. S. (1996). Short-term plasticity in primary somatosensory cortex of the rat: rapid changes in magnitudes and latencies of neuronal responses following digit denervation. *Exp. Brain Res.* 112, 505–512. doi: 10.1007/BF00227956

Dutta, A., Kambi, N., Raghunathan, P., Khushu, S., and Jain, N. (2013). Large-scale reorganization of the somatosensory cortex of adult macaque monkeys revealed by fMRI. *Brain Struct. Funct.* doi: 10.1007/s00429-013-0569-8. [Epub ahead of print].

Dykes, R. W., and Craig, A. D. (1998). Control of size and excitability of mechanosensory receptive fields in dorsal column nuclei by homolateral dorsal horn neurons. *J. Neurophysiol.* 80, 120–129.

Elbert, T., Sterr, A., Flor, H., Rockstroh, B., Knecht, S., Pantev, C., et al. (1997). Input-increase and input-decrease types of cortical reorganization after upper extremity amputation in humans. *Exp. Brain Res.* 117, 161–164. doi: 10.1007/s002210050210

Faggin, B. M., Nguyen, K. T., and Nicolelis, M. A. (1997). Immediate and simultaneous sensory reorganization at cortical and subcortical levels of the somatosensory system. *Proc. Natl. Acad. Sci. U.S.A.* 94, 9428–9433. doi: 10.1073/pnas.94.17.9428

Fang, P. C., Stepniewska, I., and Kaas, J. H. (2005). Ipsilateral cortical connections of motor, premotor, frontal eye, and posterior parietal fields in a prosimian primate, Otolemur garnetti. *J. Comp. Neurol.* 490, 305–333. doi: 10.1002/cne.20665

Fawcett, J. W., Schwab, M. E., Montani, L., Brazda, N., and Muller, H. W. (2012). Defeating inhibition of regeneration by scar and myelin components. *Handb. Clin. Neurol.* 109, 503–522. doi: 10.1016/B978-0-444-52137-8.00031-0

Flor, H., Elbert, T., Knecht, S., Wienbruch, C., Pantev, C., Birbaumer, N., et al. (1995). Phantom-limb pain as a perceptual correlate of cortical reorganization following arm amputation. *Nature* 375, 482–484. doi: 10.1038/375482a0

Flor, H., Elbert, T., Muhlnickel, W., Pantev, C., Wienbruch, C., and Taub, E. (1998). Cortical reorganization and phantom phenomena in congenital and traumatic upper-extremity amputees. *Exp. Brain Res.* 119, 205–212. doi: 10.1007/s002210050334

Florence, S. L., Hackett, T. A., and Strata, F. (2000). Thalamic and cortical contributions to neural plasticity after limb amputation. *J. Neurophysiol.* 83, 3154–3159.

Florence, S. L., and Kaas, J. H. (1995). Large-scale reorganization at multiple levels of the somatosensory pathway follows therapeutic amputation of the hand in monkeys. *J. Neurosci.* 15, 8083–8095.

Florence, S. L., Taub, H. B., and Kaas, J. H. (1998). Large-scale sprouting of cortical connections after peripheral injury in adult macaque monkeys. *Science* 282, 1117–1121. doi: 10.1126/science.282.5391.1117

Garcia-Alias, G., and Fawcett, J. W. (2012). Training and anti-CSPG combination therapy for spinal cord injury. *Exp. Neurol.* 235, 26–32. doi: 10.1016/j.expneurol.2011.09.009

Garraghty, P. E., Arnold, L. L., Wellman, C. L., and Mowery, T. M. (2006). Receptor autoradiographic correlates of deafferentation-induced reorganization in adult primate somatosensory cortex. *J. Comp. Neurol.* 497, 636–645. doi: 10.1002/cne.21018

Garraghty, P. E., Florence, S. L., and Kaas, J. H. (1990a). Ablations of areas 3a and 3b of monkey somatosensory cortex abolish cutaneous responsivity in area 1. *Brain Res.* 528, 165–169. doi: 10.1016/0006-8993(90)90213-U

Garraghty, P. E., Lachica, E. A., and Kaas, J. H. (1991). Injury-induced reorganization of somatosensory cortex is accompanied by reductions in GABA staining. *Somatosens Mot. Res.* 8, 347–354. doi: 10.3109/08990229109144757

Garraghty, P. E., Pons, T. P., and Kaas, J. H. (1990b). Ablations of areas 3b (SI proper) and 3a of somatosensory cortex in marmosets deactivate the second and parietal ventral somatosensory areas. *Somatosens Mot. Res.* 7, 125–135. doi: 10.3109/08990229009144703

Ghosh, A., Sydekum, E., Haiss, F., Peduzzi, S., Zorner, B., Schneider, R., et al. (2009). Functional and anatomical reorganization of the sensory-motor cortex after incomplete spinal cord injury in adult rats. *J. Neurosci.* 29, 12210–12219. doi: 10.1523/JNEUROSCI.1828-09.2009

Giger, R. J., Hollis, E. R. 2nd., and Tuszynski, M. H. (2010). Guidance molecules in axon regeneration. *Cold Spring Harb. Perspect. Biol.* 2, a001867. doi: 10.1101/cshperspect.a001867

Glendinning, D. S., Cooper, B. Y., Vierck, C. J. Jr., and Leonard, C. M. (1992). Altered precision grasping in stumptail macaques after fasciculus cuneatus lesions. *Somatosens Mot. Res.* 9, 61–73. doi: 10.3109/08990229209144763

Graziano, A., Foffani, G., Knudsen, E. B., Shumsky, J., and Moxon, K. A. (2013). Passive exercise of the hind limbs after complete thoracic transection of the spinal cord promotes cortical reorganization. *PLoS ONE* 8:e54350. doi: 10.1371/journal.pone.0054350

Graziano, A., and Jones, E. G. (2009). Early withdrawal of axons from higher centers in response to peripheral somatosensory denervation. *J. Neurosci.* 29, 3738–3748. doi: 10.1523/JNEUROSCI.5388-08.2009

He, Z., and Koprivica, V. (2004). The Nogo signaling pathway for regeneration block. *Annu. Rev. Neurosci.* 27, 341–368. doi: 10.1146/annurev.neuro.27.070203.144340

Hickmott, P. W., and Steen, P. A. (2005). Large-scale changes in dendritic structure during reorganization of adult somatosensory cortex. *Nat. Neurosci.* 8, 140–142. doi: 10.1038/nn1384

Hicks, S. P., and D'Amato, C. J. (1975). Motor-sensory cortex-corticospinal system and developing locomotion and placing in rats. *Am. J. Anat.* 143, 1–42. doi: 10.1002/aja.1001430102

Humanes-Valera, D., Aguilar, J., and Foffani, G. (2013). Reorganization of the intact somatosensory cortex immediately after spinal cord injury. *PLoS ONE* 8:e69655. doi: 10.1371/journal.pone.0069655

Jain, N., Catania, K. C., and Kaas, J. H. (1997). Deactivation and reactivation of somatosensory cortex after dorsal spinal cord injury. *Nature* 386, 495–498. doi: 10.1038/386495a0

Jain, N., Catania, K. C., and Kaas, J. H. (1998). A histologically visible representation of the fingers and palm in primate area 3b and its immutability following long-term deafferentations. *Cereb. Cortex* 8, 227–236. doi: 10.1093/cercor/8.3.227

Jain, N., Florence, S. L., Qi, H. X., and Kaas, J. H. (2000). Growth of new brainstem connections in adult monkeys with massive sensory loss. *Proc. Natl. Acad. Sci. U.S.A.* 97, 5546–5550. doi: 10.1073/pnas.090572597

Jain, N., Qi, H. X., Catania, K. C., and Kaas, J. H. (2001). Anatomic correlates of the face and oral cavity representations in the somatosensory cortical area 3b of monkeys. *J. Comp. Neurol.* 429, 455–468. doi: 10.1002/1096-9861(20010115)429:3%3C455::AID-CNE7%3E3.0.CO;2-F

Jain, N., Qi, H. X., Collins, C. E., and Kaas, J. H. (2008). Large-scale reorganization in the somatosensory cortex and thalamus after sensory loss in macaque monkeys. *J. Neurosci.* 28, 11042–11060. doi: 10.1523/JNEUROSCI.2334-08.2008

Jones, E. G. (2000). Cortical and subcortical contributions to activity-dependent plasticity in primate somatosensory cortex. *Annu. Rev. Neurosci.* 23, 1–37. doi: 10.1146/annurev.neuro.23.1.1

Jones, E. G., Friedman, D. P., and Hendry, S. H. (1982). Thalamic basis of place- and modality-specific columns in monkey somatosensory cortex: a correlative anatomical and physiological study. *J. Neurophysiol.* 48, 545–568.

Jones, E. G., and Pons, T. P. (1998). Thalamic and brainstem contributions to large-scale plasticity of primate somatosensory cortex. *Science* 282, 1121–1125. doi: 10.1126/science.282.5391.1121

Kaas, J. H. (2012). "Somatosensory system," in *The Human Nervous System*. 3rd Edn, eds J. K. Mai and G. Paxinos. (London: ElsevierAcademic Press), 1064–1099.

Kaas, J. H., Nelson, R. J., Sur, M., Dykes, R. W., and Merzenich, M. M. (1984). The somatotopic organization of the ventroposterior thalamus of the squirrel monkey, Saimiri sciureus. *J. Comp. Neurol.* 226, 111–140. doi: 10.1002/cne.902260109

Kaas, J. H., Nelson, R. J., Sur, M., Lin, C. S., and Merzenich, M. M. (1979). Multiple representations of the body within the primary somatosensory cortex of primates. *Science* 204, 521–523. doi: 10.1126/science.107591

Kaas, J. H., Qi, H. X., Burish, M. J., Gharbawie, O. A., Onifer, S. M., and Massey, J. M. (2008). Cortical and subcortical plasticity in the brains of humans, primates, and rats after damage to sensory afferents in the dorsal columns of the spinal cord. *Exp. Neurol.* 209, 407–416. doi: 10.1016/j.expneurol.2007.06.014

Kaas, J. H., Qi, H. X., and Iyengar, S. (2006). Cortical network for representing the teeth and tongue in primates. *Anat. Rec. A Discov. Mol. Cell Evol. Biol.* 288, 182–190. doi: 10.1002/ar.a.20267

Kambi, N., Tandon, S., Mohammed, H., Lazar, L., and Jain, N. (2011). Reorganization of the primary motor cortex of adult macaque monkeys after sensory loss resulting from partial spinal cord injuries. *J. Neurosci.* 31, 3696–3707. doi: 10.1523/JNEUROSCI.5187-10.2011

Kao, T., Shumsky, J. S., Murray, M., and Moxon, K. A. (2009). Exercise induces cortical plasticity after neonatal spinal cord injury in the rat. *J. Neurosci.* 29, 7549–7557. doi: 10.1523/JNEUROSCI.2474-08.2009

Kelahan, A. M., and Doetsch, G. S. (1984). Time-dependent changes in the functional organization of somatosensory cerebral cortex following digit amputation in adult raccoons. *Somatosens Res.* 2, 49–81.

Krajacic, A., Weishaupt, N., Girgis, J., Tetzlaff, W., and Fouad, K. (2010). Training-induced plasticity in rats with cervical spinal cord injury: effects and side effects. *Behav. Brain Res.* 214, 323–331. doi: 10.1016/j.bbr.2010.05.053

Krubitzer, L. A., and Kaas, J. H. (1990). The organization and connections of somatosensory cortex in marmosets. *J. Neurosci.* 10, 952–974.

Krupa, D. J., Ghazanfar, A. A., and Nicolelis, M. A. (1999). Immediate thalamic sensory plasticity depends on corticothalamic feedback. *Proc. Natl. Acad. Sci. U.S.A.* 96, 8200–8205. doi: 10.1073/pnas.96.14.8200

Leonard, C. M., Glendinning, D. S., Wilfong, T., Cooper, B. Y., and Vierck, C. J. Jr. (1992). Alterations of natural hand movements after interruption of fasciculus cuneatus in the macaque. *Somatosens Mot. Res.* 9, 75–89. doi: 10.3109/08990229209144764

Li, C. X., Yang, Q., Vemulapalli, S., and Waters, R. S. (2013). Forelimb amputation-induced reorganization in the cuneate nucleus (CN) is not reflected in large-scale reorganization in rat forepaw barrel subfield cortex (FBS). *Brain Res.* 1526, 26–43. doi: 10.1016/j.brainres.2013.05.049

Liao, C. C., Gharbawie, O. A., Qi, H., and Kaas, J. H. (2013). Cortical connections to single digit representations in area 3b of somatosensory cortex in squirrel monkeys and prosimian galagos. *J. Comp. Neurol.* 521, 3768–3790. doi: 10.1002/cne.23377

Lotze, M., Grodd, W., Birbaumer, N., Erb, M., Huse, E., and Flor, H. (1999). Does use of a myoelectric prosthesis prevent cortical reorganization and phantom limb pain? *Nat. Neurosci.* 2, 501–502. doi: 10.1038/9145

Marik, S. A., Yamahachi, H., McManus, J. N., Szabo, G., and Gilbert, C. D. (2010). Axonal dynamics of excitatory and inhibitory neurons in somatosensory cortex. *PLoS Biol.* 8:e1000395. doi: 10.1371/journal.pbio.1000395

Marik, S. A., Yamahachi, H., Meyer Zum Alten Borgloh, S., and Gilbert, C. D. (2014). Large-Scale Axonal Reorganization of Inhibitory Neurons following Retinal Lesions. *J. Neurosci.* 34, 1625–1632. doi: 10.1523/JNEUROSCI.4345-13.2014.

Massey, J. M., Hubscher, C. H., Wagoner, M. R., Decker, J. A., Amps, J., Silver, J., et al. (2006). Chondroitinase ABC digestion of the perineuronal net promotes functional collateral sprouting in the cuneate nucleus after cervical spinal cord injury. *J. Neurosci.* 26, 4406–4414. doi: 10.1523/JNEUROSCI.5467-05.2006

McKenna, J. E., and Whishaw, I. Q. (1999). Complete compensation in skilled reaching success with associated impairments in limb synergies, after dorsal column lesion in the rat. *J. Neurosci.* 19, 1885–1894.

Merzenich, M. M., Kaas, J. H., Sur, M., and Lin, C. S. (1978). Double representation of the body surface within cytoarchitectonic areas 3b and 1 in "SI" in the owl monkey (*Aotus trivirgatus*). *J. Comp. Neurol.* 181, 41–73. doi: 10.1002/cne.901810104

Merzenich, M. M., Kaas, J. H., Wall, J., Nelson, R. J., Sur, M., and Felleman, D. (1983a). Topographic reorganization of somatosensory cortical areas 3b and 1 in adult monkeys following restricted deafferentation. *Neuroscience* 8, 33–55. doi: 10.1016/0306-4522(83)90024-6

Merzenich, M. M., Kaas, J. H., Wall, J. T., Sur, M., Nelson, R. J., and Felleman, D. J. (1983b). Progression of change following median nerve section in the cortical representation of the hand in areas 3b and 1 in adult owl and squirrel monkeys. *Neuroscience* 10, 639–665. doi: 10.1016/0306-4522(83)90208-7

Moore, C. I., Stern, C. E., Dunbar, C., Kostyk, S. K., Gehi, A., and Corkin, S. (2000). Referred phantom sensations and cortical reorganization after spinal cord injury in humans. *Proc. Natl. Acad. Sci. U.S.A.* 97, 14703–14708. doi: 10.1073/pnas.250348997

Mountcastle, V. B., and Darian-Smith, I. (1968). "Neural mechanisms in somesthesia," in *Medical Physiology,* ed V. B. Mountcastle (St. Louis, MO: C. V. Mosby), 1372–1423.

Nathan, P. W., Smith, M. C., and Cook, A. W. (1986). Sensory effects in man of lesions of the posterior columns and of some other afferent pathways. *Brain* 109(Pt. 5), 1003–1041.

Nelson, R. J., and Kaas, J. H. (1981). Connections of the ventroposterior nucleus of the thalamus with the body surface representations in cortical areas 3b and 1 of the cynomolgus macaque, (*Macaca fascicularis*). *J. Comp. Neurol.* 199, 29–64. doi: 10.1002/cne.901990104

Nelson, R. J., Sur, M., Felleman, D. J., and Kaas, J. H. (1980). Representations of the body surface in postcentral parietal cortex of Macaca fascicularis. *J. Comp. Neurol.* 192, 611–643. doi: 10.1002/cne.901920402

Nout, Y. S., Ferguson, A. R., Strand, S. C., Moseanko, R., Hawbecker, S., Zdunowski, S., et al. (2012b). Methods for functional assessment after C7 spinal cord hemisection in the rhesus monkey. *Neurorehabil. Neural Repair* 26, 556–569. doi: 10.1177/1545968311421934

Nout, Y. S., Rosenzweig, E. S., Brock, J. H., Strand, S. C., Moseanko, R., Hawbecker, S., et al. (2012a). Animal models of neurologic disorders: a nonhuman primate model of spinal cord injury. *Neurotherapeutics* 9, 380–392. doi: 10.1007/s13311-012-0114-0

Onifer, S. M., Smith, G. M., and Fouad, K. (2011). Plasticity after spinal cord injury: relevance to recovery and approaches to facilitate it. *Neurotherapeutics* 8, 283–293. doi: 10.1007/s13311-011-0034-4

Paxino, G., and Watson, C. (2007). *The Rat Brain in Stereotaxic Coordinates.* Amsterdam: Elsevier.

Pei, Y. C., Denchev, P. V., Hsiao, S. S., Craig, J. C., and Bensmaia, S. J. (2009). Convergence of submodality-specific input onto neurons in primary somatosensory cortex. *J. Neurophysiol.* 102, 1843–1853. doi: 10.1152/jn.00235.2009

Perl, E. R., Whitlock, D. G., and Gentry, J. R. (1962). Cutaneous projection to second-order neurons of the dorsal column system. *J. Neurophysiol.* 25, 337–358.

Pons, T. P., Garraghty, P. E., Friedman, D. P., and Mishkin, M. (1987). Physiological evidence for serial processing in somatosensory cortex. *Science* 237, 417–420. doi: 10.1126/science.3603028

Pons, T. P., Garraghty, P. E., and Mishkin, M. (1992). Serial and parallel processing of tactual information in somatosensory cortex of rhesus monkeys. *J. Neurophysiol.* 68, 518–527.

Pons, T. P., Garraghty, P. E., Ommaya, A. K., Kaas, J. H., Taub, E., and Mishkin, M. (1991). Massive cortical reorganization after sensory deafferentation in adult macaques. *Science* 252, 1857–1860. doi: 10.1126/science.1843843

Qi, H. X., Chen, L. M., and Kaas, J. H. (2011a). Reorganization of somatosensory cortical areas 3b and 1 after unilateral section of dorsal columns of the spinal cord in squirrel monkeys. *J. Neurosci.* 31, 13662–13675. doi: 10.1523/JNEUROSCI.2366-11.2011

Qi, H. X., Gharbawie, O. A., Wong, P., and Kaas, J. H. (2011b). Cell-poor septa separate representations of digits in the ventroposterior nucleus of the thalamus in monkeys and prosimian galagos. *J. Comp. Neurol.* 519, 738–758. doi: 10.1002/cne.22545

Qi, H. X., Gharbawie, O. A., Wynne, K. W., and Kaas, J. H. (2013). Impairment and recovery of hand use after unilateral section of the dorsal columns of the spinal cord in squirrel monkeys. *Behav. Brain Res.* 252, 363–376. doi: 10.1016/j.bbr.2013.05.058

Qi, H. X., Jain, N., Collins, C. E., Lyon, D. C., and Kaas, J. H. (2010). Functional organization of motor cortex of adult macaque monkeys is altered by sensory loss in infancy. *Proc. Natl. Acad. Sci. U.S.A.* 107, 3192–3197. doi: 10.1073/pnas.0914962107

Qi, H. X., and Kaas, J. H. (2004). Myelin stains reveal an anatomical framework for the representation of the digits in somatosensory area 3b of macaque monkeys. *J. Comp. Neurol.* 477, 172–187. doi: 10.1002/cne.20247

Qi, H. X., Reed, J. L., Bui, T., Chen, L. M., and Kaas, J. H. (2012). Longitudinal fMRI and behavioral recovery after sensory loss from the hand of adult monkeys. *Fed. Euro. Neurosci. Soc. Forum Abstr.* A-471-0142-02394.

Qi, H. X., Reed, J. L., Gharbawie, O. A., Burish, M. J., and Kaas, J. H. (2014). Cortical neuron response properties are related to lesion extent and behavioral recovery after sensory loss from spinal cord injury in monkeys. *J. Neurosci.* 34, 4345–4363. doi: 10.1523/JNEUROSCI.4954-13.2014

Ramachandran, V. S. (1993). Behavioral and magnetoencephalographic correlates of plasticity in the adult human brain. *Proc. Natl. Acad. Sci. U.S.A.* 90, 10413–10420. doi: 10.1073/pnas.90.22.10413

Ramachandran, V. S., and Rogers-Ramachandran, D. (2000). Phantom limbs and neural plasticity. *Arch. Neurol.* 57, 317–320. doi: 10.1001/archneur.57.3.317

Rasmusson, D. D. (1996). Changes in the response properties of neurons in the ventroposterior lateral thalamic nucleus of the raccoon after peripheral deafferentation. *J. Neurophysiol.* 75, 2441–2450.

Rasmusson, D. D., and Northgrave, S. A. (1997). Reorganization of the raccoon cuneate nucleus after peripheral denervation. *J. Neurophysiol.* 78, 2924–2936.

Reed, J. L., Qi, H. X., and Kaas, J. H. (2012). Ipsilateral responses and interhemispheric interactions in area 3b after dorsal column spinal cord injury in New World monkeys. *Soc. Neurosci. Abstr.* 42.

Reed, J. L., Qi, H. X., Zhou, Z., Bernard, M. R., Burish, M. J., Bonds, A. B., et al. (2010). Response properties of neurons in primary somatosensory cortex of owl monkeys reflect widespread spatiotemporal integration. *J. Neurophysiol.* 103, 2139–2157. doi: 10.1152/jn.00709.2009

Rose, J. E., and Mountcastle, V. B. (1959). "Touch and kinesthesis," in *Handbook of Physilogy,* ed H. W. Magoun (Washington, DC: American Physiology Society), 387–429.

Rustioni, A., Hayes, N. L., and O'Neill, S. (1979). Dorsal column nuclei and ascending spinal afferents in macaques. *Brain* 102, 95–125. doi: 10.1093/brain/102.1.95

Schmidlin, E., Kaeser, M., Gindrat, A. D., Savidan, J., Chatagny, P., Badoud, S., et al. (2011). Behavioral assessment of manual dexterity in non-human primates. *J. Vis. Exp.* 57, 3258–3270. doi: 10.3791/3258

Schnell, L., Schneider, R., Kolbeck, R., Barde, Y. A., and Schwab, M. E. (1994). Neurotrophin-3 enhances sprouting of corticospinal tract during development and after adult spinal cord lesion. *Nature* 367, 170–173. doi: 10.1038/367170a0

Sengelaub, D. R., Muja, N., Mills, A. C., Myers, W. A., Churchill, J. D., and Garraghty, P. E. (1997). Denervation-induced sprouting of intact peripheral afferents into the cuneate nucleus of adult rats. *Brain Res.* 769, 256–262. doi: 10.1016/S0006-8993(97)00708-7

Silva, A. C., Rasey, S. K., Wu, X., and Wall, J. T. (1996). Initial cortical reactions to injury of the median and radial nerves to the hands of adult primates. *J. Comp. Neurol.* 366, 700–716. doi: 10.1002/(SICI)1096-9861(19960318)366:4<700::AID-CNE9>3.0.CO;2-8

Silva, N. A., Sousa, N., Reis, R. L., and Salgado, A. J. (2014). From basics to clinical: a comprehensive review on spinal cord injury. *Prog. Neurobiol.* 114, 25–57. doi: 10.1016/j.pneurobio.2013.11.002

Stepniewska, I., Preuss, T. M., and Kaas, J. H. (1993). Architectonics, somatotopic organization, and ipsilateral cortical connections of the primary motor area (M1) of owl monkeys. *J. Comp. Neurol.* 330, 238–271. doi: 10.1002/cne.903300207

Sur, M., Nelson, R. J., and Kaas, J. H. (1982). Representations of the body surface in cortical areas 3b and 1 of squirrel monkeys: comparisons with other primates. *J. Comp. Neurol.* 211, 177–192. doi: 10.1002/cne.902110207

Sur, M., Wall, J. T., and Kaas, J. H. (1984). Modular distribution of neurons with slowly adapting and rapidly adapting responses in area 3b of somatosensory cortex in monkeys. *J. Neurophysiol.* 51, 724–744.

Tandon, S., Kambi, N., Lazar, L., Mohammed, H., and Jain, N. (2009). Large-scale expansion of the face representation in somatosensory areas of the lateral sulcus after spinal cord injuries in monkeys. *J. Neurosci.* 29, 12009–12019. doi: 10.1523/JNEUROSCI.2118-09.2009

Tetzlaff, W., Fouad, K., and Kwon, B. (2009). Be careful what you train for. *Nat. Neurosci.* 12, 1077–1079. doi: 10.1038/nn0909-1077

Tommerdahl, M., Whitsel, B. L., Vierck, C. J. Jr., Favorov, O., Juliano, S., Cooper, B., et al. (1996). Effects of spinal dorsal column transection on the response of monkey anterior parietal cortex to repetitive skin stimulation. *Cereb. Cortex* 6, 131–155. doi: 10.1093/cercor/6.2.131

Turrigiano, G. G. (1999). Homeostatic plasticity in neuronal networks: the more things change, the more they stay the same. *Trends Neurosci.* 22, 221–227. doi: 10.1016/S0166-2236(98)01341-1

Vahlsing, H. L., and Feringa, E. R. (1980). A ventral uncrossed corticospinal tract in the rat. *Exp. Neurol.* 70, 282–287. doi: 10.1016/0014-4886(80)90027-8

Vierck, C. J. Jr. (1973). Alterations of spatio-tactile discrimination after lesions of primate spinal cord. *Brain Res.* 58, 69–79. doi: 10.1016/0006-8993(73)90824-X

Vierck, C. J. Jr. (1974). Tactile movement detection and discrimination following dorsal column lesions in monkeys. *Exp. Brain Res.* 20, 331–346. doi: 10.1007/BF00237379

Vierck, C. J. Jr. (1998). Impaired detection of repetitive stimulation following interruption of the dorsal spinal column in primates. *Somatosens Mot. Res.* 15, 157–163. doi: 10.1080/08990229870880

Vierck, C. J. Jr., and Cooper, B. Y. (1998). Cutaneous texture discrimination following transection of the dorsal spinal column in monkeys. *Somatosens Mot. Res.* 15, 309–315. doi: 10.1080/08990229870718

Wall, J. T., Xu, J., and Wang, X. (2002). Human brain plasticity: an emerging view of the multiple substrates and mechanisms that cause cortical changes and related sensory dysfunctions after injuries of sensory inputs from the body. *Brain Res. Brain Res. Rev.* 39, 181–215. doi: 10.1016/S0165-0173(02)00192-3

Wall, P. D. (1970). The sensory and motor role of impulses travelling in the dorsal columns towards cerebral cortex. *Brain* 93, 505–524. doi: 10.1093/brain/93.3.505

Wall, P. D. (1977). The presence of ineffective synapses and the circumstances which unmask them. *Philos. Trans. R. Soc. Lond. B Biol. Sci.* 278, 361–372. doi: 10.1098/rstb.1977.0048

Wang, Z., Qi, H. X., Kaas, J. H., Roe, A. W., and Chen, L. M. (2013). Functional signature of recovering cortex: dissociation of local field potentials and spiking activity in somatosensory cortices of spinal cord injured monkeys. *Exp. Neurol.* 249, 132–143. doi: 10.1016/j.expneurol.2013.08.013

Welker, W. I. (1973). Principles of organization of the ventrobasal complex in mammals. *Brain Behav. Evol.* 7, 253–336. doi: 10.1159/000124417

Wellman, C. L., Arnold, L. L., Garman, E. E., and Garraghty, P. E. (2002). Acute reductions in GABAA receptor binding in layer IV of adult primate somatosensory cortex after peripheral nerve injury. *Brain Res.* 954, 68–72. doi: 10.1016/S0006-8993(02)03343-7

Weng, H. R., Lenz, F. A., Vierck, C., and Dougherty, P. M. (2003). Physiological changes in primate somatosensory thalamus induced by deafferentation are dependent on the spinal funiculi that are sectioned and time following injury. *Neuroscience* 116, 1149–1160. doi: 10.1016/S0306-4522(02)00796-0

Willis, W. D., and Coggeshall, R. E. (2004). "Sensory pathways in the Dorsal Funiculus," in *Sensory Mechanisms of the Spinal cord: Ascending Sensory Tracts And Their Descending Control.* 3rd Edn, eds W. D. Willis and R. E. Coggeshall (New York, NY: Kluwer Academy/Plenum Publisher), 597–664. doi: 10.1007/978-1-4615-0035-3_9

Wise, S. P., Boussaoud, D., Johnson, P. B., and Caminiti, R. (1997). Premotor and parietal cortex: corticocortical connectivity and combinatorial computations. *Annu. Rev. Neurosci.* 20, 25–42. doi: 10.1146/annurev.neuro.20.1.25

Witham, C. L., and Baker, S. N. (2011). Modulation and transmission of peripheral inputs in monkey cuneate and external cuneate nuclei. *J. Neurophysiol.* 106, 2764–2775. doi: 10.1152/jn.00449.2011

Wu, C. W., and Kaas, J. H. (1999). Reorganization in primary motor cortex of primates with long-standing therapeutic amputations. *J. Neurosci.* 19, 7679–7697.

Xerri, C. (2012). Plasticity of cortical maps: multiple triggers for adaptive reorganization following brain damage and spinal cord injury. *Neuroscientist* 18, 133–148. doi: 10.1177/1073858410397894

Xu, J., and Wall, J. T. (1997). Rapid changes in brainstem maps of adult primates after peripheral injury. *Brain Res.* 774, 211–215. doi: 10.1016/S0006-8993(97)81706-4

Xu, J., and Wall, J. T. (1999). Evidence for brainstem and supra-brainstem contributions to rapid cortical plasticity in adult monkeys. *J. Neurosci.* 19, 7578–7590.

Yamahachi, H., Marik, S. A., McManus, J. N., Denk, W., and Gilbert, C. D. (2009). Rapid axonal sprouting and pruning accompany functional reorganization in primary visual cortex. *Neuron* 64, 719–729. doi: 10.1016/j.neuron.2009.11.026

Zhao, R. R., Andrews, M. R., Wang, D., Warren, P., Gullo, M., Schnell, L., et al. (2013). Combination treatment with anti-Nogo-A and chondroitinase ABC is more effective than single treatments at enhancing functional recovery after spinal cord injury. *Eur. J. Neurosci.* 38, 2946–2961. doi: 10.1111/ejn.12276

Zorner, B., Filli, L., Starkey, M. L., Gonzenbach, R., Kasper, H., Rothlisberger, M., et al. (2010). Profiling locomotor recovery: comprehensive quantification of impairments after CNS damage in rodents. *Nat. Methods* 7, 701–708. doi: 10.1038/nmeth.1484

13

Effects of non-pharmacological or pharmacological interventions on cognition and brain plasticity of aging individuals

Valentina Pieramico[1†], Roberto Esposito[2†], Stefano Cesinaro[1], Valerio Frazzini[1] and Stefano L. Sensi[1,2,3]*

[1] Molecular Neurology Unit, Center of Excellence on Aging, University "G. d'Annunzio," Chieti-Pescara, Chieti, Italy
[2] Department of Neuroscience, Imaging and Clinical Sciences, University "G. d'Annunzio," Chieti-Pescara, Chieti, Italy
[3] Departments of Neurology and Pharmacology, Institute for Memory Impairments and Neurological Disorders, University of California-Irvine, Irvine, CA, USA

Edited by:
Ioan Opris, Wake Forest University, USA

Reviewed by:
Preston E. Garraghty, Indiana University, USA
Mark John Ferris, Wake Forest School of Medicine, USA

****Correspondence:***
Stefano L. Sensi, Molecular Neurology Unit, Center of Excellence on Aging, University "G. d'Annunzio," Via dei Vestini, 31 Chieti-Pescara, Chieti 66100, Italy
e-mail: ssensi@uci.edu

† These authors have contributed equally to this work.

Brain aging and aging-related neurodegenerative disorders are major health challenges faced by modern societies. Brain aging is associated with cognitive and functional decline and represents the favourable background for the onset and development of dementia. Brain aging is associated with early and subtle anatomo-functional physiological changes that often precede the appearance of clinical signs of cognitive decline. Neuroimaging approaches unveiled the functional correlates of these alterations and helped in the identification of therapeutic targets that can be potentially useful in counteracting age-dependent cognitive decline. A growing body of evidence supports the notion that cognitive stimulation and aerobic training can preserve and enhance operational skills in elderly individuals as well as reduce the incidence of dementia. This review aims at providing an extensive and critical overview of the most recent data that support the efficacy of non-pharmacological and pharmacological interventions aimed at enhancing cognition and brain plasticity in healthy elderly individuals as well as delaying the cognitive decline associated with dementia.

Keywords: brain aging, neuronal plasticity, cognitive enhancing drugs, non-pharmacological interventions, cognitive enrichment

INTRODUCTION

Brain aging is associated with cognitive and functional decline and represents the favorable background for the onset and development of Alzheimer's disease (AD). AD is becoming a major socio-economical challenge for society (Hurd et al., 2013). Early use of imaging and biological markers can identify at-risk for AD subjects decades before the appearance of cognitive decline. It is therefore imperative to act during this extended pre-clinical phase and promote endogenous responses in brains that still have a large cognitive reserve and optimal levels of neural plasticity. Beside pharmacological intervention, a great deal of interest resides on ways that allow modulation of brain plasticity in the elderly by acting on cognitive stimulation and/or aerobic exercise. Cognitive enrichment as well as physical activity can in fact promote neural plasticity, increase neurotrofism and reduce AD incidence. This review aims at providing an extensive and critical overview of the most recent data that support the efficacy of non-pharmacological and pharmacological interventions aimed at enhancing cognition in healthy elderly individuals. This line of intervention can be also critical in delaying the cognitive decline associated with dementia or other widespread neurodegenerative conditions like Parkinson's disease (PD).

COGNITIVE AND NEURAL RESERVE

The central nervous system (CNS) is a highly dynamic structure that undergoes continuous functional remodeling. Salient experience promotes widespread changes within neuronal circuits and brain areas, a process that results in the harmonization of cognitive skills that are set to meet and cope with demands of everyday life. In this context, CNS plasticity is the ability to adopt functional or structural responses (Ganguly and Poo, 2013) aimed at promoting successful adaptive behavior (Xerri, 2008; Wittenberg, 2010). Activity-dependent neural plasticity is not only required for optimal brain development but is also occurring through adulthood and senescence (Buonomano and Merzenich, 1998; Feldman and Brecht, 2005; Feldman, 2009). Plasticity requires a complex process of molecular, structural, and functional integrations that are carried out in neurons, glia, and subcellular compartments like dendrites, spines, and synapses. These biochemical and morphological changes go along with spatiotemporal synchronization of large neuronal populations across different brain regions. While neuronal plasticity has been studied mostly in the neocortex and hippocampus, it is important to underline that the phenomenon is common to almost all the CNS structures. The last two decades have produced a dramatic increase in the availability of techniques that allow the extensive investigation of CNS from its subcellular components to neural circuits.

Advancements in fluorescent microscopy, molecular biology, and electrophysiological techniques have helped to unravel many molecular determinants of neuronal plasticity. On the other hand, the availability of neuroimaging tools such as functional magnetic resonance imaging (fMRI), positron emission tomography (PET), and magnetoencephalography (MEG) have enhanced the capability to detect spatiotemporal patterns of brain activation that occur within networks, nodes, and neuronal pathways (Pascual-Leone et al., 2005; Raichle and Mintun, 2006; Grefkes and Ward, 2014). These technical advancements, along with the notion that the aging brain retains the capacity to reorganize its morphological and functional architecture, have promoted strong interest and leaps forward in the knowledge of the physiology of the aging brain and aging-related cognitive processes as well as in the exploration of strategies aimed at enhancing or maintaining cognitive skills in the elderly. This area of investigation is particularly relevant as molecular, structural and functional derangement of physiological aging represents the pathological pabulum for the onset and development of neurodegenerative processes that underlay conditions like dementia or PD.

Cognitive reserve is the concept that has been proposed to explain the functional adaptation occurring in conditions that are associated with brain damage, but where structural impairment does not translate in patent cognitive deficits. When discussing this process, a clear distinction should be made between brain reserve and cognitive reserve. Brain reserve refers to the amount of preserved CNS "hardware", namely the integrity of synapses, dendrites, neurons, glia, and pathways while cognitive reserve indicates the CNS "software", in short the brain capability to reorganize its activity by setting in motion compensatory cognitive mechanisms. Thus, the cognitive reserve concept imposes to shift the attention from brain morphological integrity to functioning (Stern, 2009).

Despite recent great progress occurring in the field, the relative contribution of cognitive and brain reserve to the maintaining of brain functioning throughout aging is not completely clear. The two processes interplay and it is well known that rehabilitative interventions can positively act on both phenomena (Voss et al., 2013).

Cognitive reserve is positively influenced by educational, environmental, nutritional as well as genetic factors (Mora, 2013). The modulation of cognitive reserve greatly influences the vulnerability to dementia and affects the clinical course of the disease. Cognitive reserve has been indicated as a resource to be has tapped on in AD patients who despite the presence of large amount of AD-related pathology show relative paucity of clinical symptoms and signs. The process is thought to require the formation of new synapses as well as the plastic remodelling and functioning of brain networks (Amieva et al., 2014).

The drawback is that these patients can go undetected for long time and then, when exhaustion of the cognitive reserve occurs, eventually show a precipitous cognitive decline (Amieva et al., 2014). This rapid progression is considered to be related to high pathological loads that were compensated by a high cognitive reserve that eventually have been subdued and collapsed (Wilson et al., 2004; Amieva et al., 2014).

Neuroimaging evidence support this idea and indicate that AD patients with greater cognitive reserve often show underlying greater AD-related pathology. In a subset of AD patients, PET measurements of resting regional cerebral blood flow (rCBF) have shown an inverse relationship between resting cerebral blood volume (rCBV) and years of education (Friedland et al., 1985; McGeer et al., 1990). These studies indicate that patients with high levels of education manifest more pronounced reductions in parieto-temporal rCBV when compared to less educated subjects presenting similar clinical features. Similar results were observed in studies evaluating protective effects of rehabilitative activities (Stern et al., 1995; Scarmeas et al., 2003). fMRI studies have revealed patterns of brain network activity that supports the concept of cognitive reserve (Stern et al., 2005). Neuroimaging studies revealed that elderly people engage additional brain regions to compensate for impaired functioning (Fjell et al., 2014). For instance, upon completion of a memory task, experimental data indicate that, compared to young people, elderly individuals show increased recruitment of the prefrontal cortex (PFC), a process that possibly compensates for the reduced activity of brain regions that support visual processing of information (Ansado et al., 2013). The phenomenon has been labelled as "age-related posterior-anterior shift", or PASA (Davis et al., 2008). PASA seems to optimize cognition by inducing the inhibition of pre-potent responses (Corbetta et al., 2008; Vincent et al., 2008; Vallesi et al., 2011). Moreover, a recent study indicates that subjects performing attention tasks show an increased activity in bilateral PFC that positively correlates with enhanced performance (Davis et al., 2012).

NON-PHARMACOLOGICAL INTERVENTIONS

Age-related modulations and variations of cognitive and neural systems are dynamic and not irreversible processes. Physical or cognitive training can promote positive and lasting cognitive effects in elderly people and behavioral gains that may translate in more efficient procedural skills that help to cope with daily life activities. Non-pharmacological intervention can be divided in two approaches: aerobic training and cognitive stimulation (Jack, 2011; Vaughan et al., 2012).

AEROBIC TRAINING

Aerobic exercise is associated with increased preservation of cognitive functions (Colcombe et al., 2004). Exercise induces a cascade of molecular and sub/cellular processes that favor angiogenesis, neurogenesis, synaptogenesis as well as enhanced production of neurotrophins specially, the increased synthesis and release of brain-derived neurotrophic factor, BDNF (Deslandes et al., 2009; Coelho et al., 2013). The role of neurotrophins is crucial as decreases in BDNF levels are associated with age-related neuronal loss and BDNF reduction is also observed in patients affected by neurodegenerative or psychiatric disorders. Aerobic exercise elevates BDNF concentrations, increases hippocampal volumes (with the control group showing a reduction of volume of $\sim$1.4% while the trained group showed a volume increase of $\sim$2% over a 1-year period), and promotes better cognitive functioning in terms of executive functions, thereby suggesting that the trophin is a critical factor in mediating the protective and cognitive effects of this type of training (Erickson et al., 2013). Regular aerobic exercise improves executive function, attention, processing speed, memory, learning processes, and helps to preserve mental abilities throughout life span (Colcombe and Kramer, 2003; Curlik and Shors, 2013; Dresler et al., 2013). Exercise is also beneficial for subjects suffering from Mild Cognitive Impairment (MCI) or early-stage dementia (Smith et al., 2010).

Longitudinal studies suggest that engagement in exercise at young age leads to better cognitive performance upon senescence. The process seems to follow a dose- response effect as, in analogy with pharmacological intervention, more robust effects are obtained in individuals who in their youth have exercised more intensively (Middleton et al., 2010). Exercise appears to preferentially target selected brain regions and/or cognitive domains (Kramer et al., 2003; Colcombe et al., 2006; Erickson et al., 2013). Neuroimaging supports the idea of greater effects of exercise in the prefrontal and medial temporal cortices (Berchicci et al., 2013). The hippocampus appears to be particularly sensitive to exercise with trophic responses leading to increased hippocampal volume by ~2% in subjects undergoing training (Kerr et al., 2010; Erickson et al., 2011, 2013).

Overall, exercise-driven effects on specific cognitive domains like executive functions match morpho-functional changes in related brain regions (hippocampus, PFC, and basal ganglia) and neural networks. Elderly people who regularly exercise show brain volumes increases by ~2% in these critical areas while age-matched individuals who are less physically active undergo a 1.4% decrease in volumes (Erickson et al., 2010, 2011; Esposito et al., 2013).

COGNITIVE TRAINING

Cognitive stimulation by employing interventions that make use of ecological or virtual environments is also effective to compensate age-related cognitive decline (Curlik and Shors, 2013; Park and Bischof, 2013). To date, several types of cognitive trainings are available. Several programs are aimed at improving memory (Richmond et al., 2011; Dresler et al., 2013), learning (Bailey et al., 2010), attention (Mozolic et al., 2011), executive functions (Basak et al., 2008), fluid intelligence (Jaeggi et al., 2008), mnemonic techniques, or global cognition (Klusmann et al., 2010).

Shedding some light on the molecular targets of cognitive stimulation, preclinical models have shown that enriched environments improve cognitive performances by inducing enhanced expression of genes encoding for neurotrophins or promoting synaptogenesis, dendrite formation and arborization (van Praag et al., 2000; Fratiglioni et al., 2004). The same mechanisms also occur in brains of elderly people (Mora, 2013).

Neuroimaging data show that memory-targeted training can induce positive fMRI changes as well as modification in cortical thickness of hippocampal subfields and increases in the volumetry of left hippocampal subregions like the CA3, CA4, and dentate gyrus (Engvig et al., 2012). Memory training also increases the thickness of the right fusiform and lateral orbitofrontal cortex, a phenomenon that has been positively correlated with enhanced memory performances (Engvig et al., 2010). Unfortunately, only few fMRI studies have unveil functional connectivity effects associated with cognitive intervention (Burhan et al., 2012; Engvig et al., 2014).

PC-BASED TRAINING

Video games are not just teenager leisure material, they are gaining a place in the field of rehabilitation as tools to improve cognition in the elderly (Clark et al., 1987; Dustman et al., 1992; Goldstein et al., 1997; Basak et al., 2008). Results in this area of intervention are, however, often contradictory. Computer-based cognitive training for 6 months has been shown to stimulate multi-domain abilities like immediate memory and delayed memory or language (Miller et al., 2013). Game-based cognitive training, on the other hand, has shown no group effects on visuo-spatial navigational abilities and memory, though attention improvements have been found (Whitlock et al., 2012).

Interestingly, a recent study showed that computerized training targeted at amelioration of reaction times, inspection times, short-term memory for words, executive functions, visuo-spatial acuity, arithmetic competence, visuo-spatial memory, visual scanning, visual discrimination, and n-back working memory promoted no enhancement in these domains, but resulted in global improvement of processing speed (Simpson et al., 2012). The phenomenon is known as transfer effect. Moreover, evidence suggest that computer games designed to improve processing speed can enhance short-term memory and attention (Szelag and Skolimowska, 2012).

A very intriguing recent study has shown that cognitive capabilities can be significantly rejuvenated in the elderly (Anguera et al., 2013). Upon playing a video game targeted at increasing multitasking performance (a domain that show a physiological age-dependent decline), study subjects showed benefits not just in multitasking but also in untrained domains like sustained attention and working memory. The behavioral result was associated EEG evidence that show enhanced midline frontal theta power and frontal–posterior theta coherence in the trained group. More importantly, by simply undergoing a training period that spanned for just 12 h over a 4 week period, elderly subjects showed improved multitasking capability and matched performance levels of untrained young (20-year-old) subjects. Improved cognitive performances were maintained for 6 months after suspension of training, thereby suggesting long-lasting functional effects. Thus, the study supports the idea that age-related decline can be, not only halted, but actually reversed.

The field of PC-based cognitive training is still in its infancy, but, nevertheless, promising. Studies have started to analyze and debug areas that can potentially hamper the efficacy of this type of intervention. For instance, off the shelf, commercially available games appear to be less effective than personalized games (Peretz et al., 2011). Unfortunately, online games designed to enhance cognition in the elderly have generally failed mostly because of lack of motivation or ceiling effects in trainees who were already highly functioning and/or highly exposed to digital settings like virtual reality environments and games (Bozoki et al., 2013). Factors greatly affecting the cognitive outcome of PC-based trainings are the intensity and frequency of exposure to the training; however, a clear cut linear relationship between these factors and the cognitive output has, surprisingly, been difficult to be drawn

(Whitlock et al., 2012; Wild-Wall et al., 2012). Better study designs are therefore needed (Green and Bavelier, 2008; Nouchi et al., 2012; Whitlock et al., 2012). Finally, in a recent comparative study, a custom-made computerized intervention was found to improve overall memory and attention performances in a group of elderly subjects. The study showed that training effects were still present 3 month after training withdraw (Zelinski et al., 2011).

COMBINED TRAINING

Interest in multimodal interventions has been increased in recent years. Evidence, unfortunately still too few, suggest that strategies that combine aerobic training and cognitive stimulation have a significant synergistic value (Schneider and Yvon, 2013).

In a recent study, healthy elderly subjects were exposed to four different training conditions (Shatil, 2013). The first group was exposed to cognitive training, the second group engaged itself in moderate aerobic activity, the third group followed a combination of cognitive and aerobic training, while the control group was simply exposed to book-reading. Results of the study indicated that the third group, exposed to combined training, showed the best improvement in eye-hand coordination, working memory, long-term memory, and reaction times.

Interesting effects were also found in case of PC-based training combined with exercise. Cycling sessions performed in a virtual reality environment enhanced executive functions more effectively that regular cycling in a gym on stationary bikes (Anderson-Hanley et al., 2012). Positive effects of trained cybercyclists correlated with increase of BDNF. Important effects, in the cybercycling group, were also seen in MCI subjects. In this group, training reduced by 23% AD conversion (Anderson-Hanley et al., 2012). Another study (Maillot et al., 2012) found a significant improvement in executive control and processing speed after a 12 week aerobic training that employed the Nintendo Wii sports software console.

Other studies have supported the idea of the synergistic value of combining exercise and cognitive trainings to promote memory performance (Fabre et al., 2002; Oswald et al., 2006). Unfortunately, no data are available to verify whether these training-driven benefits translate in better performances in daily living activities. A previous study, from our group, has tried to fill the gap (Pieramico et al., 2012). We evaluated effects of 6-month combination training on cognition, functional connectivity and daily living activities. Thirty healthy elderly divided in two groups of 15 subjects were exposed to either no changes in their daily living routine (control group) or to a combination training consisting in exposure to cognitive, motor, and sensorial stimulations (trained group). Groups were evaluated, before and after the end of the training period, with neuropsychological and occupational tests, resting state fMRI and analysis of cortical thickness. Combination training improved cognitive and occupational performances, reorganized the functional connectivity of Default Mode (DMN) and Dorsal Attention (DAN) networks, and promoted lower cortical thinning in several brain regions (Pieramico et al., 2012). Interestingly, analysis of dopamine-related genes indicated that carriers of DRD3 ser9gly and catechol-O-methyltransferase (COMT) val158met polymorphisms had the greatest benefits from exposure to training, thereby suggesting a genetically-driven susceptibility to the positive effects of this type of combined intervention.

CRITICAL POINTS IN NON-PHARMACOLOGICAL INTERVENTIONS

Many unknowns are still present when dealing with training programs. For instance, the role played by intensity of intervention and knowledge on which is the most beneficial set of exercises to be employed are still largely unclear and missing. Also uncertain is what concerns the specificity and selectivity of factors that can promote significant, reproducible, and durable effects on cognition. Few studies have investigated correlations between frequency and duration of aerobic and cognitive trainings along with the overall morpho-functional changes and effects on brain functioning upon aging.

Furthermore, still not completely defined is for how long positive effects are maintained and therefore, robust well-designed longitudinal studies are needed.

A limiting factor that should be not overlooked is individual variability, an aspect that mandates more accurate customization of any given set of intervention. For instance, in analogy with the field of pharmacogenomics, a "cognitogenomic" approach, in which genetic differences are explored in relation to response to cognitive trainings, is definitely necessary (Pieramico et al., 2012).

PHARMACOLOGICAL INTERVENTIONS

Pharmacological intervention aimed at enhancing or maintaining cognitive functions has been the focus of intensive research in recent years (Lanni et al., 2008; Hussain and Mehta, 2011; Lynch et al., 2011; Lynch and Mills, 2012; Wood et al., 2013; Urban and Gao, 2014). An intuitive definition of Cognitive Enhancer Drugs (CEDs) qualifies these molecules as able to enhance cognitive skills; however, an exhaustive definition of CEDs is, perhaps, not so simple. According to Lynch et coll., there is a need for a "dimensional" system to successfully define and classify CED candidates (Lynch and Gall, 2006; Lynch et al., 2011).

The first level, or dimension, is the target of action. Does the CED candidate mainly act on "general" psychological states like arousal or attentional level or does it work by potentiating single and/or selective cognitive domains? If the action is global, CED effects should be obtained through an optimization of the processing and information flux that operate within several brain nodes and networks. In case of selective activity, the drug should instead affect only specific and distinct subsets of cognitive domains.

Another important CED level/dimension is the neurobiological one or, in other words, the molecular mechanisms of action. Which neurotransmitter systems, receptor subpopulations, neuronal circuits, and/or brain structures are modified by CED activity?

Finally, a third dimensional level is represented by the distinction between drugs that enable to perform complex tasks in a more rapid or efficient way (efficiency augmentation) vs. molecules that promote enhanced performances (cognitive capability augmentation; Lynch, 2004; Lynch et al., 2011).

In accordance with this systematization, CEDs can be classified as drugs mainly acting on general or psychological aspects of cognition, compounds aimed at potentiating more specific cognitive domains or, at least in theory, drugs that are aiming at enhancing the global cognitive capability of healthy and already well performing individuals.

Most CED candidates are evaluated in preclinical models, sets where standardized behavioral outcomes are easily assessed. Although the translation of preclinical data in valid clinical outputs poses several limitations (see Sarter, 2006), animal models remain extremely valuable to identify CED neurobiology (Roesler, 2011).

In that respect, methylphenidate and modafinil, are good examples of a category of molecules that, across the board, induces changes of psychological variables such as vigilance, attention, and memory. Drug effects on arousal have been extensively described; however, a recent study that examined human subjects required to discriminate significant stimuli from distractors raised some question about the validity of the mechanism (Agay et al., 2010). Methylphenidate increases attention or "vigilance" by stimulating the cortical dopaminergic and noradrenergic transmission systems, a mechanism of action first described in preclinical settings and then confirmed by PET in human studies. Oral methylphenidate administration (0.25 mg/Kg) has been shown to promote a 50% blockage of the dopamine transporter (Volkow et al., 1998; Hannestad et al., 2010) and significantly increase extracellular dopamine concentrations. However, oral methylphenidate (at therapeutic ranges; 0.14 mg/kg) was also shown to bind with high affinity to the norepinephrine transporter. Methylphenidate-mediated effects on attention seem quite specific for tasks that need sustained vigilance; however, the drug appears to be less efficient when subjects are dealing with situations with levels of complexity that require selective attention (Advokat, 2010; Advokat et al., 2011). The compound can also improve spatial working memory in healthy individuals in conditions in which subjects are challenged with ex novo spatial problems (Elliott et al., 1997). Interestingly, experimental data confirmed drug-dependent improvements in spatial working memory. However, the study indicated that such benefits only occurred in subjects who were poorly performing at baseline, thereby suggesting that the drug can work only when significant amounts of cognitive reserve are available to be recruited (McGeer et al., 1990).

Modafinil is another example of drugs operating on vigilance or "attentional" states. The compound was first introduced as agent that counteracts excessive sleepiness associated with narcolepsy. Modafinil binds to forebrain dopamine transporters (Volkow et al., 2009; Zolkowska et al., 2009; Andersen et al., 2010) and promotes an increase in extracellular dopamine concentrations. The molecule can also bind to norepinephrine transporters in the human thalamus (Madras et al., 2006) and modulate orexinergic neurons in the hypothalamus (Ishizuka et al., 2010). Modafinil has been shown to promote marked increases in motor activity in mice (Simon et al., 1995; Stone et al., 2002), however, the effects are modest in rats and monkeys (Edgar and Seidel, 1997; Andersen et al., 2010). Finally, some studies have indicated drug-dependent improvement in sustained attention in modafinil-treated healthy subjects (Randall et al., 2005; Esposito et al., 2013).

An important bias to be considered when evaluating CEDs is represented by the fact that most studies, in animal models (Béracochéa et al., 2002) or humans (Turner et al., 2003; Baranski et al., 2004; Muller et al., 2004; Randall et al., 2005), are focused on effects on attention and working memory while other cognitive domains (such as long-term memory) are often neglected (Minzenberg and Carter, 2008). CEDs that selectively act on specific cognitive domains (memory and attention) belong to two classes of drugs that target the fast excitatory synaptic transmission responsible for communication within cortical networks. The first class acts on nicotinic receptors (alpha7 and alpha4 agonists) and modulates glutamate release while the second one, the ampakine family, facilitates fast glutamatergic transmission by acting on α-Amino-3-hydroxy-5-methyl-4-isoxazolepropionic acid receptors (AMPAR).

The cholinergic system is involved in several important aspects of cognitive functions including attention, learning, and memory. Classical CEDs enhance brain cholinergic tone by inhibiting acetylcolinecolinesterases (AChEIs), the enzymes responsible of acetylcholine degradation. AChEIs (rivastigmine, donepezil, galantamine) are approved for the treatment of AD patients; however, these compounds have failed in patients suffering from MCI (Raschetti et al., 2007), and very little data are available on cognitive effects on healthy adults. Rivastigmine has been shown to negatively affect episodic memory and improve motor learning and visuospatial functions in healthy elderly subjects (Wezenberg et al., 2005). Donepezil has produced mixed results, the drug improves cognitive performance in healthy young subjects (Yesavage et al., 2002) but has also been shown to cause attention and short-term memory deficits in healthy elderly subjects (Beglinger et al., 2005). Selective α4β2 nicotinic receptor agonists represent a new class of drugs acting on the cholinergic system and found to induce attentional and cognitive improvements in animal models (Howe et al., 2010). Agonists of α4β2 and α7 nicotinic receptors represent interesting examples of drugs that can potentiate the prefrontal cholinergic activity. These drugs promote an increase in fast glutamatergic transmission in the cortex, thereby enhancing attentional processes (Dunbar et al., 2007; Jiang and Role, 2008; Loughead et al., 2010). The proposed mechanism of action for α4β2 agonists is based on the hypothesis that the prefrontal cholinergic system plays a crucial role in the detection of novel and relevant stimuli, thereby increasing attentional performances (Bloem et al., 2014). The drug leads to amplitude augmentation of signal-evoked cholinergic transients when a relevant stimulus is administered to a subject.

Ampakines are positive allosteric AMPAR modulators that enhance fast excitatory transmission, promote induction and enhanced strength of long-term potentiation (LTP; Lynch, 2002). These compounds also increase the production of BDNF and related proteins (Lauterborn et al., 2000, 2003; Legutko et al., 2001; Lynch, 2002; O'Neill et al., 2004, 2005; Wezenberg et al., 2007). A recent study has described a role for the CX546 ampakine in promoting the proliferation and neuronal differentiation of stem/progenitor cells originating from the subventricular zone

(Schitine et al., 2012), thereby underlying the role of these molecules in the differentiation of newborn neurons and in the shaping of neuronal circuits. The CX929 ampakine has been reported to promote LTP and counteract learning impairments in mice models of neurodevelopmental disorders. In one study, a 5 day treatment with CX929 in a mouse model of the Angelman syndrome, was reported to enhance fast EPSCs in hippocampal slices and increase long-term memory scores by 50% (Baudry et al., 2012). Ampakine are reported to improve performance in monkeys challenged with complex cognitive tasks (Porrino et al., 2005; Hampson et al., 2009) and brain imaging has demonstrated increased activity in the frontal and temporal cortices upon treatment (Porrino et al., 2005). The study revealed drug-induced activation of the precuneus, a cortical area usually less involved in task response (Porrino et al., 2005). This observation strongly suggests that ampakine administration may promote functional recruitment of additional brain areas, thereby modifying the neural substrates of cognition. Unfortunately, no ampakines are currently approved by FDA. The only molecule that reached clinical trials is CX-717. The compound was evaluated in Phase I for AD treatment but withdraw upon additional controversial results. Potential novel candidates are nevertheless being investigated for treatment of several neurologic and psychiatric disorders such as PD, schizophrenia, autism, and Attention Deficit Hyperactivity Disorder (ADHD).

Pharmaco-genomic approaches to be implemented for CED development and administration represent a promising new avenue in the field of cognitive augmentation. Traditionally these approaches have been mainly focused on the identification of genetic polymorphisms that can predict more effective drug responses in subjects already affected by neuropsychiatric disorders. However, in the past few years, studies have started to unravel the pharmacogenomic basis of individual response to CEDs occurring in healthy subjects. Factors to be considered are polymorphisms of genes regulating drug metabolizing enzymes, transporters, and receptors. These factors may profoundly influence the dose–response relationship to drugs (Roses, 2008). Differences in COMT genotypes (Val-Val vs. Met-Met) have been associated with variability in working memory performances and cognitive responses following amphetamine administration (Bilder et al., 2004). Apoliprotein E4 (apoE4), an allele of apolipoprotein E, and a risk factor for AD, is an interesting case. Quite paradoxically, ApoE polymorphism in young healthy carriers (i.e., subjects who have therefore a higher risk of developing AD later on in life) have the tendency to perform decision-making and prospective memory tasks better than, ApoE3 carriers (who are instead protected, by virtue of this genotype, from AD; Marchant et al., 2010).

CRITICAL POINTS IN PHARMACOLOGICAL INTERVENTIONS

A critical point in the clinical output of CEDs is represented by the great variability of cognitive or behavioral responses of healthy individuals to these drugs. Several studies have begun to question whether such differences depend on genotypes and/or baseline levels of cognitive function (Kimberg et al., 1997; Mehta et al., 2000; Gibbs and D'Esposito, 2005; Frank and O'Reilly, 2006; Cools et al., 2007). For example, dopaminergic drugs have been shown to improve working memory only low performing subjects (Gibbs and D'Esposito, 2006). Methylphenidate or bromocriptine seem to improve working memory in low performers but impair performance in subjects with high baseline spans (Kimberg et al., 1997; Gibbs and D'Esposito, 2006). These contradictory results have been explained by the presence of an inverted U-shaped relationship between cognitive performance and dopamine receptor stimulation (Yerkes and Dodson, 1908). Indicating some potential neurobiological determinant of the phenomenon, dopamine synthesis has been shown to be lower in in the caudate nucleus of individuals with low working memory spans when compared to synthesis in subjects with high spans (Cools et al., 2008). Accordingly, subjects with low dopamine synthesis in the basal ganglia performed better in reversal learning tasks after bromocriptine administration when compared to treated subjects who were already showing high basal ganglia synthesis (Cools et al., 2009). Modafinil administration has also been shown to have most effective cognitive effects in low performing subjects at baseline (Randall et al., 2005; Finke et al., 2010; Esposito et al., 2013).

Baseline cognitive levels also affect the cholinergic modulation of cognition in healthy individuals. Donepezil increases cognition of healthy subjects whose performance declined after sleep deprivation but the drug induced cognitive impairments in subject without sleep loss (Chuah and Chee, 2008; Chuah et al., 2009).

Finally, it should be underlined that optimal brain functioning results from a tight control of synaptic function, circuits remodeling, and connectivity modulation. In response to extrinsic stimuli, neurons accordingly change the strength of their connections in order to avoid excessive excitation or inhibition (Pozo and Goda, 2010). Therefore, CED-driven excessive connectivity can be sometimes potentially problematic. In theory, increased excitatory synaptic transmission, along with reduced synaptic pruning, may induce unregulated synaptic plasticity and neuronal circuit overactivation, thereby promoting a low signal-to-noise ratio that actually may lead to impaired cognition (Belmonte and Yurgelun-Todd, 2003).

CONCLUSION AND FUTURE DIRECTIONS

In this review, we have summarized effects on cognition and brain plasticity of non-pharmacological and pharmacological interventions targeted on elderly individuals. The field is blooming but many issues remain unresolved. Areas that are in great need of advancement concern a better understanding of the role played by genes in the modulation of senescence and/or response to intervention. Disclosure of more detailed genetic and epigenetic roadmaps will help the design and implementation of tailored and personalized training programs. A more extensive implementation of "omics" (proteomics, lipidomics, metabolomics) approaches in combination with neuroimaging will also promote a better assessment of morpho-functional changes that are occurring in the trained brain as well as whole body.

Recent progress in digital technologies leads to foresee, in the near future, a more user-friendly implementation of trainings that can avoid personal computers and make instead use of smartphones, virtual or augmented reality portable devices. In that respect, the come of age of digitally-native generations will undoubtedly promote an extraordinary acceleration in that direction.

All these, pharmacological and non pharmacological, interventions can be envisioned to be effective not only in maintaining optimal levels of cognitive capabilities in healthy elderly individuals, but also as preventive measures to counteract the development of AD or PD as well as therapeutic tools that can be employed in the early stage of these neurodegenerative conditions.

ACKNOWLEDGMENTS

Stefano L. Sensi is supported by funds from the Italian Department of Education (PRIN 2011) and the "Marisa Trampuz von Langendorf" Fellowship for Neuroscience.

REFERENCES

Advokat, C. (2010). What are the cognitive effects of stimulant medications? Emphasis on adults with attention-deficit/hyperactivity disorder (ADHD). *Neurosci. Biobehav. Rev.* 34, 1256–1266. doi: 10.1016/j.neubiorev.2010.03.006

Advokat, C., Lane, S. M., and Luo, C. (2011). College students with and without ADHD: comparison of self-report of medication usage, study habits and academic achievement. *J. Atten. Disord.* 15, 656–666. doi: 10.1177/1087054710371168

Agay, N., Yechiam, E., Carmel, Z., and Levkovitz, Y. (2010). Non-specific effects of methylphenidate (Ritalin) on cognitive ability and decision-making of ADHD and healthy adults. *Psychopharmacology (Berl)* 210, 511–519. doi: 10.1007/s00213-010-1853-4

Amieva, H., Mokri, H., Le Goff, M., Meillon, C., Jacqmin-Gadda, H., Foubert-Samier, A., et al. (2014). Compensatory mechanisms in higher-educated subjects with Alzheimer's disease: a study of 20 years of cognitive decline. *Brain.* 137(Pt 4), 1167–1175. doi: 10.1093/brain/awu035

Andersen, M. L., Kessler, E., Murnane, K. S., McClung, J. C., Tufik, S., and Howell, L. L. (2010). Dopamine transporter-related effects of modafinil in rhesus monkeys. *Psychopharmacology (Berl)* 210, 439–448. doi: 10.1007/s00213-010-1839-2

Anderson-Hanley, C., Arciero, P. J., Brickman, A. M., Nimon, J. P., Okuma, N., Westen, S. C., et al. (2012). Exergaming and older adult cognition: a cluster randomized clinical trial. *Am. J. Prev. Med.* 42, 109–119. doi: 10.1016/j.amepre.2011.10.016

Anguera, J. A., Boccanfuso, J., Rintoul, J. L., Al-Hashimi, O., Faraji, F., Janowich, J., et al. (2013). Video game training enhances cognitive control in older adults. *Nature* 501, 97–101. doi: 10.1038/nature12486

Ansado, J., Marsolais, Y., Methqal, I., Alary, F., and Joanette, Y. (2013). The adaptive aging brain: evidence from the preservation of communication abilities with age. *Eur. J. Neurosci.* 37, 1887–1895. doi: 10.1111/ejn.12252

Bailey, H., Dunlosky, J., and Hertzog, C. (2010). Metacognitive training at home: does it improve older adults' learning? *Gerontology* 56, 414–420. doi: 10.1159/000266030

Baranski, J. V., Pigeau, R., Dinich, P., and Jacobs, I. (2004). Effects of modafinil on cognitive and metacognitive performance. *Hum. Psychopharmacol.* 19, 323–332. doi: 10.1002/hup.596

Basak, C., Boot, W. R., Voss, M. W., and Kramer, A. F. (2008). Can training in a real-time strategy video game attenuate cognitive decline in older adults? *Psychol. Aging* 23, 765–777. doi: 10.1037/a0013494

Baudry, M., Kramar, E., Xu, X., Zadran, H., Moreno, S., Lynch, G., et al. (2012). Ampakines promote spine actin polymerization, long-term potentiation and learning in a mouse model of Angelman syndrome. *Neurobiol. Dis.* 47, 210–215. doi: 10.1016/j.nbd.2012.04.002

Beglinger, L. J., Tangphao-Daniels, O., Kareken, D. A., Zhang, L., Mohs, R., and Siemers, E. R. (2005). Neuropsychological test performance in healthy elderly volunteers before and after donepezil administration: a randomized, controlled study. *J. Clin. Psychopharmacol.* 25, 159–165. doi: 10.1097/01.jcp.0000155822.51962.b4

Belmonte, M. K., and Yurgelun-Todd, D. A. (2003). Functional anatomy of impaired selective attention and compensatory processing in autism. *Brain Res. Cogn. Brain Res.* 17, 651–664. doi: 10.1016/s0926-6410(03)00189-7

Béracochéa, D., Celerier, A., Borde, N., Valleau, M., Peres, M., and Pierard, C. (2002). Improvement of learning processes following chronic systemic administration of modafinil in mice. *Pharmacol. Biochem. Behav.* 73, 723–728. doi: 10.1016/s0091-3057(02)00877-8

Berchicci, M., Lucci, G., and Di Russo, F. (2013). Benefits of physical exercise on the aging brain: the role of the prefrontal cortex. *J. Gerontol. A Biol. Sci. Med. Sci.* 68, 1337–1341. doi: 10.1093/gerona/glt094

Bilder, R. M., Volavka, J., Lachman, H. M., and Grace, A. A. (2004). The catechol-O-methyltransferase polymorphism: relations to the tonic-phasic dopamine hypothesis and neuropsychiatric phenotypes. *Neuropsychopharmacology* 29, 1943–1961. doi: 10.1038/sj.npp.1300542

Bloem, B., Poorthuis, R. B., and Mansvelder, H. D. (2014). Cholinergic modulation of the medial prefrontal cortex: the role of nicotinic receptors in attention and regulation of neuronal activity. *Front Neural Circuits* 8:17. doi: 10.3389/fncir.2014.00017

Bozoki, A., Radovanovic, M., Winn, B., Heeter, C., and Anthony, J. C. (2013). Effects of a computer-based cognitive exercise program on age-related cognitive decline. *Arch. Gerontol. Geriatr.* 57, 1–7. doi: 10.1016/j.archger.2013.02.009

Buonomano, D. V., and Merzenich, M. M. (1998). Cortical plasticity: from synapses to maps. *Annu. Rev. Neurosci.* 21, 149–186. doi: 10.1146/annurev.neuro.21.1.149

Burhan, A. M., Bartha, R., Bocti, C., Borrie, M., Laforce, R., Rosa-Neto, P., et al. (2012). Role of emerging neuroimaging modalities in patients with cognitive impairment: a review from the Canadian Consensus Conference on the Diagnosis and Treatment of Dementia. *Alzheimers Res. Ther.* 5(Suppl. 1):S4. doi: 10.1186/alzrt200

Chuah, L. Y. M., and Chee, M. W. L. (2008). Cholinergic augmentation modulates visual task performance in sleep-deprived young adults. *J. Neurosci.* 28, 11369–11377. doi: 10.1523/jneurosci.4045-08.2008

Chuah, L. Y., Chong, D. L., Chen, A. K., Rekshan, W. R., Tan, J. C., Zheng, H., et al. (2009). Donepezil improves episodic memory in young individuals vulnerable to the effects of sleep deprivation. *Sleep* 32, 999–1010.

Clark, J. E., Lanphear, A. K., and Riddick, C. C. (1987). The effects of videogame playing on the response selection processing of elderly adults. *J. Gerontol.* 42, 82–85. doi: 10.1093/geronj/42.1.82

Coelho, F. G., Gobbi, S., Andreatto, C. A., Corazza, D. I., Pedroso, R. V., and Santos-Galduróz, R. F. (2013). Physical exercise modulates peripheral levels of brain-derived neurotrophic factor (BDNF): a systematic review of experimental studies in the elderly. *Arch. Gerontol. Geriatr.* 56, 10–15. doi: 10.1016/j.archger.2012.06.003

Colcombe, S. J., Erickson, K. I., Scalf, P. E., Kim, J. S., Prakash, R., McAuley, E., et al. (2006). Aerobic exercise training increases brain volume in aging humans. *J. Gerontol. A Biol. Sci. Med. Sci.* 61, 1166–1170. doi: 10.1093/gerona/61.11.1166

Colcombe, S., and Kramer, A. F. (2003). Fitness effects on the cognitive function of older adults: a meta-analytic study. *Psychol. Sci.* 14, 125–130. doi: 10.1111/1467-9280.t01-1-01430

Colcombe, S. J., Kramer, A. F., Erickson, K. I., Scalf, P., McAuley, E., Cohen, N. J., et al. (2004). Cardiovascular fitness, cortical plasticity and aging. *Proc. Natl. Acad. Sci. U S A* 101, 3316–3321. doi: 10.1073/pnas.0400266101

Cools, R., Frank, M. J., Gibbs, S. E., Miyakawa, A., Jagust, W., and D'Esposito, M. (2009). Striatal dopamine predicts outcome-specific reversal learning and its sensitivity to dopaminergic drug administration. *J. Neurosci.* 29, 1538–1543. doi: 10.1523/jneurosci.4467-08.2009

Cools, R., Gibbs, S. E., Miyakawa, A., Jagust, W., and D'Esposito, M. (2008). Working memory capacity predicts dopamine synthesis capacity in the human striatum. *J. Neurosci.* 28, 1208–1212. doi: 10.1523/JNEUROSCI.4475-07.2008

Cools, R., Sheridan, M., Jacobs, E., and D'Esposito, M. (2007). Impulsive personality predicts dopamine-dependent changes in frontostriatal activity during component processes of working memory. *J. Neurosci.* 27, 5506–5514. doi: 10.1523/jneurosci.0601-07.2007

Corbetta, M., Patel, G., and Shulman, G. L. (2008). The reorienting system of the human brain: from environment to theory of mind. *Neuron* 58, 306–324. doi: 10.1016/j.neuron.2008.04.017

Curlik, D. M., and Shors, T. J. (2013). Training your brain: do mental and physical (MAP) training enhance cognition through the process of neurogenesis in the hippocampus? *Neuropharmacology* 64, 506–514. doi: 10.1016/j.neuropharm.2012.07.027

Davis, S. W., Dennis, N. A., Daselaar, S. M., Fleck, M. S., and Cabeza, R. (2008). Que PASA? The posterior-anterior shift in aging. *Cereb. Cortex* 18, 1201–1209. doi: 10.1093/cercor/bhm155

Davis, S. W., Kragel, J. E., Madden, D. J., and Cabeza, R. (2012). The architecture of cross-hemispheric communication in the aging brain: linking behavior to functional and structural connectivity. *Cereb. Cortex* 22, 232–242. doi: 10.1093/cercor/bhr123

Deslandes, A., Moraes, H., Ferreira, C., Veiga, H., Silveira, H., Mouta, R., et al. (2009). Exercise and mental health: many reasons to move. *Neuropsychobiology* 59, 191–198. doi: 10.1159/000223730

Dresler, M., Sandberg, A., Ohla, K., Bublitz, C., Trenado, C., Mroczko-Wasowicz, A., et al. (2013). Non-pharmacological cognitive enhancement. *Neuropharmacology* 64, 529–543. doi: 10.1016/j.neuropharm.2012.07.002

Dunbar, G. C., Inglis, F., Kuchibhatla, R., Sharma, T., Tomlinson, M., and Wamsley, J. (2007). Effect of ispronicline, a neuronal nicotinic acetylcholine receptor partial agonist, in subjects with age associated memory impairment (AAMI). *J. Psychopharmacol.* 21, 171–178. doi: 10.1177/0269881107066855

Dustman, R. E., Emmerson, R. Y., Steinhaus, L. A., Shearer, D. E., and Dustman, T. J. (1992). The effects of videogame playing on neuropsychological performance of elderly individuals. *J. Gerontol.* 47, 168–171. doi: 10.1093/geronj/47.3.p168

Edgar, D. M., and Seidel, W. F. (1997). Modafinil induces wakefulness without intensifying motor activity or subsequent rebound hypersomnolence in the rat. *J. Pharmacol. Exp. Ther.* 283, 757–769.

Elliott, R., Sahakian, B. J., Matthews, K., Bannerjea, A., Rimmer, J., and Robbins, T. W. (1997). Effects of methylphenidate on spatial working memory and planning in healthy young adults. *Psychopharmacology (Berl)* 131, 196–206. doi: 10.1007/s002130050284

Engvig, A., Fjell, A. M., Westlye, L. T., Moberget, T., Sundseth, Ø., Larsen, V. A., et al. (2010). Effects of memory training on corticalthickness in the elderly. *Neuroimage* 52, 1667–1676. doi: 10.1016/j.neuroimage.2010.05.041

Engvig, A., Fjell, A. M., Westlye, L. T., Skaane, N. V., Dale, A. M., Holland, D., et al. (2014). Effects of cognitive training on gray matter volumes in memory clinic patients with subjective memory impairment. *J. Alzheimers Dis.* 41, 779–791. doi: 10.3233/JAD-131889

Engvig, A., Fjell, A. M., Westlye, L. T., Skaane, N. V., Sundseth, Ø., and Walhovd, K. B. (2012). Hippocampal subfield volumes correlate with memory training benefit in subjective memory impairment. *Neuroimage* 61, 188–194. doi: 10.1016/j.neuroimage.2012.02.072

Erickson, K. I., Gildengers, A. G., and Butters, M. A. (2013). Physical activity and brain plasticity in late adulthood. *Dialogues Clin. Neurosci.* 15, 99–108.

Erickson, K. I., Raji, C. A., Lopez, O. L., Becker, J. T., Rosano, C., Newman, A. B., et al. (2010). Physical activity predicts grey matter volume in late adulthood: the Cardiovascular Health Study. *Neurology* 75, 1415–1422. doi: 10.1212/wnl.0b013e3181f88359

Erickson, K. I., Voss, M. W., Prakash, R. S., Basak, C., Szabo, A., Chaddock, L., et al. (2011). Exercise training increases size of hippocampus and improves memory. *Proc. Natl. Acad. Sci. U S A* 108, 3017–3022. doi: 10.1073/pnas.1015950108

Esposito, R., Cilli, F., Pieramico, V., Ferretti, A., Macchia, A., Tommasi, M., et al. (2013). Acute effects of modafinil on brain resting state networks in young healthy subjects. *PLoS One* 8:e69224. doi: 10.1371/journal.pone.0069224

Fabre, C., Chamari, K., and Mucci, P. (2002). Improvement of cognitive function via mental and/or individualised aerobic training in healthy elderly subject. *Int. J. Sports Med.* 23, 415–421. doi: 10.1055/s-2002-33735

Feldman, D. E. (2009). Synaptic mechanisms for plasticity in neocortex. *Annu. Rev. Neurosci.* 32, 33–55. doi: 10.1146/annurev.neuro.051508.135516

Feldman, D. E., and Brecht, M. (2005). Map plasticity in somatosensory cortex. *Science* 310, 810–815. doi: 10.1126/science.1115807

Finke, K., Dodds, C. M., Bublak, P., Regenthal, R., Baumann, F., Manly, T., et al. (2010). Effects of modafinil and methylphenidate on visual attention capacity: a TVA-based study. *Psychopharmacology (Berl)* 210, 317–329. doi: 10.1007/s00213-010-1823-x

Fjell, A. M., McEvoy, L., Holland, D., Dale, A. M., and Walhovd, K. B. (2014). Alzheimer's disease neuroimaging initiative. What is normal in normal aging? Effects of aging, amyloid and Alzheimer's disease on the cerebral cortex and the hippocampus. *Prog. Neurobiol.* 117, 20–40. doi: 10.1016/j.pneurobio.2014.02.004

Frank, M. J., and O'Reilly, R. C. (2006). A mechanistic account of striatal dopamine function in human cognition: psychopharmacological studies with cabergoline and haloperidol. *Behav. Neurosci.* 120, 497–517. doi: 10.1037/0735-7044.120.3.497

Fratiglioni, L., Paillard-Borg, S., and Winblad, B. (2004). An active and socially integrated lifestyle in late life might protect against dementia. *Lancet Neurol.* 3, 343–353. doi: 10.1016/s1474-4422(04)00767-7

Friedland, R. P., Brun, A., and Budinger, T. F. (1985). Pathological and positron emission tomographic correlations in Alzheimer's disease. *Lancet* 1, 228. doi: 10.1016/s0140-6736(85)92074-4

Ganguly, K., and Poo, M. M. (2013). Activity-dependent neural plasticity from bench to bedside. *Neuron* 80, 729–741. doi: 10.1016/j.neuron.2013.10.028

Gibbs, S. E. B., and D'Esposito, M. (2005). Individual capacity differences predict working memory performance and prefrontal activity following dopamine receptor stimulation. *Cogn. Affect Behav. Neurosci.* 5, 212–221. doi: 10.3758/cabn.5.2.212

Gibbs, S. E., and D'Esposito, M. (2006). A functional magnetic resonance imaging study of the effects of pergolide, a dopamine receptor agonist, on component processes of working memory. *Neuroscience* 139, 359–371. doi: 10.1016/j.neuroscience.2005.11.055

Goldstein, J., Cajko, L., Oosterbroek, M., Michielsen, M., and Van Houten, O. (1997). Video game and the elderly. *Soc. Behav. Pers. Int. J.* 25, 345–352.

Green, C. S., and Bavelier, D. (2008). Exercising your brain: a review of human brain plasticity and training-induced learning. *Psychol. Aging* 23, 692–701. doi: 10.1037/a0014345

Grefkes, C., and Ward, N. S. (2014). Cortical reorganization after stroke: how much and how functional? *Neuroscientist* 20, 56–70. doi: 10.1177/1073858413491147

Hampson, R. E., España, R. A., Rogers, G. A., Porrino, L. J., and Deadwyler, S. A. (2009). Mechanisms underlying cognitive enhancement and reversal of cognitive deficits in nonhuman primates by the ampakine CX717. *Psychopharmacology (Berl)* 202, 355–369. doi: 10.1007/s00213-008-1360-z

Hannestad, J., Gallezot, J. D., Planeta-Wilson, B., Lin, S. F., Williams, W. A., van Dyck, C. H., et al. (2010). Clinically relevant doses of methylphenidate significantly occupy norepinephrine transporters in humans in vivo. *Biol. Psychiatry* 68, 854–860. doi: 10.1016/j.biopsych.2010.06.017

Howe, W. M., Ji, J., Parikh, V., Williams, S., Mocaër, E., Trocmé-Thibierge, C., et al. (2010). Enhancement of attentional performance by selective stimulation of alpha4beta2(*) nAChRs: underlying cholinergic mechanisms. *Neuropsychopharmacology* 35, 1391–1401. doi: 10.1038/npp.2010.9

Hurd, M. D., Martorell, P., and Langa, K. M. (2013). Monetary costs of dementia in the United States. *N. Engl. J. Med.* 369, 489–490. doi: 10.1056/nejmc1305541

Hussain, M., and Mehta, M. A. (2011). Cognitive enhancement by drugs in health and disease. *Trends Cogn. Sci.* 15, 28–36. doi: 10.1016/j.tics.2010.11.002

Ishizuka, T., Murotani, T., and Yamatodani, A. (2010). Modanifil activates the histaminergic system through the orexinergic neurons. *Neurosci. Lett.* 483, 193–196. doi: 10.1016/j.neulet.2010.08.005

Jack, A. J. (2011). The impact of physical and mental activity on cognitive aging. *Curr. Top. Behav. Neurosci.* 10, 273–291. doi: 10.1007/7854_2011_141

Jaeggi, S. M., Buschkuehl, M., Jonides, J., and Perrig, W. J. (2008). Improving fluid intelligence with training on working memory. *Proc. Natl. Acad. Sci. U S A* 105, 6829–6833. doi: 10.1073/pnas.0801268105

Jiang, L., and Role, L. W. (2008). Facilitation of cortico-amygdala synapses by nicotine: activitydependent modulation of glutamatergic transmission. *J. Neurophysiol.* 99, 1988–1999. doi: 10.1152/jn.00933.2007

Kerr, A. L., Steuer, E. L., Pochtarev, V., and Swain, R. A. (2010). Angiogenesis but not neurogenesis is critical for normal learning and memory acquisition. *Neuroscience* 171, 214–226. doi: 10.1016/j.neuroscience.2010.08.008

Kimberg, D. Y., D'Esposito, M., and Farah, M. J. (1997). Effects of bromocriptine on human subjects depend on working memory capacity. *Neuroreport* 8, 3581–3585. doi: 10.1097/00001756-199711100-00032

Klusmann, V., Evers, A., Schwarzer, R., Schlattmann, P., Reischies, F. M., Heuser, I., et al. (2010). Complex mental and physical activity in older women and cognitive performance: a 6-month randomized controlled trial. *J. Gerontol. A Biol. Sci. Med. Sci.* 65, 680–688. doi: 10.1093/gerona/glq053

Kramer, A. F., Colcombe, S. J., McAuley, E., Eriksen, K. I., Scalf, P., Jerome, G. J., et al. (2003). Enhancing brain and cognitive function of older adults through fitness training. *J. Mol. Neurosci.* 20, 213–221. doi: 10.1385/jmn:20:3:213

Lanni, C., Racchi, M., Uberti, D., Mazzini, G., Stanga, S., Sinforiani, E., et al. (2008). Pharmacogenetics and pharmagenomics, trends in normal and pathological aging studies: focus on p53. *Curr. Pharm. Des.* 14, 2665–2671. doi: 10.2174/138161208786264133

Lauterborn, J. C., Lynch, G., Vanderklish, P., Arai, A., and Gall, C. M. (2000). Positive modulation of AMPA receptors increases neurotrophin expression by hippocampal and cortical neurons. *J. Neurosci.* 20, 8–21.

Lauterborn, J. C., Truong, G. S., Baudry, M., Bi, X., Lynch, G., and Gall, C. M. (2003). Chronic elevation of brain-derived neurotrophic factor by ampakines. *J. Pharmacol. Exp. Ther.* 307, 297–305. doi: 10.1124/jpet.103.053694

Legutko, B., Li, X., and Skolnick, P. (2001). Regulation of BDNF expression in primary neuron culture by LY392098, a novel AMPA receptor potentiator. *Neuropharmacology* 40, 1019–1027. doi: 10.1016/s0028-3908(01)00006-5

Loughead, J., Ray, R., Wileyto, E. P., Ruparel, K., Sanborn, P., Siegel, S., et al. (2010). Effects of the alpha4beta2 partial agonist varenicline on brain activity and working memory in abstinent smokers. *Biol. Psychiatry* 67, 715–721. doi: 10.1016/j.biopsych.2010.01.016

Lynch, G. (2002). Memory enhancement: the search for mechanism-based drugs. *Nat. Neurosci.* 5(Suppl. 1), 1035–1038. doi: 10.1038/nn935

Lynch, G. (2004). AMPA receptor modulators as cognitive enhancers. *Curr. Opin. Pharmacol.* 4, 4–11. doi: 10.1016/j.coph.2003.09.009

Lynch, G., and Gall, C. M. (2006). Ampakines and the threefold path to cognitive enhancement. *Trends Neurosci.* 29, 554–562. doi: 10.1016/j.tins.2006.07.007

Lynch, M. A., and Mills, K. H. (2012). Immunology meets neuroscience–opportunities for immune intervention in neurodegenerative diseases. *Brain Behav. Immun.* 26, 1–10. doi: 10.1016/j.bbi.2011.05.013

Lynch, G., Palmer, L. C., and Gall, C. M. (2011). The likelihood of cognitive enhancement. *Pharmacol. Biochem. Behav.* 99, 116–129. doi: 10.1016/j.pbb.2010.12.024

Madras, B. K., Xie, Z., Lin, Z., Jassen, A., Panas, H., Lynch, L., et al. (2006). Modafinil occupies dopamine and norepinephrine transporters in vivo and modulates the transporters and trace amine activity in vitro. *J. Pharmacol. Exp. Ther.* 319, 561–569. doi: 10.1124/jpet.106.106583

Maillot, P., Perrot, A., and Hartley, A. (2012). Effects of interactive physical-activity video-game training on physical and cognitive function in older adults. *Psychol. Aging* 27, 589–600. doi: 10.1037/a0026268

Marchant, N. L., King, S. L., Tabet, N., and Rusted, J. M. (2010). Positive effects of cholinergic stimulation favor young APOE epsilon4 carriers. *Neuropsychopharmacology* 35, 1090–1096. doi: 10.1038/npp.2009.214

McGeer, E. G., Peppard, R. P., McGeer, P. L., Tuokko, H., Crockett, D., Parks, R., et al. (1990). 18Fluorodeoxyglucose positron emission tomography studies in presumed Alzheimer cases, including 13 serial scans. *Can. J. Neurol. Sci.* 17, 1–11.

Mehta, M. A., Owen, A. M., Sahakian, B. J., Mavaddat, N., Pickard, J. D., and Robbins, T. W. (2000). Methylphenidate enhances working memory by modulating discrete frontal and parietal lobe regions in the human brain. *J. Neurosci.* 20:RC65.

Middleton, L. E., Barnes, D. E., Lui, L. Y., and Yaffe, K. (2010). Physical activity over the life course and its association with cognitive performance and impairment in old age. *J. Am. Geriatr. Soc.* 58, 1322–1326. doi: 10.1111/j.1532-5415.2010.02903.x

Miller, K. J., Dye, R. V., Kim, J., Jennings, J. L., O'Toole, E., Wong, J., et al. (2013). Effect of a computerized brain exercise program on cognitive performance in older adults. *Am. J. Geriatr. Psychiatry* 21, 655–663. doi: 10.1016/j.jagp.2013.01.077

Minzenberg, M. J., and Carter, C. S. (2008). Modafinil: a review of neurochemical actions and effects on cognition. *Neuropsychopharmacology* 33, 1477–1502. doi: 10.1038/sj.npp.1301534

Mora, F. (2013). Successful brain aging: plasticity, environmental enrichment and lifestyle. *Dialogues Clin. Neurosci.* 15, 45–52.

Mozolic, J. L., Long, A. B., Morgan, A. R., Rawley-Payne, M., and Laurienti, P. J. (2011). A cognitive training intervention improves modality-specific attention in a randomized controlled trial of healthy older adults. *Neurobiol. Aging* 32, 655–668. doi: 10.1016/j.neurobiolaging.2009.04.013

Muller, U., Steffenhagen, N., Regenthal, R., and Bublak, P. (2004). Effects of modafinil on working memory processes in humans. *Psychopharmacology (Berl)* 177, 161–169. doi: 10.1007/s00213-004-1926-3

Nouchi, R., Taki, Y., Takeuchi, H., Hashizume, H., Nozawa, T., Kambara, T., et al. (2012). Brain training game improves executive functions and processing speed in the elderly: a randomized controlled trial. *PLoS One* 7:e29676. doi: 10.1371/journal.pone.0029676

O'Neill, M. J., Bleakman, D., Zimmerman, D. M., and Nisenbaum, E. S. (2004). AMPA receptor potentiators for the treatment of CNS disorders. *Curr. Drug Targets CNS Neurol. Disord.* 3, 181–194. doi: 10.2174/1568007043337508

O'Neill, M. J., Murray, T. K., Clay, M. P., Lindstrom, T., Yang, C. R., and Nisenbaum, E. S. (2005). LY503430: pharmacology, pharmacokinetics and effects in rodent models of Parkinson's disease. *CNS Drug Rev.* 11, 77–96. doi: 10.1111/j.1527-3458.2005.tb00037.x

Oswald, W., Gunzelmann, T., Rupprecht, R., and Hagen, B. (2006). Differential effects of single versus combined cognitive and physical training with older adults: the SimA study in a 5-year perspective. *Eur. J. Ageing* 3, 179–192. doi: 10.1007/s10433-006-0035-z

Park, D. C., and Bischof, G. N. (2013). The aging mind: neuroplasticity in response to cognitive training. *Dialogues Clin. Neurosci.* 15, 109–119. doi: 10.1016/b978-0-12-380882-0.00007-3

Pascual-Leone, A., Amedi, A., Fregni, F., and Merabet, L. B. (2005). The plastic human brain cortex. *Annu. Rev. Neurosci.* 28, 377–401. doi: 10.1016/j.cortex.2014.06.001

Peretz, C., Korczyn, A. D., Shatil, E., Aharonson, V., Birnboim, S., and Giladi, N. (2011). Computer-based, personalized cognitive training versus classical computer games: a randomized double-blind prospective trial of cognitive stimulation. *Neuroepidemiology* 36, 91–99. doi: 10.1159/000323950

Pieramico, V., Esposito, R., Sensi, F., Cilli, F., Mantini, D., Mattei, P. A., et al. (2012). Combination training in aging individuals modifies functional connectivity and cognition and is potentially affected by dopamine-related genes. *PLoS One* 7:e43901. doi: 10.1371/journal.pone.0043901

Porrino, L. J., Daunais, J. B., Rogers, G. A., Hampson, R. E., and Deadwyler, S. A. (2005). Facilitation of task performance and removal of the effects of sleep deprivation by an ampakine (CX717) in nonhuman primates. *PLoS Biol.* 3:e299. doi: 10.1371/journal.pbio.0030299

Pozo, K., and Goda, Y. (2010). Unraveling mechanisms of homeostatic synaptic plasticity. *Neuron* 66, 337–351. doi: 10.1016/j.neuron.2010.04.028

Raichle, M. E., and Mintun, M. A. (2006). Brain work and brain imaging. *Annu. Rev. Neurosci.* 29, 449–476. doi: 10.1146/annurev.neuro.29.051605.112819

Randall, D. C., Shneerson, J. M., and File, S. E. (2005). Cognitive effects of modafinil in student volunteers may depend on IQ. *Pharmacol. Biochem. Behav.* 82, 133–139. doi: 10.1016/j.pbb.2005.07.019

Raschetti, R., Albanese, E., Vanacore, N., and Maggini, M. (2007). Cholinesterase inhibitors in mild cognitive impairment: a systematic review of randomised trials. *PLoS Med.* 4:e338. doi: 10.1371/journal.pmed.0040338

Richmond, L. L., Morrison, A. B., Chein, J. M., and Olson, I. R. (2011). Working memory training and transfer in older adults. *Psychol. Aging* 26, 813–822. doi: 10.1037/a0023631

Roesler, R. (2011). Cognitive enhancers: focus on modulatory signaling influencing memory consolidation. *Pharmacol. Biochem. Behav.* 99, 155–163. doi: 10.1016/j.pbb.2010.12.028

Roses, A. D. (2008). Pharmacogenetics in drug discovery and development: a translational perspective. *Nat. Rev. Drug Discov.* 7, 807–817. doi: 10.1038/nrd2593

Sarter, M. (2006). Preclinical research into cognition enhancers. *Trends Pharmacol. Sci.* 27, 602–608. doi: 10.1016/j.tips.2006.09.004

Scarmeas, N., Zarahn, E., Anderson, K. E., Habeck, C. G., Hilton, J., Flynn, J., et al. (2003). Association of life activities with cerebral blood flow in Alzheimer disease: implications for the cognitive reserve hypothesis. *Arch. Neurol.* 60, 359–365. doi: 10.1001/archneur.60.3.359

Schitine, C., Xapelli, S., Agasse, F., Sardà-Arroyo, L., Silva, A. P., De Melo Reis, R. A., et al. (2012). Ampakine CX546 increases proliferation and neuronal differentiation in subventricular zone stem/progenitor cell cultures. *Eur. J. Neurosci.* 35, 1672–1683. doi: 10.1111/j.1460-9568.2012.08072.x

Schneider, N., and Yvon, C. (2013). A review of multidomain interventions to support healthy cognitive ageing. *J. Nutr. Health Aging* 17, 252–257. doi: 10.1007/s12603-012-0402-8

Shatil, E. (2013). Does combined cognitive training and physical activity training enhance cognitive abilities more than either alone? A four-condition randomized controlled trial among healthy older adults. *Front. Aging Neurosci.* 5:8. doi: 10.3389/fnagi.2013.00008

Simon, P., Hémet, C., Ramassamy, C., and Costentin, J. (1995). Non-amphetaminic mechanism of stimulant locomotor effect of modafinil in mice. *Eur. Neuropsychopharmacol.* 5, 509–514. doi: 10.1016/0924-977x(95)00041-m

Simpson, T., Camfield, D., Pipingas, A., Macpherson, H., and Stough, C. (2012). Improved processing speed: online computer-based cognitive training in older adults. *Educ. Gerontol.* 38, 445–458. doi: 10.1080/03601277.2011.559858

Smith, P. J., Blumenthal, J. A., Hoffman, B. M., Cooper, H., Strauman, T. A., Welsh-Bohmer, K., et al. (2010). Aerobic exercise and neurocognitive performance: a meta-analytic review of randomized controlled trials. *Psychosom. Med.* 72, 239–252. doi: 10.1097/psy.0b013e3181d14633

Stern, Y. (2009). Cognitive reserve. *Neuropsychologia* 47, 2015–2028. doi: 10.1016/j.neuropsychologia.2009.03.004

Stern, Y., Alexander, G. E., Prohovnik, I., Stricks, L., Link, B., Lennon, M. C., et al. (1995). Relationship between lifetime occupation and parietal flow: implications for a reserve against Alzheimer's disease pathology. *Neurology* 45, 55–60. doi: 10.1212/wnl.45.1.55

Stern, Y., Habeck, C., Moeller, J., Scarmeas, N., Anderson, K. E., Hilton, H. J., et al. (2005). Brain networks associated with cognitive reserve in healthy young and old adults. *Cereb. Cortex* 15, 394–402. doi: 10.1093/cercor/bhh142

Stone, E. A., Cotecchia, S., Lin, Y., and Quartermain, D. (2002). Role of brain alpha 1B-adrenoceptors in modafinil-induced behavioral activity. *Synapse* 46, 269–270. doi: 10.1002/syn.10127

Szelag, E., and Skolimowska, J. (2012). Cognitive function in elderly can be ameliorated by training in temporal information processing. *Restor. Neurol. Neurosci.* 30, 419–434. doi: 10.3233/RNN-2012-120240

Turner, D. C., Robbins, T. W., Clark, L., Aron, A. R., Dowson, J., and Sahakian, B. J. (2003). Cognitive enhancing effects of modafinil in healthy volunteers. *Psychopharmacology (Berl)* 165, 260–269.

Urban, K. R., and Gao, W. J. (2014). Performance enhancement at the cost of potential brain plasticity: neural ramifications of nootropic drugs in the healthy developing brain. *Front. Syst. Neurosci.* 8:38. doi: 10.3389/fnsys.2014.00038

Vallesi, A., McIntosh, A. R., and Stuss, D. T. (2011). Overrecruitment in the aging brain as a function of task demands: evidence for a compensatory view. *J. Cogn. Neurosci.* 23, 801–815. doi: 10.1162/jocn.2010.21490

van Praag, H., Kempermann, G., and Gage, F. H. (2000). Neural consequences of environmental enrichment. *Nat. Rev. Neurosci.* 1, 191–198. doi: 10.1038/35044558

Vaughan, S., Morris, N., Shum, D., O'Dwyer, S., and Polit, D. (2012). Study protocol: a randomised controlled trial of the effects of a multi-modal exercise program on cognition and physical functioning in older women. *BMC Geriatr.* 12:60. doi: 10.1186/1471-2318-12-60

Vincent, J. L., Kahn, I., Snyder, A. Z., Raichle, M. E., and Buckner, R. L. (2008). Evidence for a frontoparietal control system revealed by intrinsic functional connectivity. *J. Neurophysiol.* 100, 3328–3342. doi: 10.1152/jn.90355.2008

Volkow, N. D., Fowler, J. S., Logan, J., Alexoff, D., Zhu, W., Telang, F., et al. (2009). Effects of modafinil on dopamine and dopamine transporters in the male human brain: clinical implications. *JAMA* 301, 1148–1154. doi: 10.1001/jama.2009.351

Volkow, N. D., Wang, G. J., Fowler, J. S., Gatley, S. J., Logan, J., Ding, Y. S., et al. (1998). Dopamine transporter occupancies in the human brain induced by therapeutic doses of oral methylphenidate. *Am. J. Psychiatry.* 155, 1325–1331.

Voss, M. W., Vivar, C., Kramer, A. F., and van Praag, H. (2013). Bridging animal and human models of exercise-induced brain plasticity. *Trends Cogn. Sci.* 17, 525–544. doi: 10.1016/j.tics.2013.08.001

Wezenberg, E., Verkes, R. J., Ruigt, G. S., Hulstijn, W., and Sabbe, B. G. (2007). Acute effects of the ampakinefarampator on memory and information processing in healthy elderly volunteers. *Neuropsychopharmacology* 32, 1272–1283. doi: 10.1038/sj.npp.1301257

Wezenberg, E., Verkes, R. J., Sabbe, B. G., Ruigt, G. S., and Hulstijn, W. (2005). Modulation of memory and visuospatial processes by biperiden and rivastigmine in elderly healthy subjects. *Psychopharmacology (Berl)* 181, 582–594. doi: 10.1007/s00213-005-0083-7

Whitlock, L. A., Collins, A. C., and Allaire, J. C. (2012). Individual differences in response to cognitive training: using a multi-modal, attentionally demanding game-based intervention for older adults. *Comput. Human Behav.* 28, 1091–1096. doi: 10.1016/j.chb.2012.01.012

Wild-Wall, N., Falkenstein, M., and Gajewski, P. D. (2012). Neural correlates of changes in a visual search task due to cognitive training in seniors. *Neural Plast.* 2012:529057. doi: 10.1155/2012/529057

Wilson, R. S., Li, Y., Aggarwal, N. T., Barnes, L. L., McCann, J. J., Gilley, D. W., et al. (2004). Education and the course of cognitive decline in Alzheimer disease. *Neurology* 63, 1198–1202. doi: 10.1212/01.wnl.0000140488.65299.53

Wittenberg, G. F. (2010). Experience, cortical remapping and recovery in brain disease. *Neurobiol. Dis.* 37, 252–258. doi: 10.1016/j.nbd.2009.09.007

Wood, S., Sage, J. R., Shuman, T., and Anagnostaras, S. G. (2013). Psychostimulants and cognition: a continuum of behavioral and cognitive activation. *Pharmacol. Rev.* 66, 193–221. doi: 10.1124/pr.112.007054

Xerri, C. (2008). Imprinting of idiosyncratic experience in cortical sensory maps: neural substrates of representational remodeling and correlative perceptual changes. *Behav. Brain Res.* 192, 26–141. doi: 10.1016/j.bbr.2008.02.038

Yerkes, R. M., and Dodson, J. D. (1908). The relation of strength of stimulus to rapidity of habit-formation. *J. Comp. Neurol. Psychol.* 18, 459–482. doi: 10.1002/cne.920180503

Yesavage, J. A., Mumenthaler, M. S., Taylor, J. L., Friedman, L., O'Hara, R., Sheikh, J., et al. (2002). Donepezil and flight simulator performance: effects on retention of complex skills. *Neurology* 59, 123–125. doi: 10.1212/wnl.59.1.123

Zelinski, E. M., Spina, L. M., Yaffe, K., Ruff, R., Kennison, R. F., Mahncke, H. W., et al. (2011). Improvement in memory with plasticity-based adaptive cognitive training: results of the 3-month follow-up. *J. Am. Geriatr. Soc.* 59, 258–265. doi: 10.1111/j.1532-5415.2010.03277.x

Zolkowska, D., Jain, R., Rothman, R. B., Partilla, J. S., Roth, B. L., Setola, V., et al. (2009). Evidence for the involvement of dopamine transporters in behavioral stimulant effects of modafinil. *J. Pharmacol. Exp. Ther.* 329, 738–746. doi: 10.1124/jpet.108.146142

14

Large-scale resting state network correlates of cognitive impairment in Parkinson's disease and related dopaminergic deficits

Alexander V. Lebedev[1]*, Eric Westman[2], Andrew Simmons[3,4], Aleksandra Lebedeva[2], Françoise J. Siepel[1], Joana B. Pereira[2] and Dag Aarsland[1,2]

[1] *Department of Psychiatry, Centre for Age-Related Medicine, Stavanger University Hospital, Stavanger, Norway*
[2] *Department of Neurobiology, Care Sciences and Society, Karolinska Institutet, Stockholm, Sweden*
[3] *Department of Neuroimaging, Institute of Psychiatry, King's College London, London, UK*
[4] *NIHR Biomedical Research Centre for Mental Health and Biomedical Research Unit for Dementia, London, UK*

Edited by:
Mikhail Lebedev, Duke University, USA

Reviewed by:
Nicola B. Mercuri, University of Rome, Italy
Simon J. G. Lewis, Brain and Mind Research Institute, Australia
Andrew V. Poliakov, Seattle Children's Hospital, USA

***Correspondence:**
Alexander V. Lebedev, Department of Psychiatry, Centre for Age-Related Medicine, Stavanger University Hospital, Armauer Hansens vei 20, 4011 Stavanger, Norway
e-mail: alexander.vl.lebedev@gmail.com

Cognitive impairment is a common non-motor feature of Parkinson's disease (PD). Understanding the neural mechanisms of this deficit is crucial for the development of efficient methods for treatment monitoring and augmentation of cognitive functions in PD patients. The current study aimed to investigate resting state fMRI correlates of cognitive impairment in PD from a large-scale network perspective, and to assess the impact of dopamine deficiency on these networks. Thirty PD patients with resting state fMRI were included from the Parkinson's Progression Marker Initiative (PPMI) database. Eighteen patients from this sample were also scanned with ^{123}I-FP-CIT SPECT. A standardized neuropsychological battery was administered, evaluating verbal memory, visuospatial, and executive cognitive domains. Image preprocessing was performed using an SPM8-based workflow, obtaining time-series from 90 regions-of-interest (ROIs) defined from the AAL brain atlas. The Brain Connectivity Toolbox (BCT) was used to extract nodal strength from all ROIs, and modularity of the cognitive circuitry determined using the meta-analytical software Neurosynth. Brain-behavior covariance patterns between cognitive functions and nodal strength were estimated using Partial Least Squares. Extracted latent variable (LV) scores were matched with the performances in the three cognitive domains (memory, visuospatial, and executive) and striatal dopamine transporter binding ratios (SBR) using linear modeling. Finally, influence of nigrostriatal dopaminergic deficiency on the modularity of the "cognitive network" was analyzed. For the range of deficits studied, better executive performance was associated with increased dorsal fronto-parietal cortical processing and inhibited subcortical and primary sensory involvement. This profile was also characterized by a relative preservation of nigrostriatal dopaminergic function. The profile associated with better memory performance correlated with increased prefronto-limbic processing, and was not associated with presynaptic striatal dopamine uptake. SBR ratios were negatively correlated with modularity of the "cognitive network," suggesting integrative effects of the preserved nigrostriatal dopamine system on this circuitry.

Keywords: parkinson's disease, cognition, dopamine, resting state fMRI, SPECT, graph theory, nodal strength, modularity

INTRODUCTION

Cognitive impairment is a very important and common non-motor feature of Parkinson's disease (PD) with a major impact on patients' and caregivers' quality of life, as well as healthcare costs (Muslimovic et al., 2005; Vossius et al., 2011; Svenningsson et al., 2012). Approximately one-fifth of newly diagnosed PD patients fulfill clinical criteria for mild cognitive impairment (PD-MCI) (Aarsland et al., 2009) and about one-sixth develop dementia after 5 years (Williams-Gray et al., 2009).

Although the exact role and mechanisms of the dopaminergic system in cognition are still a matter of debate, there is no doubt that its preservation is crucial for cognitive functioning of PD patients. Thus, there is strong evidence suggesting that the impairment of at least 3 major dopaminergic pathways (nigrostriatal, mesocortical, mesolimbic) originating in the brainstem play a very important role in cognitive dysfunction associated with PD (Narayanan et al., 2013).

Previous neuroimaging studies assessing brain networks *in vivo* have shown impairment of the dopaminergic pathways and related neural circuits in PD. Numerous studies on cognitive dysfunction associated with PD have revealed structural and functional abnormalities within the cortico-strio-thalamo-cortical circuits, known to be largely modulated by the dopaminergic system (Hirano et al., 2012; Christopher and Strafella, 2013).

Decreased 6-[^{18}F]-fluorodopa (^{18}F-DOPA) uptake in the anterior cingulate cortex, ventral striatum and right caudate nucleus has been found in PD patients with dementia (PDD) compared to PD (Ito et al., 2002). Studies employing Single Photon Emission Computed Tomography (SPECT) with the dopamine transporter-binding ligands (DaTSCAN) also suggest more severe striatal presynaptic dopaminergic deficiency in PDD compared to PD patients, especially in the caudate nuclei (O'Brien et al., 2004). In addition, there is also evidence suggesting an association between striatal ^{18}F-DOPA uptake and executive performance in PD patients (Bruck et al., 2001; Cheesman et al., 2005; Cropley et al., 2008).

Several ^{18}F-fludeoxyglucose Positron Emission Tomography (FDG-PET) studies analyzing brain networks in PD have identified partially overlapping patterns of brain metabolic changes associated with cognitive impairment in multiple domains, suggesting that the PD-related profile of cognitive impairment is associated with reduced glucose metabolism mainly in prefrontal, parietal, hippocampal, and striatal regions (Mentis et al., 2002; Huang et al., 2007a,b; Eidelberg, 2009). $H_2^{15}O$-PET studies have shown an impaired basal ganglia and dorsolateral prefrontal response during executive task performance in PD (Owen et al., 1998; Dagher et al., 2001; Cools et al., 2002).

Functional MRI studies have also revealed abnormalities within the frontal-subcortical circuits in patients with PD. For instance, an abnormal fronto-striatal response during executive task performance has been found in cognitively impaired PD patients compared to non-impaired ones (Lewis et al., 2003). Another fMRI study assessing working memory and motor functions in ON and OFF dopaminergic medication states in PD patients (Mattay et al., 2002) found increased prefrontal and parietal activations during the working memory task performance in the OFF state, which were positively correlated with errors during the task. Studies focusing on set-shifting paradigms have found a PD-associated pattern of prefrontal and parietal response characterized by either reduced or increased activation depending on whether the caudate nucleus was involved in the task (Monchi et al., 2004, 2007).

Notably, a pharmacological fMRI study in healthy subjects revealed a significant effect of L-dopa administration on striatal functional connectivity (Kelly et al., 2009). In addition to its effects on motor networks, L-dopa increased functional connectivity between the ventral striatum and ventrolateral prefrontal cortex, and disrupted connectivity of the striatum with components of the default mode network (Kelly et al., 2009). Impaired deactivation of the default mode network during executive task performance has been reported in several fMRI studies of PD (Tinaz et al., 2008; Van Eimeren et al., 2009). Resting state fMRI studies have reported abnormal cortico-striatal connectivity in PD (Wu et al., 2009; Helmich et al., 2010; Kwak et al., 2010), while L-DOPA administration has been shown to enhance functional connectivity in the frontal areas of the sensorimotor network (Esposito et al., 2013).

The brain is a complex biological system that demonstrates emergent network properties on different scales, even at a cellular and single-structure level (Welsh et al., 2010). At the cellular scale, neocortical neurons are organized into sets of structurally and physiologically merged modules (Mountcastle, 1997), which in turn, are grouped into functionally segregated hypercolumns, wired with inter-modular connections. At the larger scale, system-wide coordination of the brain networks give rise to the coherent dynamic states that support cognitive functions and behavior (Sporns, 2013). Large-scale network architecture of the human brain appears to combine two principles of structural and functional organization. On the one hand, densely connected network modules or communities promote specialized processing and *functional segregation*. On the other hand, these specialized communities are interconnected via long-distance pathways that ensure efficient *functional integration* across multiple functional domains. Maintaining the balance between segregation and integration is thought to be essential for establishing complex network dynamics that support cognition (Sporns, 2010).

Recent advances in neuroscience and mathematical modeling have made it possible to apply classical concepts of graph theory to the analysis of brain network structure and dynamics (Rubinov and Sporns, 2010; Sporns, 2010). Graph-theoretical studies of structural and functional networks of the brain have revealed "small-world" properties (Achard and Bullmore, 2007), i.e., the coexistence of dense local connectivity with relatively sparse long-range connections. Such small-world networks combine high clustering with a relatively short path length between any pair of the elements (e.g., brain regions). The "small-world" model may be of functional importance as it balances functional segregation (high modularity or clustering) and functional integration (short path length) and thus offers a network architecture that may be well-suited for neuronal information processing (Sporns and Zwi, 2004).

To date, there are very few studies of PD employing graph theoretical framework for fMRI data analysis. Skidmore et al. found reduced whole-brain global efficiency in PD (Skidmore et al., 2011). Compared to healthy controls, 14 PD patients included in the study demonstrated reduced local efficiency (nodal level) in the precentral regions, primary and secondary visual cortex. Another recent study found global reduction of network-level processing efficacy in PD. Analysis of network modules indicated decreased interaction of the visual network with other brain modules, but abnormally increased connectivity within the sensorimotor network. The authors interpreted the latter as a compensatory mechanism aimed at overcoming the striato-cortical functional deficit within the motor loops, which may also be associated with loss of mutual inhibition between brain networks (Gottlich et al., 2013).

To the best of our knowledge, there are no previous studies assessing brain correlates of PD-related cognitive impairment employing both dopamine transporter imaging and fMRI with graph theory metrics.

In the present study, we assessed global and local network-level correlates of cognitive dysfunction and related dopaminergic impairment in PD using the graph theory metrics of nodal strength and modularity.

We hypothesized that the PD-related profile of cognitive impairment would be associated mainly with abnormalities within the fronto-subcortical (impaired cortico-striatal connectivity) and fronto-parietal circuits, which are closely related to nigrostriatal deficiency.

METHODS

The main workflow steps are illustrated in **Figure S1**.

INCLUSION AND EXCLUSION CRITERIA

We included all 30 subjects (31 minus one subject excluded during quality control due to "cuts" of dorsal cortical areas) with rs-fMRI enrolled in the Parkinson's Progression Marker Initiative (PPMI) (in total 452 PD patients), a multicenter study launched in 2010 designed to identify progression biomarkers in newly diagnosed PD patients (www.ppmi-info.org/data).

Inclusion criteria required that subjects must have at least two of the following symptoms: resting tremor, bradykinesia, rigidity or either asymmetric resting tremor or asymmetric bradykinesia. In addition, the subjects had to be drug naïve, Hoehn and Yahr stage I or II at baseline, and a screening ^{123}I-FP-CIT SPECT scan, sensitive to the loss of striatal dopamine transporter (DaT) binding.

Exclusion criteria were atypical PD syndromes due to drugs or metabolic disorders, encephalitis, or other degenerative diseases. In addition, it was required that the subject was not taking levodopa, DA agonists, MAO-B inhibitors, amantadine, or other PD medication; or had taken levodopa or dopamine agonists prior to baseline for more than a total of 60 days.

NEUROPSYCHOLOGICAL ASSESSMENT

In addition to a cognitive screening test, the Montreal Cognitive Assessment (MoCA), all subjects underwent a neuropsychological test battery developed to assess major cognitive domains affected by PD.

Visuospatial function was evaluated using the 15-item version of the Benton's Judgment of Line Orientation Test, which examines the ability of a subject to estimate angular relationships between line segments by visually matching angled line pairs to 11 numbered radii forming a semi-circle (Benton et al., 1978).

Verbal memory was assessed using the Hopkins Verbal Learning Test-Revised (HVLT-R) (Shapiro et al., 1999), which consists of presenting a list of 12 words over three learning trials. With each repetition, subjects are expected to learn additional words on the list and increase their performance with each trial. Total immediate recall or encoding (sum of trial 1–3) and delayed recall (after 20–25 min) scores were included in this study.

Executive functions were evaluated using three semantic fluency tests (names of animals, fruits, and vegetables, in 1 min each), the MoCA subtests of phonemic fluency (words that start from the letter "F," in 1 min) and alternating trail making (drawing a line, going from a number to a letter, in ascending order; score 0–1).

Attention was assessed by the Letter-Number Sequencing Test (LNST), in which a combination of numbers and letters is read to the subject who is then asked to recall the numbers, first in ascending order and then the letters in alphabetical order. The Symbol Digit Modalities Test (SDMT) was also used to assess attention, in which specific numbers had to be paired with geometric figures based on a reference key within 90 s.

COGNITIVE DOMAINS

Three cognitive domains were calculated based on the standardized tests for memory, visuospatial, and attention/executive functioning. Raw values were converted to z-scores using the mean and standard deviation of the healthy control group. Domain composite scores were calculated by averaging z-scores of the standardized tests in each cognitive domain.

In the *memory domain*, three learning trials and the delayed recall of HVLT-R were included. The *visuospatial domain* included the Benton judgment of line orientation. The *attention/executive domain* included the LNST, SDMT, semantic fluency, and the phonemic fluency test. No corrections were performed to adjust the tests scores for age or gender given that the subsequent analyses included these variables as nuisances.

Since the calculated composite scores for cognitive domains were scaled and reflected positive cognitive performance (the higher the score, the better functioning in a corresponding domain), we defined the "motor" domain by inverting and scaling UPDRS-III raw scores in order to achieve the same variable scale and direction (higher scores correspond to better motor function) when assessing and plotting the results.

AUTOMATED META-ANALYSIS IN NEUROSYNTH

In order to support our hypotheses and to objectively identify regions that are relevant for cognitive functions, an automated search using the meta-analytical software Neurosynth (http://neurosynth.org) was undertaken. This approach utilizes text-mining and machine-learning techniques to perform probabilistic mapping between neural and cognitive states (Yarkoni et al., 2011). In the present study, the Python-based version (https://github.com/neurosynth/neurosynth) was used. The database was accessed on 24.10.13, searching for the key-words "executive" (237 studies), "visuospatial" ($n = 116$) and "memory" ($n = 1470$).

After the search overlapping patterns were found between cognitive domains. They were in line with the regions that have revealed an association with cognitive impairment in PD highlighted in the introduction. Thus, the profile of visuospatial functions included prefrontal, parietal, and occipital regions. The "executive" pattern contained prefrontal [with more extended involvement of dorsolateral prefrontal cortex (DLPFC)], cingulate, superior parietal, temporo-occipital, basal ganglia, and cerebellar regions. Finally, the "memory" profile, in addition to prefrontal and parietal regions, also included hippocampus, temporal areas, and basal ganglia.

Due to the observed overlap, the resulting statistical maps were merged and overlaid with the Automated Anatomical Labeling (AAL) atlas in order to have an unbiased definition of ROIs associated with cognitive functions for further network analysis. The main steps of the meta-analysis and the resulting maps are illustrated in **Figure S2**.

MRI

Image acquisition

A standardized MRI protocol included acquisition of whole-brain structural and functional scans on 3 Tesla Siemens Trio Tim MR system. More details can be found in the MRI technical operations manual at http://www.ppmi-info.org/.

3D T1 structural images were acquired in a sagittal orientation using a MPRAGE GRAPPA protocol with Repetition Time (TR) = 2300 ms, Echo Time (TE) = 2.98 ms, Field of View (FoV) = 256 mm, Flip Angle (FA) = 9° and 1 mm^3 isotropic voxel.

For each subject, 212 BOLD echo-planar rs-fMRI images (40 slices each, ascending direction) were acquired during a 8 min, 29 s scanning session (acquisition parameters: $TR = 2400$ ms, $TE = 25$ ms, $FoV = 222$ mm, $FA = 80°$ and 3.3 mm^3 isotropic voxels). Subjects were instructed to rest quietly, keeping their eyes open and not to fall asleep.

^{123}I-FP-CIT SPECT

In the fMRI + DaTSCAN subgroup ($n = 18$), only those PD patients who had both fMRI and DaTSCAN acquired within less than a week interval were included.

Image acquisition was performed 4 ± 0.5 h after injection of ^{123}I-FP-CIT, a time-point at which striatal specific binding ratios are stable (Booij et al., 1999) with a target dose of 185 MBq. The radiopharmaceutical was provided as a unit dose and filled to a standard volume, which was re-assayed.

Raw projection data were acquired into a 128 × 128 matrix with steps of 3 or 4 degrees for the total projections. Image preprocessing (reconstruction, attenuation correction, spatial normalization) was performed using the Hermes software (Medical Solutions, Stockholm, Sweden) at a central SPECT Core lab in New Haven (Connecticut, United States). Specific binding ratios were calculated for the left and right caudate nuclei according to specific binding ratio = (L/R Caudate)/(Occipital area) − 1 and then averaged for further analysis.

IMAGE PREPROCESSING

As a first step, a population template was generated from the bias-corrected T1 structural images using the Diffeomorphic Anatomical Registration Through Exponentiated Lie Algebra (DARTEL) algorithm (Ashburner, 2007) in order to improve normalization quality.

For the fMRI data, two initial echo-planar volumes were automatically removed by the scanner software to minimize T1 effects on the T2* echo-planar images, and the remaining 210 volumes underwent preprocessing in the SPM8-based (http://www.fil.ion.ucl.ac.uk/spm) pipeline implemented in the Data Processing Assistant for Resting-State fMRI: Advanced Edition (DPARSFA, version 2.3) (Chao-Gan and Yu-Feng, 2010), installed within the MATLAB environment (Matlab 8.0 and Statistics Toolbox, 2012).

Next, functional images underwent the following preprocessing steps: spatial realignment and slice-timing correction, co-registration with the high-resolution structural scans. Finally, the co-registered BOLD volumes were normalized into standardized Montreal Neurological Institute (MNI) space using the DARTEL template and resampled to 3 mm^3 isotropic voxels. Spurious variance was reduced by a voxel-specific head motion correction (Satterthwaite et al., 2013) and by regressing-out time-series from the white matter and cerebrospinal fluid. Next, the images were band-pass filtered to eliminate biologically non-relevant signals (Biswal et al., 1995; Lowe et al., 1998) (it was not necessary to use large smoothing kernels due to a ROI-based framework implemented in the study), and the resulting low-frequency fluctuations were extracted from 90 regions-of-interest (ROIs) defined in the AAL atlas (Tzourio-Mazoyer et al., 2002) and were used in the subsequent network analysis (Rubinov and Sporns, 2010).

DATA ANALYSIS

Network analysis

The data analysis workflow was developed in order to assess both regional and global network-level correlates of presynaptic DAT uptake and cognitive functions. To do this, two metrics were selected: *nodal strength* (local measure) and *modularity* of a network (global measure).

Generalization of nodal strength and modularity for positive and negative connections

In binarized networks, the number of edges emanating from a particular node is known as its degree. For non-binarized networks, this metric has generalization called nodal strength (weighted degree), defined as the sum of neighboring link weights (Rubinov and Sporns, 2010).

Although the source of negative correlations in rs-fMRI is still a matter of debate (Fox et al., 2009; Murphy et al., 2009), there is strong evidence supporting a biological origin (Chang and Glover, 2009). In light of this, generalizations of several weighted graph theory metrics have been developed taking into account negative correlations (Rubinov and Sporns, 2011).

Thus, nodal strength can be calculated for positive and negative connections. The corresponding definition is straightforward:

$$S_i^{\pm} = \sum_{j \in N} w_{ij}^{\pm} \tag{1}$$

[Equation (1), adopted from Rubinov and Sporns, 2011] Where:

N—set of all nodes in the network;

(i, j)—link between nodes i and j $(i, j \in N)$, associated with connection weights w_{ij} $(0 < |w| < 1)$

Nodal strength can therefore be computed for both positive and negative weights (±). In our analysis, the total strength of both positive and negative weights was used.

A widely used metric for network modularity is formally defined as the fraction of the edges that are within a given set of communities minus the expected fraction of edges if the network was randomly wired (Newman, 2006). The metric therefore serves as a global large-scale network measure that allows quantification of the community structure of the brain. Higher modularity values for a particular network are generally associated with denser within-modular connections, but sparser connections between nodes that are in different modules.

Generalization of the modularity to both positive and negative correlations is more complex than nodal strength due to the differences in significance of positive and negative weights when determining modularity-partitions. Therefore, a non-symmetric generalization of network modularity has been proposed as:

$$Q^* = Q^+ + \frac{v^-}{v^+ + v^-} Q^- \quad (2a)$$

or more complete definition:

$$Q^* = \frac{1}{v^+} \sum_{ij} \left(w_{ij}^+ - e_{ij}^+ \right) \delta_{M_i M_j} - \frac{v^-}{v^+ + v^-} \sum_{ij} \left(w_{ij}^- - e_{ij}^- \right) \delta_{M_i M_j} \quad (2b)$$

Both equations are adopted from Rubinov and Sporns (2011)

Where:

$Q^{\pm}$—modularity;

$\left(w_{ij}^{\pm} - e_{ij}^{\pm} \right)$—difference between present within-module connection weights w and chance-expected within-module connection weights e;

$\delta_{M_i M_j} = 1$, when i and j are in the same module and $\delta_{M_i M_j} = 0$ otherwise.

$v^{\pm} = \sum_{i \in N} s_i^{\pm}$—total weight (the sum of all positive or negative weights)

The Brain Connectivity Toolbox (BCT, http://www.brain-connectivity-toolbox.net) (Rubinov and Sporns, 2010) was used to compute the described measures. Of note, connectivity matrices were neither thresholded nor binarized. Instead we employed a strategy that aimed to analyze weighted graphs by taking into account both positive and negative weights.

Next, the analysis proceeded in two directions with the aim of assessing local and global network-level correlates of cognitive functioning in PD and the impact of nigrostriatal dopaminergic deficiency on these networks.

All statistical analyses were performed using the R programming language, version 3.0.1 (R Core Team, 2013).

Dimensionality reduction: covariance patterns between nodal strength and cognitive functions

Partial Least Squares Regression (PLSR) was performed to reduce the dimensionality of the data, estimating latent components associated with composite scores for each domain (executive, memory, visuospatial).

PLSR is an effective data-driven method that allows high-dimensional associations between explanatory and response variables to be reduced into a small set of latent variables (LVs) (Wold et al., 1984). After decomposition, each of the LVs represents a distinct pattern of brain–behavior associations.

The following elements of these components were of particular interest in our study: (1) eigenvector (loadings) showing the degree to which a given LV contributes to the variance within the X-matrix (in our case, brain network measures), and (2) a set of scores representing a transform of a particular data-point into a latent component's space (the degree to which a given component is "represented" in a particular subject).

The models were assessed with leave-one-out cross-validation. As a result, 3 LVs minimizing total Root Mean Squared Error Prediction (RMSEP) for all 3 domains were selected. For details, see **Figure S3**. Individual LV scores were subsequently correlated with 3 cognitive domains using motor function, age, and sex as nuisance covariates.

GLM formula:

$$\begin{aligned} LV_N\text{−score} \sim & \text{(executive domain)} + \text{(memory domain)} \\ & + \text{(visuospatial domain)} + \text{(motor domain)} \\ & + \text{(age)} + \text{(sex)}. \end{aligned} \quad (3)$$

Finally, the scores were correlated with mean caudate DaT binding ratios in order to investigate which of them were influenced by nigrostriatal dopamine deficiency. The analysis was focused only on the caudate nuclei (without putamen), as this striatal structure is well-documented to be involved in cognition.

Due to the concerns regarding potential influence of motion artifacts, in addition to a voxel-specific correction strategy (Satterthwaite et al., 2013), analysis of motion with respect to the variables of interest (cognitive, motor domains, and age) was also performed. For this purpose, first principal component extracted from the absolute mean displacement values (x, y, and z axes) as well as relative displacements were used.

None of our variables of interest (executive, memory, and visuospatial domains) demonstrated significant association. The only significant associations were found for the motor domain ($p_{\text{mean displacement}} = 0.036$; $p_{\text{relative displacement}} = 0.035$) and age ($p_{\text{mean displacement}} = 0.026$), as expected. These variables were included in the modes as nuisance covariates.

Impact of nigrostriatal deficiency on the modularity of cognitive brain circuitry

For the second part, adjacency matrices were constructed using 60 AAL ROIs identified during the meta-analysis step (see Meta-Analysis section and **Figure S2**). Next, modularity was estimated based on both negative and positive weights [as described in Equations 2a and 2b].

Finally, an association between network modularity and mean DaT uptake in the caudate nuclei was analyzed using linear modeling.

RESULTS

DEMOGRAPHICS AND CLINICAL DATA

Demographics and clinical characteristics are shown in **Table 1**.

The data were representative of the entire DaTSCAN cohort of PD patients (results not shown). Of note, visuospatial functions were relatively less affected than executive and memory domains.

GRAPH THEORETICAL ANALYSIS

Brain-behavior covariance patterns

The analysis was performed with PLS LV-scores determined after the dimensionality reduction step (see corresponding Methods section).

Nodal strength

The first PLS LV captured global effects. Its higher scores were associated with higher strength of all 90 nodes with largest effects on motor, prefrontal cortices, and striatum. On a behavioral level,

Table 1 | Demographics and clinical data.

	Complete sample ($n = 30$)		Subsample* ($n = 18$)	
	Mean [±SD]	Median (range)	Mean [±SD]	Median (range)
Age	61.67 [±9.46]	62 (40–75)	60.11 [±9.04]	61 (44–75)
MoCA	26.67 [±3]	27 (15–30)	26.72 [±3.5]	27 (15–30)
ExecDom	−0.254 [±0.73]	−0.125 (−1.37–1.26)	−0.297 [±0.67]	−0.125 (−1.35–0.99)
MemDom	−0.51 [±1.2]	−0.41 (−2.81–1.47)	−0.73 [±1.26]	−0.51 (−2.81–1.25)
VspDom	0.06 [±0.78]	−0.06 (−1.57–0.95)	0.08 [±0.84]	0.44 (−1.57–0.95)
UPDRS III	20.2 [±10.6]	17 (7–47)	19.83 [±10.9]	17 (7–47)

Male/Female ratio was 2:1.

**Subsample of subjects who had both fMRI and DaTSCAN acquired within less than a week interval.*

MoCA, the Montreal Cognitive Assessment; ExecDom, "Executive" domain; MemDom, "Memory" domain; VspDom, "Visuospatial" domain; UPDRS III, part III of the Unified Parkinson's Disease Rating Scale.

Table 2 | Associations between component scores and behavioral data: nodal strength.

	Executive			Memory			Visuospatial			Motor		
	T	DOF	*p*	*T*	DOF	*p*	*T*	DOF	*p*	*T*	DOF	*p*
LV I	0.782	29	0.442	1.35	29	0.19	−0.89	29	0.383	3	29	0.006
LV II	−0.656	29	0.518	−2.45	29	0.022	−1.74	29	0.094	1.327	29	0.127
LV III	3.21	29	0.004	−1.74	29	0.096	1.65	29	0.113	−2.02	29	0.055

The table shows associations between latent variable (LV) scores extracted from the nodal strength data and performance in 3 cognitive (executive, memory, visuospatial) and motor domains. Positive significant associations are depicted in red and negative ones in blue.

In total, 3 models were fitted with component scores as dependent variables, cognitive domains as independent variables (other covariates: motor domain score [also shown here as an important confounder], age and sex).

***T**, t-statistics; **DOF**, degrees of freedom.*

this component was positively associated with motor function (see **Table 2**, **Figure 1**).

The second LV was associated with higher degree of posterior (supramarginal, superior parietal, posterior cingulate, occipital regions) and striatal nodes, and lower prefronto-limbic (orbitofrontal, anterior cingulate, parahippocampal, temporopolar regions) nodal strength (except for operculo-triangular, middle frontal areas, and left hippocampus, which demonstrated positive associations). Behaviorally, this component displayed a negative association with memory function, that is to say that better memory performance was associated with reversed component pattern, favoring the involvement of prefronto-limbic nodes (see **Table 2**, **Figure 1**).

The third LV, in turn, favored cortical-subcortical segregation with positive associations found in dorsal cortical nodes (dorsolateral prefrontal, frontal and parietal areas) and negative in subcortical structures (hippocampi, striatum, globus pallidus), primary visual, middle temporal, and paralimbic (ventral prefrontal) areas. Higher scores of this component were associated with better executive performance (see **Table 2**, **Figure 1**).

Latent variable scores and caudate DaT uptake

Analysis of the effects of nigrostriatal dopaminergic deficiency on the LVs estimated from the nodal strength revealed significant positive associations of mean caudate SBR ratios with I and III LV-scores (See **Table 3**, **Figure 2**).

This means that higher caudate DaT binding is associated with global increase of nodal strength and segregation toward more active dorsal cortical processing when the subject is at rest.

Modularity of the cognitive circuitry and caudate DaT binding

The analysis revealed negative effects of the preserved dopaminergic function on modularity of the cognitive circuit ($T = -3.6$, 17 DOF, $p = 0.002$), suggesting greater integration among regions within this network (see **Figure 3**).

DISCUSSION

To the best of our knowledge, this is the first study to assess large-scale network correlates of PD-related cognitive impairment and presynaptic dopaminergic deficiency, combining rs-fMRI and DaTSCAN. Higher executive functional scores were associated with higher nodal strength of dorsal cortical nodes (predominantly in dorsolateral prefrontal, premotor, and superior parietal regions) and lower involvement of subcortical, occipital, temporal, and ventral cortical nodes, suggesting that relative preservation of executive functions in PD is linked to the dominance of dorsal cortical processing with inhibition of subcortical, paralimbic, and primary sensory circuitry when the subject is at resting state with eyes open. This pattern was positively influenced by higher nigrostriatal dopaminergic function.

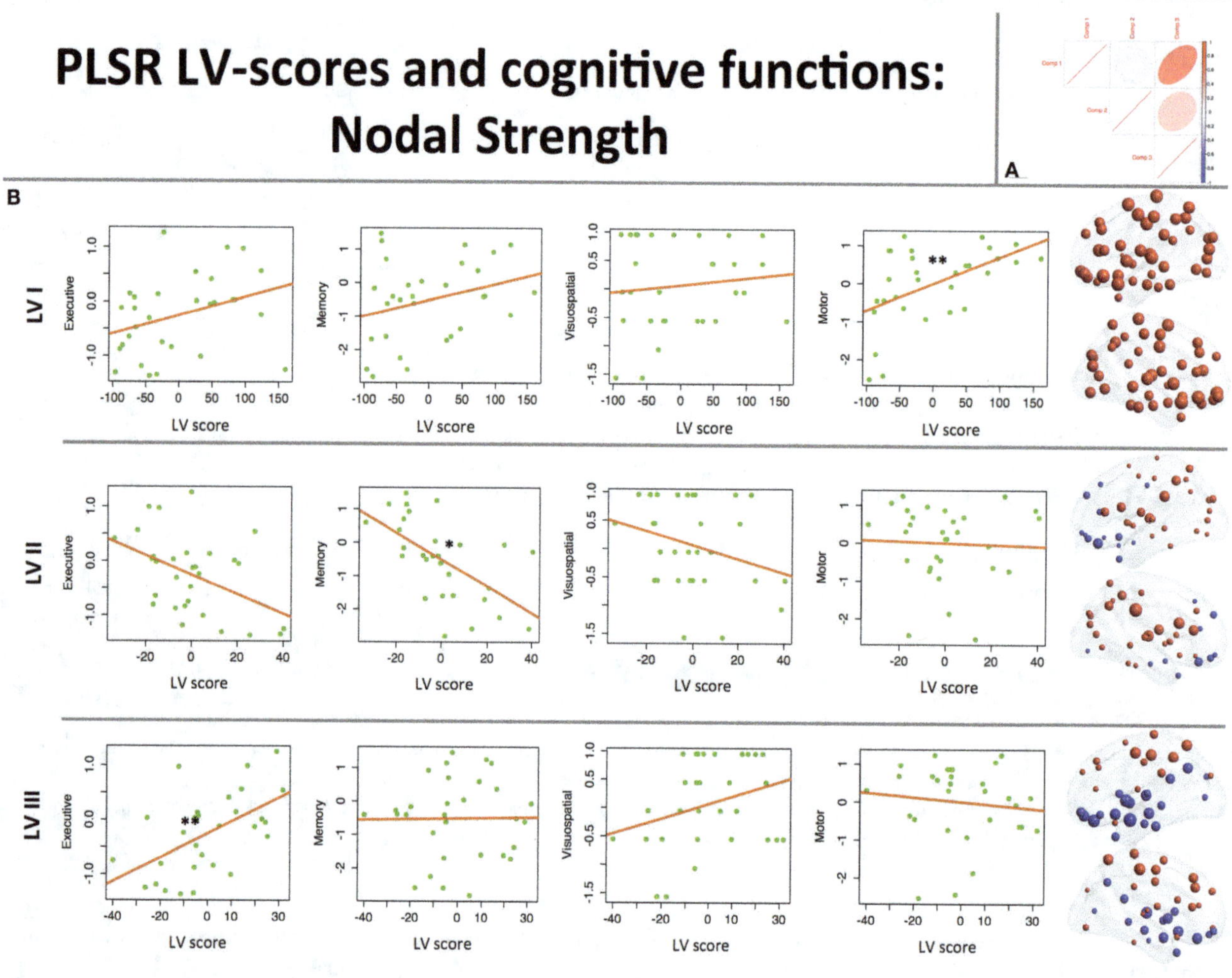

FIGURE 1 | Associations between component scores and behavioral data: nodal strength. (A) Between-component correlation plot. Positive association ($r = 0.5$) was found between latent variables (LVs) I and III. **(B)** Associations between LV scores extracted from the nodal strength data and performance in 3 cognitive (executive, memory, visuospatial) and motor domains. On the right-hand side of the graph, corresponding loading maps are depicted in brain space, reflecting the relevance of the nodes (spheres) for a particular LV, the magnitude of which is represented by nodal size. Positive loading values are depicted as red spheres, whereas negative ones are shown in blue. $^{*}p < 0.05$, $^{**}p < 0.01$.

Our results are consistent with an abnormally increased fronto-striatal connectivity found in a single-blind placebo-controlled rs-fMRI study of PD patients (Kwak et al., 2010), in which this hyperconnectivity was down-regulated by L-DOPA administration. Further analysis in this study revealed PD-related increase of power in the low-frequency band (0.02–0.05 Hz) in the striatum, which was also reduced after L-DOPA administration. Of note, this reduction correlated with L-DOPA-associated cognitive improvement. Apart from this, an increase in spontaneous oscillatory activity in the 10–35 Hz range (beta frequency band), occurring within the basal ganglia-thalamocortical networks and suppressed by dopaminergic treatment, is a well-replicated pathophysiological finding in PD (Brown et al., 2001; Levy et al., 2002; Gatev et al., 2006; Hammond et al., 2007), which provides additional support of our results converging from other imaging modalities.

The pattern associated with higher scores in the memory domain favoring prefronto-limbic processing did not reveal associations with presynaptic striatal dopamine uptake in the present study. The latter suggests that other mechanisms may be involved in the development of memory impairment associated with PD. The most likely ones are mesocortical dopaminergic deficiency (Narayanan et al., 2013) and impaired cortical cholinergic function (Bohnen et al., 2003), which in turn may at least be partly associated with concomitant cortical atrophy (Weintraub et al., 2012).

Of note, our study did not find any correlates of visuospatial impairment. However, this finding may be influenced by small sample size and due to the fact that visuospatial function was only mildly affected in the present cohort.

According to Mink's hypothesis (Mink, 1996), the basal ganglia play a crucial role in sustaining the balance between facilitation and suppression of movements. If we consider executive functions as the "movement of thoughts" a similar analogy can be drawn within this context. Indeed, cognitive frontal-subcortical loops is a widely accepted notion, where the DLPFC circuit has been documented to mediate set-shifting, complex problem-solving, retrieval abilities, organizational strategies, concept-formation, working memory (Zgaljardic et al., 2006), and other executive functions that are known to be affected in PD. Preserved nigrostriatal dopamine function therefore not only allows effective execution and termination of motor activity, but may also implement smooth switching between cognitive patterns, controlling mutual inhibition and/or facilitation of fronto-subcortical circuits. This is also supported by computational models of the basal ganglia that highlight their routing role in various cognitive functions, such as for example action-selection (Stocco et al., 2010).

In general, higher DaT binding values were associated with global integrative effects on the brain (global increase of nodal strength). This was also confirmed for the cognitive circuitry (defined during meta-analysis), where higher DaT SBR ratios (relative preservation of dopaminergic function) were associated with lower network-level modularity, suggesting that dopamine favors integration of the cognitive network when the subject is at rest. These results are in line with previous fMRI studies that indicated globally impaired network-level processing in PD (Skidmore et al., 2011; Gottlich et al., 2013). Negative effects of the preserved dopaminergic function on the modularity of cognitive circuitry are also in line with previous literature. Thus, a recent randomized double-blind rs-fMRI study of healthy subjects with bromocriptine administration (dopamine agonist) revealed drug-induced decreases in modularity, estimated for the whole brain (White et al., 2013). Our results also suggest that preserved nigrostriatal dopaminergic system allows supporting integrity of the cognitive network when a subject is at rest. In

Table 3 | Latent variable scores and mean caudate DaT binding.

	CN DaT binding		
	T	**DOF**	***p***
LV I	2.87	17	0.011
LV II	−0.096	17	0.925
LV III	2.281	17	0.037

The table shows associations of the PLS latent variables (LVs) extracted during the dimensionality reduction step with nigrostriatal dopaminergic function measured by ^{123}I-FP-CIT SPECT (mean caudate SBR ratios). Positive significant associations (depicted in red) were found for LVs I ("global/motor") and III ("executive").

CN, Caudate Nucleus; DaT, Dopamine Transporter; ***T****, t-statistics;* ***DOF****, degrees of freedom.*

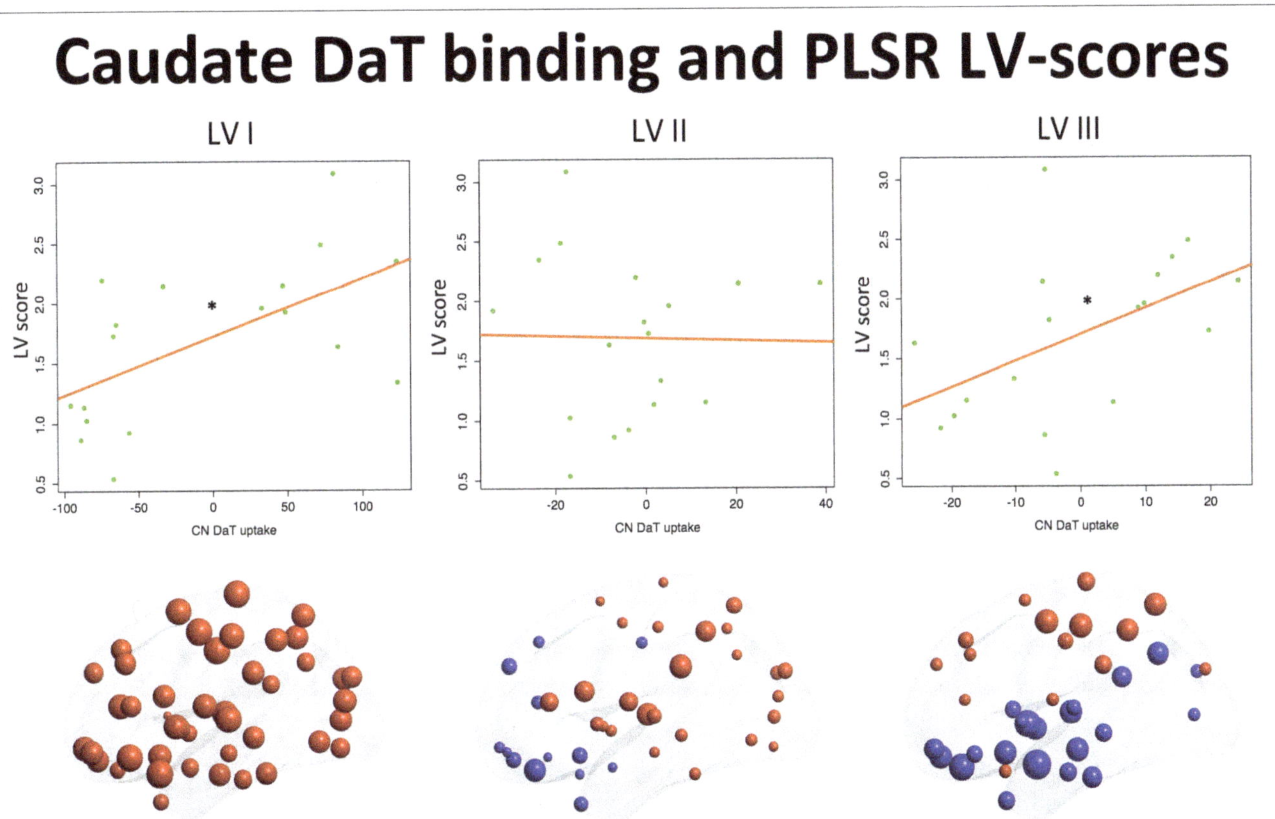

FIGURE 2 | Associations between component scores and mean caudate DaT binding. Associations of latent variable (LV) scores extracted from the nodal strength data with nigrostriatal dopaminergic function measured by ^{123}I-FP-CIT SPECT (mean caudate SBR ratios). Positive associations (*$p < 0.05$) were found for the Ist ("global/motor") and IIIrd ("executive") LVs. Corresponding loading maps are depicted in brain space, reflecting the relevance of the nodes (spheres) for a particular LV, the magnitude of which is represented by nodal size. Positive loading values are depicted as red spheres, whereas negative ones are shown in blue.

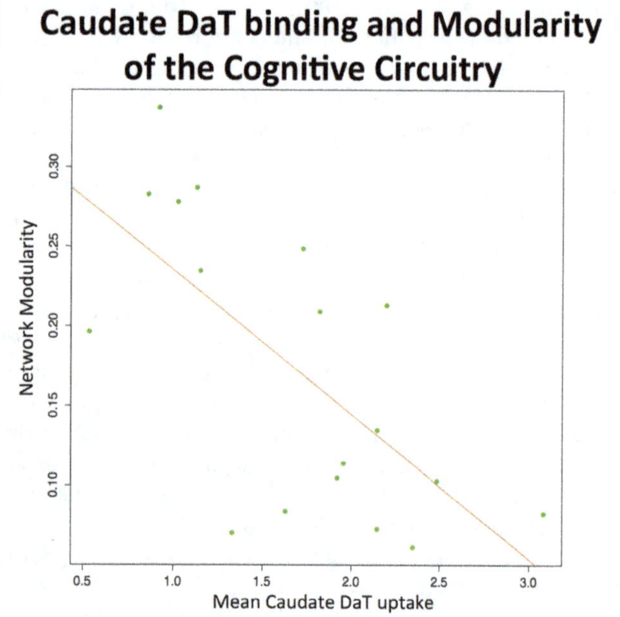

FIGURE 3 | Caudate DaT uptake and modularity of the cognitive circuitry at rest. The figure shows significant ($p < 0.01$) negative association between modularity of the cognitive circuitry (identified with automated meta-analysis) and nigrostriatal dopaminergic function measured by ^{123}I-FP-CIT SPECT (mean caudate SBR ratios).

the light of this, it would be interesting to assess the dynamics of cognitive circuitry during performance of particular executive tasks or multi-tasking, where dopamine may have different or even opposite effects on network modularity. This is supported by previous functional imaging studies of executive functions in PD, revealing that hypodopaminergic states are associated with increased prefrontal cortical responses during performance of corresponding tasks (Mattay et al., 2002), whereas L-dopa administration, in contrast, decreases it (Cools et al., 2002). In this context, it is also worth mentioning an event-related fMRI study that found PD-related brain abnormalities during performance of the set-shifting task specifically developed to elicit caudate responses (Monchi et al., 2007). Compared to the control group, patients demonstrated increased cortical activation in the condition not specifically requiring the caudate nucleus, whereas decreased cortical activation was observed in the task that involved the caudate nucleus. These studies, however, are not focused on any specific dopaminergic system, looking at general dopamine-related effects instead, and therefore do not necessarily confirm the role of exactly nigrostriatal dopaminergic system in these phenomena.

Finally, a recently published graph theoretical MEG study with longitudinal design found that progression of PD is associated with growing impairment of local integration (measured by clustering coefficient) in multiple frequency bands and loss of global brain network efficiency (based on path length) in the alpha2 frequency band. This deterioration was, in turn, correlated with cognitive and motor impairment observed during disease progression (Olde Dubbelink et al., 2014). These findings provide additional support for our results, also suggesting global positive effects of dopaminergic preservation on efficient functioning of the brain networks.

The main limitation of the present study is a relatively small sample size. In addition, the cross-sectional design complicates causal interpretation of the results. Apart from this, the resting state setting itself hampers direct interpretation of the findings with regard to the role of brain networks in cognitive task performance. Active cognitive processing is likely associated with patterns of brain dynamics that are different compared to the ones occurring when the subject is at rest. These patterns in turn may have different associations with altered dopaminergic function in PD. Therefore, this presents a need for further studies of brain dynamics underlying cognitive processing in PD and related dopaminergic deficits.

The main strengths are a multimodal approach and graph theoretical setting that have not yet been implemented together for clarifying brain mechanisms of PD-related cognitive impairment. Further strengths are a relatively broad cognitive evaluation combining multiple tests to assess three major functional domains and the drug-naïve status of the participants. Of note, although the present study specifically investigated the nigrostriatal system, the deficiency measured by ^{123}I-FP-CIT SPECT might also reflect indirect effects of neurodegeneration of dopaminergic neurons within other pathways, since the severity of dopaminergic deficits may correlate across different systems. Therefore, the results should be interpreted with caution.

To summarize, our study found that PD-related executive impairment is associated with altered balance between cortical and subcortical processing at rest, when contribution of the dorsal cortex is getting abnormally suppressed, and subcortical processing is disinhibited. This pattern (unlike brain profiles of visuospatial and memory impairment) is linked to nigrostriatal deficiency, which also has disruptive effects on cognitive circuitry at the network scale.

The results provide evidence for the contribution of the nigrostrital dopaminergic system in human cognition, and the described concept can potentially be utilized in future interventional studies to monitor the effects of treatments, including the approaches that augment cognitive functions.

ACKNOWLEDGMENTS

Data used in the preparation of this article were obtained from the Parkinson's Progression Markers Initiative (PPMI) database (www.ppmi-info.org/data). For up-to-date information on the study, visit www.ppmi-info.org. PPMI—a public-private partnership—is funded by the Michael J. Fox Foundation for Parkinson's Research and funding partners, including Abbott, Avid, Biogen Idec, Bristol-Myers Squibb, Covance, Elan, GlaxoSmithKline, Lilly, Merck, UCB, F. Hoffman-La Roche Ltd., GE Healthcare, Genentech, and Pfizer Inc. The authors are grateful to Dr. Olaf Sporns (Indiana University, USA) for the valuable discussions we had when working on the manuscript. Alexander V. Lebedev was supported by the Helse Vest Strategic Funding 2013 and MoodNet. Joana B. Pereira was funded by a Marie Curie fellowship for postdoctoral researchers (call FP7-PEOPLE-2012-IEF).

SUPPLEMENTARY MATERIAL

Figure S1 | Study Workflow. The study workflow consisted of IV main steps: (I) Selection of 30 PD subjects with fMRI data from the complete PPMI cohort and an fMRI + DaTSCAN subsample of 18 subjects; (II) Preparation of the data for further analysis that, in turn, included (IIa) calculation of composite scores for 3 cognitive domains, (IIb) automated meta-analysis to define "cognitive network," (IIc) image preprocessing and network measure extraction; (III) Dimensionality reduction with PLS followed by parametric tests evaluating associations between latent variable (LV) scores and cognitive functions; (IV) Final analysis assessing influence of caudate dopamine transporter (DaT) uptake on LV scores and modularity of the "cognitive network.

Figure S2 | Automated meta-analysis workflow. An automated search using the meta-analytical software Neurosynth (http://neurosynth.org) was undertaken in order to identify regions that are relevant for cognitive functions. The key-words "executive" (237 studies), "visuospatial" ($n = 116$) and "memory" ($n = 1470$). The profile of visuospatial functions included prefrontal, parietal, and occipital regions. The "executive" pattern contained prefrontal (with more extended involvement of DLPFC), cingulate, superior parietal, temporo-occipital, basal ganglia, and cerebellar regions. Finally, the "memory" profile, in addition to prefrontal and parietal regions, also included hippocampus, temporal areas, and basal ganglia. Due to the observed overlap, the resulting statistical maps were merged and overlaid with the Automated Anatomical Labeling (AAL) atlas defining cognitive circuitry, the modularity of which was then correlated with nigrostriatal function measured by ^{123}I-FP-CIT Single-Photon Emission Computed Tomography.

Figure S3 | Latent variable selection. The figure shows Root Mean Squared Error Prediction (RMSEP) as a function of a number of PLS latent variables (LVs). The maximum number of LVs was selected that minimized total training (red dashed line) and leave-one-out cross-validation (green solid line) errors for all the domains ($n = 3$).

REFERENCES

Aarsland, D., Bronnick, K., Larsen, J. P., Tysnes, O. B., Alves, G., and Norwegian Parkwest Study, G. (2009). Cognitive impairment in incident, untreated Parkinson disease: the Norwegian ParkWest study. *Neurology* 72, 1121–1126. doi: 10.1212/01.wnl.0000338632.00552.cb

Achard, S., and Bullmore, E. (2007). Efficiency and cost of economical brain functional networks. *PLoS Comput. Biol.* 3:e17. doi: 10.1371/journal.pcbi.0030017

Ashburner, J. (2007). A fast diffeomorphic image registration algorithm. *Neuroimage* 38, 95–113. doi: 10.1016/j.neuroimage.2007.07.007

Benton, A. L., Varney, N. R., and Hamsher, K. D. (1978). Visuospatial judgment. A clinical test. *Arch. Neurol.* 35, 364–367. doi: 10.1001/archneur.1978.00500300038006

Biswal, B., Yetkin, F. Z., Haughton, V. M., and Hyde, J. S. (1995). Functional connectivity in the motor cortex of resting human brain using echo-planar MRI. *Magn. Reson. Med.* 34, 537–541. doi: 10.1002/mrm.1910340409

Bohnen, N. I., Kaufer, D. I., Ivanco, L. S., Lopresti, B., Koeppe, R. A., Davis, J. G., et al. (2003). Cortical cholinergic function is more severely affected in parkinsonian dementia than in Alzheimer disease: an *in vivo* positron emission tomographic study. *Arch. Neurol.* 60, 1745–1748. doi: 10.1001/archneur.60.12.1745

Booij, J., Hemelaar, T. G., Speelman, J. D., De Bruin, K., Janssen, A. G., and Van Royen, E. A. (1999). One-day protocol for imaging of the nigrostriatal dopaminergic pathway in Parkinson's disease by [123I]FPCIT SPECT. *J. Nucl. Med.* 40, 753–761.

Brown, P., Oliviero, A., Mazzone, P., Insola, A., Tonali, P., and Di Lazzaro, V. (2001). Dopamine dependency of oscillations between subthalamic nucleus and pallidum in Parkinson's disease. *J. Neurosci.* 21, 1033–1038.

Bruck, A., Portin, R., Lindell, A., Laihinen, A., Bergman, J., Haaparanta, M., et al. (2001). Positron emission tomography shows that impaired frontal lobe functioning in Parkinson's disease is related to dopaminergic hypofunction in the caudate nucleus. *Neurosci. Lett.* 311, 81–84. doi: 10.1016/S0304-3940(01)02124-3

Chang, C., and Glover, G. H. (2009). Effects of model-based physiological noise correction on default mode network anti-correlations and correlations. *Neuroimage* 47, 1448–1459. doi: 10.1016/j.neuroimage.2009.05.012

Chao-Gan, Y., and Yu-Feng, Z. (2010). DPARSF: a MATLAB toolbox for "pipeline" data analysis of resting-state fMRI. *Front. Syst. Neurosci.* 4:13. doi: 10.3389/fnsys.2010.00013

Cheesman, A. L., Barker, R. A., Lewis, S. J., Robbins, T. W., Owen, A. M., and Brooks, D. J. (2005). Lateralisation of striatal function: evidence from 18F-dopa PET in Parkinson's disease. *J. Neurol. Neurosurg. Psychiatry* 76, 1204–1210. doi: 10.1136/jnnp.2004.055079

Christopher, L., and Strafella, A. P. (2013). Neuroimaging of brain changes associated with cognitive impairment in Parkinson's disease. *J. Neuropsychol.* 7, 225–240. doi: 10.1111/jnp.12015

Cools, R., Stefanova, E., Barker, R. A., Robbins, T. W., and Owen, A. M. (2002). Dopaminergic modulation of high-level cognition in Parkinson's disease: the role of the prefrontal cortex revealed by PET. *Brain* 125, 584–594. doi: 10.1093/brain/awf052

Cropley, V. L., Fujita, M., Bara-Jimenez, W., Brown, A. K., Zhang, X. Y., Sangare, J., et al. (2008). Pre- and post-synaptic dopamine imaging and its relation with frontostriatal cognitive function in Parkinson disease: PET studies with [11C]NNC 112 and [18F]FDOPA. *Psychiatry Res.* 163, 171–182. doi: 10.1016/j.pscychresns.2007.11.003

Dagher, A., Owen, A. M., Boecker, H., and Brooks, D. J. (2001). The role of the striatum and hippocampus in planning: a PET activation study in Parkinson's disease. *Brain* 124, 1020–1032. doi: 10.1093/brain/124.5.1020

Eidelberg, D. (2009). Metabolic brain networks in neurodegenerative disorders: a functional imaging approach. *Trends Neurosci.* 32, 548–557. doi: 10.1016/j.tins.2009.06.003

Esposito, F., Tessitore, A., Giordano, A., De Micco, R., Paccone, A., Conforti, R., et al. (2013). Rhythm-specific modulation of the sensorimotor network in drug-naive patients with Parkinson's disease by levodopa. *Brain* 136, 710–725. doi: 10.1093/brain/awt007

Fox, M. D., Zhang, D., Snyder, A. Z., and Raichle, M. E. (2009). The global signal and observed anticorrelated resting state brain networks. *J. Neurophysiol.* 101, 3270–3283. doi: 10.1152/jn.90777.2008

Gatev, P., Darbin, O., and Wichmann, T. (2006). Oscillations in the basal ganglia under normal conditions and in movement disorders. *Mov. Disord.* 21, 1566–1577. doi: 10.1002/mds.21033

Gottlich, M., Munte, T. F., Heldmann, M., Kasten, M., Hagenah, J., and Kramer, U. M. (2013). Altered resting state brain networks in Parkinson's disease. *PLoS ONE* 8:e77336. doi: 10.1371/journal.pone.0077336

Hammond, C., Bergman, H., and Brown, P. (2007). Pathological synchronization in Parkinson's disease: networks, models and treatments. *Trends Neurosci.* 30, 357–364. doi: 10.1016/j.tins.2007.05.004

Helmich, R. C., Derikx, L. C., Bakker, M., Scheeringa, R., Bloem, B. R., and Toni, I. (2010). Spatial remapping of cortico-striatal connectivity in Parkinson's disease. *Cereb. Cortex* 20, 1175–1186. doi: 10.1093/cercor/bhp178

Hirano, S., Shinotoh, H., and Eidelberg, D. (2012). Functional brain imaging of cognitive dysfunction in Parkinson's disease. *J. Neurol. Neurosurg. Psychiatry* 83, 963–969. doi: 10.1136/jnnp-2011-301818

Huang, C., Mattis, P., Tang, C., Perrine, K., Carbon, M., and Eidelberg, D. (2007a). Metabolic brain networks associated with cognitive function in Parkinson's disease. *Neuroimage* 34, 714–723. doi: 10.1016/j.neuroimage.2006.09.003

Huang, C., Tang, C., Feigin, A., Lesser, M., Ma, Y., Pourfar, M., et al. (2007b). Changes in network activity with the progression of Parkinson's disease. *Brain* 130, 1834–1846. doi: 10.1093/brain/awm086

Ito, K., Nagano-Saito, A., Kato, T., Arahata, Y., Nakamura, A., Kawasumi, Y., et al. (2002). Striatal and extrastriatal dysfunction in Parkinson's disease with dementia: a 6-[18F]fluoro-L-dopa PET study. *Brain* 125, 1358–1365. doi: 10.1093/brain/awf134

Kelly, C., De Zubicaray, G., Di Martino, A., Copland, D. A., Reiss, P. T., Klein, D. F., et al. (2009). L-dopa modulates functional connectivity in striatal cognitive and motor networks: a double-blind placebo-controlled study. *J. Neurosci.* 29, 7364–7378. doi: 10.1523/JNEUROSCI.0810-09.2009

Kwak, Y., Peltier, S., Bohnen, N. I., Muller, M. L., Dayalu, P., and Seidler, R. D. (2010). Altered resting state cortico-striatal connectivity in mild to moderate stage Parkinson's disease. *Front. Syst. Neurosci.* 4:143. doi: 10.3389/fnsys.2010.00143

Levy, R., Ashby, P., Hutchison, W. D., Lang, A. E., Lozano, A. M., and Dostrovsky, J. O. (2002). Dependence of subthalamic nucleus oscillations on movement and dopamine in Parkinson's disease. *Brain* 125, 1196–1209. doi: 10.1093/brain/awf128

Lewis, S. J., Dove, A., Robbins, T. W., Barker, R. A., and Owen, A. M. (2003). Cognitive impairments in early Parkinson's disease are accompanied by reductions in activity in frontostriatal neural circuitry. *J. Neurosci.* 23, 6351–6356.

Lowe, M. J., Mock, B. J., and Sorenson, J. A. (1998). Functional connectivity in single and multislice echoplanar imaging using resting-state fluctuations. *Neuroimage* 7, 119–132. doi: 10.1006/nimg.1997.0315

Matlab 8.0 and Statistics Toolbox 8.1. (2012). T. M., Inc., Natick, MA, USA.

Mattay, V. S., Tessitore, A., Callicott, J. H., Bertolino, A., Goldberg, T. E., Chase, T. N., et al. (2002). Dopaminergic modulation of cortical function in patients with Parkinson's disease. *Ann. Neurol.* 51, 156–164. doi: 10.1002/ana.10078

Mentis, M. J., McIntosh, A. R., Perrine, K., Dhawan, V., Berlin, B., Feigin, A., et al. (2002). Relationships among the metabolic patterns that correlate with mnemonic, visuospatial, and mood symptoms in Parkinson's disease. *Am. J. Psychiatry* 159, 746–754. doi: 10.1176/appi.ajp.159.5.746

Mink, J. W. (1996). The basal ganglia: focused selection and inhibition of competing motor programs. *Prog. Neurobiol.* 50, 381–425. doi: 10.1016/S0301-0082(96)00042-1

Monchi, O., Petrides, M., Doyon, J., Postuma, R. B., Worsley, K., and Dagher, A. (2004). Neural bases of set-shifting deficits in Parkinson's disease. *J. Neurosci.* 24, 702–710. doi: 10.1523/JNEUROSCI.4860-03.2004

Monchi, O., Petrides, M., Mejia-Constain, B., and Strafella, A. P. (2007). Cortical activity in Parkinson's disease during executive processing depends on striatal involvement. *Brain* 130, 233–244. doi: 10.1093/brain/awl326

Mountcastle, V. B. (1997). The columnar organization of the neocortex. *Brain* 120(Pt 4), 701–722. doi: 10.1093/brain/120.4.701

Murphy, K., Birn, R. M., Handwerker, D. A., Jones, T. B., and Bandettini, P. A. (2009). The impact of global signal regression on resting state correlations: are anti-correlated networks introduced? *Neuroimage* 44, 893–905. doi: 10.1016/j.neuroimage.2008.09.036

Muslimovic, D., Post, B., Speelman, J. D., and Schmand, B. (2005). Cognitive profile of patients with newly diagnosed Parkinson disease. *Neurology* 65, 1239–1245. doi: 10.1212/01.wnl.0000180516.69442.95

Narayanan, N. S., Rodnitzky, R. L., and Uc, E. Y. (2013). Prefrontal dopamine signaling and cognitive symptoms of Parkinson's disease. *Rev. Neurosci.* 24, 267–278. doi: 10.1515/revneuro-2013-0004

Newman, M. E. (2006). Modularity and community structure in networks. *Proc. Natl. Acad. Sci. U.S.A.* 103, 8577–8582. doi: 10.1073/pnas.0601602103

O'Brien, J. T., Colloby, S., Fenwick, J., Williams, E. D., Firbank, M., Burn, D., et al. (2004). Dopamine transporter loss visualized with FP-CIT SPECT in the differential diagnosis of dementia with Lewy bodies. *Arch. Neurol.* 61, 919–925. doi: 10.1001/archneur.61.6.919

Olde Dubbelink, K. T., Hillebrand, A., Stoffers, D., Deijen, J. B., Twisk, J. W., Stam, C. J., et al. (2014). Disrupted brain network topology in Parkinson's disease: a longitudinal magnetoencephalography study. *Brain.* 137(Pt 1), 197–207. doi: 10.1093/brain/awt316

Owen, A. M., Doyon, J., Dagher, A., Sadikot, A., and Evans, A. C. (1998). Abnormal basal ganglia outflow in Parkinson's disease identified with PET. Implications for higher cortical functions. *Brain* 121(Pt 5), 949–965. doi: 10.1093/brain/121.5.949

R Core Team. (2013). *R: A Language and Environment for Statistical Computing.* Version 3.0.1. Vienna: R Foundation for Statistical Computing. ISBN: 3-900051-07-0. Available online at: http://www.R-project.org/ [Online] [Accessed].

Rubinov, M., and Sporns, O. (2010). Complex network measures of brain connectivity: uses and interpretations. *Neuroimage* 52, 1059–1069. doi: 10.1016/j.neuroimage.2009.10.003

Rubinov, M., and Sporns, O. (2011). Weight-conserving characterization of complex functional brain networks. *Neuroimage* 56, 2068–2079. doi: 10.1016/j.neuroimage.2011.03.069

Satterthwaite, T. D., Elliott, M. A., Gerraty, R. T., Ruparel, K., Loughead, J., Calkins, M. E., et al. (2013). An improved framework for confound regression and filtering for control of motion artifact in the preprocessing of resting-state functional connectivity data. *Neuroimage* 64, 240–256. doi: 10.1016/j.neuroimage.2012.08.052

Shapiro, A. M., Benedict, R. H., Schretlen, D., and Brandt, J. (1999). Construct and concurrent validity of the Hopkins Verbal Learning Test-revised. *Clin. Neuropsychol.* 13, 348–358. doi: 10.1076/clin.13.3.348.1749

Skidmore, F., Korenkevych, D., Liu, Y., He, G., Bullmore, E., and Pardalos, P. M. (2011). Connectivity brain networks based on wavelet correlation analysis in Parkinson fMRI data. *Neurosci. Lett.* 499, 47–51. doi: 10.1016/j.neulet.2011.05.030

Sporns, O. (2010). *Networks of the Brain, 1st Edn.* Cambridge, MA: The MIT Press.

Sporns, O. (2013). Network attributes for segregation and integration in the human brain. *Curr. Opin. Neurobiol.* 23, 162–171. doi: 10.1016/j.conb.2012.11.015

Sporns, O., and Zwi, J. D. (2004). The small world of the cerebral cortex. *Neuroinformatics* 2, 145–162. doi: 10.1385/NI:2:2:145

Stocco, A., Lebiere, C., and Anderson, J. R. (2010). Conditional routing of information to the cortex: a model of the basal ganglia's role in cognitive coordination. *Psychol. Rev.* 117, 541–574. doi: 10.1037/a0019077

Svenningsson, P., Westman, E., Ballard, C., and Aarsland, D. (2012). Cognitive impairment in patients with Parkinson's disease: diagnosis, biomarkers, and treatment. *Lancet Neurol.* 11, 697–707. doi: 10.1016/S1474-4422(12)70152-7

Tinaz, S., Schendan, H. E., and Stern, C. E. (2008). Fronto-striatal deficit in Parkinson's disease during semantic event sequencing. *Neurobiol. Aging* 29, 397–407. doi: 10.1016/j.neurobiolaging.2006.10.025

Tzourio-Mazoyer, N., Landeau, B., Papathanassiou, D., Crivello, F., Etard, O., Delcroix, N., et al. (2002). Automated anatomical labeling of activations in SPM using a macroscopic anatomical parcellation of the MNI MRI single-subject brain. *Neuroimage* 15, 273–289. doi: 10.1006/nimg.2001.0978

Van Eimeren, T., Monchi, O., Ballanger, B., and Strafella, A. P. (2009). Dysfunction of the default mode network in Parkinson disease: a functional magnetic resonance imaging study. *Arch. Neurol.* 66, 877–883. doi: 10.1001/archneurol.2009.97

Vossius, C., Larsen, J. P., Janvin, C., and Aarsland, D. (2011). The economic impact of cognitive impairment in Parkinson's disease. *Mov. Disord.* 26, 1541–1544. doi: 10.1002/mds.23661

Weintraub, D., Dietz, N., Duda, J. E., Wolk, D. A., Doshi, J., Xie, S. X., et al. (2012). Alzheimer's disease pattern of brain atrophy predicts cognitive decline in Parkinson's disease. *Brain* 135, 170–180. doi: 10.1093/brain/awr277

Welsh, D. K., Takahashi, J. S., and Kay, S. A. (2010). Suprachiasmatic nucleus: cell autonomy and network properties. *Annu. Rev. Physiol.* 72, 551–577. doi: 10.1146/annurev-physiol-021909-135919

White, R., Esther Aarts, E., and D'Esposito, M. (2013). Interactions of resting state brain networks, dopamine, and working memory behavior: a resting state functional MRI study. *Neurology* 80(Meeting Abstr. 1):S54.003.

Parkinson's disease. *Neurosci. Lett.* 460, 6–10. doi: 10.1016/j.neulet.2009.05.046

Yarkoni, T., Poldrack, R. A., Nichols, T. E., Van Essen, D. C., and Wager, T. D. (2011). Large-scale automated synthesis of human functional neuroimaging data. *Nat. Methods* 8, 665–670. doi: 10.1038/nmeth.1635

Zgaljardic, D. J., Borod, J. C., Foldi, N. S., Mattis, P. J., Gordon, M. F., Feigin, A., et al. (2006). An examination of executive dysfunction associated with frontostriatal circuitry in Parkinson's disease. *J. Clin. Exp. Neuropsychol.* 28, 1127–1144. doi: 10.1080/13803390500246910

Williams-Gray, C. H., Evans, J. R., Goris, A., Foltynie, T., Ban, M., Robbins, T. W., et al. (2009). The distinct cognitive syndromes of Parkinson's disease: 5 year follow-up of the CamPaIGN cohort. *Brain* 132, 2958–2969. doi: 10.1093/brain/awp245

Wold, S., Ruhe, A., Wold, H., and Dunn, W. J. III. (1984). The collinearity problem in linear regression. The Partial Least Squares (PLS) approach to generalized inverses. *SIAM J. Sci. Stat. Comput.* 5, 735–743. doi: 10.1137/0905052

Wu, T., Wang, L., Chen, Y., Zhao, C., Li, K., and Chan, P. (2009). Changes of functional connectivity of the motor network in the resting state in

15

An electrocorticographic BCI using code-based VEP for control in video applications: a single-subject study

Christoph Kapeller[1,2,3], Kyousuke Kamada[4], Hiroshi Ogawa[4], Robert Prueckl[1,2,3], Josef Scharinger[3] and Christoph Guger[1,2]*

[1] *Guger Technologies OG, Graz, Austria*
[2] *g.tec medical engineering GmbH, Schiedlberg, Austria*
[3] *Department of Computational Perception, Johannes Kepler University, Linz, Austria*
[4] *Department of Neurosurgery, Asahikawa Medical University, Asahikawa, Japan*

Edited by:
Mikhail Lebedev, Duke University, USA

Reviewed by:
Duk Shin, Tokyo Institute of Technology, Japan
Martin Spüler, University of Tübingen, Germany

****Correspondence:***
Christoph Guger, g.tec medical engineering GmbH, Sierningstrasse 14, Schiedlberg 4521, Austria
e-mail: guger@gtec.at

A brain-computer-interface (BCI) allows the user to control a device or software with brain activity. Many BCIs rely on visual stimuli with constant stimulation cycles that elicit steady-state visual evoked potentials (SSVEP) in the electroencephalogram (EEG). This EEG response can be generated with a LED or a computer screen flashing at a constant frequency, and similar EEG activity can be elicited with pseudo-random stimulation sequences on a screen (code-based BCI). Using electrocorticography (ECoG) instead of EEG promises higher spatial and temporal resolution and leads to more dominant evoked potentials due to visual stimulation. This work is focused on BCIs based on visual evoked potentials (VEP) and its capability as a continuous control interface for augmentation of video applications. One 35 year old female subject with implanted subdural grids participated in the study. The task was to select one out of four visual targets, while each was flickering with a code sequence. After a calibration run including 200 code sequences, a linear classifier was used during an evaluation run to identify the selected visual target based on the generated code-based VEPs over 20 trials. Multiple ECoG buffer lengths were tested and the subject reached a mean online classification accuracy of 99.21% for a window length of 3.15 s. Finally, the subject performed an unsupervised free run in combination with visual feedback of the current selection. Additionally, an algorithm was implemented that allowed to suppress false positive selections and this allowed the subject to start and stop the BCI at any time. The code-based BCI system attained very high online accuracy, which makes this approach very promising for control applications where a continuous control signal is needed.

Keywords: electrocorticography, brain-computer-interface, code-based stimulation, VEP, augmented control

INTRODUCTION

People have long sought to extract users' intentions from brain signals to give impaired persons a communication channel or optimize interaction between users and their environments. Such a brain-computer-interface (BCI) allows the user to control a device or software with brain activity (Wolpaw et al., 2002). People can use a BCI to interact with their environments even if they have limited or no muscle control. Various data acquisition techniques like electroencephalography (EEG) (Wolpaw et al., 2002), electrocorticography (ECoG) (Leuthardt et al., 2004), functional magnetic resonance imaging (fMRI) (Weiskopf et al., 2004), and near infrared spectroscopy (NIRS) (Coyle et al., 2004) can be used as a BCI system.

The EEG is the most common brain imaging method in BCI research because it is inexpensive, portable, non-invasive, and has excellent temporal resolution (Mason et al., 2007). However, the EEG has only a limited spatial resolution, as each channel is influenced by the activation of millions of neurons, and the signal is smeared and filtered during passage through the scalp. ECoG signals recorded from the brain's surface are more robust against electromyographic (EMG) artifacts and provide a higher spatial and temporal resolution compared to EEG signals (Leuthardt et al., 2004). Several groups investigated the reliability of electrocorticographic signals for real-time applications, like 2D movement control based on motor imagery tasks (Schalk et al., 2008) or a P300 spelling device (Brunner et al., 2011).

Most BCIs rely on one of three kinds of brain signals: event related desynchronization (ERD) associated with motor-imagery, P300 and steady-state visual evoked potentials (SSVEP) (Wolpaw et al., 2002). While P300 based systems typically rely on discrete control, which is excellent for selecting commands to control a spelling device (Mason et al., 2007; Guger et al., 2009), the motor imagery and SSVEP based systems often give a continuous control signal that could be used to steer a wheelchair in different directions. The performance of a BCI relying on motor imagery has already been comprehensively investigated using EEG (Müller-Gerking et al., 1999; Guger et al., 2000, 2003; Krausz et al., 2003; Blankertz et al., 2010) and ECoG recordings (Leuthardt et al., 2004; Schalk et al., 2008; Miller et al., 2010). Recently, an ECoG BCI was presented that decoded attempted arm and hand movements for 3D cursor control using activation of the high-frequency band between 40 and 200 Hz, which were mapped to velocity control signals (Wang et al., 2013).

This work is focused on BCIs based on visual evoked potentials (VEP) derived from subdural ECoG signals over the visual cortex. Two methods are generally used to distinguish different visual targets: phase coding and frequency coding (Wang et al., 2008). In SSVEPs, the brain waves derived from the scalp contain sinusoidal signals with the same frequency as the visual stimuli. The so called Bremen BCI used a minimum energy based feature extraction applied on EEG data including SSVEPs and reached a mean ITR of 61.70 bits/min and a mean accuracy of 96.79% (Volosyak, 2011). Another SSVEP BCI study presented a grand average accuracy of 95.50% for EEG recordings from 53 subjects (Guger et al., 2012). An alternative type of stimulation that combines the phase and frequency coded VEPs is based on code sequences, producing code-based VEPs (c-VEP) (Bin et al., 2009). This type of BCI was initially proposed by Erich Sutter as a spelling device and tested with an ALS patient having epidural implants over 11 months (Sutter, 1992). The subject achieved a spelling rate of 10–12 words per minute. In a more recent paper, a multi-channel c-VEP BCI was tested with EEG signals (Bin et al., 2011). A spatial filter was computed from a canonical correlation analysis (CCA) and then applied on multiple EEG channels over the visual cortex. The authors developed a 32 target system with a stimulation sequence of 1.05 s. The resulting mean online accuracy was 85.00%, which led to an ITR of 108 bits/min. An even faster version of this c-VEP speller application led to an average accuracy of 96.00% and an ITR of 144 bit/min (Spüler et al., 2012). Although the code-based stimulation approach is not the same as a conventional steady state stimulus, BCIs based on c-VEP are often grouped together with SSVEP BCIs for convenience.

BCIs relying on VEPs could benefit from on-screen solutions, which do not need additional hardware like LEDs and can be embedded into a virtual environment. This was achieved inside a 2D or 3D gaming environments, as well as virtual reality scenarios (Lalor et al., 2005; Martinez et al., 2007; Faller et al., 2010). In a previous study we tested a c-VEP BCI for robotic control with EEG on 11 subjects showing a grand average online accuracy of 98.18% (Kapeller et al., 2013). Specifically, the control interface was embedded inside a video application showing the moving robot, while the user was steering the robot along a given path.

The main goal of this study is to investigate an intracranial c-VEP BCI designed as a continuous control interface for augmentation of video applications.

MATERIALS AND METHODS

SUBJECT DESCRIPTION

The subject, a 35 year old woman suffering from intractable epilepsy underwent subdural grid implantation prior to resective brain surgery, which was part of the clinical treatment. After full explanation of the experimental procedure and its possible risks, a written informed consent was obtained from the subject. This work was approved by the institutional review board of the Asahikawa Medical University (No. 693) before the study. She had corrected-to-normal vision and a Japanese Wechsler Memory Scale—Revised Edition (WMS-R) test showed normal memory function (average score 100, $SD = 15$). As the epileptic focus did not overlap with the visual cortex, there was no reason to reject the subject from the study.

In order to localize epileptic foci, four grids and five strips containing 100 subdural electrodes were temporarily implanted widely across the right hemisphere. **Figure 1** shows the grid alignment on the cortex and the numbering of the electrodes. The clinical electrodes were made of platinum and had an inter-electrode distance of 10 mm and a conductive area of about 7.1 mm^2.

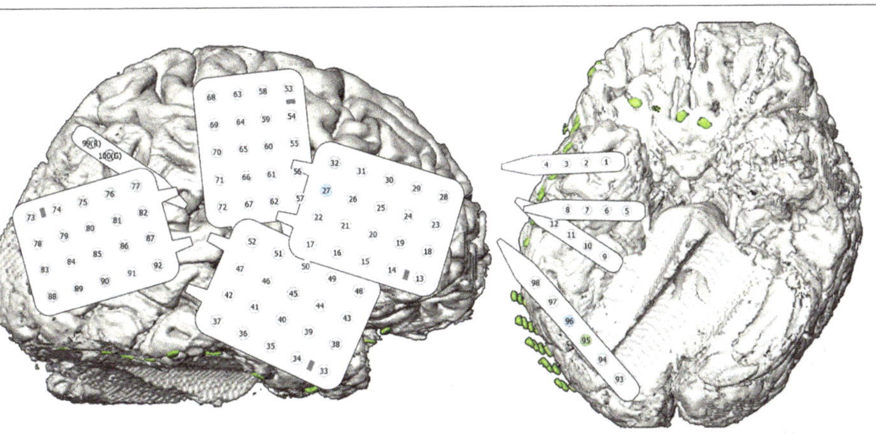

FIGURE 1 | Implanted electrodes. The subject had 100 electrodes on **four** grids and **five** strips located implanted over the frontal, temporal, parietal, and occipital lobe of the right hemisphere. The schematic views of the grids and strips contain electrodes represented by a circle and their number in the montage. An additional strip on the frontal base region was not recorded and is not included into the electrode numbering. The gray highlighted electrodes represent very noisy channels which were recorded, but not considered for signal processing. The green/blue colored channels indicate high/medium contribution during feature extraction.

DATA ACQUISITION

The electrodes were connected to a g.HIamp (g.tec medical engineering GmbH, Austria) biosignal data acquisition device, which digitized the data with 24 bit resolution and 256 Hz sampling frequency. The data were band-pass filtered between 1 and 30 Hz and notch filtered at 50 Hz to suppress power line interference. This pass band was designed to maximize the signal-to-noise ratio (SNR) of the recorded VEPs for a maximum stimulation frequency of 30 Hz using a monitor with a refresh rate of 60 Hz. The grounding strip covering the superior parietal lobule contained the electrodes number 99 and 100, which were used as reference (REF) and ground (GND) electrode, respectively. Therefore, 98 signal channels were recorded during the experiment.

The biosignal data acquisition device transferred the data via USB to the computer system, which was used for data acquisition, online processing, experimental paradigm control, data visualization and data storage.

SYSTEM CONFIGURATION

The design of the BCI system is based on the work of Bin et al. (2011) and modified for continuous control input from the user. The stimulation unit, a 60 Hz LCD monitor, presents visual targets that each occupy 4.2 × 2.4 cm of the screen. These targets are embedded inside an OpenGL based video application and remotely connected with the BCI system, which controls the visual stimulation and the feedback to the user.

The stimulus definition is based on a pseudo-random binary code sequence, a so called m-sequence. These binary sequences are used for nonlinear signal analysis and also in multi input systems (Golomb et al., 1982). Therefore, black and white stimulation is applied using a 63 bit m-sequence, where 1 and 0 are represented by white and black, respectively. Due to the stimulation rate of 60 Hz, one stimulation sequence lasts 1.05 s. The BCI presented in this work contains four visual targets (C1, C2, C3, and C4), which can be selected by the user. This is a well-suited number of classes for a continuous control task, e.g., moving a robotic device or a virtual avatar forward, backward, left or right (Kapeller et al., 2013). As the autocorrelation function of the m-sequence is approximating the unit impulse function (Zierler, 1959), we can use the same modulation sequence for all visual targets. Only a phase shift of the sequence onset is necessary to distinguish between the resultant VEPs inside the synchronized processing unit of the BCI. The phase shift for each target is equally distributed along the m-sequence and then rounded to the next lower integer value. This leads to a phase shift in bits of $\rho_1 = 0$, $\rho_2 = 15$, $\rho_3 = 30$, and $\rho_4 = 45$ for class C1 to C4, respectively.

In order to synchronize the visual stimulation with the recorded ECoG signals, a trigger signal representing the sequence onset of C1 is sent via UDP connection to the BCI system. Once the stimulation is synchronized, the BCI is processing the resultant VEPs using a signal buffer that is updated each 51 samples (~200 ms). The processing system is running in the MATLAB/Simulink rapid prototyping environment.

SCREEN OVERLAY CONTROL INTERFACE (SOCI)

The visual targets are presented on the monitor through the SOCI module. The SOCI module is a C++ library based on OpenGL that is loadable at runtime and can be used by OpenGL based host applications to embed visual stimulation. The host applications could be virtual reality environments or simple real-world videos that are acquired from a camera. The SOCI works as a remote visual stimulator and provides a network interface that can be used to load visual targets, start or stop the flickering, and synchronize the stimulation with the signal processing. Since it is a multi-threaded application, the communication with the BCI model and the OpenGL drawing commands are handled within separate threads. The host graphics application has to initialize and control the SOCI. This utilizes an abstract interface class that provides public functions to embed the module.

The visual targets can be configured very flexibly using an XML description provided from a configuration file or an external application (Putz et al., 2011). Users can change the number, position, size, and content of the icons and modify other parameters.

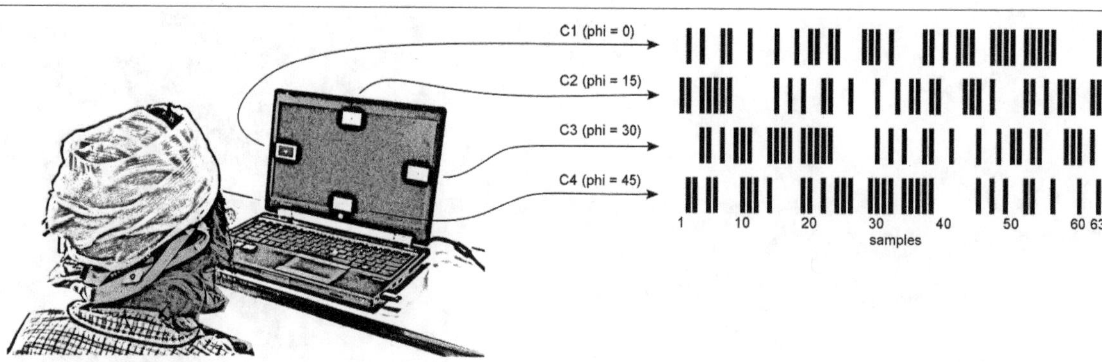

FIGURE 2 | Experimental design. A notebook presented **four** visual targets to the subject, who sat around 80 cm in front of the monitor. The size of **one** target was 4.2 × 2.4 cm leading to a visual angle of 3.0 × 1.7°. Each visual target (C1, C2, C3, and C4) was flickering with a phase shifted version of the same m-sequence. The subject was asked to focus the cued target or to choose an arbitrary target if the cue was disabled. In unsupervised mode, the selected target was surrounded by a green border.

EXPERIMENTAL DESIGN

The subject was seated ~80 cm in front of the stimulation monitor visualizing the BCI targets during the experiment (see **Figure 2**), which was separated into three phases. Specifically, the subject participated in a calibration run to compute a classifier, an evaluation run to estimate the accuracy of the BCI and a free run to let the subject experience unsupervised interaction with the system in combination with online feedback of the selected target.

After a pre-run delay of 10 s (to avoid settling effects of the filters), the subject performed the calibration run. The subject's task was to focus on target C1 for 200 stimulation cycles, while all other targets were not visible. Since one cycle lasts 1.05 s, the entire calibration took less than 4 min.

In the evaluation run, all targets were displayed on the monitor and the online accuracy of the BCI system was tested across 20 trials. Specifically, the SOCI displayed four rectangles on the top, bottom, left, and right of the monitor (see **Figure 2**). During each trial, the subject focused on the target that was highlighted by a visual cue (green border around the target). Each trial consisted of a 3.0 s long resting phase with no visual stimulation, followed by a 7.0 s long stimulation period showing all targets flickering simultaneously. This trial definition was based on previous studies about BCIs using SSVEP or c-VEP (Guger et al., 2012; Kapeller et al., 2013). Since the stimulation period exceeded the longest buffer size and the signal buffer was updated each 200 ms, we decided to keep a trial duration that is not a multiple of the stimulation sequence. No feedback about the classification result was given to the subject at any time during the evaluation run.

Finally, the subject performed the free run to experience the interaction with the BCI by getting feedback about the selected target. Again, all four targets were flickering simultaneously with the m-sequence and corresponding phase shift. No cue was presented on the screen to indicate the current target, and all targets continued flickering throughout the free run. The subject could select any target at any time. Feedback reflecting the current selection was presented as a green border around the selected target. After the free run, the subject was asked about her impression of the system's accuracy.

OFFLINE ANALYSES

The recorded data set from the calibration run was used for offline analyses. As we had to exclude bad channels from the offline analyses, all channels that did not pass visual inspection of the raw data were set to zero. After checking the signal quality, the 200 recorded sequences were epoched and DC corrected for each trial. Then the trials were averaged to a set of templates for each signal channel and phase shift. These templates were used for waveform detection of the c-VEP inside the ECoG signals. Therefore, a CCA was used to maximize the correlation coefficient of all templates and the raw data.

Compared to ordinary correlation, the CCA is independent from the used coordinate system. It provides the maximum correlation of the variables, which is also called the canonical correlation (Borga, 2001). The correlation coefficient ρ is maximized, with respect to the normalized base vectors for canonical correlation ($\hat{w}_x$ and $\hat{w}_y$):

$$\max_{\widehat{w}_x\widehat{w}_y} \rho = \max_{\widehat{w}_x\widehat{w}_y} \left(\frac{E\left[\widehat{w}_x^T XY^T \widehat{w}_y\right]}{E\left[\widehat{w}_x^T XX^T \widehat{w}_x\right] E\left[\widehat{w}_y^T YY^T \widehat{w}_y\right]} \right)$$

X and Y are the analyzed multidimensional variables. In our case, X contained the raw ECoG data of 200 sequences and Y consisted of 200 concatenated templates for each channel.

The calculation of the maximum correlation is based on the eigenvalue equations below, where C is the covariance matrix of the multidimensional variables. In these equations, multiple non-zero eigenvalues are possible. As the eigenvalues represent the squared correlation coefficients, the highest eigenvalue leads to the canonical correlation. The corresponding eigenvectors are the base vectors from:

$$C_{xx}^{-1} C_{xy} C_{yy}^{-1} C_{yx} \widehat{w}_x = \rho^2 \widehat{w}_x$$

$$C_{yy}^{-1} C_{yx} C_{xx}^{-1} C_{xy} \widehat{w}_y = \rho^2 \widehat{w}_y.$$

The resultant vectors $\hat{w}_x$ and $\hat{w}_y$ were interpreted as spatial filters, where $\hat{w}_x$ was applied on the raw ECoG signals and $\hat{w}_y$ was applied on the template data. **Figure 3** shows the averaged c-VEP templates for each channel together with the weight for the individual channel.

The spatial filtered calibration data was then used for computing a linear classifier using a multi-class linear discriminant analysis (m-LDA) (Duda et al., 2000). The features were extracted by computing the correlation coefficients of the spatially filtered templates and the spatially filtered raw data. In order to extract features for each class, the data set of the calibration run was epoched four times. Before each epoching step, the signals were shifted with respect to the trigger channel and the phase shift of the current class. Hence, the correlation coefficients were maximized for the corresponding phase shift.

A zero class provided an idle state that occurred when no target was selected by the user. Based on the classification scores only, it is not possible to determine whether the user has selected any target. This entails rejecting any classification result for which the residual error probability is larger than a predefined limit. A Softmax function is used, which transforms the output of the discrimination function into a value p between 0 and 1:

$$p_i = \frac{e^{q_i/\tau}}{\sum_{b=1}^{N} e^{q_b/\tau}}$$

Where q_i is the distance to class i and τ is called the temperature, which is used to adjust the gap between the resultant probabilities (Sutton and Barto, 1998). N is the total number of possible classes.

SETUP FOR THE ONLINE EXPERIMENT

During the online experiments a Simulink model was processing incoming data with an update rate of 256 Hz driven by the data acquisition device. After the preprocessing step described in Section Data Acquisition, the recorded ECoG signals were buffered and DC corrected. The size of the signal buffer was set to a multiple of the template length and was updated every 51 processing steps. In order to extract characteristic features for each individual class, this buffer was then compared with the templates for each phase shift. Therefore, two processing steps were required. First, the spatial filter from the offline analysis was applied to the signal buffer and the templates and led to a combined channel with maximized correlation with respect to the spatially filtered templates. Second, the spatially filtered signal was correlated with each spatially filtered template leading to one feature channel for each class.

Before starting the free run, the data from the evaluation run was used to investigate the system's accuracy and latency. Different settings were tested to provide the best configuration for the free run.

As the length of the ECoG signal buffer could heavily influence the performance of the BCI, we tested the system accuracy for multiple buffer lengths. The signal buffer has to be a multiple of the m-sequence length, where the minimum length is the duration of one m-sequence cycle. We explored buffer lengths of 1.05, 2.10, and 3.15 s. Longer buffer lengths were not considered in this work, since this would not proper to our previously proposed BCI applications.

In order to stabilize the features, a 1.0 s moving window filter was used before applying the linear classifier. If the classification result was below a 97–100% confidence interval, the output was assigned to the zero class.

The mean online accuracy of the BCI was determined by averaging all classifier outputs at the last 2 s of each trial. This gives a measure about the performance of the BCI, when the feature values reached their maximum with respect to the selected target.

RESULTS

CLASSIFICATION ACCURACY

Figure 4A shows the mean on-line accuracy for three buffer lengths (1.05, 2.10, and 3.15 s) after 20 trials. The shortest window length resulted in the lowest accuracy, but fastest reaction of the BCI system. The classification accuracies for growing buffer length were 86.76, 92.96, and 99.21%, respectively. **Figure 4B** illustrates the BCI latency that was necessary to reach 80% classification accuracy. Specifically, this latency consisted of the moving average window length (1.0 s), the signal buffer length and the time that was necessary for the user to locate and focus on the

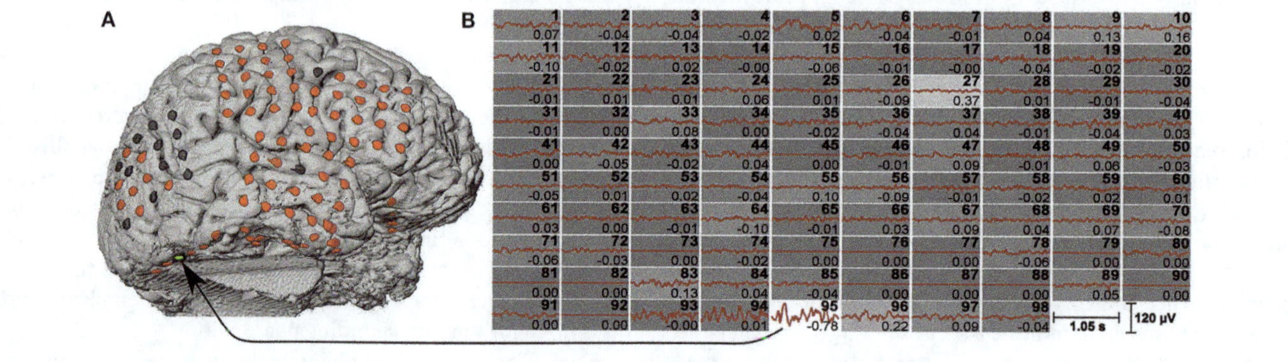

FIGURE 3 | c-VEP templates and spatial filter. (A) Co-registered brain model of a pre-surgical T1-weighted MRI and a post-implantation CT scan. The channels are highlighted in different colors (bad channels are gray, normal channels are red, and the maximum weighted channel of the CCA is green). **(B)** Signals of all 98 channels were averaged over 200 stimulation sequences. Channel numbers are shown on the top right corner of each plot, while the spatial filter coefficients are shown on the bottom right corner. Beside the numeric value, the spatial filter coefficients are also represented by the background intensity of each channel (the highest weight is plotted on white background). Bad channels were set to zero.

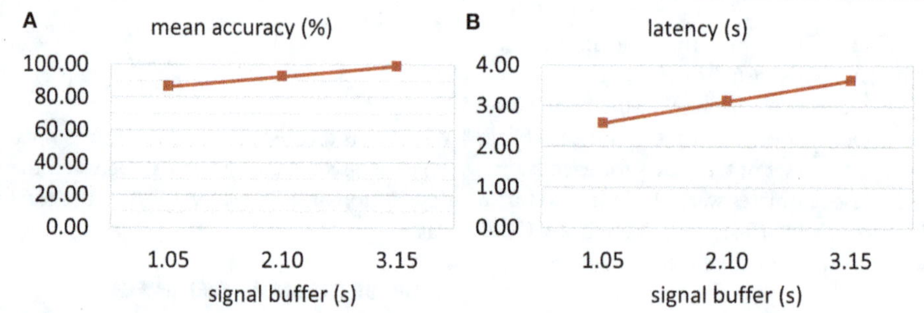

FIGURE 4 | Optimization of the signal buffer. The classification accuracy for **three** different signal buffer sizes was tested. **(A)** Increasing the buffer size from **one** to **three** stimulation sequence lengths (1.05–3.15 s) led to an increase in mean accuracy from 86.76 to 99.21%. **(B)** Of course, the latency of the system depends on the signal buffer length. However, small buffer might reduce the quality of the extracted features. Hence, the latency presented here shows the time that is necessary to achieve classification accuracy above 80%. Increasing the signal buffer size increased the latency from 2.59 to 3.65 s.

target and then produce clear ECoG activity. The exact latencies were 2.59, 3.14, and 3.65 s for a buffer length of 1.05, 2.10, and 3.15 s, respectively.

EVALUATION OF THE ZERO CLASS

Figure 5 shows as an example the effect of the zero class for a signal buffer window length of 2.10 s. The highest classification accuracy could be reached when no zero class was applied. However, if the subject was not attending to any target, the resultant false positive (FP) rate was very high and showed random target selection. If the threshold for the zero class was set to a confidence level of 97%, then the classification accuracy was about 30–40% lower, but also FP rate dropped down to less than 5% if the subject was not attending to one of the targets (second 0.0 to 3.0 in **Figure 5**). Once the subject was focusing a target and the signal buffer contained the corresponding c-VEPs, the FP rate even dropped down to 0%, which means that only reliable features were accepted for classification. The period from second −3.0 to 0.0 represented a period, in which the subject was intended to stop the selection of the previous target. From second −3.0 to −2.0 the FP rate rose up to 50–60%. This period was characterized by high feature values from the last classification leading to an FP rate similar to the classification accuracy with enabled zero class. After another 1.5 s the signal buffer did not contain any target related VEPs anymore.

UNSUPERVISED ONLINE EXPERIMENT

During the free run, the subject performed 17 unsupervised selections. She reported that the feedback of the selected targets was correct throughout the whole run.

DISCUSSION

This work successfully showed that a continuous control signal can be extracted from ECoG data with c-VEPs. The c-VEP approach has an advantage over SSVEPs: there is no single frequency that flashes. Instead, a certain code is embedded, and therefore the risk of inducing seizures is reduced, which is especially important for subjects with increased photosensitivity. SSVEP studies showed that the area of the flashing item, the intensity and the frequency are important parameters for improving the performance. But increasing area and intensity are especially problematic for these persons. SSVEP BCIs work best in a frequency range between about 8–25 Hz, which is a sensitive range for inducing seizures. The c-VEPs contain a mixture of frequencies with lower intensity, comparable to watching TV, and are therefore better suited for these persons.

A big problem of ECoG BCI studies is the rapid selection of appropriate channels coding the necessary information. This can either be done offline with channel selection algorithms like distinction sensitive learning vector quantization (DSLVQ) (Pregenzer and Pfurtscheller, 1995) or by observing reactive frequency spectra or similar parameters. But all these procedures require manual optimization and are time consuming. In the presented work, a spatial filter was automatically obtained using the calibration data during the offline analyses. The result is a spatial filter that selects the most important channels according to their importance for the discrimination task. This is comparable to common spatial patterns (CSP) that are used for motor imagery based BCI system to automatically weight the channels (Guger et al., 2000). For this patient, one of the electrodes (channel 95) mostly contributed to the classification task, two more channels showed medium weights for the spatial filter (channel number

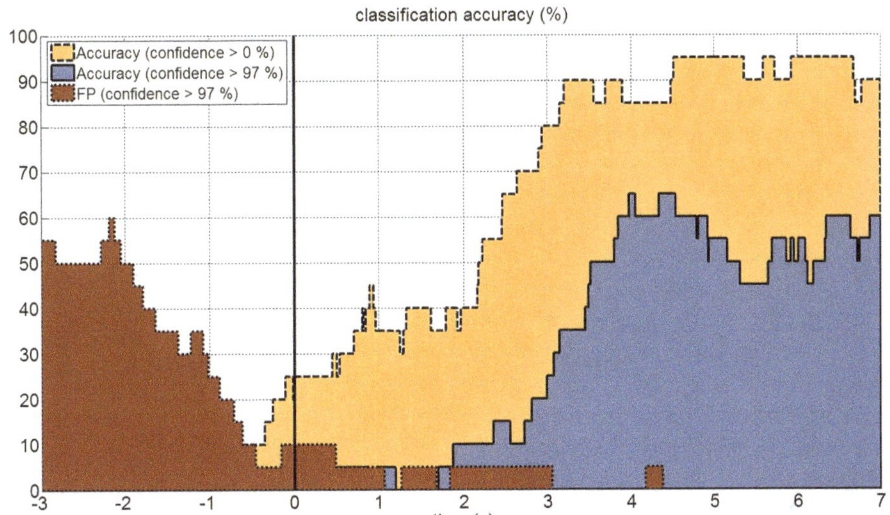

FIGURE 5 | Online accuracy and zero class. The figure shows the online classification accuracy for a 10 s long trial. The black vertical line indicates the onset of the visual stimulation for each trial. Classification was performed using a 2.10 s signal buffer and a confidence interval for classification of 0–100% (yellow area with dashed line) and 97–100% (blue area with solid line). The false positive rate (red area with dotted line) was very high before the stimulation onset, because of the buffer overlap from previous trials. Once the signal buffer did not contain any c-VEPs anymore, the false positive rate dropped down to around 5% and then to 0%, when the signal buffer was again filled with c-VEPs.

27 and 96 ordered by priority). This is similar to CSP, where the weights of the electrodes are also ordered according to the eigenvalues obtained with the algorithm (Müller-Gerking et al., 1999). Interestingly, electrodes 95 and 96 were neighbors located at occipital base (green/blue channel in **Figure 1**), but electrode 27 was located at lateral frontal lobe (blue channel in **Figure 1**). However, as the amplitude of the VEPs of the electrodes 95 and 96 were much higher than for electrode 27, the contribution of electrode 27 to the feature values was very small.

The spatial filter also allows easy system configuration updating with new calibration data. Previous publications with EEG data showed that subjects were trained multiple times to increase the classification accuracy (Guger et al., 2012). In an SSVEP group study with EEG recordings from 53 subjects, the classification accuracy could be increased from a grand average accuracy of 87.9–95.5% after only 20 min of training (Guger et al., 2012). In the current study the used c-VEP algorithm showed a high mean classification accuracy of 99.21% that was achieved with only 200 s of calibration data and after only a single training run lasting less than 4 min in total.

In comparison, the group study of Guger et al. (2012) showed that 27 out of 53 subjects achieved perfect accuracy of 100% and only seven subjects achieved less than 90% accuracy. Another study with a c-VEP BCI including 11 subjects reported a grand average classification accuracy of 98.18% with nobody below 90% accuracy (Kapeller et al., 2013). This study showed that a BCI using c-VEPs works even for subjects who could not use an SSVEP BCI. The c-VEP BCI using ECoG showed similar results compared to the EEG study. This might be an indicator that the SNR of the recorded VEPs was similar in both setups. However, it is important to note that the ECoG setup is much more robust against eye blinks or EMG artifacts. Moreover, in this study the signals were recorded from the right hemisphere only and it is unclear if the electrode positions were optimal with respect to the amplitude of the VEPs.

Notably, the mean classification accuracy from second 5 to 7 is 99.21%, which shows that the subject could continue attending to a certain target for a longer time window. This is important for generating a continuous control signal, unlike discrete selection BCI systems such as a typical P300 BCI. Sutter tested an approach similar to the present system with ECoG data in 1992. He used also c-VEPs with 64 icons on a screen for a spelling system. The study showed that 64 targets could be successfully selected by the ALS patient, who reached about 10–12 words a minute with this setup. Nowadays, the P300 is used for most BCI spellers because these BCI systems support a very high number of targets and can work even better if more targets are used (Allison and Pineda, 2003; Sellers et al., 2006; Guger et al., 2009; Brunner et al., 2011). The SSVEP and c-VEP principles are limited by the number of different targets that can be generated. While the screen refresh rate is a limiting factor for an SSVEP BCI, the sequence length defines the number of possible targets in a c-VEP BCI.

Although, the c-VEP principle allows fast switching from one target to another target, the latency of at least 1.05 s requires anticipation of the user, e.g., while steering an avatar or a robotic system in real-time. Previous studies using ECoG showed very short latencies during 3D cursor control (Wang et al., 2013) or movement of a prosthetic arm (Yanagisawa et al., 2012). In these studies the subjects either performed real or attempted movements in order to detect changes in power of different frequency bands, especially in the frequency band >70 Hz. However, such a BCI system that is independent from motor execution usually requires a much longer training period than the calibration time presented in this work. While using the c-VEP BCI, the subject learned very easily and quickly how to control the system. She was able perform a calibration run, a testing run and a free run within 30 min.

In combination with a goal-oriented BCI system, this allows for full control of humanoid robotic systems. For such applications, it is important to embed the BCI controls into a control display that is either a computer screen or a head-mounted display. Such a humanoid robotic system might have also cameras with 2D or 3D vision embedded for online transmission of a video stream to the BCI feedback monitor, so that the BCI user is also embedded in its avatar for optimizing the control behavior (Gergondet et al., 2012). In this case a big advantage is the zero class property, because it ensures that the humanoid robotic system does not make movements if the user is not attending to one of the controls.

We plan to integrate and test different target shapes and patterns and increase the number of targets. Since the number of targets for the c-VEP configuration is only limited by the sequence length and the minimum phase shift between the sequences, the system can be optimized in terms of number of decisions and reaction time.

ACKNOWLEDGMENT

This research is supported by the European Union FP7 integrated project VERE (No. 257695) and the ENIAC JU project DeNeCor (No. 324257).

REFERENCES

Allison, B. Z., and Pineda, J. A. (2003). ERPs evoked by different matrix sizes: implications for a brain computer interface (BCI) system. *IEEE Trans. Neural Syst. Rehabil. Eng.* 11, 110–113. doi: 10.1109/TNSRE.2003.814448

Bin, G., Gao, X., Wang, Y., Hong, B., and Gao, S. (2009). VEP-based brain-computer interfaces: time, frequency, and code modulations [Research Frontier]. *IEEE Comput. Intell. Mag.* 4, 22–26. doi: 10.1109/MCI.2009.934562

Bin, G., Gao, X., Wang, Y., Li, Y., Hong, B., and Gao, S. (2011). A high-speed BCI based on code modulation VEP. *J. Neural Eng.* 8:025015. doi: 10.1088/1741-2560/8/2/025015

Blankertz, B., Tangermann, M., Vidaurre, C., Fazli, S., Sannelli, C., Haufe, S., et al. (2010). The Berlin brain–computer interface: non-medical uses of BCI technology. *Front. Neurosci.* 4:198. doi: 10.3389/fnins.2010.00198

Borga, M. (2001). *Canonical Correlation: A Tutorial.* On line tutorial. Available online at: http://people.imt.liu.se/magnus/cca

Brunner, P., Ritaccio, A. L., Emrich, J. F., Bischof, H., and Schalk, G. (2011). Rapid communication with a "P300" matrix speller using electrocorticographic signals (ECoG). *Front. Neurosci.* 5:5. doi: 10.3389/fnins.2011.00005

Coyle, S., Ward, T., Markham, C., and McDarby, G. (2004). On the suitability of near-infrared (NIR) systems for next-generation brain–computer interfaces. *Physiol. Meas.* 25:815. doi: 10.1088/0967-3334/25/4/003

Duda, R. O., Hart, P. E., and Stork, D. G. (2000). "Component analysis and discriminations," in *Pattern Classification* (New York, NY: John Wiley & Sons), 117–124.

Faller, J., Müller-Putz, G., Schmalstieg, D., and Pfurtscheller, G. (2010). An application framework for controlling an avatar in a desktop-based virtual environment via a software ssvep brain-computer interface. *Presence Teleoper. Virtual Environ.* 19, 25–34. doi: 10.1162/pres.19.1.25

Gergondet, P., Petit, D., and Kheddar, A. (2012). "Steering a robot with a brain-computer interface: impact of video feedback on BCI performance," in *RO-MAN, 2012 International Symposium on Robot and Human Interactive Communication* (Paris), 271–276.

Golomb, S. W., Welch, L. R., Goldstein, R. M., and Hales, A. W. (1982). *Shift Register Sequences,* Vol. 78. Laguna Hills, CA: Aegean Park Press.

Guger, C., Allison, B. Z., Grosswindhager, B., Prückl, R., Hintermüller, C., Kapeller, C., et al. (2012). How many people could use an SSVEP BCI? *Front. Neurosci.* 6:169. doi: 10.3389/fnins.2012.00169

Guger, C., Daban, S., Sellers, E., Holzner, C., Krausz, G., Carabalona, R., et al. (2009). How many people are able to control a P300-based brain–computer interface (BCI)? *Neurosci. Lett.* 462, 94–98. doi: 10.1016/j.neulet.2009.06.045

Guger, C., Edlinger, G., Harkam, W., Niedermayer, I., and Pfurtscheller, G. (2003). How many people are able to operate an EEG-based brain-computer interface (BCI)? *IEEE Trans. Neural Syst. Rehabil. Eng.* 11, 145–147. doi: 10.1109/TNSRE.2003.814481

Guger, C., Ramoser, H., and Pfurtscheller, G. (2000). Real-time EEG analysis with subject-specific spatial patterns for a brain-computer interface (BCI). *IEEE Trans. Rehabil. Eng.* 8, 447–456. doi: 10.1109/86.895947

Kapeller, C., Hintermuller, C., Abu-Alqumsan, M., Pruckl, R., Peer, A., and Guger, C. (2013). "A BCI using VEP for continuous control of a mobile robot," in *2013 35th Annual International Conference of the IEEE Engineering in Medicine and Biology Society (EMBC)* (Osaka), 5254–5257. doi: 10.1109/EMBC.2013.6610734

Krausz, G., Scherer, R., Korisek, G., and Pfurtscheller, G. (2003). Critical decision-speed and information transfer in the "Graz Brain–Computer Interface." *Appl. Psychophysiol. Biofeedb.* 28, 233–240. doi: 10.1023/A:1024637331493

Lalor, E. C., Kelly, S. P., Finucane, C., Burke, R., Smith, R., Reilly, R. B., et al. (2005). Steady-state VEP-based brain-computer interface control in an immersive 3D gaming environment. *EURASIP J. Appl. Signal Process.* 2005, 3156–3164. doi: 10.1155/ASP.2005.3156

Leuthardt, E. C., Schalk, G., Wolpaw, J. R., Ojemann, J. G., and Moran, D. W. (2004). A brain–computer interface using electrocorticographic signals in humans. *J. Neural Eng.* 1:63. doi: 10.1088/1741-2560/1/2/001

Martinez, P., Bakardjian, H., and Cichocki, A. (2007). Fully online multicommand brain-computer interface with visual neurofeedback using SSVEP paradigm. *Comput. Intell. Neurosci.* 2007:13. doi: 10.1155/2007/94561

Mason, S. G., Bashashati, A., Fatourechi, M., Navarro, K. F., and Birch, G. E. (2007). A comprehensive survey of brain interface technology designs. *Ann. Biomed. Eng.* 35, 137–169. doi: 10.1007/s10439-006-9170-0

Miller, K. J., Schalk, G., Fetz, E. E., den Nijs, M., Ojemann, J. G., and Rao, R. P. (2010). Cortical activity during motor execution, motor imagery, and imagery-based online feedback. *Proc. Natl. Acad. Sci. U.S.A.* 107, 4430–4435. doi: 10.1073/pnas.0913697107

Müller-Gerking, J., Pfurtscheller, G., and Flyvbjerg, H. (1999). Designing optimal spatial filters for single-trial EEG classification in a movement task. *Clin. Neurophysiol.* 110, 787–798. doi: 10.1016/S1388-2457(98)00038-8

Pregenzer, M., and Pfurtscheller, G. (1995). "Distinction Sensitive Learning Vector Quantization (DSLVQ) application as a classifier based feature selection method for a brain computer interface," in *Fourth International Conference on Artificial Neural Networks* (Cambridge), 433–436.

Putz, V., Guger, C., Holzner, C., Torrellas, S., and Miralles, F. (2011). "A unified XML based description of the contents of brain computer interfaces," in *Proceedings of the 5th International BCI Conference* (Graz), 22–24.

Schalk, G., Miller, K. J., Anderson, N. R., Wilson, J. A., Smyth, M. D., Ojemann, J. G., et al. (2008). Two-dimensional movement control using electrocorticographic signals in humans. *J. Neural. Eng.* 5, 75–84. doi: 10.1088/1741-2560/5/1/008

Sellers, E. W., Krusienski, D. J., McFarland, D. J., Vaughan, T. M., and Wolpaw, J. R. (2006). A P300 event-related potential brain–computer interface (BCI): the effects of matrix size and inter stimulus interval on performance. *Biol. Psychol.* 73, 242–252. doi: 10.1016/j.biopsycho.2006.04.007

Spüler, M., Rosenstiel, W., and Bogdan, M. (2012). Online adaptation of a c-VEP Brain-computer Interface (BCI) based on error-related potentials and unsupervised learning. *PLoS ONE* 7:e51077. doi: 10.1371/journal.pone.0051077

Sutter, E. E. (1992). The brain response interface: communication through visually-induced electrical brain responses. *J. Microcomp. Appl.* 15, 31–45. doi: 10.1016/0745-7138(92)90045-7

Sutton, R. S., and Barto, A. G. (1998). "Softmax action selection," in *Reinforcement Learning: An Introduction*, eds R. S. Sutton and A. G. Barto (Cambridge: The MIT Press), 1998.

Volosyak, I. (2011). SSVEP-based Bremen–BCI interface—boosting information transfer rates. *J. Neural Eng.* 8:036020. doi: 10.1088/1741-2560/8/3/036020

Wang, W., Collinger, J. L., Degenhart, A. D., Tyler-Kabara, E. C., Schwartz, A. B., Moran, D. W., et al. (2013). An electrocorticographic brain interface in an individual with tetraplegia. *PLoS ONE* 8:e55344. doi: 10.1371/journal.pone.0055344

Wang, Y., Gao, X., Hong, B., Jia, C., and Gao, S. (2008). Brain-computer interfaces based on visual evoked potentials. *IEEE Eng. Med. Biol. Mag.* 27, 64–71. doi: 10.1109/MEMB.2008.923958

Weiskopf, N., Mathiak, K., Bock, S. W., Scharnowski, F., Veit, R., Grodd, W., et al. (2004). Principles of a brain-computer interface (BCI) based on real-time functional magnetic resonance imaging (fMRI). *IEEE Trans. Biomed. Eng.* 51, 966–970. doi: 10.1109/TBME.2004.827063

Wolpaw, J. R., Birbaumer, N., McFarland, D. J., Pfurtscheller, G., and Vaughan, T. M. (2002). Brain–computer interfaces for communication and control. *Clin. Neurophysiol.* 113, 767–791. doi: 10.1016/S1388-2457(02)00057-3

Yanagisawa, T., Hirata, M., Saitoh, Y., Kishima, H., Matsushita, K., Goto, T., et al. (2012). Electrocorticographic control of a prosthetic arm in paralyzed patients. *Ann. Neurol.* 71, 353–361. doi: 10.1002/ana.22613

Zierler, N. (1959). Linear recurring sequences. *J. Soc. Ind. Appl. Math.* 7, 31–48. doi: 10.1137/0107003

16

Stem cell-paved biobridge facilitates neural repair in traumatic brain injury

Naoki Tajiri[1]*, Kelsey Duncan[1], Alesia Antoine[1], Mibel Pabon[1], Sandra A. Acosta[1], Ike de la Pena[1], Diana G. Hernadez-Ontiveros[1], Kazutaka Shinozuka[1], Hiroto Ishikawa[1], Yuji Kaneko[1], Ernest Yankee[2], Michael McGrogan[2], Casey Case[2] and Cesar V. Borlongan[1]*

[1] Center of Excellence for Aging and Brain Repair, Department of Neurosurgery and Brain Repair, Morsani College of Medicine, University of South Florida, Tampa, FL, USA

[2] Sanbio Inc., Mountain View, CA, USA

Edited by:
Manuel Casanova, University of Louisville, USA

Reviewed by:
Jun Takahashi, Kyoto University, Japan
Ana Bribian, Paraplegics National Hospital, Spain

***Correspondence:**
Naoki Tajiri and Cesar V. Borlongan, Department of Neurosurgery and Brain Repair, University of South Florida Morsani College of Medicine, 12901 Bruce B. Downs Blvd, Tampa, FL 33612, USA
e-mail: ntajiri@health.usf.edu; cborlong@health.usf.edu

Modified mesenchymal stromal cells (MSCs) display a unique mechanism of action during the repair phase of traumatic brain injury by exhibiting the ability to build a biobridge between the neurogenic niche and the site of injury. Immunohistochemistry and laser capture assay have visualized this biobridge in the area between the neurogenic subventricular zone and the injured cortex. This biobridge expresses high levels of extracellular matrix metalloproteinases (MMPs), which are initially co-localized with a stream of transplanted MSCs, but later this region contains only few to non-detectable grafts and becomes overgrown by newly recruited host cells. We have reported that long-distance migration of host cells from the neurogenic niche to the injured brain site can be attained via these transplanted stem cell-paved biobridges, which serve as a key regenerative process for the initiation of endogenous repair mechanisms. Thus, far the two major schools of discipline in stem cell repair mechanisms support the idea of "cell replacement" and the bystander effects of "trophic factor secretion." Our novel observation of stem cell-paved biobridges as pathways for directed migration of host cells from neurogenic niche toward the injured brain site adds another mode of action underlying stem cell therapy. More in-depth investigations on graft-host interaction will likely aid translational research focused on advancing this stem cell-paved biobridge from its current place, as an equally potent repair mechanism as cell replacement and trophic factor secretion, into a new treatment strategy for traumatic brain injury and other neurological disorders.

Keywords: trauma, cell transplantation, regenerative medicine, neurogenesis, extracellular matrix

A NOVEL BRAIN REPAIR MECHANISM OF TRANSPLANTED STEM CELLS

Stem cell research offers an avenue for an in-depth study of cell biology, as well as in the development of new strategies to treat diseases (Yasuhara et al., 2006, 2008; Tajiri et al., 2012). Nevertheless, much remains to be understood about the mechanisms underlying the beneficial effects of stem cell therapy. To date, there are two major schools of discipline in stem cell-mediated repair mechanism in brain damage caused by injury or neurodegenerative disorders (Borlongan et al., 2004; Pastori et al., 2008). The first concept supports the idea of "cell replacement," i.e., stem cells implanted into the brain directly replace dead or dying cells (**Figure 1A**), whereas the other argues that transplanted stem cells secrete growth factors that indirectly rescue the injured tissue (i.e., bystander effects of stem cells) (Lee et al., 2007; Redmond et al., 2007) (**Figure 1B**).

Stem cells exist through adulthood (Ma et al., 2010), and possess the capacity for self-renewal and differentiation into multiple lineages. They have also been shown to contribute to the maintenance of homeostasis (Kim et al., 2011), exert therapeutic benefits both endogenously (Barha et al., 2011; Borlongan, 2011; Jaskelioff et al., 2011; Wang et al., 2011) and following transplantation into injured organs, e.g., the brain (Mazzocchi-Jones et al., 2009; Hargus et al., 2010; Lee et al., 2010; Andres et al., 2011; Liu et al., 2011; Mezey, 2011; Yasuda et al., 2011). There are two major stem cell niches in the brain namely, the subventricular zone (SVZ) of the lateral ventricles and the subgranular zone of the hippocampus dentate gyrus (DG) (Carlén et al., 2009; Sanai et al., 2011), although quiescent neural stem cells (NSCs) have been found in other brain regions (Robel et al., 2011). The discovery that stem cells are activated following injury opened up new research frontiers in regenerative medicine (Yasuhara et al., 2006; Mazzocchi-Jones et al., 2009; Hargus et al., 2010; Lee et al., 2010; Andres et al., 2011; Barha et al., 2011; Borlongan, 2011; Jaskelioff et al., 2011; Liu et al., 2011; Mezey, 2011; Wang et al., 2011; Yasuda et al., 2011; Tajiri et al., 2012). Consequently, this research paved the way for translation of laboratory studies on stem cells into limited clinical trials for brain disorders (Pollock et al., 2006; Yasuhara et al., 2009; Seol et al., 2011). Despite these scientific advances and clinical applications, the mechanisms underlying

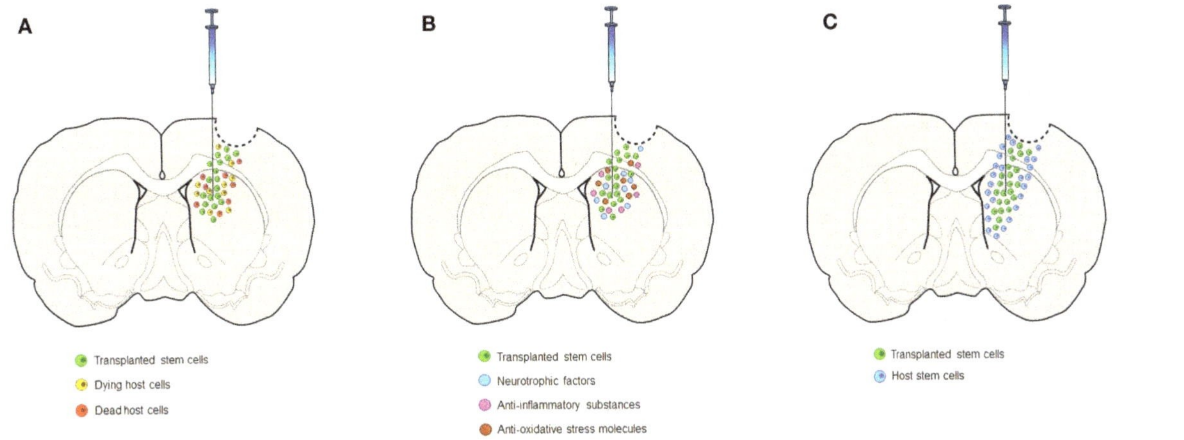

FIGURE 1 | Multiple mechanisms underlying stem cell therapy. **(A)** Cell replacement entails that transplanted cells replace dead or dying host cells, which would require neuronal differentiation of stem cells and reconstruction of the damaged synaptic circuitry. **(B)** By-stander effects involve secretion of neurotrophic factors, anti-inflammatory substances, and anti-oxidative stress molecules by the transplanted cells, which subsequently rescue spared host cells or stimulate neurogenesis. **(C)** Stem cell-paved biobridges show that transplanted cells form a biological pathway, enriched in MMPs, and ferries newly born host stem cells from the neurogenic niche SVZ to the injured host tissue.

stem cell-mediated repair in brain injury are not yet completely understood.

In a recent study, we demonstrated motor and neurological improvements in rats subjected to traumatic brain injury (TBI) and transplanted intracerebrally with cultured Notch-induced human bone marrow-derived mesenchymal stromal cells (referred to as SB623, supplied by SanBio Inc.) While we obtained important results that corroborate the putative therapeutic benefits of stem cell transplantation for TBI, our research on the mechanism of action of SB623 revealed breakthrough findings which support the discovery of a novel stem-cell mediated repair mechanism in brain injury. Accordingly, we observed the capacity of transplanted stem cells to harness a "biobridge" between the neurogenic niche and the site of brain injury, enabling long-distance migration of host neurogenic cells and consequently, initiating endogenous repair mechanisms. In this paper, we discuss the properties and characteristics of these stem cell paved-biobridges, elaborate on the unique mechanism by which these biobridges facilitate repair in a rat model of TBI, and importantly, suggest the clinical significance of exploiting this novel stem cell-mediated concept of brain repair for the treatment of brain injury and other neurological disorders.

BREAKTHROUGH DISCOVERY: STEM CELL-PAVED FORMATION OF "BIOBRIDGES" IN EXPERIMENTAL MODELS OF TBI

Rats subjected to TBI were intracerebrally transplanted with SB623 (gene-modified human mesenchymal stromal cells) (Zhao et al., 2007; Yasuhara et al., 2009). Thereafter, the motor and neurological functions of these rats were evaluated at 1, 2, and 3 months post-TBI, and histological studies were performed to assess the therapeutic effects of SB623 transplantation. The behavioral studies showed significant motor and neurological improvement in TBI rats which received SB623. Histological studies also showed profound reduction in TBI-induced damages to the cortical core and the peri-injured cortical areas in SB623-transplanted TBI rats. The behavioral and histological improvements, however, were achieved despite minimal graft survival—0.60 and 0.16% at 1 and 3 months, respectively. These findings led us to examine the condition of the host tissue, in view of functional recovery despite lack of graft persistence.

At 1 month post-TBI, we observed notable increases in endogenous cellular proliferation (Ki67) as well as immature neural differentiation (nestin) in the peri-injured cortical areas and SVZ, along with a stream of migrating cells along the corpus callosum (CC) of SB623 transplanted TBI animals. Furthermore, at 3 months post-TBI, we observed enhanced cellular proliferation and neural differentiation in the peri-injured cortical (CTX) areas of SB623 transplanted TBI animals, accompanied by a solid stream of neuronally-labeled cells (nestin and DCX) migrating not only along but also across the CC from the SVZ to the impacted CTX. Contrastingly, TBI rats which received vehicle infusion exhibited elevated cellular proliferation; however the newly formed cells were "trapped" within the SVZ and CTX and did not migrate to the impacted CTX.

We next analyzed the formation of the biobridge by means of the cells leaving the SVZ and moving toward the site of injury was laser captured in the animals receiving the SB623 cells.

The biobridge between the SVZ and the impacted cortex was composed of highly proliferative, neutrally committed, and migratory cells. These animals showed a 2 and 9-fold upregulation of the matrix metalloproteinase-9 (MMP) activity and expression at 1 and 3 months post-TBI, respectively. Further *in vitro* studies also showed the ability of SB623 cells to enhance cell migration via this MMP-rich signaling cues. These signals are crucial to the migration of endogenous cells which can then assist with functional recovery of damaged tissue. Merely 1 month post-TBI, a surge of proliferative Ki67 positive cells and neurally immature nestin labeled cells in the peri-injured areas and SVZ were discerned. The high level of MMP-9 in the biobridge indicates the importance of this neurovascular proteinase. Interestingly, this proteinase was upregulated in the vehicle group, but reverted back to control-sham levels at 3 months post-TBI. This illustrates the role of MMP in long-term recovery and adds another facet to the mechanism through which stem cells aid in recovery of damaged tissue.

To provide further evidence that the implanted SB623 cells facilitated the formation of the biobridge, thus enabling the migration of host stem cells from the SVZ to the site of injury and the up-regulation of endogenous cells, an *in vitro* study was performed with primary rat cortical cells grown both alone and co-cultured with SB623 cells. These were grown either in the presence or absence of the MMP-9 inhibitor Cyclosporin-A. Migratory cell assay revealed noticeably enhanced migration of primary rat cortical cells in the chamber containing SB623, which was then significantly suppressed by treatment with the MMP-9 inhibitor. Treatment with the inhibitor alone, combined treatment with SB623 and the inhibitor, and absence of both SB623 and the inhibitor did not significantly alter migratory potential.

Although endogenous repair mechanisms are initiated post-TBI, these effects are typically limited to the neurogenic SVZ and quiescent neurogenic resident cells around the impacted cortex. Accordingly, these endogenous mechanisms are not robust enough to provide a solid defense against TBI or other disease-induced cell death cascades necessitating introduction of exogenous cells to aid migration of endogenous stem cells from the neurogenic niche to the site of injury. Stem cell transplantation into the peri-injured cortical areas purportedly creates a biobridge comprised of a neurovascular matrix which allows newly formed endogenous cells to migrate efficiently to the site of injury. Moreover, biobridge is established, exogenous cells slowly fade away, supplanted by newly formed endogenous cells that can maintain recovery even in the absence of transplanted stem cells.

A BIOBRIDGE BETWEEN THE NEUROGENIC NICHE AND THE ISCHEMIC TISSUE

The results show SB623 transplants aid in regeneration of the traumatically injured brain by constructing a biobridge between the SVZ and the peri-injured cortex (**Figure 1C**). This novel mechanism opens new doors for cell therapy by allowing the creation of similar biobridges between neurogenic and non-neurogenic sites to aid in injury-specific migration of cells across tissues that are barriers to cellular motility.

A phase I/IIa study of SB623 cell transplantation in chronic stroke patients has already been initiated. Transplantation of SB623 cells has been shown to mitigate histological and behavioral deficits associated with stroke, spinal cord injury, and Parkinson's Disease in both cell culture and animal models of brain disorders. The use of SB623 cells in TBI patients is an innovative concept that has already been FDA approved for a limited clinical trial based on the data presented.

Understanding SB623's role in facilitating the migration of endogenous cells via a biobridge exposes the active role of MMPs and ECMs in stroke pathology (Park et al., 2009; el Zoppo et al., 2012) and highlights their increasingly prominent role as therapeutic targets for stroke. Functions and levels of MMPs and ECMs have been shown to be influenced by a variety of cells coming from variable sources including umbilical cord blood, peripheral blood, and the adult brain (Barkho et al., 2008; Sobrino et al., 2012; Lin et al., 2013). This suggests a potential for these molecules to serve as biobridges similar to the current function of Notch-induced SB623 mesenchymal stromal cells.

While documented neurogenic niches such as the SVZ exist in the adult brain and contain cells that play a critical role in repairing the stroke brain (Ekdahl et al., 2009; Ducruet et al., 2012; Hassani et al., 2012; Wang et al., 2012; Trueman et al., 2013), it has been shown that a major limiting factor for endogenous repair is the lack of successful migration of newly formed host cells to the site of injury. Currently, results show SB623 cell transplantation boosts endogenous repair mechanisms by guiding the transition of new cells from the neurogenic SVZ, across a non-neurogenic brain area, to the site of injury. The ability of SB623 cells to form biobridges containing MMPs and ECMs which can then entice newly formed cells from the niche into the ischemic tissue appears to be a fundamental mechanism of action. Once the transplanted SB623 cells have pioneered the formation of these biobridges, they allow the endogenous stem cells to take over the remodeling process.

The precise mechanism by which the graft cells are integrated into the recipient brain tissue and subsequently interact with the host cells to result in functional restoration remains unknown. This essential interaction between the transplanted cell and host cell becomes even more obscure when graft survival is minimal. This indicates that the role of the SB623 is to set in motion robust and stable therapeutic benefits, particularly by leading the way for host cells to reach the injured site even across non-neurogenic and injured tissues. MMP has been implicated in chronic brain injury recovery through studies that inhibited MMPs, which consequently halted neurogenic migration from the SVZ into damaged tissues. The result was a noticeable retardation in neurovascular remodeling. This supports the concept that exogenously added cells can express MMPs and thereby reinforce the neurovascular unit, aiding in the transplant-mediated host cell migration toward the site of injury. This potentially allows for the formation of biobridges, thereby affording functional recovery in TBI.

BEYOND TBI: EXPLOITING STEM CELL-PAVED BIOBRIDGES FOR THE TREATMENT OF OTHER NEUROLOGICAL DISORDERS

The most adult stem cells in the brain are found in the SVZ of the lateral ventricles and the subgranular zone of the hippocampus dentate gyrus. The microenvironment of a stem cell niche is maintained by the signaling molecules, growth factors, and receptors. In adults, these stem cells typically remain in a dormant non-dividing state until activated by an insult. When an insult occurs motility ensues and the endogenous stem cells find themselves trapped and unable to reach the site of injury. The novel discovery that grafted cells can facilitate endogenous stem cell migration from the neurogenic niche to the site of injury is indeed a significant progress in the both stem cell and TBI research.

Our recent study (Tajiri et al., 2013) advances the concept of the biobridge mechanism as a cell mediated repair strategy in TBI, and opens new avenues for translational applications of cell therapy in TBI. Monitoring long term safety and efficacy of SB623 cell therapy in TBI animal models in order to optimize the conduct of clinical trials involving these cells in TBI patients is a priority. Gaining a more concrete understanding of the stem cell mechanism is the next step which will help to push forth the boundaries of stem cell research and explain the mechanism of cellular therapy in neurological disease.

In addition to TBI, a number of other neurological disorders are characterized by a "biological gap" between the site of injury and intact tissue. In this regard, disorders like stroke and Parkinson's disease may benefit from a deeper understanding on the concept of stem cell-paved biobridge because both disorders present with a site of cellular degeneration that is physically separated from the area of the brain that could aid in the recovery of dead tissue or lost cells. For example, stroke entails an ischemic core and penumbra residing next to intact tissue. While the ischemic core damage cannot be recovered, the potential for neural repair has been demonstrated by targeting the penumbra. Accordingly, a biobridge between the penumbra and the intact tissue (i.e., neurogenic niche) could potentially aid in stroke. Parkinson's disease involves the degeneration of the nigrostriatal dopaminergic pathway, which could improve drastically with directed migration of host stem cells toward this region in the form of a biobridge. Further investigations are warranted to determine how the concept of stem-cell paved biobridge could be exploited for the treatment of other neurological disorders.

MULTI-PRONGED MECHANISMS UNDERLYING STEM CELL THERAPY

As noted above, stem cell-mediated repair mechanisms have been widely purported as afforded via cell replacement and bystander effects (Snyder et al., 1997; Borlongan et al., 2004; Lee et al., 2007; Redmond et al., 2007; Pastori et al., 2008; Acosta et al., 2014). Our proposed third mechanism describes the recruitment of endogenous stem cells from the stem cell niches (Alvarez-Buylla et al., 2008) to the injured site through the transplanted stem cell-formed biobridge. This begs the question of whether the biobridge provides the scaffold or trophic factors to promote stem cell migration. Interestingly, new reports suggest candidate ECMs may serve as a scaffold or trophic factor-rich soluble molecules. For example, a study observed that the limits of interstitial cell migration depends upon scaffold porosity and deformation of the nucleus, with pericellular collagenolysis and mechanocoupling as modulators acting as scaffolds and assisting with biobridge formation (i.e., stem cell migration) (Wolf et al., 2013). Alternatively, a study found that functional analysis of mesenchymal stem cell proliferation, migration, and adhesion to ECMs revealed that IL-1β did not affect proliferation but served to induce the secretion of trophic factors and adhesion to ECM components such as collagen and laminin (Carrero et al., 2012).

In the end, stem cell functionality is a key factor to achieve clinically relevant outcomes of stem cell therapy. Of note, neurogenesis *per se* does not equate to these new neurons integrating with the damaged area, and that physiological and functional assays (e.g., synaptic circuitry reconstruction, evoked potentials, long-term potentiation, etc.) will be necessary to unequivocally reveal the contribution of these newly formed cells in the resulting behavioral recovery. Depending on the target disease of stem cell therapy, it is likely that neuronal differentiation to specific disease-phenotype (Hong et al., 2011), as in the case of Parkinson's disease and Huntington's disease, may be needed to produce functional effects. However, we caution that such neuronal differentiation may occur in both exogenously transplanted cells and the mobilized endogenous stem cells. Our concept of biobridge formation highlights the need for these stem cells to be guided toward the site of injury, which may facilitate the therapeutic effects of these newly formed cells that have committed to neuronally differentiated cells. Alternatively or a complement mechanism in the absence of neuronal differentiation, we also propose the biobridge-facilitated by-stander effects, in that with the directed migration of these stem cells toward the site of injury, the biobridge is able to harness the secretion of growth factors, anti-inflammatory substances, and/or anti-oxidative stress molecules close to the damaged area.

The concept of stem cell-paved biobridge may have some similarities with the use of olfactory ensheathing glia in spinal cord injury. Compelling evidence from animal models and clinical studies suggest that transplantation of olfactory ensheathing cells (OECs), specialized glia in the olfactory system, combined with specific training may be therapeutically useful in central nervous system (CNS) injuries and neurodegenerative diseases. The unique function of OECs could be attributed to both production of cell adhesion molecules and secretion of growth factors in OECs, which support neuron survival and neurite outgrowth (He et al., 2013). Another study showed that transplantation of OEG and Schwann cell (SCs) in a sub-acute phase can improve anatomical outcomes after a contusion injury to the spinal cord by increasing the number of spared/regenerated supraspinal fibers, reducing cavitation, and enhancing tissue integrity (Barbour et al., 2013). Most spinal cord injury models evaluating the therapeutic efficacy of OEC transplants have reported functional recovery via indirect and direct reparative pathways involving growth factor secretion, neuronal and axonal regeneration, and remyelination (Roet et al., 2013).

Although similarities exist between the biobridge seen with OECs in spinal cord injury and our observed biobridge in TBI, the biobridge seen in spinal cord injury involves the ensheating features of OECs, as well as the fabrication of scaffolds (such as laminin and fibronectin) and seeding the stem cells onto these matrices in order to create a biobridge. In contrast, our observed biobridge involves a natural process of the stem cells themselves serving as matrices in facilitating the migration of endogenous stem cells from the neurogenic niche toward the injured host tissue. With this in mind, a similar biobridge strategy was documented in Parkinson's disease whereby the transplanted dopamine-secreting cells were deposited along the nigrostriatal system (instead of merely transplanting the cells into the striatum) to closely reconstruct the major dopaminergic afferent and efferent pathways (Wang et al., 1996; Tang et al., 1998; Chiang et al., 2001). Compared to our observed biobridge formation, this bridging graft in Parkinson's disease is an artificial reconstruction of the dopaminergic system whereby micro-deposits of immature cells are undertaken along the nigrostriatal pathway, whereas our biobridge formation reveals a natural process of the transplanted stem cells homing from the neurogenic niche and forming a bridge toward the injured site, and subsequently attracting endogenous stem cells to populate the biobridge and to eventually continue the brain reparative process.

Altogether, these observations suggest that while distinct mechanisms of action may be individually facilitating the neural repair of transplanted stem cells in the injured brain, overlapping regenerative processes involving cell replacement, by-stander effects, and biobridge formation may be working in tandem in realizing the therapeutic benefits of stem cell therapy.

ACKNOWLEDGMENTS

This work was supported by NIH NINDS RO1 1R01NS071956-01 (Cesar V. Borlongan), James, and Esther King Biomedical Research Program 09KB-01-23123 (Cesar V. Borlongan) and 1KG01-33966 (Cesar V. Borlongan).

REFERENCES

Acosta, S. A., Tajiri, N., Shinozuka, K., Ishikawa, H., Sanberg, P. R., Sanchez-Ramos, J., et al. (2014). Combination therapy of human umbilical cord blood cells and granulocyte colony stimulating factor reduces histopathological and motor impairments in an experimental model of chronic traumatic brain injury. *PLoS ONE* 9:e90953. doi: 10.1371/journal.pone.0090953

Alvarez-Buylla, A., Kohwi, M., Nguyen, T. M., and Merkle, F. T. (2008). The heterogeneity of adult neural stem cells and the emerging complexity of their niche. *Cold Spring Harb. Symp. Quant. Biol.* 73, 357–365. doi: 10.1101/sqb.2008.73.019

Andres, R. H., Horie, N., Slikker, W., Keren-Gill, H., Zhan, K., Sun, G., et al. (2011). Human neural stem cells enhance structural plasticity and axonal transport in the ischaemic brain. *Brain* 134, 1777–1789. doi: 10.1093/brain/awr094

Barbour, H. R., Plant, C. D., Harvey, A. R., and Plant, G. W. (2013). Tissue sparing, behavioral recovery, supraspinal axonal sparing/regeneration following subacute glial transplantation in a model of spinal cord contusion. *BMC Neurosci.* 14:106. doi: 10.1186/1471-2202-14-106

Barha, C. K., Ishrat, T., Epp, J. R., Galea, L. A., and Stein, D. G. (2011). Progesterone treatment normalizes the levels of cell proliferation and cell death in the dentate gyrus of the hippocampus after traumatic brain injury. *Exp. Neurol.* 231, 72–81. doi: 10.1016/j.expneurol.2011.05.016

Barkho, B. Z., Munoz, A. E., Li, X., Li, L., Cunningham, L. A., and Zhao, X. (2008). Endogenous matrix metalloproteinase (MMP)-3 and MMP-9 promote the differentiation and migration of adult neural progenitor cells in response to chemokines. *Stem Cells* 26, 3139–3149. doi: 10.1634/stemcells.2008-0519

Borlongan, C. V. (2011). Bone marrow stem cell mobilization in stroke: a 'bonehead' may be good after all!. *Leukemia* 25, 1674–1686. doi: 10.1038/leu.2011.167

Borlongan, C. V., Hadman, M., Sanberg, C. D., and Sanberg, P. R. (2004). Central nervous system entry of peripherally injected umbilical cord blood cells is not required for neuroprotection in stroke. *Stroke* 35, 2385–2389. doi: 10.1161/01.STR.0000141680.49960.d7

Carlén, M., Meletis, K., Goritz, C., Darsalia, V., Evergren, E., Tanigaki, K., et al. (2009). Forebrain ependymal cells are Notch-dependent and generate neuroblasts and astrocytes after stroke. *Nat. Neurosci.* 12, 259–267. doi: 10.1038/nn.2268

Carrero, R., Cerrada, I., Lledó, E., Dopazo, J., García-García, F., Rubio, M. P., et al. (2012). IL1β induces mesenchymal stem cells migration and leucocyte chemotaxis through NF-κB. *Stem Cell Rev.* 8, 905–916. doi: 10.1007/s12015-012-9364-9

Chiang, Y., Morales, M., Zhou, F. C., Borlongan, C., Hoffer, B. J., and Wang, Y. (2001). Fetal intra-nigral ventral mesencephalon and kidney tissue bridge transplantation restores the nigrostriatal dopamine pathway in hemi-parkinsonian rats. *Brain Res.* 889, 200–207. doi: 10.1016/S0006-8993(00)03133-4

del Zoppo, G. J., Frankowski, H., Gu, Y. H., Osada, T., Kanazawa, M., Milner, R., et al. (2012). Microglial cell activation is a source of metalloproteinase generation during hemorrhagic transformation. *J. Cereb. Blood Flow Metab.* 32, 919–932. doi: 10.1038/jcbfm.2012.11

Ducruet, A. F., Zacharia. B. E., Sosunov, S. A., Gigante, P. R., Yeh, M. L., Gorski, J. W., et al. (2012). Complement inhibition promotes endogenous neurogenesis and sustained anti-inflammatory neuroprotection following reperfused stroke. *PLoS ONE* 7:e38664. doi: 10.1371/journal.pone.0038664

Ekdahl, C. T., Kokaia, Z., and Lindvall, O. (2009). Brain inflammation and adult neurogenesis: the dual role of microglia. *Neuroscience* 158, 1021–1029. doi: 10.1016/j.neuroscience.2008.06.052

Hargus, G., Cooper, O., Deleidi, M., Levy, A., Lee, K., Marlow, E., et al. (2010). Differentiated Parkinson patient-derived induced pluripotent stem cells grow in the adult rodent brain and reduce motor asymmetry in Parkinsonian rats. *Proc. Natl. Acad. Sci U.S.A.* 107, 15921–15926. doi: 10.1073/pnas.1010209107

Hassani, Z., O,Reilly, J., Pearse, Y., Stroemer, P., Tang, E., Sinden, J., et al. (2012). Human neural progenitor cell engraftment increases neurogenesis and microglial recruitment in the brain of rats with stroke. *PLoS ONE* 7:e50444. doi: 10.1371/journal.pone.0050444

He, B. R., Xie, S. T., Wu, M. M., Hao, D. J., and Yang, H. (2013). Phagocytic removal of neuronal debris by olfactory ensheathing cells enhances neuronal survival and neurite outgrowth via p38MAPK activity. *Mol. Neurobiol.* 49, 1501–1512. doi: 10.1007/s12035-013-8588-2

Hong, S. H., Rampalli, S., Lee, J. B., McNicol, J., Collins, T., Draper, J. S., et al. (2011). Cell fate potential of human pluripotent stem cells is encoded by histone modifications.*Cell Stem Cell* 9, 24–36. doi: 10.1016/j.stem.2011.06.002

Jaskelioff, M., Muller, F. L., Paik, J. H., Thomas, E., Jiang, S., Adams, A. C., et al. (2011). Telomerase reactivation reverses tissue degeneration in aged telomerase-deficient *mice. Nature* 469, 102–106. doi: 10.1038/nature09603

Kim, Y., Sharov, A. A., McDole, K., Cheng, M., Hao, H., Fan, C. M., et al. (2011). Mouse B-type lamins are required for proper organogenesis but not by embryonic stem cells. *Science* 334, 1706–1710. doi: 10.1126/science.1211222

Lee, H. S., Bae, E. J., Yi, S. H., Shim, J. W., Jo, A. Y., Kang, J. S., et al. (2010). Foxa2 and Nurr1 synergistically yield A9 nigral dopamine neurons exhibiting improved differentiation, function, and cell survival. *Stem Cells* 28, 501–512. doi: 10.1002/stem.294

Lee, J. P., Jeyakumar, M., Gonzalez, R., Takahashi, H., Lee, P. J., Baek, R. C., et al. (2007). Stem cells act through multiple mechanisms to benefit mice with neurodegenerative metabolic disease. *Nat. Med.* 13, 439–447. doi: 10.1038/nm1548

Lin, C. H., Lee, H. T., Lee, S. D., Lee, W., Cho, C. W., Lin, S. Z., et al. (2013). Role of HIF-1alpha-activated Epac1 on HSC-mediated neuroplasticity in stroke model. *Neurobiol. Dis.* 58C, 76–91. doi: 10.1016/j.nbd.2013.05.006

Liu, Z., Li, Y., Zhang, R. L., Cui, Y., and Chopp, M. (2011). Bone marrow stromal cells promote skilled motor recovery and enhance contralesional axonal connections after ischemic stroke in adult mice. *Stroke* 42, 740–744. doi: 10.1161/STROKEAHA.110.607226

Ma, D. K., Marchetto, M. C., Guo, J. U., Ming, G. L., Gage, F. H., and Song, H. (2010). Epigenetic choreographers of neurogenesis in the adult mammalian brain. *Nat. Neurosci.* 13, 1338–1344. doi: 10.1038/nn.2672

Mazzocchi-Jones, D., Döbrössy, M., and Dunnet, S. B. (2009). Embryonic striatal grafts restore bi-directional synaptic plasticity in a rodent model of Huntington's disease. *Eur. J. Neurosci.* 30, 2134–2142. doi: 10.1111/j.1460-9568.2009.07006.x

Mezey, E. (2011). The therapeutic potential of bone marrow-derived stem cells. *J. Cell. Biochem.* 112, 2683–2687. doi: 10.1002/jcb.23216

Park, K. P., Rosell, A., Foerch, C., Xing, C., Kim, W. J., Lee, S., et al. (2009). Plasma and brain matrix metalloproteinase-9 after acute focal cerebral ischemia in rats. *Stroke* 40, 2836–2842. doi: 10.1161/STROKEAHA.109.554824

Pastori, C., Librizzi, L., Breschi, G. L., Regondi, C., Frassoni, C., Panzica, F., et al. (2008). Arterially perfused neurosphere-derived cells distribute outside the ischemic core in a model of transient focal ischemia and reperfusion *in vitro*. *PLoS ONE* 3:e2754. doi: 10.1371/journal.pone.0002754

Pollock, K., Stroemer, P., Patel, S., Stevanato, L., Hope, A., Miljan, E., et al. (2006). A conditionally immortal clonal stem cell line form human cortical neuroepithelium for the treatment of ischemic stroke. *Exp. Neurol.* 199, 143–155. doi: 10.1016/j.expneurol.2005.12.011

Redmond, D. E. Jr, Bjugstad, K. B., Teng, Y. D., Ourednik, V., Ourednik, J., Wakeman, D. R., et al. (2007). Behavioral improvement in a primate Parkinson's model is associated with multiple homeostatic effects of human neural stem cells. *Proc. Natl. Acad. Sci. U.S.A.* 104, 12175–12180. doi: 10.1073/pnas.0704091104

Robel, S., Berninger, B., and Gotz, M. (2011). The stem cell potential of glia: lessons from reactive gliosis. *Nat. Rev. Neurosci.* 12, 88–104. doi: 10.1038/nrn2978

Roet, K. C., Franssen, E. H., de Bree, F. M., Essing, A. H., Zijlstra, S. J., Fagoe, N. D., et al. (2013). A multilevel screening strategy defines a molecular fingerprint of proregenerative olfactory ensheathing cells and identifies SCARB2, a protein that improves regenerative sprouting of injured sensory spinal axons. *J. Neurosci.* 33, 11116–11135. doi: 10.1523/JNEUROSCI.1002-13.2013

Sanai, N., Nguyen, T., Ihrie, R. A., Mirzadeh, Z., Tsai, H. H., Wong, M., et al. (2011). Corridors of migrating neurons in the human brain and their decline during infancy. *Nature* 478, 382–386. doi: 10.1038/nature10487

Seol, H. J., Jin, J., Seong, D. H., Joo, K. M., Kang, W., Yang, H., et al. (2011). Genetically engineered human neural stem cells with rabbit carboxyl esterase can target brain metastasis from breast cancer. *Cancer Lett.* 311, 152–159. doi: 10.1016/j.canlet.2011.07.001

Snyder, E. Y., Yoon, C., Flax, J. D., and Macklis, J. D. (1997). Multipotent neural precursors can differentiate toward replacement of neurons undergoing targeted apoptotic degeneration in adult mouse neocortex. *Proc. Natl. Acad. Sci. U.S.A.* 94, 11663–11668. doi: 10.1073/pnas.94.21.11663

Sobrino, T., Perez-Mato, M., Brea, D., Rodriguez-Yanez, M., Blanco, M., and Castillo, J. (2012). Temporal profile of molecular signatures associated with circulating endothelial progenitor cells in human ischemic stroke. *J. Neurosci. Res.* 90, 1788–1793. doi: 10.1002/jnr.23068

Tajiri, N., Acosta, S., Glover, L. E., Bickford, P. C., Jacotte Simancas, A., Yasuhara, T., et al. (2012) Intravenous grafts of amniotic fluid-derived stem cells induce endogenous cell proliferation and attenuate behavioral deficits in ischemic stroke rats. *PLoS ONE* 7:e43779. doi: 10.1371/journal.pone.0043779

Tajiri, N., Kaneko, Y., Shinozuka, K., Ishikawa, H., Yankee, E., McGrogan, M., et al. (2013). Stem cell recruitment of newly formed host cells via a successful seduction? Filling the gap between neurogenic niche and injured brain site. *PLoS ONE* 8:e74857. doi: 10.1371/journal.pone.0074857

Tang, F. I., Tien, L. T., Zhou, F. C., Hoffer, B. J., and Wang, Y. (1998). Intranigral ventral mesencephalic grafts and nigrostriatal injections of glial cell line-derived neurotrophic factor restore dopamine release in the striatum of 6-hydroxydopamine-lesioned rats. *Exp. Brain Res.* 119, 287–296. doi: 10.1007/s002210050344

Trueman, R. C., Klein, A., Lindgren, H. S., Lelos, M. J., and Dunnett, S. B. (2013). Repair of the CNS using endogenous and transplanted neural stem cells. *Curr. Top. Behav. Neurosci.* 15, 357–398. doi: 10.1007/7854_2012_223

Wang, L., Chopp, M., Teng, H., Bolz, M., Francisco, M. A., Aluigi, D. M., et al. (2011). Tumor necrosis factor α primes cerebral endothelial cells for erythropoietin-induced angiogenesis. *J. Cereb. Blood Flow Metab.* 31, 640–647. doi: 10.1038/jcbfm.2010.138

Wang, X., Mao, X., Xie, L., Sun, F., Greenberg, D. A., and Jin, K. (2012). Conditional depletion of neurogenesis inhibits long-term recovery after experimental stroke in mice. *PLoS ONE* 7:e38932. doi: 10.1371/journal.pone.0038932

Wang, Y., Tien, L. T., Lapchak, P. A., and Hoffer, B. J. (1996). GDNF triggers fiber outgrowth of fetal ventral mesencephalic grafts from nigra to striatum in 6-OHDA-lesioned rats. *Cell Tissue Res.* 286, 225–233. doi: 10.1007/s004410050691

Wolf, K., Te Lindert, M., Krause, M., Alexander, S., Te Riet, J., Willis, A. L., et al. (2013). Physical limits of cell migration: control by ECM space and nuclear deformation and tuning by proteolysis and traction force. *J. Cell Biol.* 201, 1069–1084. doi: 10.1083/jcb.201210152

Yasuda, A., Tsuji, O., Shibata, S., Nori,S., Takano, M., Kobayashi, Y., et al. (2011). Significance of remyelination by neural stem/progenitor cells transplanted into the injured spinal cord. *Stem Cell* 29, 1983–1994. doi: 10.1002/stem.767

Yasuhara, T., Hara, K., Maki, M., Mays, R. W., Deans, R. J., Hess, D. C., et al. (2008). Intravenous grafts recapitulate the neurorestoration afforded by intracerebrally delivered multipotent adult progenitor cells in neonatal hypoxic-ischemic rats. *J. Cereb. Blood Flow Metab.* 28, 1804–1810. doi: 10.1038/jcbfm.2008.68

Yasuhara, T., Matsukawa, N., Hara, K., Maki, M., Ali, M. M., Yu, S. J., et al. (2009). Notch-induced rat and human bone marrow stromal cell grafts reduce ischemic cell loss and ameliorate behavioral deficits in chronic stroke animals. *Stem Cells Dev.* 18, 1501–1514. doi: 10.1089/scd.2009.0011

Yasuhara, T., Matsukawa, N., Hara, K., Yu, G., Xu, L., Maki, M., et al. (2006). Transplantation of human neural stem cells exerts neuroprotection in a rat model of Parkinson's disease. *J. Neurosci.* 26, 12497–12511. doi: 10.1523/JNEUROSCI.3719-06.2006

Zhao, B. Q., Tejima, E., and Lo, E. H. (2007). Neurovascular proteases in brain injury, hemorrhage and remodeling after stroke. *Stroke* 38, 748–752. doi: 10.1161/01.STR.0000253500.32979.d1

17

Enhancing multiple object tracking performance with noninvasive brain stimulation: a causal role for the anterior intraparietal sulcus

Eric J. Blumberg *, Matthew S. Peterson and Raja Parasuraman

Arch Lab, Department of Psychology, George Mason University, Fairfax, VA, USA

Edited by:
Mikhail Lebedev, Duke University, USA

Reviewed by:
Shalini Narayana, University of Tennessee Health Science Center at Memphis, USA
Richard Andrew McKinley, Air Force Research Laboratory, USA
Ruyuan Zhang, University of Rochester, China

***Correspondence:**
Eric J. Blumberg, Arch Lab, Department of Psychology, George Mason University, David King Hall 2083, MSN 3F5, 4400 University Drive, Fairfax, VA 22030-4444, USA
e-mail: ericjoshua@gmail.com

Multiple object tracking (MOT) is a complex task recruiting a distributed network of brain regions. There are also marked individual differences in MOT performance. A positive causal relationship between the anterior intraparietal sulcus (AIPS), an integral region in the MOT attention network and inter-individual variation in MOT performance has not been previously established. The present study used transcranial direct current stimulation (tDCS), a form of non-invasive brain stimulation, in order to examine such a causal link. Active anodal stimulation was applied to the right AIPS and the left dorsolateral prefrontal cortex (DLPFC) (and sham stimulation), an area associated with working memory (but not MOT) while participants completed a MOT task. Stimulation to the right AIPS significantly improved MOT accuracy more than the other two conditions. The results confirm a causal role of the AIPS in the MOT task and illustrate that tDCS has the ability to improve MOT performance.

Keywords: tDCS, brain stimulation, multiple object tracking, anterior intraparietal sulcus, spatial attention

INTRODUCTION

Multiple object tracking (MOT) is a dynamic, effortful task that assesses how many moving objects a person can attend to over a short period of time (Pylyshyn and Storm, 1988). In the traditional MOT paradigm, participants are presented with multiple objects (e.g., circles) on a monitor and are instructed to track a subset of those objects. The objects move independently and continuously around the screen, and after they stop, participants attempt to indicate which objects they had been tracking. Accuracy, or the proportion of correctly identified targets, is generally used to measure MOT performance.

MOT tasks have been used to evaluate attention capacity (Alvarez and Franconeri, 2007; Horowitz and Cohen, 2010), mechanisms of perceptual organization (Yantis, 1992; Scholl et al., 2001), and distributed attention (Sears and Pylyshyn, 2000). While MOT is a process-intensive task involving attention, object selection, object tracking, memory, and multiple types of eye movements, a number of studies (Pylyshyn and Storm, 1988; Cavanagh and Alvarez, 2005) have illustrated that on average, individuals have a tracking accuracy of 85% for two objects, and as the number of items to track increases, accuracy decreases sharply. In addition, there are marked inter-individual differences in MOT tracking capacity, reflecting inter-individual variation in spatial ability (Oksama and Hyönä, 2004). Given such variability, it is important to understand the underlying neural mechanisms involved in performance of dynamic attentional tasks such as the MOT.

Several researchers (Culham et al., 1998, 2001; Jovicich et al., 2001; Howe et al., 2009) have used functional magnetic resonance imaging (fMRI) to identify the brain areas associated with MOT. Given the number of perceptual and attentional processes involved in MOT, it is not surprising that the fMRI studies have implicated 12 unique brain areas recruited during MOT. Culham et al. (1998) concluded that 11 different brain areas were recruited during MOT whereas Jovicich et al. (2001) identified 12 areas, 9 of which were consistent with the previous work by Culham et al. These studies identified brain regions sensitive to attention, motion, and areas involved in eye movements. However, Howe et al. (2009) identified a number of issues with the previous fMRI and MOT studies, the greatest of which was that the studies did not correctly differentiate brain areas specifically related to tracking objects vs. attending to objects, a critical differentiation in analysis of MOT performance.

After controlling for the effects of attention, Howe et al. (2009) concluded that the frontal eye fields (FEF), anterior intraparietal sulcus (AIPS), the superior parietal lobule (SPL), posterior intraparietal sulcus (PIPS), and the human motion areas (MT+) were all consistently activated during MOT. The FEF and SPL are involved with the generation and execution of eye movements and spatial attention, processes clearly involved with visually tracking objects (Nobre et al., 1997; Donner et al., 2000). Area MT+ plays a critical role in motion-based tasks, and might potentially be responsible for updating location information (d'Avossa et al., 2007). Recent evidence has suggested that the PIPS plays a role in attention to both stationary and moving objects, and may be responsible for managing pointers to the spatial locations of attended objects. PIPS and MT+ may also interact to support MOT with the PIPS involved in attending to the items and MT+ associated with updating of locations (Howe et al., 2009). The AIPS was identified to be active only when objects were moving, suggesting a dissociation between tracking moving objects and attending to stationary ones, and indicating that it plays a crucial role within the identified attention network. In addition, AIPS has been shown to be sensitive to tracking load, with greater activation associated with increased number of items to be tracked (Culham et al., 2001; Jovicich et al., 2001). Supporting this view, a lesion study conducted by Battelli et al. (2001) showed that individuals with a unilateral right parietal lesion were significantly worse at tracking objects in the contralateral field even when only one object was presented in each visual field. Furthermore, Battelli et al. (2009) provided initial evidence supporting the causal role of the AIPS in MOT performance by demonstrating that MOT performance was inhibited by transcranial magnetic stimulation (TMS) over the right and left intraparietal sulcus but not MT+.

A method that can provide evidence for a positive causal relationship between the AIPS and MOT is transcranial direct current stimulation (tDCS). It involves the application of small amounts of constant direct electric current (1–2 mA) with electrodes attached to the scalp. A positive polarity (anode) is typically used to stimulate neuronal function and enhance performance, while a negative polarity (cathode) is used to inhibit neuronal activity. The electric current is thought to affect the resting potential of cortical neurons (Bindman et al., 1964; Antal et al., 2001) and also synaptic efficacy (Rahman et al., 2013), which in turn increases their sensitivity, leading to an increased likelihood of firing while performing a task. (See Bikson et al., 2004, for a deeper explanation on the neural affects of tDCS). The standard current values for active stimulation conditions can fluctuate up to 2 mA while control/sham levels are either 0.1 mA or a 2 mA ramp-up and immediate ramp-down (Clark et al., 2012). No serious side effects have been associated with normal tDCS operations for 30 min or less of prolonged stimulation (Bikson et al., 2009).

Research by Andrews et al. (2011) has indicated that the effects of tDCS are not global, and only occur when administered in a specific manner: the stimulation must be applied so that stimulation targets areas that are involved in the task being trained on. tDCS is thought to facilitate changes in active neurons and pathways, and those pathways must be active while the stimulation is being administered in order to show a benefit. Through the excitatory (anodal) and inhibitory (cathodal) affects on cell membranes, tDCS can improve our understanding of brain function and its corresponding behavioral correlates.

The present study used tDCS to provide a unique approach to investigating the causal role of the AIPS and of evaluating the plasticity of MOT. To demonstrate that the effects of stimulation are focal rather than global in nature both a target and a control site for stimulation were chosen. As discussed previously, the right AIPS was chosen as the targeted experimental site for potential enhancement of MOT performance. The left dorsolateral prefrontal cortex (DLPFC) was chosen as a control stimulation site because previous fMRI studies have shown that it is minimally involved, if at all, in MOT performance (Howe et al., 2009). In contrast, data from Culham et al., 2001 suggests a right lateralized recruitment in frontal brain areas during MOT. Stimulation of this area may lead to inadvertent affects on MOT performance, and because we focused on the right AIPS in the present study, we used the left DLPFC for the control stimulation condition. In addition to the active stimulation control, we also included a sham stimulation of the left DLPFC (to control for a placebo effect). The sham condition is included to control for placebo effects as previous studies have failed to identify meaningful effects of sham stimulation on task performance (Berryhill et al., 2014). Participants were naïve as to the relationship between scalp location and its corresponding behavioral outcomes, making the sham stimulation location unimportant.

We hypothesized that tDCS would improve performance in the right AIPS stimulation condition and that there would be differences in performance between participants stimulated over the right AIPS compared to those stimulated over the left DLPFC in both active and sham conditions. To assess the possible interaction of stimulation with the processing demand associated with attentional tracking, we administered both a low and a high tracking load version of the MOT. We anticipated that an effect of tDCS would be greatest for the high tracking load and may even be absent in the low load condition due to ceiling effects for tasks already at or near ceiling in performance (Ball et al., 2007; Schmiedek et al., 2010; Jaeggi et al., 2011). In addition, previous researchers have suggested that tDCS may be more beneficial for novices/lower performers than for experts/higher performers (Bullard et al., 2011; Tseng et al., 2012; Blumberg et al., 2014; Foroughi et al., 2015) and that tDCS may be more effective in difficult tasks (Berryhill et al., 2014), suggesting that both task difficulty and individual abilities may play a critical role in the effectiveness of stimulation.

MATERIALS AND METHODS

PARTICIPANTS

Forty-eight undergraduates participated in the experiment (28 females) with an average age of 19 years (range from 18–32). Participants met the following conditions: (1) right handed; (2) normal or corrected to normal vision; and (3) English as a first language. Participants were randomly assigned to one of the three between-subject stimulation conditions while they performed the MOT task under two tracking loads. Sixteen subjects were assigned to each condition. Participants were given course credit for the their participation. All participants gave written informed consent to participate in a protocol approved by the George Mason Institutional Review Board.

TASK AND EQUIPMENT

MOT task

Participants engaged in a computer-based MOT task on a Dell 15" inch LCD monitor at a distance of 40 cm from the screen. The experimental stimuli consisted of eight green circles (two or four of the circles were targets). The circles were 1° of visual angle in size. Each trial consisted of three steps. The eight circles initially appeared as static images (no movement) while the target circles flashed for 1 s. Then the circles moved continuously and independently for 8 s, and could overlap as they traveled across the screen. The circles moved at a constant rate of 13°/sec and in constant directions (when they encountered the border of the screen they were redirected in another direction based upon the angle of impact with the border). After the circles stopped, participants selected the target circles with mouse clicks. The experimental sequence can be seen below in **Figure 1**. Participants tracked two circles (25% of all the circles) in the low load condition and four (50% of all the circles) in the high load condition.

tDCS

tDCS was applied using an ActivaDose II Iontophoresis Delivery Unit. Current was constantly supplied to two electrode pads with 11 cm^2 saline soaked sponges that were attached (with self-adhesive bandage strips) to the participant's scalp and shoulder. The anode was placed on the scalp while the cathode was placed on the contralateral upper arm, consistent with a non-cephalic montage (Falcone et al., 2012; McKinley et al., 2013). Subjects were randomly assigned to one of three stimulation conditions: AIPS active anodal stimulation, DLPFC active anodal stimulation, and DLPFC sham stimulation. In the AIPS experimental condition the anode was placed near CP4 in the 10–20 EEG system while the cathode was placed on the contralateral upper arm. We used Soterix Medical's HDExplore software to identify an appropriate montage to best target the AIPS. A standard adult male head was incorporated for the model; therefore, a single current flow model was identified and applied for all participants. We modeled a number of different montages before identifying scalp site CP4 as the site that best activated AIPS. In both the active and sham control conditions the anode was placed near electrode site F3 in the 10–20 EEG system with the cathode placed on the contralateral upper arm (right). F3 is a commonly used site when modulating the DLPFC (Coffman et al., 2014). Participants in both experimental conditions were given 2.0 mA of stimulation for 30 min. Participants in the sham condition received a 2.0 mA ramp-up and immediate ramp-down to 0 mA lasting 30 s. The brief amount of stimulation provided participants with the full sensation of tDCS.

DESIGN

A 3 × 2 mixed design was employed. The between-subjects variable (stimulation site) had the following levels: AIPS active, DLPFC active, and DLPFC sham. The within-subjects variable was tracking load (low or high). Each participant completed six blocks of 44 trials (three blocks during baseline testing and three blocks while stimulation was administered). The trials in each block were randomized with an equal representation of low and high tracking trials.

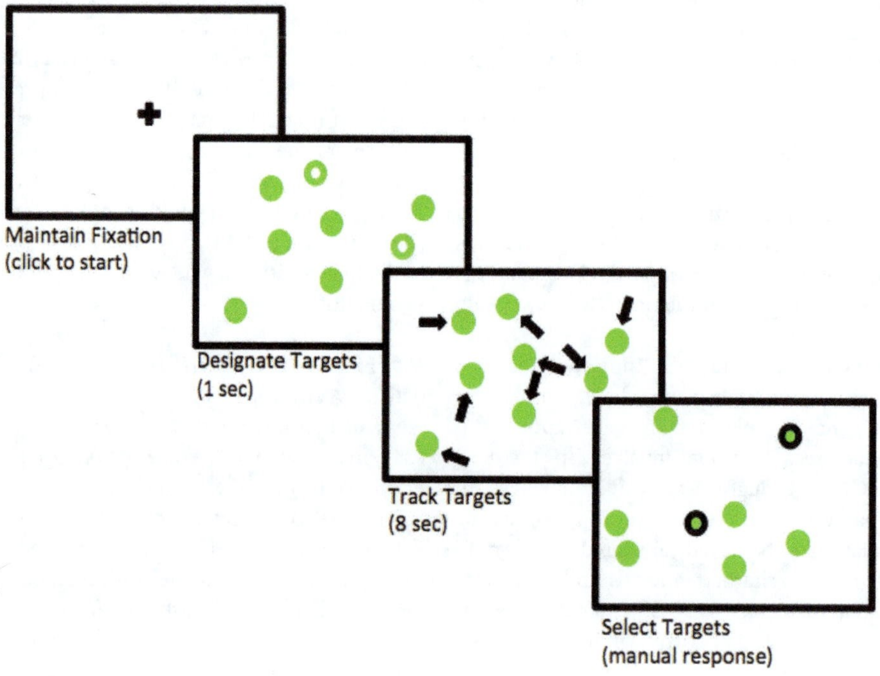

FIGURE 1 | Sequence of actions within the MOT task.

PROCEDURE

Upon arrival participants were asked to read and sign the informed consent form outlining the nature of the task and any risks/benefits they may receive for participating. The Snellen near-sightedness exam was administered to test vision (20–30 or better vision required). Participants were then instructed on how to perform the MOT task. Participants completed a baseline of three blocks of 44 trials to test their baseline performance. The three blocks were completed back-to-back without any breaks.

Following baseline testing, the experimenter prepared the tDCS setup. Participants were given the DCS Sensation Questionnaire (Scheldrup et al., 2014) at three time points throughout the stimulation subsession (approximately 1-, 10-, and 30 min post stimulation onset) measuring how much itching, heat/burning, and tingling the participant felt at that moment. Immediately following the first administration of the sensation questionnaire participants completed a demographic and video game questionnaire. After they finished the questionnaires they completed the second sensation questionnaire. Participants then completed the final three blocks of the MOT task (132 total trials) while tDCS was being administered. After completing the trials the tDCS unit was turned off and the electrodes were removed. Finally, each participant completed the third sensation questionnaire and then was debriefed about the experiment.

RESULTS

MOT ACCURACY

The primary goal of this experiment was to investigate whether a relatively short period of brain stimulation (30 min) could be used to improve MOT performance, thereby establishing a positive causal role of the right AIPS in MOT performance. The behavioral and dependent variable in the experiment was MOT accuracy. Accuracy was calculated by dividing the number of correctly identified targets by the total possible targets for each trial. Accuracy scores were then created for both the baseline and stimulation subsessions by averaging the accuracy scores across trials and blocks within each subsession. Separate accuracy scores were created for both load conditions leaving each participant with four different accuracy scores (see **Figure 2**).

BASELINE COMPARISON

We initially tested whether baseline performance across stimulation conditions was significantly different from one another. Two separate (low and high tracking loads) one-way analysis of variance (ANOVA) were conducted because we did not want a potential ceiling effect in the low tracking load condition (hypothesized *a priori*) to reduce the likelihood of finding an effect in the high tracking load condition. The ANOVA for the low tracking load condition failed to identify a significant main effect of stimulation condition ($F_{(2,45)} = 0.87$, $p > 0.20$). The ANOVA for the high tracking load condition also did not reveal a significant main effect of stimulation condition ($F_{(2,45)} = 1.34$, $p > 0.20$) suggesting that baseline performance was not significantly different across stimulation groups in either tracking load condition.

CONDITION SPECIFIC STIMULATION EFFECT

We then conducted a 2 × 2 × 3 mixed-design ANOVA with subsession and tracking load as the within-subjects factors, stimulation site as the between-subjects factor, and MOT accuracy as the independent variable. A self-assessment of first person shooter video game experience was initially included in the analysis as a covariate because prior research (Green and Bavelier, 2006) suggested it predicts MOT performance, however, this effect was not significant in the present study and was therefore removed from the subsequent analyses. The analysis revealed a 2-way interaction between tracking load and subsession ($F_{(1,45)} = 5.24$, $p < 0.05$, $\eta^2_{partial} = 0.10$), a main effect for subsession ($F_{(1,45)} = 351.14$, $p < 0.01$), and a main effect for tracking load ($F_{(1,45)} = 4.34$, $p < 0.05$). Tests of simple main effects for the two-way interaction using a Bonferroni correction ($\alpha = 0.05$) revealed that within the high tracking load condition, MOT performance was significantly greater in the stimulation subsession compared to baseline, ($F_{(1,45)} = 9.5$, $p < 0.01$, $\eta^2_{partial} = 0.17$). The three-way interaction was not significant ($p > 0.10$).

To better test our initial hypothesis about whether tDCS stimulation applied to the AIPS can improve MOT performance, a series of planned paired samples *t*-tests were conducted to identify if stimulation improved MOT accuracy beyond that of baseline. Six, separate paired samples *t*-test using a Ŝidák correction ($\alpha = 0.0063$, given six related tests) were conducted comparing each baseline score to its corresponding stimulation score (low and high tracking load for each stimulation site). A significant difference in performance was identified in the high tracking load condition between AIPS baseline ($M = 76.42\%$, $SE = 1.66$) and AIPS stimulation ($M = 72.54\%$, $SE = 1.86$), $t_{(15)} = 4.10$, $p = 0.00047$, $d = 1.03$ illustrating a 4% improvement in MOT accuracy, see **Figure 2**. No other *t*-test reached significance (largest $t = 1.0$; smallest $p = 0.33$). Given that stimulation did not affect performance in the low tracking load condition across any stimulation condition and we did not make any *a priori*

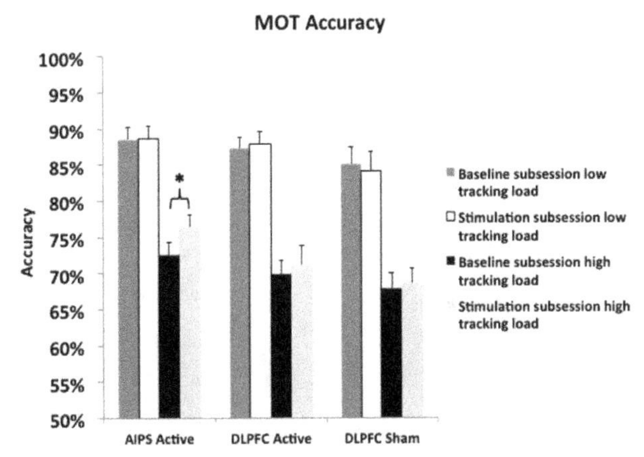

FIGURE 2 | MOT accuracy ± SEM (standard error of the mean) across stimulation sites broken down by time point (baseline and stimulation) and tracking load (low and high). * indicates significant difference.

predictions, the low tracking load condition was excluded from the following analyses.

COMPARISON OF STIMULATION EFFECTS ACROSS CONDITIONS

In addition to testing for changes in performance due to stimulation, we also examined whether stimulation led to group differences. Given the *a priori* hypothesis that in the high tracking load condition the AIPS stimulation condition would be significantly different from the two DLPFC control conditions, the DLPFC active (M = 71.16%, SE = 2.67) and DLPFC sham (M = 68.56%, SE = 2.12) groups were initially compared against one another to identify any differences. An independent samples t-test using a Šidák correction ($\alpha = 0.025$, given two related tests) was conducted to compare performance across the two control conditions in the stimulation subsession. The analysis did not reveal a significant difference between the two control groups, $t_{(30)} = 0.45$, $p = 0.41$. The two DLPFC control conditions were therefore collapsed into one control condition in the subsequent analysis, leaving two levels of the stimulation variable (AIPS active and DLPFC control).

We then tested if performance in the AIPS active and DLPFC control condition were significantly different from one another in the stimulation subsession, examining if AIPS stimulation led to better MOT performance compared to the DLPFC control. An independent samples t-test using a Šidák correction ($\alpha = 0.025$) was conducted to compare performance between the AIPS active (M = 76.42%, SE = 1.67) and DLPFC control (M = 69.86%, SE = 1.69) conditions. The analysis revealed a significant difference $t_{(46)} = 2.45$, $p = 0.009$, $d = 0.80$. The data suggests that in the high tracking load condition, right AIPS stimulation improved MOT accuracy significantly more than in the combined control condition, see **Figures 2, 3**.

MOT CAPACITY

Due to the high accuracy scores in the low tracking load condition, an important question becomes: is accuracy a sensitive enough measure to detect performance changes close to ceiling? To answer this question, we non-linearly transformed the accuracy scores into capacity measures (k) according to Horowitz et al. (2007) and Scholl et al. (2001). The capacity measure did not lead to any significantly different outcomes compared to the accuracy measure, therefore, the analyses will not be included in this manuscript, see **Table 1** for means.

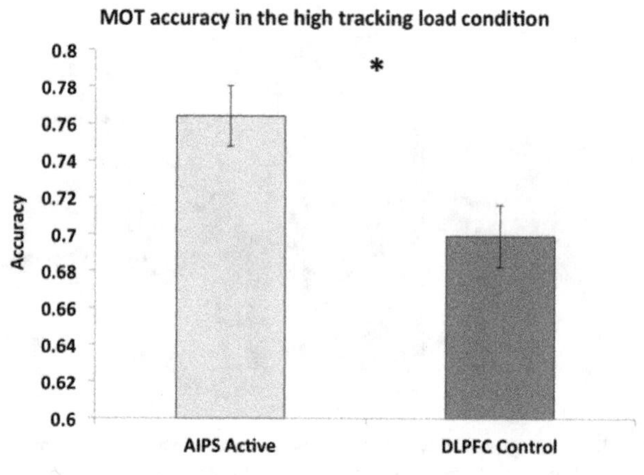

FIGURE 3 | MOT accuracy in the high tracking load condition + SEM (standard error of the mean). * indicates significant difference.

BASELINE VS. CHANGE IN MOT PERFORMANCE

We also examined whether baseline MOT accuracy predicted the amount of improvement exhibited in the right AIPS stimulation condition (high tracking load trials). To accomplish this we compared participants' baseline MOT accuracy to their change in MOT accuracy (stimulation minus baseline). The two scores were negatively correlated, $r_{(16)} = -0.45$, $p < 0.05$, see **Figure 4**. This significant association suggests that tDCS may be more beneficial to individuals with lower baseline MOT abilities. Note also, that all but two of the participants, irrespective of their baseline performance, showed improvement in MOT accuracy with tDCS.

RATE OF MOT IMPROVEMENT

Additionally, we examined the rate at which stimulation impacted MOT performance in the AIPS stimulation high tracking load condition. We ran a repeated measure ANOVA with block (only in the stimulation subsession) as the within-subjects factor. Block was not significant ($F_{(2,30)} = 0.04$, $p > 0.10$) indicating that stimulation led to an immediate boost in MOT performance that was sustained across the three blocks (see **Figure 5**—Blocks 4,5,6).

DISCUSSION

The present study evaluated the efficacy of using targeted non-invasive brain stimulation to improve understanding of the causal role of the right AIPS in MOT performance through improved learning and skill acquisition of MOT. tDCS was targeted to the right AIPS, a brain area that plays a unique and integral role for tracking multiple objects (Howe et al., 2009). Active anodal stimulation to the right AIPS improved MOT performance in the high tracking load condition but not in the low tracking load condition. Active and sham stimulation of the left DLPFC had no effect in either tracking load condition. This finding suggests that: (1) the right AIPS plays an active role in MOT; (2) modulation of this area by tDCS directly leads to changes in MOT performance; and (3) the effects of the tDCS were focal in nature and not a global enhancement due to stimulation of the entire cortex.

Right AIPS stimulation improved performance in the more difficult tracking load condition where participants' accuracy was relatively low (~70%) whereas stimulation did not affect performance in the easier tracking load condition (85–90%) where participants were performing at or close to ceiling. These results are consistent with the *a priori* hypotheses and are in line with the previous literature that suggests that tDCS is more beneficial to novices (Bullard et al., 2011) and lower performers (Tseng et al., 2012; Blumberg et al., 2014; Foroughi et al., 2015) and may be more effective when paired with difficult tasks (Jones and Berryhill, 2012; Berryhill et al., 2014). Additionally, cognitive training is not beneficial for individuals already performing at

Table 1 | Means for both accuracy and capacity measure across stimulation condition, tracking load, and subsession.

		Low		High	
		Baseline	Stimulation	Baseline	Stimulation
Accuracy	AIPS Active	88.59	88.64	72.54	76.42
DLPFC Active		87.26	87.97	69.89	71.16
DLPFC Sham		85.09	84.14	67.80	68.56
Capacity	AIPS Active	1.77	1.77	2.88	3.04
DLPFC Active		1.74	1.76	2.77	2.82
DLPFC Sham		1.70	1.68	2.68	2.72

ceiling (Ball et al., 2007; Schmiedek et al., 2010; Jaeggi et al., 2011).

We also identified that in the high tracking load condition, the amount of improvement in MOT was negatively correlated with a participant's baseline MOT ability. On average, individuals with lower baseline MOT accuracies exhibited greater increases in accuracy compared to those with higher baseline abilities. Tseng et al. (2012) found a similar inverse effect in change-detection ability stimulating a posterior parietal location.

Additionally, we identified that stimulation had an immediate effect on MOT performance in the right AIPS high tracking load condition. Performances across the three blocks in the stimulation subsession were similar, illustrating a constant positive impact of stimulation. We believe this is due to the fact that MOT is a very simple task with little to no learning curve, therefore, stimulation immediately modulated the relationship between the right AIPS and MOT performance.

While research (Green and Bavelier, 2006; Boot et al., 2008) has previously shown that specific types of training such as playing action video games can improve MOT performance, this is the first study to show that brain stimulation can do so too, but in a much shorter time. If used as a tool for accelerated training, tDCS may offer a number of benefits compared to traditional training paradigms. Video game training can take extended periods of time (Green and Bavelier, 2006; Feng et al., 2007; Basak et al., 2008), whereas in this study, tDCS immediately improved spatial tracking performance. Also, specific subsets of the population cannot or do not enjoy playing video games because the games can be difficult to learn, can cause frustration, and can require fine motor control. On the other hand, tDCS requires little or no additional effort from the user apart from the task being performed, making it ideally suited to a larger segment of the population. tDCS focused on the right AIPS, a brain area integral to the attention network (Howe et al.,

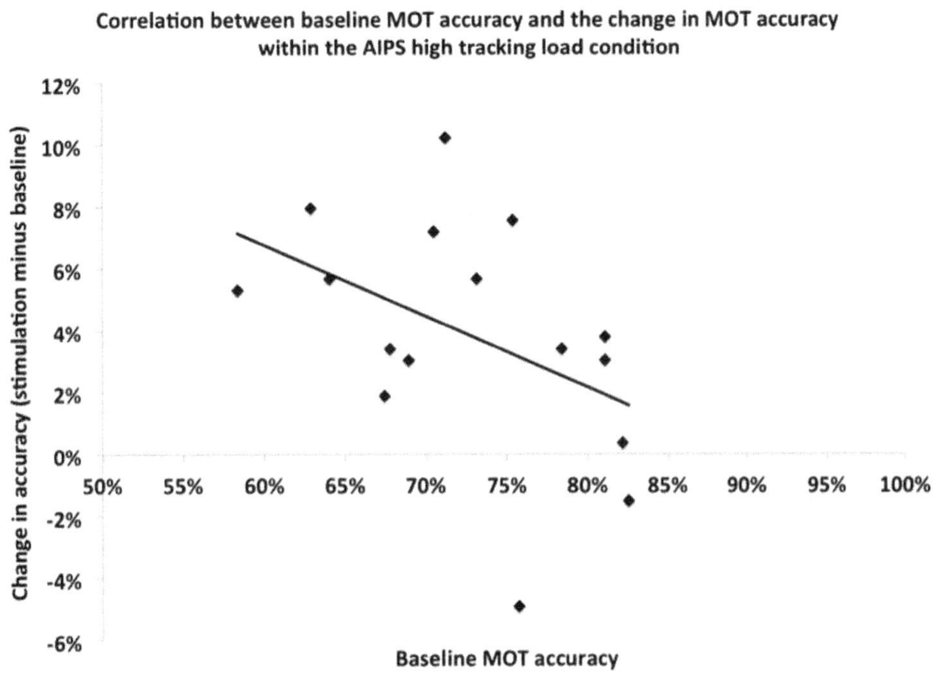

FIGURE 4 | Correlation between baseline MOT accuracy and the change in MOT accuracy within the AIPS high tracking load condition.

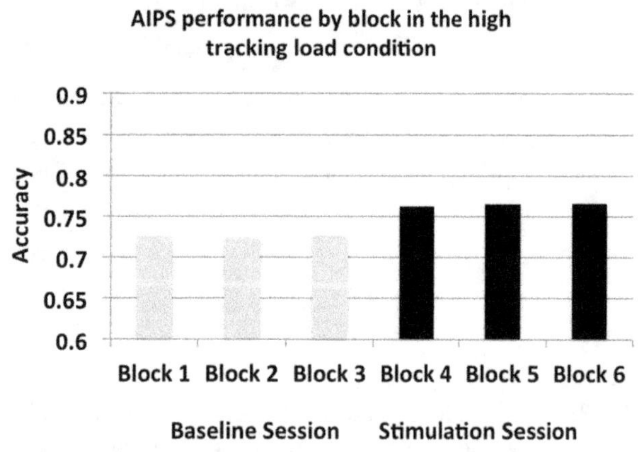

FIGURE 5 | Accuracy per block in the AIPS stimulation high tracking load condition, subsession differentiated by bar color.

2009) immediately improved MOT performance, this transient improvement was accomplished in a substantially shorter amount of time than through traditional training programs, however, the effects may not be as significant or as long lasting. While this study provides initial evidence that tDCS can rapidly improve MOT performance, further research should identify if these effects are transferable to other spatial tracking tasks in both basic and complex settings. Brain stimulation over the right AIPS offers a unique method to better understand the function of this area as it relates to MOT. This study adds to the existing literature that the right AIPS plays an active role in MOT and that the neural substrates recruited for MOT exhibit significant plasticity.

Our findings mirror previous tDCS studies that have found effects on perception, attention, and memory abilities (Coffman et al., 2014). For example, Clark et al. (2012) showed increased perceptual learning when tDCS electrodes were targeted to brain areas related to perceptual learning, with the benefit of tDCS being retained for at least 24 h (Falcone et al., 2012). Of particular note is the study by Moos et al. (2012), in which they observed that cathodal stimulation over the right AIPS increased top-down attentional selection. While they applied cathodal stimulation to the same area we did, the two studies measured different aspects of attentional selection. Additionally, TMS has previously been applied to support a causal mechanism between modulation of the IPS and MOT (Battelli et al., 2009). They inhibited IPS function, leading to decreased MOT accuracy. However, our study is the first to illustrate that the causal mechanism is in the positive direction as well. We used tDCS to illustrate the facilitative effects of AIPS stimulation on MOT ability, finding increased MOT accuracy. tDCS is also less invasive and more easily applied making it a more practical tool to accelerate MOT abilities.

This study had some limitations. Although current modeling was used to identify the electrode montage that would best lead to stimulation of AIPS, such modeling involves a number of assumptions that may not always be met, and modeling must be considered as a hypothesis to be tested rather than definitive. That the empirical evidence confirmed the hypothesis and showed that other stimulation sites did not lead to improvement in MOT performance is consistent with the predicted results. Furthermore, we did not directly measure cortical activation in AIPS or other parietal regions as a result of tDCS. However, previous research has illustrated that tDCS does affect neuronal firing (Radman et al., 2009). Additionally, the tDCS electrode montage used in the experiment may have resulted in stimulation of the posterior parietal cortex in general.

Another possible concern involves the baseline performance of the different stimulation/sham groups. While statistically significant differences between groups in MOT baseline performance were not found, one could argue that individuals in the AIPS condition were somewhat better to begin with, so that the difference identified in the stimulation subsession could just reflect these initial differences in performance and random variation or potentially a small tDCS effect. However, it would be highly unlikely that random noise would increase performance in individuals that were already performing at high levels and not for individuals performing poorly. Additionally, it is unlikely given that individuals with the lowest baseline MOT abilities saw the largest increases in MOT performance. If baseline averages were identical (decreasing initial AIPS accuracy) potentially more individuals would see greater benefits in their MOT performance. Task difficulty can also modulate the beneficial effects of tDCS (Jones and Berryhill, 2012; Berryhill et al., 2014). While AIPS stimulation significantly improved MOT accuracy in the four ball tracking condition (an amount at or close to our attention capacity) and not the two ball tracking condition, an even more difficult MOT condition (i.e., tracking six objects) may have resulted in larger effects. Therefore, the findings in this paper may be underestimating the beneficial effect of tDCS on MOT performance. Future research should investigate the limitations of applying tDCS to the intraparietal sulcus, how cathodal stimulation may affect spatial tracking performance, and how tDCS could be used in conjunction with other training programs to improve spatial tracking beyond that of just video game play or tDCS alone. Additionally, it will be very important to identify how long the tDCS effects last, especially if tDCS is used for long-term enhancement of spatial abilities.

The current study is the first to illustrate that brain stimulation can improve MOT accuracy. Stimulation to the AIPS, a central location in the attention network improved MOT accuracy while stimulation to the DLPFC did not. Accelerated training techniques like tDCS can be used to improve perceptual, attention, and memory training programs and to identify the causal relationships between brain and behavior.

ACKNOWLEDGMENTS

This research was supported by Air Force Office of Scientific Research Grant FA9550-10-1-0385 to RP and the Center of Excellence in Neuroergonomics, Technology, and Cognition (CENTEC). We would like to acknowledge Amanda Hanelli and Juliane Holmblad for helping with the experiment.

REFERENCES

Alvarez, G. A., and Franconeri, S. L. (2007). How many objects can you track?: evidence for a resource-limited attentive tracking mechanism. *J. Vis.* 7:14. doi: 10.1167/7.13.14

Andrews, S. C., Hoy, K. E., Enticott, P. G., Daskalakis, Z. J., and Fitzgerald, P. B. (2011). Improving working memory: the effect of combining cognitive activity and anodal transcranial direct current stimulation to the left dorsolateral prefrontal cortex. *Brain Stimul.* 4, 84–89. doi: 10.1016/j.brs.2010.06.004

Antal, A., Nitsche, M. A., and Paulus, W. (2001). External modulation of visual perception in humans. *Neuroreport* 12, 3553–3555. doi: 10.1097/00001756-200111160-00036

Ball, K., Edwards, J. D., and Ross, L. A. (2007). The impact of speed of processing training on cognitive and everyday functions. *J. Gerontol. B Psychol. Sci. Soc. Sci.* 62, 19–31. doi: 10.1093/geronb/62.special_issue_1.19

Basak, C., Boot, W. R., Voss, M. W., and Kramer, A. F. (2008). Can training in a real-time strategy video game attenuate cognitive decline in older adults?. *Psychol. Aging* 23, 765–777. doi: 10.1037/a0013494

Battelli, L., Alvarez, G. A., Carlson, T., and Pascual-Leone, A. (2009). The role of the parietal lobe in visual extinction studied with transcranial magnetic stimulation. *J. Cogn. Neurosci.* 21, 1946–1955. doi: 10.1162/jocn.2008.21149

Battelli, L., Cavanagh, P., Intriligator, J., Tramo, M. J., Hénaff, M. A., Michèl, F., et al. (2001). Unilateral right parietal damage leads to bilateral deficit for high-level motion. *Neuron* 32, 985–995. doi: 10.1016/s0896-6273(01)00536-0

Berryhill, M. E., Peterson, D. J., Jones, K. T., and Stephens, J. A. (2014). Hits and misses: leveraging tDCS to advance cognitive research. *Front. Psychol.* 5:800. doi: 10.3389/fpsyg.2014.00800

Bikson, M., Datta, A., and Elwassif, M. (2009). Establishing safety limits for transcranial direct current stimulation. *Clin. Neurophysiol.* 120, 1033–1034. doi: 10.1016/j.clinph.2009.03.018

Bikson, M., Inoue, M., Akiyama, H., Deans, J. K., Fox, J. E., Miyakawa, H., et al. (2004). Effects of uniform extracellular DC electric fields on excitability in rat hippocampal slices in vitro. *J. Physiol.* 557, 175–190. doi: 10.1113/jphysiol.2003.055772

Bindman, L. J., Lippold, O. C. J., and Redfearn, J. W. T. (1964). The action of brief polarizing currents on the cerebral cortex of the rat (1) during current flow and (2) in the production of long-lasting after-effects. *J. Physiol.* 172, 369–382. doi: 10.1113/jphysiol.1964.sp007425

Blumberg, E. J., Foroughi, C. K., Scheldrup, M. R., Peterson, M. S., Boehm-Davis, D. A., and Parasuraman, R. (2014). Reducing the disruptive effect of interruptions with noninvasive brain stimulation. *Hum. Factors.* doi: 10.1177/0018720814565189

Boot, W. R., Kramer, A. F., Simons, D. J., Fabiani, M., and Gratton, G. (2008). The effects of video game playing on attention, memory and executive control. *Acta Psychol. (Amst)* 129, 387–398. doi: 10.1016/j.actpsy.2008.09.005

Bullard, L. M., Browning, E. S., Clark, V. P., Coffman, B. A., Garcia, C. M., Jung, R. E., et al. (2011). Transcranial direct current stimulation's effect on novice versus experienced learning. *Exp. Brain Res.* 213, 9–14. doi: 10.1007/s00221-011-2764-2

Cavanagh, P., and Alvarez, G. A. (2005). Tracking multiple targets with multifocal attention. *Trends Cogn. Sci.* 9, 349–354. doi: 10.1016/j.tics.2005.05.009

Clark, V. P., Coffman, B. A., Mayer, A. R., Weisend, M. P., Lane, T. D., Calhoun, V. D., et al. (2012). tDCS guided using fMRI significantly accelerates learning to identify concealed objects. *Neuroimage* 59, 117–128. doi: 10.1016/j.neuroimage.2010.11.036

Coffman, B. A., Clark, V. P., and Parasuraman, R. (2014). Battery powered thought: enhancement of attention, learning and memory in healthy adults using transcranial direct current stimulation. *Neuroimage* 85, 895–908. doi: 10.1016/j.neuroimage.2013.07.083

Culham, J. C., Brandt, S. A., Cavanagh, P., Kanwisher, N. G., Dale, A. M., and Tootell, R. B. (1998). Cortical fMRI activation produced by attentive tracking of moving targets. *J. Neurophysiol.* 80, 2657–2670.

Culham, J. C., Cavanagh, P., and Kanwisher, N. G. (2001). Attention response functions: characterizing brain areas using fMRI activation during parametric variations of attentional load. *Neuron* 32, 737–745. doi: 10.1016/s0896-6273(01)00499-8

d'Avossa, G., Tosetti, M., Crespi, S., Biagi, L., Burr, D. C., and Morrone, M. C. (2007). Spatiotopic selectivity of BOLD responses to visual motion in human area MT. *Nat. Neurosci.* 10, 249–255. doi: 10.1038/nn1824

Donner, T., Kettermann, A., Diesch, E., Ostendorf, F., Villringer, A., and Brandt, S. A. (2000). Involvement of the human frontal eye field and multiple parietal areas in covert visual selection during conjunction search. *Eur. J. Neurosci.* 12, 3407–3414. doi: 10.1046/j.1460-9568.2000.00223.x

Falcone, B., Coffman, B. A., Clark, V. P., and Parasuraman, R. (2012). Transcranial direct current stimulation augments perceptual sensitivity and 24-hour retention in a complex threat detection task. *PLoS One* 7:e34993. doi: 10.1371/journal.pone.0034993

Feng, J., Spence, I., and Pratt, J. (2007). Playing an action video game reduces gender differences in spatial cognition. *Psychol. Sci.* 18, 850–855. doi: 10.1111/j.1467-9280.2007.01990.x

Foroughi, C. K., Blumberg, E. J., and Parasuraman, R. (2015). Activation and inhibition of posterior parietal cortex have bi-directional effects following interruptions. *Front. Syst. Neurosci.* 8:245. doi: 10.3389/fnsys.2014.00245

Green, C. S., and Bavelier, D. (2006). Enumeration versus multiple object tracking: the case of action video game players. *Cognition* 101, 217–245. doi: 10.1016/j.cognition.2005.10.004

Horowitz, T. S., and Cohen, M. A. (2010). Direction information in multiple object tracking is limited by a graded resource. *Atten. Percept. Psychophys.* 72, 1765–1775. doi: 10.3758/APP.72.7.1765

Horowitz, T. S., Klieger, S. B., Fencsik, D. E., Yang, K. K., Alvarez, G. A., and Wolfe, J. M. (2007). Tracking unique objects. *Percept. Psychophys.* 69, 172–184. doi: 10.3758/bf03193740

Howe, P. D., Horowitz, T. S., Morocz, I. A., Wolfe, J., and Livingstone, M. S. (2009). Using fMRI to distinguish components of the multiple object tracking task. *J. Vis.* 9:10. doi: 10.1167/9.4.10

Jaeggi, S. M., Buschkuehl, M., Jonides, J., and Shah, P. (2011). Short-and long-term benefits of cognitive training. *Proc. Natl. Acad. Sci. U S A* 108, 10081–10086. doi: 10.1073/pnas.1103228108

Jones, K. T., and Berryhill, M. E. (2012). Parietal contributions to visual working memory depend on task difficulty. *Front. Psychiatry* 3:81. doi: 10.3389/fpsyt.2012.00081

Jovicich, J., Peters, R. J., Koch, C., Braun, J., Chang, L., and Ernst, T. (2001). Brain areas specific for attentional load in a motion-tracking task. *J. Cogn. Neurosci.* 13, 1048–1058. doi: 10.1162/089892901753294347

McKinley, R. A., McIntire, L., Bridges, N., Goodyear, C., and Weisend, M. P. (2013). Acceleration of image analyst training with transcranial direct current stimulation. *Behav. Neurosci.* 127, 936–946. doi: 10.1037/a0034975

Moos, K., Vossel, S., Weidner, R., Sparing, R., and Fink, G. R. (2012). Modulation of top-down control of visual attention by cathodal tDCS over right IPS. *J. Neurosci.* 32, 16360–16368. doi: 10.1523/JNEUROSCI.6233-11.2012

Nobre, A. C., Sebestyen, G. N., Gitelman, D. R., Mesulam, M. M., Frackowiak, R. S., and Frith, C. D. (1997). Functional localization of the system for visuospatial attention using positron emission tomography. *Brain* 120, 515–533. doi: 10.1093/brain/120.3.515

Oksama, L., and Hyönä, J. (2004). Is multiple object tracking carried out automatically by an early vision mechanism independent of higher-order cognition? An individual difference approach. *Vis. Cogn.* 11, 631–671. doi: 10.1080/13506280344000473

Pylyshyn, Z. W., and Storm, R. W. (1988). Tracking multiple independent targets: evidence for a parallel tracking mechanism. *Spat. Vis.* 3, 179–197. doi: 10.1163/156856888x00122

Radman, T., Datta, A., Ramos, R. L., Brumberg, J. C., and Bikson, M. (2009). "One-dimensional representation of a neuron in a uniform electric field," in *Engineering in Medicine and Biology Society, 2009. EMBC 2009. Annual International Conference of the IEEE* (Minneapolis, MN: IEEE), 6481–6484.

Rahman, A., Reato, D., Arlotti, M., Gasca, F., Datta, A., Parra, L. C., et al. (2013). Cellular effects of acute direct current stimulation: somatic and synaptic terminal effects. *J. Physiol.* 591, 2563–2578. doi: 10.1113/jphysiol.2012.247171

Scheldrup, M., Greenwood, P. M., McKendrick, R., Strohl, J., Bikson, M., Alam, M., et al. (2014). Transcranial direct current stimulation facilitates cognitive multi-task performance differentially depending on anode location and subtask. *Front. Hum. Neurosci.* 8:665. doi: 10.3389/fnhum.2014.00665

Schmiedek, F., Lövdén, M., and Lindenberger, U. (2010). Hundred days of cognitive training enhance broad cognitive abilities in adulthood: findings from the COGITO study. *Front. Aging Neurosci.* 2:27. doi: 10.3389/fnagi.2010.00027

Scholl, B. J., Pylyshyn, Z. W., and Feldman, J. (2001). What is a visual object? Evidence from target merging in multiple object tracking. *Cognition* 80, 159–177. doi: 10.1016/s0010-0277(00)00157-8

Sears, C. R., and Pylyshyn, Z. W. (2000). Multiple object tracking and attentional processing. *Can. J. Exp. Psychol.* 54, 1–14. doi: 10.1037/h0087326

Tseng, P., Hsu, T. Y., Chang, C. F., Tzeng, O. J., Hung, D. L., Muggleton, N. G., et al. (2012). Unleashing potential: transcranial direct current stimulation over the right posterior parietal cortex improves change detection in low-performing individuals. *J. Neurosci.* 32, 10554–10561. doi: 10.1523/jneurosci.0362-12.2012

Yantis, S. (1992). Multielement visual tracking: attention and perceptual organization. *Cogn. Psychol.* 24, 295–340. doi: 10.1016/0010-0285(92)90010-y

18

Gaze-independent ERP-BCIs: augmenting performance through location-congruent bimodal stimuli

Marieke E. Thurlings[1,2]*, Anne-Marie Brouwer[2], Jan B. F. Van Erp[2] and Peter Werkhoven[1]

[1] Information and Computing Sciences, Utrecht University, Utrecht, Netherlands
[2] Perceptual and Cognitive Systems, TNO, Soesterberg, Netherlands

Edited by:
Mikhail Lebedev, Duke University, USA

Reviewed by:
Dewen Hu, National University of Defense Technology, China
Betts Peters, Oregon Health and Science University, USA

***Correspondence:**
Marieke E. Thurlings, Information and Computing Sciences, Utrecht University, P. O. Box 80.089, 3508 TB Utrecht, Netherlands
e-mail: marieke.thurlings@gmail.com

Gaze-independent event-related potential (ERP) based brain-computer interfaces (BCIs) yield relatively low BCI performance and traditionally employ unimodal stimuli. Bimodal ERP-BCIs may increase BCI performance due to multisensory integration or summation in the brain. An additional advantage of bimodal BCIs may be that the user can choose which modality or modalities to attend to. We studied bimodal, visual-tactile, gaze-independent BCIs and investigated whether or not ERP components' tAUCs and subsequent classification accuracies are increased for (1) bimodal vs. unimodal stimuli; (2) location-congruent vs. location-incongruent bimodal stimuli; and (3) attending to both modalities vs. to either one modality. We observed an enhanced bimodal (compared to unimodal) P300 tAUC, which appeared to be positively affected by location-congruency (p = 0.056) and resulted in higher classification accuracies. Attending either to one or to both modalities of the bimodal location-congruent stimuli resulted in differences between ERP components, but not in classification performance. We conclude that location-congruent bimodal stimuli improve ERP-BCIs, and offer the user the possibility to switch the attended modality without losing performance.

Keywords: BCI, ERP, gaze-independent, bimodal, tactile, multisensory, location-congruency, selective attention

INTRODUCTION

Event-related potential (ERP) based brain-computer interfaces (BCIs) can be used to actively and voluntarily control a system, e.g., for communication (Farwell and Donchin, 1988) or navigation (Bell et al., 2008; Thurlings et al., 2010). ERP-BCIs make use of stimuli that correspond to control options (e.g., "left" or "right"). The user can select an option by attending to the corresponding stimulus (target) while ignoring other stimuli (nontargets). Stimulus-locked brain responses (ERPs) differ between the attended targets and ignored nontargets.

Most ERP-BCIs employ visual stimuli and require the user to gaze at the target stimulus, i.e., such a BCI is *gaze-dependent*. When the user does not directly gaze at the target but only covertly attends to it, the high-level endogenous ERP components but not the low-level perceptual ERP-components differ from those of nontargets. This results in a reduced BCI performance in terms of classification accuracy (and hence bitrate) (Brunner et al., 2010; Treder and Blankertz, 2010). BCIs for which users do not have to gaze at the stimuli or to shift focus (alter viewing direction) in order to control it are called *gaze-independent*. An example is the Hex-o-Spell of Treder and Blankertz (2010). The importance of developing BCIs independent of the ability to shift focus has been expressed in studies investigating the rapid serial visual presentation paradigm (Orhan et al., 2012; Acqualagna and Blankertz, 2013). Yet, in that paradigm participants are required to directly focus at the visual stimuli.

When users cannot reliably direct their gaze, or when other tasks interfere with gaze, stimuli can also be presented in other modalities like the auditory modality (Schreuder et al., 2010, 2011; Höhne et al., 2011). In application domains such as driving and gaming, BCIs must be gaze-independent as gaze is required for control and navigation tasks and the visual (and auditory) channel is already heavily loaded (Van Erp and Van Veen, 2004). The tactile channel has also been suggested as a viable alternative for these situations, and Brouwer and Van Erp (2010) demonstrated the feasibility of employing tactile stimuli around the waist in a tactile ERP-BCI. The natural correspondence of tactile stimuli around the waist with navigation directions (Van Erp, 2005) makes a tactile ERP-BCI especially interesting for navigation applications.

BCI performance of tactile ERP-BCIs (Brouwer et al., 2010; Thurlings et al., 2012a,b) is generally lower than that of gaze-dependent BCIs (Thurlings et al., 2012a,b). In addition, when a BCI is used as a control device in the context of a dual-task, for example to navigate in a game, BCI performance is even lower than in BCI-only tasks (Thurlings et al., 2013). Therefore, in order to achieve effective use of BCI outside the lab, it is highly important to increase BCI performance of gaze-independent BCIs.

This study focusses on potential benefits regarding brain activity resulting from stimulus presentation in multiple sensory modalities, using a gaze-independent setup, and addresses three main research questions which are introduced in the next sections.

THE BIMODAL ERP-BCI

The processing and integration of multisensory stimuli is likely to cause additional neuronal activity (Ernst and Bülthoff, 2004; Driver and Noesselt, 2008; Stein and Stanford, 2008). Integration may take place at perceptual stages (Molholm et al., 2002; Philippi et al., 2008), higher cognitive stages (Schröger and Widmann, 1998), and/or during motor preparation and execution (Giray and Ulrich, 1993). Bimodal stimuli generally yield faster behavioral responses and more accurate perceptual discrimination (Gondan et al., 2005; Teder-Sälejärvi et al., 2005; Philippi et al., 2008).

Multisensory integration has extensively been investigated in cognitive science, but has barely received attention in the field of BCI. In a recent BCI-study, we showed that an additional (early) ERP component was present when participants were presented with and attended to stimuli in two modalities rather than one, due to multisensory interaction (Thurlings et al., 2012a). To the best of our knowledge, only two other BCI-related studies investigated bimodal stimuli: visual-tactile stimuli (Brouwer et al., 2010), and audio-visual stimuli (Belitski et al., 2011). In both studies the authors reported increased classification accuracies (i.e., the percentage of correctly classified target responses) for bimodal compared to unimodal conditions, which is in line with the trend we reported in Thurlings et al. (2012a).

Multisensory or bimodal ERP-BCIs can be regarded as a type of hybrid BCIs (Pfurtscheller et al., 2010a). Hybrid BCIs are BCIs that "can either process their inputs simultaneously, or operate two systems sequentially". By allowing the processing of two inputs simultaneously, the second input could improve the classification accuracy of the first BCI (Pfurtscheller et al., 2010a; Yin et al., 2013).

As motivated in the beginning of the introduction, we are interested in multisensory BCIs, as a way to potentially increase BCI performance of (traditional) unimodal ERP-BCIs, in particularly the gaze-independent variants. From the three above mentioned bimodal studies, only Brouwer and Van Erp (2010) used a gaze-independent setup with visual-tactile stimuli. However in that study the effects on target and non-target responses of endogenous (voluntary) attention and exogenous (stimulus driven) attention were confound. Both endogenous and exogenous attention can affect ERP components (Woldorff and Hillyard, 1991), but only endogenous attention is relevant for BCI operation. Thus, the question whether or not gaze-independent ERP-BCIs benefit from bimodal stimulus presentation remains unanswered.

Multisensory integration has been shown to start as early as 80–120 ms after stimulus onset for visual-tactile stimuli (Sambo and Forster, 2009), but is modulated by endogenous attention at different stages of processing (Talsma and Woldorff, 2005). As reported in Thurlings et al. (2012a), positive effects of bimodal stimulus attending have been shown on an early stage of processing, i.e., early negative activity (N1) in the difference ERP (target minus nontarget ERP) was stronger for the bimodal compared to the unimodal conditions. However, we observed negative effects of bimodal stimulus attending on a late stage of the ERP, i.e., positive late activity (P300) in the difference ERP was stronger for one of the unimodal conditions (visual) compared to the bimodal condition. We hypothesized that the latter effect was caused by the spatial relation of the two unimodal stimuli that formed a bimodal stimulus pair. More specifically, although the spatial relation unambiguously indicated which unimodal stimuli formed a pair, those stimuli were not co-located. Possibly, this affected spatial attention and top-down stimulus processing. Therefore in the present study we focus on co-located (i.e., location-congruent) bimodal stimuli, with the expectation to lose the negative effects on late ERP components.

Thus, our first research question is: Are ERP components (quantified in the topographic Area Under the Curve or tAUC; Thurlings et al., 2012a,b) and corresponding classification accuracies of a bimodal visual-tactile ERP-BCI enhanced compared to its unimodal counterparts? We hypothesize enhanced bimodal ERP tAUCs both on early and late stages of processing when employing location-congruent bimodal stimuli in a gaze-independent setup, which should result in enhanced classification accuracies.

EFFECTS OF LOCATION-CONGRUENCY ON THE BIMODAL ERP-BCI

In case we find a benefit of bimodal compared to unimodal stimulus presentation and attending, as hypothesized in the previous section, it is relevant to know whether or not that effect depends (partly) on the spatial relation within the bimodal stimulus pairs. This is important for the designing of bimodal ERP-BCIs, especially since the most straightforward design might employ location incongruent bimodal stimulus pairs as in Thurlings et al. (2012a). In that study, a display presented visual navigation information and included visual stimuli located at the possible navigation directions. Tactile stimuli were presented around the waist, corresponding with navigation directions around us. To make the spatial relation as congruent as possible in that setup, the display was oriented in the horizontal plane, to match the horizontal lay-out of the tactile stimuli (Thurlings et al., 2012b). Therefore the bimodal stimulus pairs were directional-congruent, but not location-congruent. We showed in Thurlings et al. (2012a) that location-incongruency resulted in negative effects of bimodal (compared to unimodal) stimulus attending on a late stage, while effects on the early stage were positive (see previous section).

Literature on the effects of location-congruency is not unequivocal. According to the spatial rule (Meredith and Stein, 1986), stimuli from different modalities are only integrated when stimuli are spatially co-located (or proximate). Stein et al. (1989) showed for example that the performance of animals that were trained to approach visual stimuli is improved when matched with (unattended) auditory stimuli, but only if the visual-auditory stimulus pairs were spatially co-located (or proximate). Frassinetti et al. (2002) replicated these results in humans. However, also when bimodal stimulus-pairs are not location-congruent, behavior performance has been found to be enhanced (Gondan et al., 2005; Teder-Sälejärvi et al., 2005; Philippi et al., 2008). These studies differ in tasks, but have in common that the task does not enforce selective attention to one modality (as in the studies of Meredith and Stein), but rather both modalities need to be attended. Apparently the role of the spatial relation within multisensory information and if and how it affects multisensory integration depends on the specific circumstances (We address the role of selective attention to modality in the next section). Nevertheless, also when bimodal benefits are found for location-incongruent bimodal stimuli, behavioral performance may be further improved by location-congruency (Gondan et al., 2005). Teder-Sälejärvi et al. (2005) did not observe such a behavioral benefit, but did report differences in the ERP for location-congruent and location-incongruent bimodal stimuli after 100 ms. They concluded that there are overlapping and distinct processes involved in processing of location-congruent and incongruent stimuli.

Multisensory studies typically involve a task that requires participants to distinguish targets from nontargets based on physical stimulus characteristics, instead of on (only) spatial differences such as is the case in a BCI-setup (which uses spatial selective attention). Possibly, the role of the spatial relation is larger when the task is only based on spatial discrimination. Therefore it is important to study the role of the spatial relation of bimodal stimuli in ERP-BCIs.

Our second research question is: What is the effect of location-congruent compared to location-incongruent bimodal stimuli on the ERP tAUCs and corresponding classification accuracies in an ERP-BCI? We hypothesize positive effects for location congruent bimodal stimuli at late stages (e.g., P300 tAUC) of stimulus processing, which should correspond to enhanced classification accuracies.

EFFECTS OF SELECTIVE ATTENTION TO MODALITY ON THE BIMODAL ERP-BCI

Both exogenous and endogenous attention affect the ERP (Eimer et al., 2001). When participants are presented with bimodal stimuli, but they endogenously attend to either one or both modalities, exogenous attention involved in both cases is the same (as the physical characteristics have not changed). However, the amount of attentional resources allocated endogenously for processing the stimulus information of the two modalities involved differs between these cases (Macaluso, 2010). For example, when participants are precued and (pre)attending to the visual rather than the auditory modality, audio-visual stimuli are processed differently, resulting in enhanced early activity starting around 110 ms and peaking around 150 ms (Foxe and Simpson, 2005). Talsma et al. (2007) showed that for the earliest multisensory integration effect (a superadditive effect) of audiovisual stimuli to occur, both modalities need to be attended. Nevertheless, if only a single modality was attended integration still occurred but the process appeared to start later (after 250 ms after stimulus onset) and was dependent on which modality was attended.

Users of a bimodal ERP-BCI could choose to attend to either one or both modalities, which could affect the resulting ERP and may require modality-specific trained classifiers for optimal performance. In this study, we investigated the trade-off between possibly affected classification accuracies (when a bimodal classifier trained with attending to both modalities is used also when only one modality is attended to) and the advantage of the flexibility offered to the user to choose the modality to attend to.

Our third research question is: Does, and if so how does, attending to the visual or tactile modality, or both modalities affect ERP components' tAUCs and corresponding classification accuracies in a bimodal ERP-BCI? We hypothesize that when both modalities (as opposed to either one alone) of bimodal (location-congruent) stimuli are attended, the early stage of the bimodal ERP tAUC is enhanced. Such an enhancement of the ERP tAUC could also result in enhanced classification accuracies.

Following up on the third main research question, a sub-question is: (3a) How do these classification accuracies depend on the degree of overlap in the attended modalities of the datasets during training and classification. That is, would it be possible to switch the attended modality during use, or does the classifier then need to be retrained? We hypothesize that classification accuracies are negatively affected if the applied classifier is trained on data with a different attended modality than the data that are being classified. When attended modalities during training and classifying partly overlap (i.e., visual and bimodal, or tactile and bimodal) higher classification accuracies are expected than when they do not overlap (i.e., visual and tactile).

MATERIALS AND METHODS

PARTICIPANTS

Ten students voluntarily participated in this study. Participants were aged between 22 and 26 years (mean age 23.5 years). All participants were male and had normal or corrected-to-normal vision. None had previously participated in a BCI-experiment and one was left-handed. The participants signed informed consent forms.

TASK

The task was to select one of two possible control options: left or right. In this study we used the index fingers to present stimulus information, in contrast to locations around the waist (corresponding to navigation directions around us) used in our previous tactile studies. The reason is that we here focus on a gaze-independent and location-congruent setup of bimodal stimuli, and participants should be able to comfortably perceive visual and tactile information from the same location(s). Because the bimodal stimuli should in addition be located at equal distances and angles from fixation, we opted to only employ two bimodal stimuli.

The two control options were presented sequentially in random order, at the left and right index finger through a tactile actuator, an LED, or both. To select an option, participants had to attend to a target stimulus location and modality, and count the number of tactile, visual or visual–tactile activations at that location. At the beginning of each trial the current target (i.e., a combination of finger and modality) was indicated by means of a short activation of the particular target stimulus. Participants were instructed to attend to all targets (and count them internally), and ignore nontargets. Within one trial, each control option (target and nontarget) was activated 10 times.

Note that although ERP-BCIs typically make use of more than two control options (i.e., more than one nontarget), Brouwer and Van Erp (2010) have shown that the P300 is also elicited in a 2-class tactile BCI and operation is not significantly reduced compared to a 4- or 6-class BCI.

DESIGN

The experiment involved six conditions, named after the type of stimuli and attended modality involved. In four conditions targets had to be attended in the modalities that the stimuli of that condition were presented in (no selective attention to modality): Visual, Tactile, Bimodal, Bimodal-Incongr (i.e., short for "Incongruent"). In the Bimodal condition a control option consisted of the simultaneous activation of a visual and tactile actuator at the same finger, while for Bimodal-Incongr a visual and tactile actuator of opposite fingers were matched. In the two other conditions, only one modality had to be attended, while bimodal (location-congruent) stimuli were presented. For attending the visual or tactile modality, the conditions were named: Bimodal-Att-V and Bimodal-Att-T, respectively. The order of the conditions was counterbalanced over participants.

Each condition consisted of three sets. In each set, each of the two control options was designated as the target three times, i.e., there were six trials. Each trial consisted of 10 consecutive repetitions of the control options in random order, i.e., in each set there were 60 target and 60 nontarget activations. The data of the first two sets (the training sets) were used for the training of a classifier, which was applied to classify the data in the third set (the test set). Online BCI-feedback was given to participants in the test set about which stimulus was classified as the target. The training (but not the test) set was also used for the analysis of participants' ERP components.

MATERIALS

General

An actuator pair, consisting of a tactile vibrator and a visual LED, was attached with Velcro to each index finger (22 degrees from a fixation cross). The target and nontarget stimuli consisted of a single pulse with a pulse duration of 187.5 ms. The interval between pulses was 437.5 ms. To indicate the designated target control option at the beginning of a trial and the classified control option for BCI-feedback at the end of a trial, a 2 s and a 1 s single pulse were presented, respectively.

Stimuli

Tactile stimuli: The tactile stimuli were presented through a vibrating element called a tactor. The tactors were custom built and consisted of a plastic case with a contact area of 1 × 2 cm containing a 160 Hz electromotor (TNO, The Netherlands, model JHJ-3, see: Van Erp et al., 2007). To prevent participants from perceiving auditory information from the tactors, they listened to pink noise via speakers during the experiment in all conditions.

Visual stimuli: Visual stimuli were presented through two white LEDs of 5 mm, 3.2 V.

Bimodal stimuli: For all bimodal conditions, except for Bimodal-Incongr, bimodal stimuli consisted of the simultaneous activation of the visual and tactile stimulus on the same index finger (location-congruent). For the Bimodal-Incongr condition, the visual stimulus of one index finger and the tactile stimulus of the other index finger were activated simultaneously.

EEG recording equipment

EEG was recorded from eight linked-mastoids-referenced scalp electrodes (F_Z, C_Z, P_Z, O_Z, P_3, P_4, PO_7, PO_8) that used a common forehead ground (g.Tec medical engineering, GmbH). The impedance of each electrode was below 5 kΩ, as was confirmed prior to and during the measurements. EEG data were recorded with a hardware filter (bandpass 0.1–60 Hz, notch at 50 Hz) and sampled at a frequency of 256 Hz.

DATA ANALYSIS

EEG preprocessing and selection

To prepare the recorded EEG for ERP-analysis, we followed similar procedures as taken in Thurlings et al. (2012a,b): selecting (non)target responses, baseline correction, threshold rejection of responses, and computation of a difference ERP. However, the data were not additionally low-pass filtered (the relatively large band was chosen because of potential multisensory effects in the 30–60 Hz band).

Selecting (non)target responses: For ERP-analysis, both target and nontarget responses were used when preceded by a nontarget. Responses preceded by a target were discarded (i.e., there were no (other) targets presented between −625 and 625 ms relative to (non)target onset) (see also Treder and Blankertz, 2010).

Baseline correction: For the selected targets and nontargets, epochs from all electrodes were extracted from −100 to 625 ms relative to stimulus onset and baseline corrected relative to the average voltage during the 100 ms preceding the stimulus onset.

Threshold rejection of responses: We discarded epochs from all electrodes belonging to a certain stimulus, if any epoch contained amplitude differences exceeding 100 μV, indicating movement artifacts. On average, the previous steps left us with 58.8 target epochs (with a range over participants and conditions from 35 to 70) and 54.0 nontarget epochs (with a range over participants and conditions from 32 to 67). Subsequently, the selected target and nontarget epochs were averaged per participant, per condition and per electrode.

Difference ERP: We subtracted the averaged clean nontarget epochs from the averaged clean target epochs for each participant, each condition and each electrode. With this step, we removed exogenous (involuntary or automatic) attention effects. Further analyses were performed regarding this difference ERP (or endogenous ERP).

Identifying and quantifying ERP components

To identify and quantify ERP components triggered by endogenously attended stimuli, we applied the detection method as reported in Thurlings et al. (2012a,b). Only data of the training set was used, to prevent influence of BCI feedback. We identified significant effects of attending stimuli by performing a sample-by-sample *t*-test on the difference ERP (between 0 and 625 ms relative to (non)target onset) for each electrode and condition and clustered the stable segments (i.e., in this case at least seven consecutive significant samples; see also: Guthrie and Buchwald,

1991). Clusters were considered robust if they contained segments of at least two electrodes. These robust clusters defined the topographic distribution and the interval of the endogenous ERP components, taking the beginning of the earliest segment and the ending of the latest segment in the clusters as ERP component intervals.

We quantified the endogenous ERP components by using the tAUC-value (topographic Area Under the Curve), as described in Thurlings et al. (2012a,b). The tAUC reflects the magnitude of an ERP component not only by taking the averaged amplitude and duration of the component into account but also by considering the topographic distribution.

Online and offline BCI performance

Classification accuracies were calculated both online and offline. Online analysis was performed using BCI2000 (Schalk et al., 2004), which made use of SWLDA (stepwise linear discriminant analysis) on epochs from 0–797 ms after stimulus onset, decimation factor 4 (i.e., 64 Hz), and other standard parameters (maximum of 60 features, *p*-values initially included and backward excluded from the model <0.1 and >0.15 respectively; see Krusienski et al., 2008). The classifier was trained using the training set for each participant and for each condition.

We investigated classification accuracies more detailed offline. Standard classification parameters are based on visual ERP-BCI research. We established potentially more appropriate parameters for bimodal BCIs, and using those parameters assessed the results of the research questions in practical use. To this end, for all conditions we executed a parameter sweep with all combinations of decimation factors (between 4 and 26), and the number of blocks of downsampled windows (between 1 block and the maximum number of blocks approaching a correspondence of 800 ms). The parameter-pair resulting in the highest overall classification accuracies (averaged over all six conditions) after 10 repetitions was selected for further analyses. Then for each condition, we calculated accuracies after each repetition and established the number of repetitions which is expected most appropriate in practical use. We considered the number of repetitions the most appropriate, when classification accuracies of 70% or higher were achieved using a minimal number of repetitions (Kubler et al., 2004; Birbaumer and Cohen, 2007; Pfurtscheller et al., 2010b).

For all conditions, classification accuracies were determined by classifying the test set using a classifier trained on the training set. Additionally, to assess what the costs on BCI performance are of switching attended modality during BCI operation, analysis was done cross-conditionally: that is, for each of the conditions Bimodal, Bimodal-Att-V, and Bimodal-Att-T, the test set was classified using a classifier trained on the test set of each of the other two conditions. From the nine resulting classes of responses, we clustered three categories: (1) trained and tested on data of the same condition ("Equal"); (2) trained and tested on data of two different conditions, but with an overlap in the attended modality (e.g., trained on Bimodal, tested on Bimodal-Att-V; attending of the visual modality is overlapping) ("Overlap"); and (3) trained and tested on data of two different conditions, but without an overlap in the attended modality (e.g., trained on Bimodal-Att-V, tested on Bimodal-Att-T ("No Overlap"). Within each category the included classes were averaged per participant.

Statistical analysis

ERP components' tAUC-values and classification accuracies were statistically analyzed using Statistica 8.0 (StatSoft, Tulsa, USA). To test for normality Shapiro-Wilk tests were applied, and when normality could not be assumed the data were log-transformed. We used separate one-way repeated-measures ANOVAs to examine different subsets of data appropriate to answer each of the three research questions when comparing three conditions, and paired *t*-tests when comparing two conditions. The dependent variables were tAUCs and classification accuracies. For the three main research questions, the independent variables were: (1) Bimodality (three levels: Visual, Tactile, Bimodal); (2) Location-Congruency (two levels: Bimodal, Bimodal-Incongr); and (3) Attending Modality (three levels: Bimodal, Bimodal-Att-V, Bimodal-Att-T). For sub-question (3a) the dependent variable was classification accuracies, and the independent variable was Cross-training (three levels: Equal, Overlap, No Overlap). Tukey *post-hoc* tests were applied when appropriate.

PROCEDURE

After the participant was verbally instructed and had read and signed the informed consent form, we attached the visual-tactile actuator pairs on his index-fingers using Velcro. The participant was seated in a dimly lit, electromagnetically shielded room and positioned his arms on the desk in front of him. We allowed the participant to become accustomed to the stimuli, by activating them for several minutes. The participant was asked to gaze at the fixation cross in front of him on the table.

During EEG preparation, we repeated the outline of the experiment and instructed the participant to move as little as possible during stimulus presentations. Before each condition, we informed the participant about the oncoming condition. When the participant indicated to be ready to begin, we started the condition. In the test sets, online BCI feedback was given after each trial (i.e., the 10th repetition). Each condition (including two training and one test recording) took approximately 3.8 min recording time. Conditions followed each other with 1–15 min breaks in between, depending on the participant's preferences.

RESULTS

First we describe the general observed results (General) considering ERP components and BCI performance for each condition. Subsequently, the effects for each of the three main research questions (regarding the effects of bimodality (The effect of Bimodality), location-congruency (The effect of Location-Congruency), and selective attention to modality (The effect of Selective Attention to Modality)) are reported both with respect to ERP components and classification accuracy. Additionally, the effect of the sub-question of the third main research (addressing the effect of Cross-training) is presented in terms of classification accuracies (Classification accuracies of Cross-training (attended modality cross classifier)).

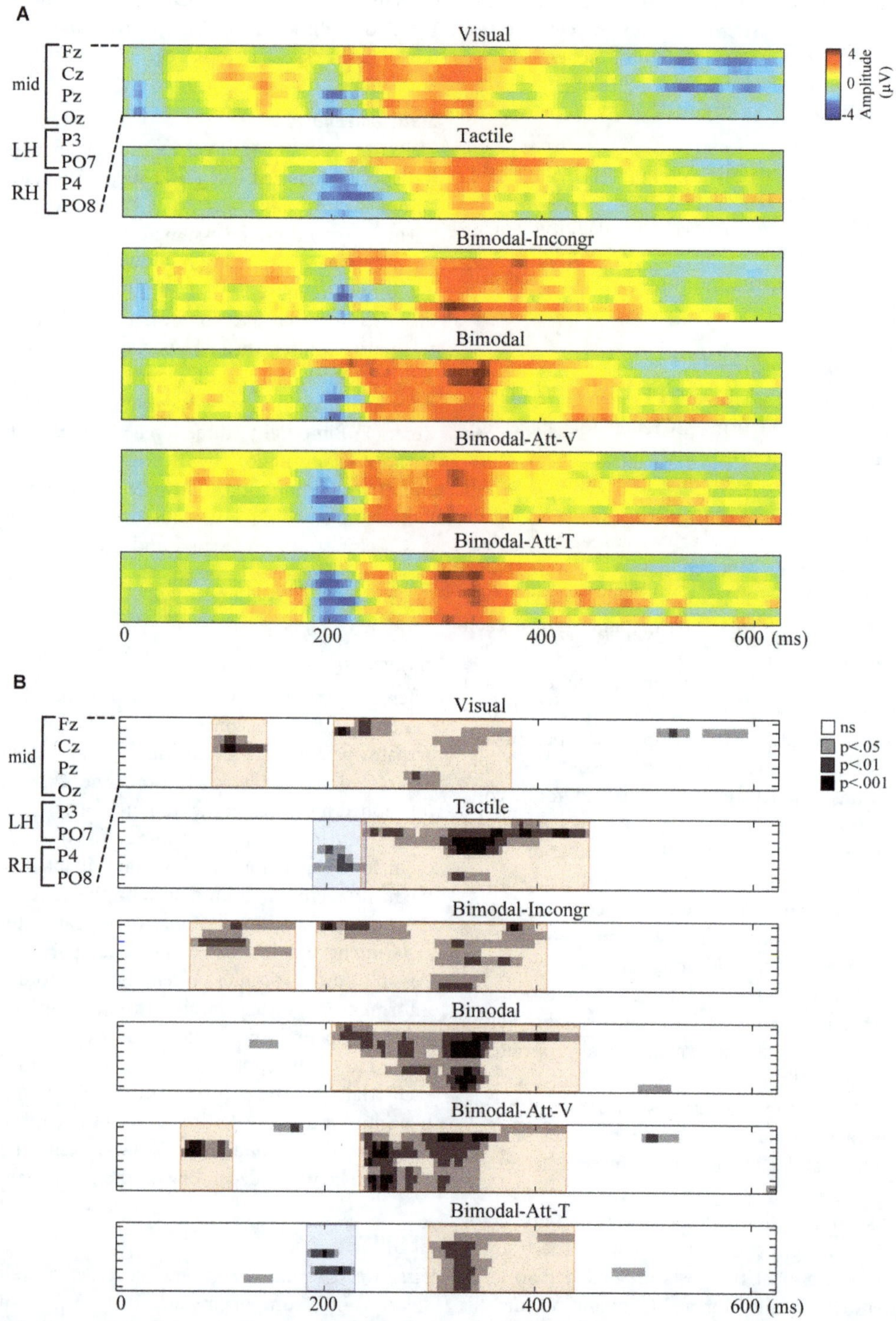

FIGURE 1 | Spatiotemporal representations of the endogenous ERP for each condition, with time (ms) on the x-axis and electrodes on the y-axis. Electrodes from top to bottom: F_Z, C_Z, P_Z, O_Z, P_3, P_4, PO_7, PO_8. **(A)** The Grand Average of the amplitudes of the endogenous ERP (µV) for each condition. **(B)** The statistical significance of the endogenous ERP (*p*-values) resulting in stable segments, clustered in ERP components. ERP components are marked by colored overlays in red and blue for positive and negative components, respectively.

GENERAL

Endogenous ERP components

Spatiotemporal presentations of the amplitudes of the endogenous ERPs are presented in **Figure 1A**. For all conditions, endogenous activity was observed during one or two periods within the analyzed interval from 0 until 625 ms after stimulus onset. In **Figure 1B**, spatiotemporal plots show the significant stable segments. The red and blue areas in that figure indicate

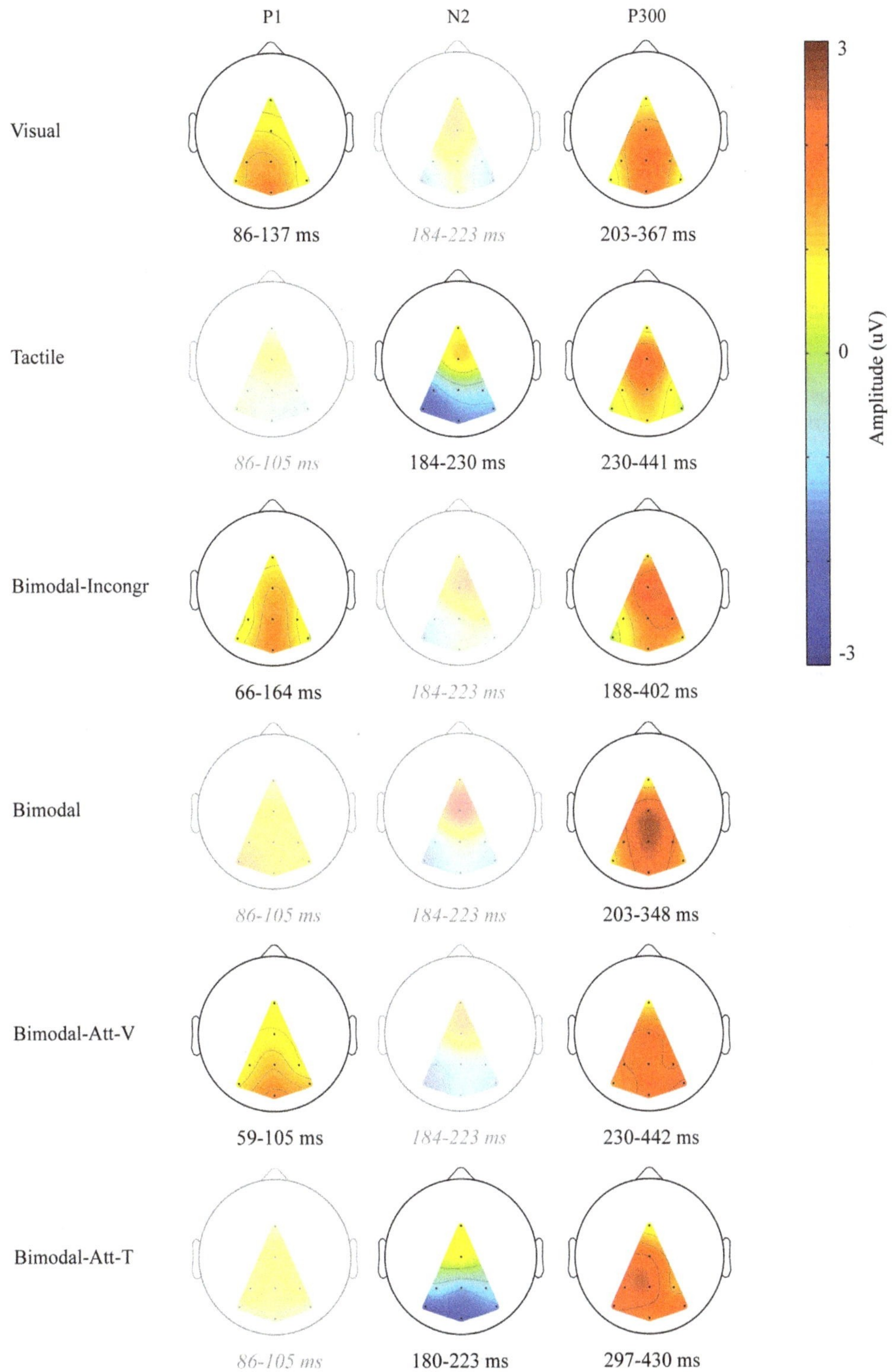

FIGURE 2 | Scalp distributions of the endogenous ERP for the identified endogenous ERP components. Only that part of the scalp is visualized, in which electrode information could be interpolated. Amplitudes (μV) are averages calculated within each ERP component's interval, averaged over participants. If no ERP component was identified, the overlapping interval (of the windows of the ERP component for conditions in which it was identified) was used to visualize that activity for comparison. In that case, the scalp plot is left semitransparent, and the corresponding interval is shown in gray and italics.

the polarities (positive and negative, respectively) of the clustered segments that were found to be robust and were thus identified as endogenous ERP components.

As apparent from **Figure 1B**, only one endogenous ERP component was identified in all six conditions: the P300. In **Figure 2**, the ERP components are visualized by means of scalp plots (averaged amplitudes of the endogenous ERP at all electrodes, within the ERP components' intervals). The P300 amplitudes were largest in the central-parietal area, it appeared to be the strongest in the Bimodal and Bimodal-Att-V conditions, and the weakest for the Visual condition. The windows in which the P300 was detected were: 203–367 ms (Visual), 230–441 ms (Tactile), 188–402 ms (Bimodal-Incongr), 203–348 ms (Bimodal), 230–442 ms (Bimodal-Att-V), and 297–430 ms (Bimodal-Att-T) after stimulus onset.

Furthermore, early positive activity was detected and identified as P1 for the Visual, Bimodal-Att-V and Bimodal-Incongr conditions, in the windows 86–137 ms, 59–105 ms, and 66–164 ms respectively, after stimulus onset. For the Tactile and Bimodal-Att-T conditions a different early component was detected. Early negative activity was identified as an N2 in the windows 184–230 ms, and 180–223 ms respectively after stimulus onset.

The complete ERPs are visualized for each condition for electrode P_z in **Figure 3** (grouped per research question). The main effect of conditions on the ERP components' tAUC-values are visualized in **Figures 5A–C**.

BCI performance

A parameter-sweep was performed for combinations of decimation factors and the length of the epoch used (divided into blocks of downsampled windows). The parameter-pair of decimation factor 5 (i.e., 51.2 Hz) and epoch length of 625 ms resulted in the highest overall classification accuracies of 82.2% (SD: 11.1) over conditions. Thus, these parameters were further used for offline analysis.

Both online and offline classification accuracies are visualized in **Figure 4**. Overall classification accuracies (averaged over participants) are highest for all bimodal conditions employing location-congruent stimuli (i.e., Bimodal, Bimodal-Att-V, and Bimodal-Att-T). For all conditions offline classification accuracies increase with each repetition, except for the Bimodal-Incongr condition. After six repetitions, the averaged classification accuracies for five out of the six conditions exceeded the threshold of 70% necessary for effective control. For the Bimodal-Incongr condition this threshold was not reached at all. Therefore the sixth repetition is considered the most appropriate to assess effects of all research questions in a practical setting, and was used for statistical analysis.

THE EFFECT OF BIMODALITY

ERP components' tAUCs

The P300 tAUC (**Table 1**) was significantly affected by Bimodality ($F_{(2,18)} = 23.93$, $p < 0.001$). The P300 tAUC was larger for the Bimodal condition compared to both unimodal conditions (both $p < 0.001$), and did not differ significantly between the unimodal conditions (**Figure 5A**).

The P1 was only identified for the Visual condition (neither for Tactile nor for Bimodal) and the P1's tAUC (**Table 1**) differed significantly from 0 ($t_{(9)} = 6.69$, $p < 0.001$).

The N2 was only identified for the Tactile condition (neither for Visual nor for Bimodal) and the N2's tAUC (**Table 1**) differed significantly from 0 ($t_{(9)} = 6.41$, $p < 0.001$).

Classification accuracies

The effect of Bimodality on classification accuracies was significant ($F_{(2,18)} = 7.30$, $p < 0.01$), with higher accuracies for Bimodal compared to Visual ($p < 0.05$) and Tactile ($p < 0.01$) (**Figure 5D**).

THE EFFECT OF LOCATION-CONGRUENCY

ERP components' tAUCs

An increased P300 tAUC (**Table 1**) for Bimodal compared to Bimodal-Incongr approached significance ($t_{(9)} = 2.19$, $p = 0.056$) (**Figure 5B**).

The P1 was only identified for the Bimodal-Incongr condition (not for Bimodal) and the P1's tAUC (**Table 1**) differed significantly from 0 ($t_{(9)} = 5.91$, $p < 0.001$).

Classification accuracies

An effect of Location-Congruency on classification accuracies was found, with higher accuracies for Bimodal compared to Bimodal-Incongr ($t_{(9)} = 3.88$, $p < 0.01$) (**Figure 5E**).

THE EFFECT OF SELECTIVE ATTENTION TO MODALITY

ERP components' tAUCs

The P300 tAUC was significantly affected by Modality ($F_{(2,18)} = 7.50$, $p < 0.01$). The P300 was stronger for the Bimodal and Bimodal-Att-V conditions compared to the Bimodal-Att-T condition ($p < 0.05$ and $p < 0.01$, respectively) (**Figure 5C**).

The P1 was only identified for the Bimodal-Att-V condition (neither for Bimodal-Att-T nor for Bimodal) and the P1's tAUC (**Table 1**) differed significantly from 0 ($t_{(9)} = 8.19$, $p < 0.001$).

The N2 was only identified for the Bimodal-Att-T condition (neither for Bimodal-Att-V nor for Bimodal) and the N2's tAUC (**Table 1**) differed significantly from 0 ($t_{(9)} = 6.20$, $p < 0.001$).

Classification accuracies (attended modality specific classifier)

For the attended modality specific classifier, the data used for training of the classifier and for the actual classification are recorded under the same attending-modality conditions (using bimodal location-congruent stimuli only).

No effect of Attending Modality on classification accuracies was found (**Figure 5F**).

Classification accuracies of Cross-training (attended modality cross classifier)

In this subsection the results of sub-question 3a are reported. For the attended modality cross classifier, training of the classifier occurred for each of the attending-modality conditions, and the resulting classifier was used to cross-classify the data of each of the attending-modality conditions.

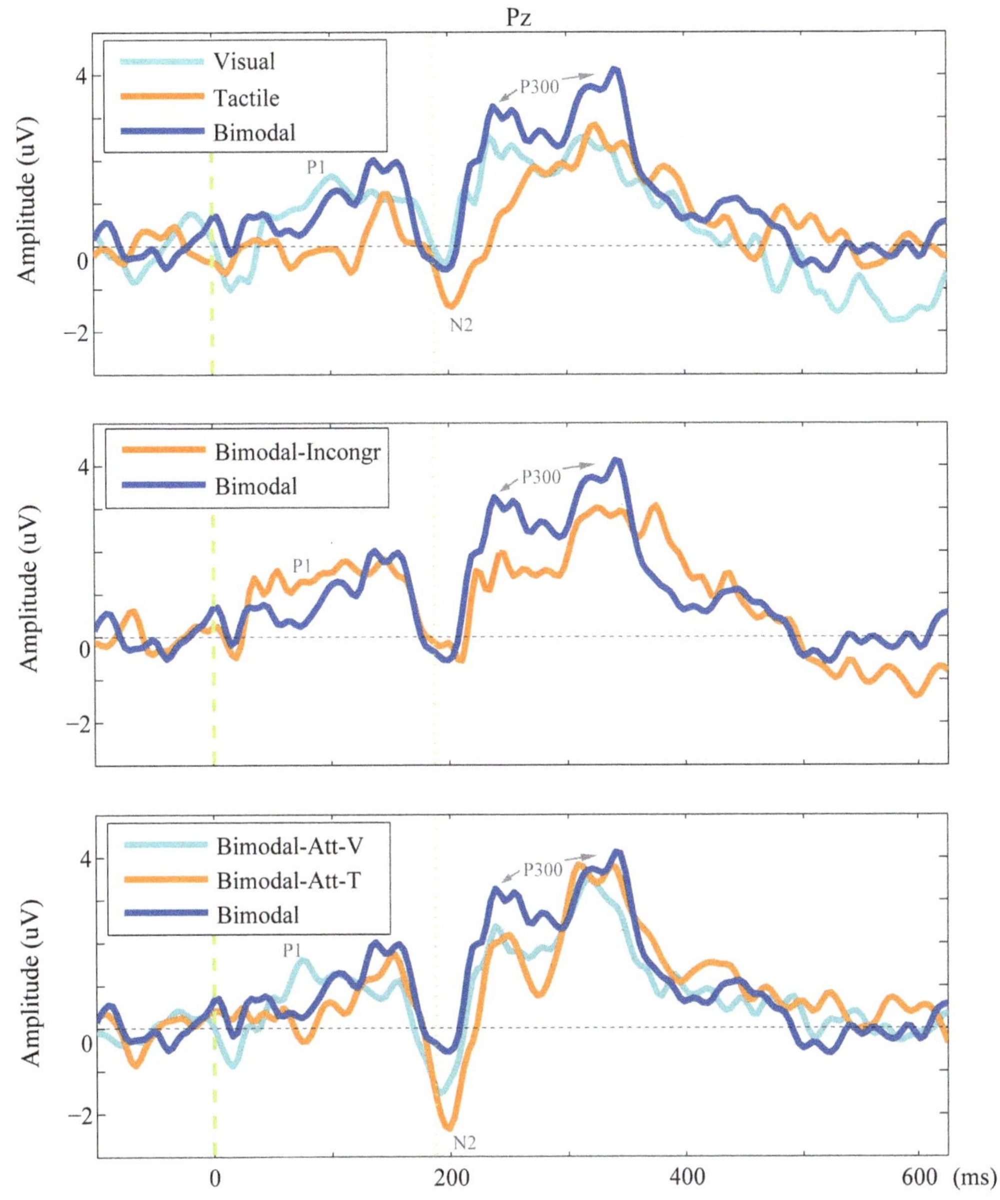

FIGURE 3 | Grand average of the endogenous ERP. The averaged endogenous ERP is visualized for electrode P_z for each condition included in the comparison for each research question.

Table 1 | Mean and standard errors averaged over participants of the tAUC-values (μV*ms) of all identified ERP components for each condition.

ERP Component	Visual	Tactile	Bimodal-Incongr	Bimodal	Bimodal-Att-V	Bimodal-Att-T
P1	37.6 (17.8)		92.3 (49.4)		36.4 (14.1)	
N2		56.5 (27.9)				44.4 (22.7)
P300	168.9 (63.5)	237.0 (73.4)	351.3 (140.9)	526.7 (223.3)	534.7 (125.4)	265.2 (168.0)

Table 2 shows the results of the cross-condition classification analyses. In **Figure 5G** the effect of Cross-training on the clustered categories is visualized. Cross-training affected classification accuracies ($F_{(2,18)} = 4.86$, $p < 0.05$), with higher accuracies for Equal compared to No Overlap ($p < 0.05$).

DISCUSSION

THE EFFECT OF BIMODALITY

The first and main research question addressed in this study was: Are ERP components' tAUCs and corresponding classification accuracies of a bimodal visual-tactile ERP-BCI enhanced

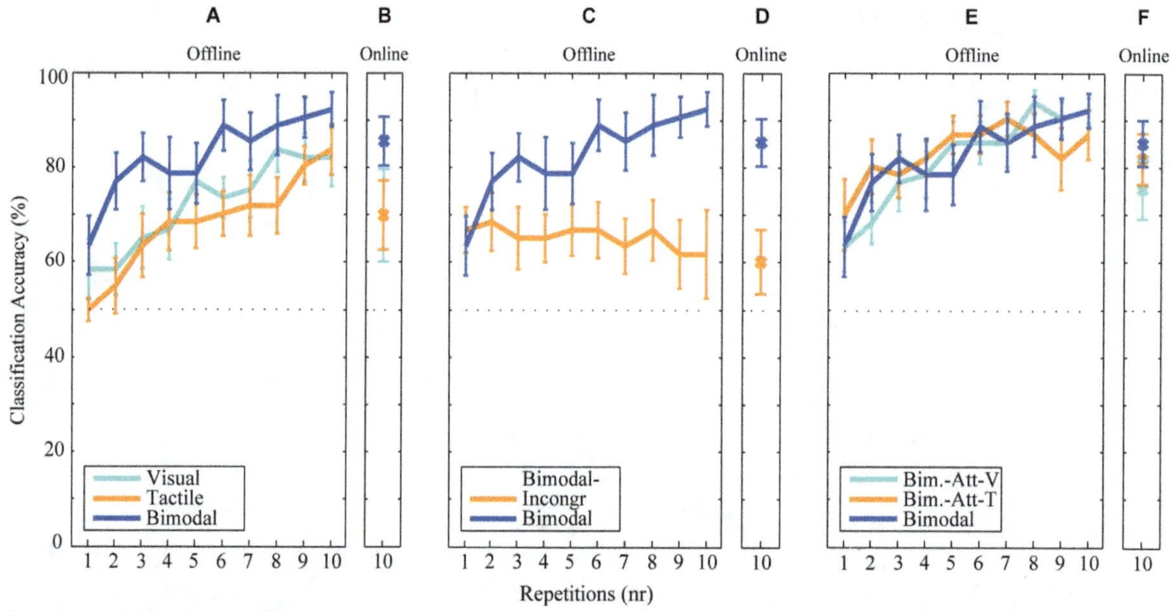

FIGURE 4 | Offline and online classification accuracies. (A) Offline and **(B)** online classification accuracies after each repetition for the conditions involved in the analysis of the first research question (the effect of Bimodality). **(C)** Offline and **(D)** online classification accuracies after each repetition for the conditions involved in the analysis of the second research question (the effect of Location Congruency). **(E)** Offline and **(F)** online classification accuracies after each repetition for the conditions involved in the analysis of the third research question (the effect of Attending Modality).

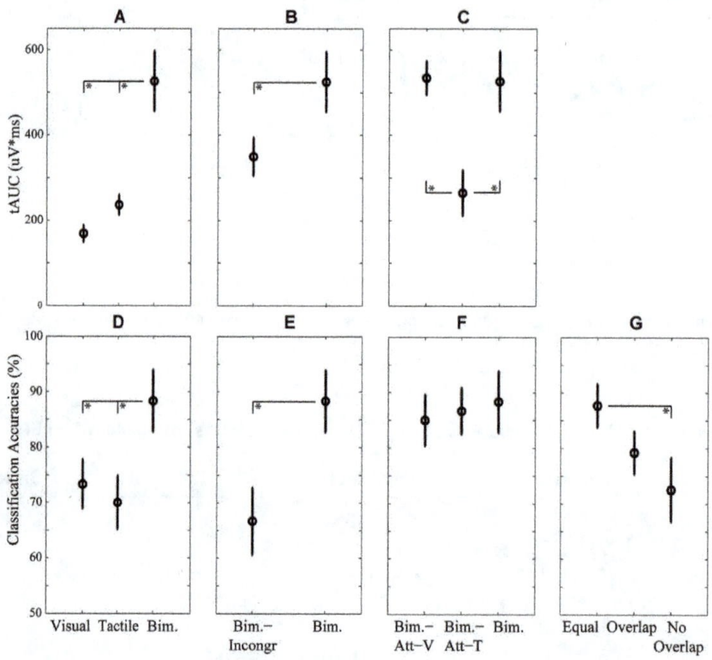

FIGURE 5 | Mean and standard errors over participants of the P300 (A–C) and classification accuracies (D–G), for each research question: the effect of modality (A,D), the effect of location-congruency (B,E), the effect of selective attention to modality (C,F), and the effect of cross-training (G). Condition pairs that significantly differed from each other are indicated by an asterisk (*) symbol.

Table 2 | Classification accuracies (averages and standard deviations) for each class of cross-conditional classification.

Tested on	Trained on Bimodal	Bimodal-Att-V	Bimodal-Att-T
Bimodal	83.33 (17.66)*	76.67 (21.08)^	80.00 (18.92)^
Bimodal-Att-V	81.67 (12.30)^	85.00 (14.59)*	73.33 (14.05)#
Bimodal-Att-T	76.67 (17.92)^	71.67 (26.12)#	86.67 (13.15)*

*Symbols *^# indicate which classes are categorized together, with * for Equal, ^ for Overlap, and # for No Overlap.*

compared to its unimodal counterparts? As we hypothesized, we found an enhanced late effect on the ERP (P300 tAUC) and corresponding enhanced classification accuracies for the location-congruent bimodal compared to the unimodal conditions, using a gaze-independent setup. In our previous bimodal work (Thurlings et al., 2012a), we did not find an enhanced bimodal P300. Instead, the bimodal P300 was even decreased compared to the visual P300. We hypothesized that effect to be a result of location-incongruent bimodal stimuli, as the P300 is affected by spatial attention (Kramer and Strayer, 1988). In this study, we showed that attending to (location-congruent) bimodal (compared to unimodal) stimuli does indeed result in an increasement of the P300 tAUC. The different findings in these two studies hint that location-congruency may indeed affect the processing of bimodal stimuli, which we will further discuss in the next section (The effect of Location-Congruency).

In contrast to our expectations, we did not find positive effects of attending to bimodal stimuli on the early stage of processing. In fact, we did not detect an early bimodal ERP component at all for location-congruent stimuli when both modalities were attended. However we did observe early ERP components for both unimodal conditions: a visual P1 and a tactile N2. Because the unimodal conditions resulted in early ERP components with opposite polarities, the lack of a bimodal early ERP component in this study may be explained by counterbalanced activity. In Thurlings et al. (2012a) we did find a bimodal early ERP component (N1), which was not detected in either of the unimodal conditions. The early ERPs of those unimodal conditions, however, appeared much more alike and already showed a slight negative drift. Also in Talsma and Woldorff (2005)—in which positive effects of audiovisual stimulus attending on early and late stages of processing are reported- the unimodal early ERPs were quite alike. The same is the case in other bimodal studies (e.g., Gondan et al., 2005; Teder-Sälejärvi et al., 2005; Philippi et al., 2008). In multisensory literature there is an on-going debate about whether or not superadded activity is elicited when multisensory integration takes place, and how integration effects can be measured (Barth et al., 1995; Gondan and Röder, 2006; Boll and Berti, 2009; Senkowski et al., 2011). Perhaps ERP summation is the driving factor behind enhanced effects of bimodal compared to unimodal ERPs in our study.

If unimodal ERP components need to be alike to elicit bimodal effects usable in BCI, it is relevant to understand why in the current study this was not the case. For the tactile condition the early ERP component (N1) resembles the tactile N2 described in Thurlings et al. (2012a), but occurred slightly (~25 ms) earlier in this study. The P1 from the visual condition also occurs ~25 ms earlier compared to the visual N2 in Thurlings et al. (2012a), but has a reversed polarity. Possibly, these visual early components do have the same generator: The polarity of the P1 can be reversed if the concerning electrode is measured in reference to for example the nose instead of linked-mastoids (Chiappa and Chiappa, 1997). Indeed in this study linked-mastoid references were used (with which a visual P1 is expected: Mangun, 1995) while in Thurlings et al. (2012a) a nose-reference was used. Not every ERP component has to be affected by such a difference: depending on the generator of a certain ERP component and the recorded electrode(s) this can affect polarity.

Attending to bimodal compared to unimodal stimuli may have increased exogenous as well as endogenous attention. Therefore the cause of the bimodality effect here could theoretically be either bottom-up, or top-down driven, or by an interaction between the two. In this study Bimodality affected the ERP positively at the late stage. Since Hopfinger and West (2006) found the P300 to be unaffected by increased exogenous attention, we think that top-down controlled endogenous attention caused the Bimodality effect. While this study does not map out the exact mechanism behind the effect, it is clear that BCI performance was much higher when congruent bimodal stimuli were used compared to unimodal stimuli. We therewith provide a way to improve performance of a gaze-independent ERP-BCI.

THE EFFECT OF LOCATION-CONGRUENCY

The second research question concerned the effect of location-congruent compared to location-incongruent bimodal stimuli on the ERP components' tAUC and corresponding classification accuracies in an ERP-BCI. As we hypothesized, we found an indication that location-congruency positively affects the late ERP component tAUC in response to bimodal stimuli ($p = 0.056$), and this trend corresponded to increased classification accuracies.

Although we only expected location-congruency to influence the late stage of the ERP, we also found a difference at the early stage: A P1 was observed for the Bimodal-Incongr condition, whereas we did not detect early ERP components for the Bimodal condition at all. This P1 resembles the P1 from the conditions in which the visual modality was relevant (Visual and Bimodal-Att-V). Therefore the occurrence of the P1 in the Bimodal-Incongr condition could be due to (stronger) attending to the visual modality. Although for that condition, participants were instructed to attend both modalities equally, the task may have been too difficult as the locations of the visual and tactile parts of the bimodal incongruent stimuli were rather far apart, and even in opposite hemifields. This could have caused participants to attend more to one of the modalities, in this case, the visual modality. The P1 seems even stronger in the Bimodal-Incongr compared to the Visual condition and compared to the Bimodal-Att-V condition, suggesting that in the Bimodal-Incongr condition participants tried to focus even more on the visual part of the stimulus to not have themselves distracted by the tactile stimulus.

BCI performance was clearly affected by location-congruency. Therefore bimodal BCIs (based on spatial attention) should be based on location-congruent bimodal stimuli for optimal performance. The performance drop caused by location-incongruent bimodal stimuli is expected to depend on the degree of incongruency.

THE EFFECT OF SELECTIVE ATTENTION TO MODALITY

The third research question was does, and if so how does, attending to the visual or tactile modality, or both modalities affect ERP components' tAUCs and corresponding classification accuracies in a bimodal ERP-BCI? We hypothesized a positive effect on the late ERP component tAUC when both modalities of bimodal (location-congruent) stimuli were attended rather than just one. Indeed attending to both modalities resulted in a stronger P300 compared to attending to the tactile modality alone, but it was equally strong as attending to the visual modality alone. Possibly, and in line with our interpretation of effects on the P1 as discussed in the previous section (processing of), the visual stimulus was dominant over (processing of) the tactile stimulus.

Selectively attending modality also had an effect on the early ERP components' tAUCs. When the visual modality was attended in a bimodal BCI, a P1 was detected, similar as in the visual BCI. Likewise, when the tactile modality was attended in a bimodal BCI, an N2 was detected, similar as for the tactile BCI. Thus, these early ERP effects appear unrelated to multisensory interaction and solely explainable by unisensory (bottom-up) effects of stimulus processing at attended locations and within attended modalities.

The effect of Cross-training

BCI performance in terms of classification accuracies was equally good for the three bimodal attention conditions. This means that users can choose a preferred modality to attend to for operating a bimodal BCI when training and classifying occurs using the same attended modalities (attended modality specific classifier). We additionally assessed the effect of switching the attended modality during BCI operation by cross-classifying each one of the three bimodal attention conditions (sub-question 3a). The results indicate that when the attended modalities are different during bimodal BCI operation and training of the bimodal classifier (attended modality cross classifier), this causes a drop in BCI performance. The size of this drop depends on the degree of overlap in the attended modalities. However, even if there is no overlap, operation of the bimodal BCI is still feasible and performance is similar to that of unimodal BCIs. That means that bimodal BCIs offer the option to be used flexibly, i.e., users can switch the modality to attend to during operation.

CONCLUSION

Multisensory effects can be used to enhance BCI performance (as reflected by classification accuracies) by employing bimodal stimuli. In this study we investigated bimodal effects in gaze-independent ERP-BCIs, using visual-tactile stimuli. The P300 tAUC and corresponding classification accuracies were enhanced when participants were attending to (location-congruent) bimodal vs. unimodal stimuli. Unexpectedly, we did not observe early bimodal effects for the specific condition where stimuli were location-congruent and both modalities were attended. This is possibly due to reversed polarities of early unimodal ERP components. We suggest that bimodal BCI performance may further be improved when the early unimodal ERP components are more similar, which may be achieved with different locations of the EEG reference electrode.

Furthermore, bimodal classification accuracies were improved when bimodal stimuli were location-congruent. Thus bimodal BCIs should be designed location-congruent for optimal performance.

Additionally, BCI performance was invariant for the specific modality attended, although the underlying ERP components' tAUCs were affected. When the bimodal classifier was not trained for the specific modality attended, the drop in BCI performance depends on the degree of overlap in attended modalities between training and classifying, but was still at least as good as for the unimodal ERP-BCIs. Thus bimodal BCIs may increase BCI performance and offer more flexibility in use. This implies that for the practical use of BCIs, people who are either restricted physically or by the context of use (e.g., sensory overload of the visual channel while driving) to attend to a certain modality may benefit from using bimodal BCIs.

ACKNOWLEDGMENTS

This research has been supported by the GATE project, funded by the Netherlands Organization for Scientific Research (NWO) and the Netherlands ICT Research and Innovation Authority (ICT Regie). The authors gratefully acknowledge the support of the BrainGain Smart Mix Programme of the Netherlands, the Ministry of Economic Affairs and the Netherlands Ministry of Education, Culture and Science.

We also like to thank the students of the elective course "Multimodal Perception and Interaction" at the Utrecht University, and Antoon Wennemers.

REFERENCES

Acqualagna, L., and Blankertz, B. (2013). Gaze-independent BCI-spelling using rapid serial visual presentation (RSVP). *Clin. Neurophysiol.* 124, 901–908. doi: 10.1016/j.clinph.2012.12.050

Barth, D. S., Goldberg, N., Brett, B., and Di, S. (1995). The spatiotemporal organization of auditory, visual and auditory-visual evoked potentials in rat cortex. *Brain Res.* 678, 177–190. doi: 10.1016/0006-8993(95)00182-p

Belitski, A., Farquhar, J., and Desain, P. (2011). P300 audio-visual speller. *J. Neural Eng.* 8:025022. doi: 10.1088/1741-2560/8/2/025022

Bell, C. J., Shenoy, P., Chalodhorn, R., and Rao, R. P. N. (2008). Control of a humanoid robot by a noninvasive brain-computer interface in humans. *J. Neural Eng.* 5, 214–220. doi: 10.1088/1741-2560/5/2/012

Birbaumer, N., and Cohen, L. G. (2007). Brain-computer interfaces: communication and restoration of movement in paralysis. *J. Physiol.* 579, 621–636. doi: 10.1113/jphysiol.2006.125633

Boll, S., and Berti, S. (2009). Distraction of task-relevant information processing by irrelevant changes in auditory, visual and bimodal stimulus features: a behavioral and event-related potential study. *Psychophysiology* 46, 645–654. doi: 10.1111/j.1469-8986.2009.00803.x

Brouwer, A.-M., and Van Erp, J. B. F. (2010). A tactile P300 brain-computer interface. *Front. Neurosci.* 4:19. doi: 10.3389/fnins.2010.00019

Brouwer, A.-M., Van Erp, J. B. F., Aloise, F., and Cincotti, F. (2010). Tactile, visual and bimodal P300s: could bimodal P300s boost BCI performance? *SRX Neurosci.* 2010. doi: 10.3814/2010/967027

Brunner, P., Joshi, S., Briskin, S., Wolpaw, J. R., Bischof, H., and Schalk, G. (2010). Does the 'P300' speller depend on eye gaze? *J. Neural Eng.* 7:056013. doi: 10.1088/1741-2560/7/5/056013

Chiappa, K. H., and Chiappa, K. H. (1997). Pattern-shift visual evoked potentials: methodology. *Evoked Potentials Clin. Med.* 2, 37–109.

Driver, J., and Noesselt, T. (2008). Multisensory interplay reveals crossmodal influences on 'sensory-specific' brain regions, neural responses and judgments. *Neuron* 57, 11–23. doi: 10.1016/j.neuron.2007.12.013

Eimer, M., Cockburn, D., Smedley, B., and Driver, J. (2001). Cross-modal links in endogenous spatial attention are mediated by common external locations: evidence from event-related brain potentials. *Exp. Brain Res.* 139, 398–411. doi: 10.1007/s002210100773

Ernst, M. O., and Bülthoff, H. H. (2004). Merging the senses into a robust percept. *Trends Cogn. Sci.* 8, 162–169. doi: 10.1016/j.tics.2004.02.002

Farwell, L. A., and Donchin, E. (1988). Talking off the top of your head—toward a mental prosthesis utilizing event-related brain potentials. *Electroencephalogr. Clin. Neurophysiol.* 70, 510–523. doi: 10.1016/0013-4694(88)90149-6

Foxe, J. J., and Simpson, G. V. (2005). Biasing the brain's attentional set: II. Effects of selective intersensory attentional deployments on subsequent sensory processing. *Exp. Brain Res.* 166, 393–401. doi: 10.1007/s00221-005-2379-6

Frassinetti, F., Bolognini, N., and Ladavas, E. (2002). Enhancement of visual perception by crossmodal visuo-auditory interaction. *Exp. Brain Res.* 147, 332–343. doi: 10.1007/s00221-002-1262-y

Giray, M., and Ulrich, R. (1993). Motor coactivation revealed by response force in divided and focused attention. *J. Exp. Psychol. Hum. Percept. Perform.* 19, 1278–1291. doi: 10.1037/0096-1523.19.6.1278

Gondan, M., Niederhaus, B., Rösler, F., and Röder, B. (2005). Multisensory processing in the redundant-target effect: a behavioral and event-related potential study. *Percept. Psychophys.* 67, 713–726. doi: 10.3758/bf03193527

Gondan, M., and Röder, B. (2006). A new method for detecting interactions between the senses in event-related potentials. *Brain Res.* 1073–1074, 389–397. doi: 10.1016/j.brainres.2005.12.050

Guthrie, D., and Buchwald, J. S. (1991). Significance testing of difference potentials. *Psychophysiology* 28, 240–244. doi: 10.1111/j.1469-8986.1991.tb00417.x

Höhne, J., Schreuder, M., Blankertz, B., and Tangermann, M. (2011). A novel 9-class auditory erp paradigm driving a predictive text entry system. *Front. Neurosci.* 5:99. doi: 10.3389/fnins.2011.00099

Hopfinger, J. B., and West, V. M. (2006). Interactions between endogenous and exogenous attention on cortical visual processing. *Neuroimage* 31, 774–789. doi: 10.1016/j.neuroimage.2005.12.049

Kramer, A. F., and Strayer, D. L. (1988). Assessing the development of automatic processing: an application of dual-task and event-related brain potential methodologies. *Biol. Psychol.* 26, 231–267. doi: 10.1016/0301-0511(88)90022-1

Krusienski, D. J., Sellers, E. W., McFarland, D. J., Vaughan, T. M., and Wolpaw, J. R. (2008). Toward enhanced P300 speller performance. *J. Neurosci. Methods* 167, 15–21. doi: 10.1016/j.jneumeth.2007.07.017

Kubler, A., Neumann, N., Wilhelm, B., Hinterberger, T., and Birbaumer, N. (2004). Brain-computer predictability of brain-computer communication. *J. Psychophysiol.* 18, 121–129. doi: 10.1027/0269-8803.18.23.121

Macaluso, E. (2010). Orienting of spatial attention and the interplay between the senses. *Cortex* 46, 282–297. doi: 10.1016/j.cortex.2009.05.010

Mangun, G. R. (1995). Neural mechanisms of visual selective attention. *Psychophysiology* 32, 4–18. doi: 10.1111/j.1469-8986.1995.tb03400.x

Meredith, M. A., and Stein, B. E. (1986). Spatial factors determine the activity of multisensory neurons in cat superior colliculus. *Brain Res.* 365, 350–354. doi: 10.1016/0006-8993(86)91648-3

Molholm, S., Ritter, W., Murray, M. M., Javitt, D. C., Schroeder, C. E., and Foxe, J. J. (2002). Multisensory auditory-visual interactions during early sensory processing in humans: a high-density electrical mapping study. *Brain Res. Cogn. Brain Res.* 14, 115–128. doi: 10.1016/s0926-6410(02)00066-6

Orhan, U., Ii, K. E. H., Erdogmus, D., Roark, B., Oken, B., and Fried-oken, M. (2012). RSVP keyboard: an EEG based typing interface. *Acoustics, Speech and Signal Processing (ICASSP), 2012 IEEE International Conference on* (Kyoto), 645–648.

Pfurtscheller, G., Allison, B. Z., Brunner, C., Bauernfeind, G., Solis-Escalante, T., Scherer, R., et al. (2010a). The hybrid BCI. *Front. Neurosci.* 4:30. doi: 10.3389/fnpro.2010.00003

Pfurtscheller, G., Solis-Escalante, T., Ortner, R., Linortner, P., and Muller-Putz, G. R. (2010b). Self-paced operation of an ssvep-based orthosis with and without an imagery-based "brain switch:" a feasibility study towards a hybrid BCI. *IEEE Trans. Neural Syst. Rehabil. Eng.* 18, 409–414. doi: 10.1109/tnsre.2010.2040837

Philippi, T. G., Van Erp, J. B. F., and Werkhoven, P. J. (2008). Multisensory temporal numerosity judgment. *Brain Res.* 1242, 116–125. doi: 10.1016/j.brainres.2008.05.056

Sambo, C. F., and Forster, B. (2009). An ERP investigation on visuotactile interactions in peripersonal and extrapersonal space: evidence for the spatial rule. *J. Cogn. Neurosci.* 21, 1550–1559. doi: 10.1162/jocn.2009.21109

Schalk, G., McFarland, D. J., Hinterberger, T., Birbaumer, N., and Wolpaw, J. R. (2004). BCI2000: a general-purpose, brain-computer interface (BCI) system. *IEEE Trans. Biomed. Eng.* 51, 1034–1043. doi: 10.1109/tbme.2004.827072

Schreuder, M., Blankertz, B., and Tangermann, M. (2010). A new auditory multi-class brain-computer interface paradigm: spatial hearing as an informative cue. *PLoS One* 5:e9813. doi: 10.1371/journal.pone.0009813

Schreuder, M., Rost, T., and Tangermann, M. (2011). Listen, you are writing! speeding up online spelling with a dynamic auditory BCI. *Front. Neurosci.* 5:112. doi: 10.3389/fnins.2011.00112

Schröger, E., and Widmann, A. (1998). Speeded responses to audiovisual signal changes result from bimodal integration. *Psychophysiology* 35, 755–759. doi: 10.1111/1469-8986.3560755

Senkowski, D., Saint-Amour, D., Hofle, M., and Foxe, J. J. (2011). Multisensory interactions in early evoked brain activity follow the principle of inverse effectiveness. *Neuroimage* 56, 2200–2208. doi: 10.1016/j.neuroimage.2011.03.075

Stein, B. E., Meredith, M. A., Huneycutt, W. S., and McDade, L. (1989). Behavioral indices of multisensory integration: orientation to visual cues is affected by auditory stimuli. *J. Cogn. Neurosci.* 1, 12–24. doi: 10.1162/jocn.1989.1.1.12

Stein, B. E., and Stanford, T. R. (2008). Multisensory integration: current issues from the perspective of the single neuron. *Nat. Rev. Neurosci.* 9, 255–266. doi: 10.1038/nrn2377

Talsma, D., Doty, T. J., and Woldorff, M. G. (2007). Selective attention and audiovisual integration: is attending to both modalities a prerequisite for early integration? *Cereb. Cortex* 17, 679–690. doi: 10.1093/cercor/bhk016

Talsma, D., and Woldorff, M. G. (2005). Selective attention and multisensory integration: multiple phases of effects on the evoked brain activity. *J. Cogn. Neurosci.* 17, 1098–1114. doi: 10.1162/0898929054475172

Teder-Sälejärvi, W. A., Di Russo, F., McDonald, J. J., and Hillyard, S. A. (2005). Effects of spatial congruity on audio-visual multimodal integration. *J. Cogn. Neurosci.* 17, 1396–1409. doi: 10.1162/0898929054985383

Thurlings, M. E., Brouwer, A. M., Van Erp, J. B. F., Blankertz, B., and Werkhoven, P. J. (2012a). Does bimodal stimulus presentation increase ERP components usable in BCIs? *J. Neural Eng.* 9:045005. doi: 10.1088/1741-2560/9/4/045005

Thurlings, M. E., Van Erp, J. B. F., Brouwer, A.-M., Blankertz, B., and Werkhoven, P. J. (2012b). Control-display mapping in brain-computer interfaces. *Ergonomics* 55, 564–580. doi: 10.1080/00140139.2012.661085

Thurlings, M. E., Van Erp, J. B. F., Brouwer, A.-M., and Werkhoven, P. J. (2010). "EEG-based navigation from a human factors perspective," in *Brain-Comput. Interfaces*, eds D. S. Tan and A. Nijholt (London: Springer), 71–86.

Thurlings, M. E., Van Erp, J. B. F., Brouwer, A.-M., and Werkhoven, P. (2013). Controlling a tactile ERP-BCI in a multimodal dual-task. *IEEE Trans. Comput. Intell. AI in Games* 5, 129–140. doi: 10.1109/tciaig.2013.2239294

Treder, M. S., and Blankertz, B. (2010). (C)overt attention and visual speller design in an ERP-based brain-computer interface. *Behav. Brain Funct.* 6:28. doi: 10.1186/1744-9081-6-28

Van Erp, J. B. F. (2005). Presenting directions with a vibrotactile torso display. *Ergonomics* 48, 302–313. doi: 10.1080/0014013042000327670

Van Erp, J. B. F., Eriksson, L., Levin, B., Carlander, O., Veltman, J. A., and Vos, W. K. (2007). Tactile cueing effects on performance in simulated aerial combat with high acceleration. *Aviat. Space Environ. Med.* 78, 1128–1134. doi: 10.3357/asem.2133.2007

Van Erp, J. B. F., and Van Veen, H. A. H. C. (2004). Vibrotactile in-vehicle navigation system. *Transp. Res. Part F Traffic Psychol. Behav.* 7, 247–256. doi: 10.1016/j.trf.2004.09.003

Van Erp, J. B. F., Veltman, J. A., and Grootjen, M. (2010). "Brain-based indices for user system symbiosis," in *Brain Computer Interfaces, Human-Computer Interaction Series*, eds D. S. Tan and A. Nijholt (London: Spinger-Verlag), 201–219.

Woldorff, M. G., and Hillyard, S. A. (1991). Modulation of early auditory processing during selective listening to rapidly presented tones. *Electroencephalogr. Clin. Neurophysiol.* 79, 170–191. doi: 10.1016/0013-4694(91)90136-r

Yin, E., Zhou, Z., Jiang, J., Chen, F., Liu, Y., and Hu, D. (2013). A novel hybrid BCI speller based on the incorporation of SSVEP into the P300 paradigm. *J. Neural Eng.* 10:026012. doi: 10.1088/1741-2560/10/2/026012

19

Treatment of visuospatial neglect with biparietal tDCS and cognitive training: a single-case study

Anna-Katharine Brem[1]*, Evelyn Unterburger[2], Irving Speight[3] and Lutz Jäncke[4,5,6,7,8]

[1] Berenson-Allen Center for Noninvasive Brain Stimulation, Division of Cognitive Neurology, Department of Neurology, Beth Israel Deaconess Medical Center, Harvard Medical School, Boston, MA, USA
[2] Department of Neuropsychology, University Hospital Zurich, Zurich, Switzerland
[3] Department of Neuropsychology, Zürcher Höhenklinik Wald ZHW, Rehabilitation Center, Faltigberg-Wald, Switzerland
[4] Division Neuropsychology, Institute of Psychology, University of Zurich, Zurich, Switzerland
[5] Center for Integrative Human Physiology, University of Zurich, Zurich, Switzerland
[6] International Normal Aging and Plasticity Imaging Center, University of Zurich, Zurich, Switzerland
[7] University Research Priority Program "Dynamic of Healthy Aging," University of Zurich, Zurich, Switzerland
[8] Department of Special Education, King Abdulaziz University, Jeddah, Saudi Arabia

Edited by:
Mikhail Lebedev, Duke University, USA

Reviewed by:
Manuel Casanova, University of Louisville, USA
Georg Kerkhoff, Saarland University, Germany

***Correspondence:**
Anna-Katharine Brem, Berenson-Allen Center for Noninvasive Brain Stimulation, Beth Israel Deaconess Medical Center, 330 Brookline Ave., Kirstein Building KS 158, Boston, MA 02215, USA
e-mail: abrem@bidmc.harvard.edu

Symptoms of visuospatial neglect occur frequently after unilateral brain damage. Neglect hampers rehabilitation progress and is associated with reduced quality of life. However, existing treatment methods show limited efficacy. Transcranial direct current stimulation (tDCS) is a neuromodulatory technique, which can be used to increase or decrease brain excitability. Its combination with conventional neglect therapy may enhance treatment efficacy. A 72-year-old male with a subacute ischemic stroke of the right posterior cerebral artery suffering from visuospatial neglect, hemianopia, and hemiparesis was treated with biparietal tDCS and cognitive neglect therapy in a double-blind, sham-controlled single-case study. Four weeks of daily treatment sessions (5 days per week, 30 min) were started 26 days post-stroke. During week 1 and 4 the patient received conventional neglect therapy, during week 2, conventional neglect therapy was combined once with sham and once with real biparietal tDCS. Week 3 consisted of daily sessions of real biparietal tDCS (1 mA, 20 min) combined with neglect therapy. Outcome measures were assessed before, immediately after, as well as 1 week and 3 months after the end of treatment. They included subtests of the Test for Attentional Performance (TAP): covert attention (main outcome), alertness, visual field; the Neglect-Test (NET): line bisection, cancelation, copying; and activities of daily living (ADL). After real stimulation, covert attention allocation toward left-sided invalid stimuli was significantly improved, and line bisection and copying improved qualitatively as compared to sham stimulation. ADL were only improved at the 3-month follow-up. This single-case study demonstrates for the first time that combined application of tDCS and cognitive training may enhance training-induced improvements in measures of visuospatial neglect and is applicable in a clinical context.

Keywords: transcranial direct current stimulation, visuospatial neglect, rehabilitation, cognitive therapy, stroke

INTRODUCTION

Neglect is a higher-order, supramodal cognitive deficit, which affects space-related behavior not caused by an elementary sensorimotor deficit (Kerkhoff, 2001), and is mainly caused by lesions in frontoparietal cortical and subcortical networks (Doricchi et al., 2008). Symptoms are heterogeneous and are expressed in different sensory-spatial modalities (visual, auditory, tactile, olfactory). Visuospatial neglect occurs in over 40% of right brain-lesioned patients and in 20% of left brain-lesioned patients (Ringman et al., 2004) and more than 60% of the patients remain impaired after the end of rehabilitation (Carod-Artal et al., 2000; Clarke et al., 2002). Importantly, visuospatial neglect also limits the success of other neurorehabilitative interventions, such as physical and occupational therapy.

Treatment options to date show limited efficiency (Bowen et al., 2013) despite being time-intense. They mostly aim to compensate (e.g., optokinetic stimulation or neck muscle vibration) or substitute functions (e.g., prism adaptation), and few aim to restitute functions (e.g., mental imagery). In the clinical setting, different therapeutic approaches are often combined and individually adapted to the needs of each patient.

In the past decade researchers started to investigate the use of non-invasive brain stimulation in the treatment of neglect. The rationale for using brain stimulation for patients with neglect is based on the "hemispheric rivalry model" proposed by Kinsbourne (1987, 1993). According to this model allocation of visuospatial attention toward both hemifields is balanced by mutual transcallosal inhibition, where each hemisphere competes to direct attention to the contralateral hemifield. Brain lesions disturb this balance, and while the unimpaired hemisphere becomes hyperexcitable, the impaired hemisphere experiences a reduction in excitability. Supporting evidence for this model was first presented by Vuilleumier et al. (1996). They described a patient who suffered from visuospatial neglect after a stroke affecting the right angular gyrus, which however improved after a second stroke affecting the left frontal eye fields. Both of these areas are important for shifting attention via connections with subcortical structures, moreover supporting the assumption of a widespread network subserving spatial attention.

Later studies using brain stimulation methods further supported Kinsbourne's model. Non-invasive brain stimulation methods can be applied to either increase brain excitability in the lesioned hemisphere or reduce hyperexcitability in the unlesioned hemisphere. Several groups applied repetitive transcranial magnetic stimulation (rTMS) during a single session (Oliveri et al., 2001; Koch et al., 2008), or over several days (Brighina et al., 2003; Shindo et al., 2006; Song et al., 2009; Lim et al., 2010; Kim et al., 2013), with the latter leading to improvements for up to 2–6 weeks after the end of treatment. Two studies reported symptom improvement after a single session of transcranial direct current stimulation (tDCS) (Ko et al., 2008; Sparing et al., 2009). Generally, studies using multiple sessions of TMS showed stronger effects that lasted over a longer period of time.

Diagnostic guidelines for neglect are limited (e.g., Duncan et al., 2005; Intercollegiate Stroke Working Party, 2008) and recommend a multidisciplinary diagnostic approach. In order to diagnose visuospatial neglect, various diagnostic tools should be combined with clinical observation, as individual deficits vary greatly between patients. Covert attention measures provide a sensitive tool to assess the impact of visuospatial neglect and are used as the main outcome measure for this study. Posner et al. (1984) stressed the importance of the parietal lobe in covert attention processes, specifically the disengagement operation, when the target is located in the contralateral hemifield. Furthermore, alertness functions are known to draw on a right-lateralized fronto-parietal network (Sturm and Willmes, 2001; Jäncke et al., 2003) and improvements in alertness are thought to contribute to neglect recovery. Alertness was therefore used as a control parameter. We furthermore applied more traditional tests such as line bisection, cancelation, and copying and furthermore assessed visual field deficits and ADL.

The rational to use bilateral tDCS in this study is based on Kinsbourne's interhemispheric rivalry model and the hypothesis that concurrent biparietal modulation would have a stronger and longer-lasting impact on interhemispheric balance than unilateral stimulation. Biparietal stimulation (anode right, cathode left) was applied to concomitantly increase brain excitability in the lesioned right posterior parietal cortex (PPC) and reduce hyperexcitability in the unlesioned left PPC. Furthermore, we hypothesized that combining stimulation with conventional neglect therapy could have synergistic effects and therefore enhance treatment efficacy.

To our knowledge, this is the first study to report the combined impact of repeated biparietal tDCS sessions and cognitive neglect therapy on rehabilitation outcome.

MATERIALS AND METHODS

PATIENT

We studied a 72-year-old, ambidextrous male who was admitted to the neurorehabilitation unit 23 days after the onset of a moderate ischemic stroke (NIHSS 11/42) of the right posterior cerebral artery of unknown etiology (TOAST 5). At admission he suffered from a left-sided hemiparesis of the arm and face, hemianopia, and severe neglect symptoms. Structural magnetic resonance imaging showed extensive lesions within the right hemisphere affecting mostly subcortical areas of the temporal, parietal and occipital lobe (**Figure 1**).

Neglect symptoms included sensory as well as motor components (directional hypokinesia). Visuospatial symptoms were more space- than object-centered and N.H. showed a gaze deviation toward the right. Imaginary spatial representation was well preserved as compared to his reduced exploratory-perceptional performance. Alertness performance was initially reduced and fluctuating. Furthermore, impairments in spontaneous speech functions (finding words, dysarthria), and a moderate impairment of verbal and non-verbal memory functions, as well as executive functions (inhibitory control, cognitive flexibility) were observed. On discharge, 12 weeks after stroke onset, he had improved attention allocation toward the left hemi-space, however, transfer to activities of daily living (ADL) was limited, specifically in situations with many external distractors. Executive functions and non-verbal memory improved during rehabilitation but were still impaired at discharge. Verbal memory as well as speech functions normalized. N.H. gave written and oral consent according to the Declaration of Helsinki (1964). Family members were informed about all study procedures and approved of his participation. The protocol was approved by the local ethics committee.

STUDY DESIGN

This double-blind, sham-controlled single-case study consisted of 4 weeks of daily treatment sessions (5 days per week, 30 min) starting 26 days post-stroke (**Figure 2**). During week 1 and 4 the patient received conventional cognitive neglect therapy, during week 2, conventional therapy was combined once with sham tDCS and once with real biparietal tDCS. Week 3 consisted of daily sessions of real biparietal tDCS (1 mA, 20 min) combined with neglect therapy and covert attention was measured immediately after every session. Outcome measures were assessed before and after baseline (week 1), single stimulation sessions (week 2), repeated stimulation sessions (week 3), as well as 1 week and 3 months after the end of treatment. After the end of combined treatment, the patient received 7 more weeks of standard neurorehabilitative care before being discharged from the hospital. Assessors and the patient were blinded with regards to stimulation protocols. During the 4-week treatment N.H. furthermore attended occupational (daily), physical (daily), and music therapy (twice per week).

ASSESSMENTS

Covert attention, alertness (intrinsic and phasic), and visual field were assessed with subtests of the Test for Attentional Performance (TAP 2.2, Zimmermann and Fimm, 2002). The

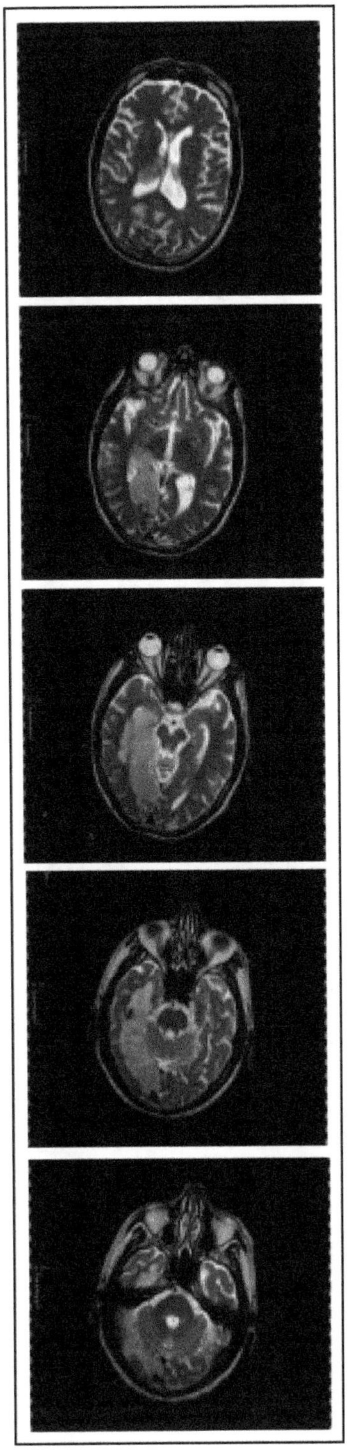

FIGURE 1 | sMRI T2 after admission to acute hospital.

subtests to assess intrinsic and phasic alertness consist of simple reaction paradigms that require keystrokes as selective reactions to non-verbal stimuli (cross displayed in the middle of the screen). Intrinsic alertness measures the general alertness of the subject, while phasic alertness measures the ability to increase and maintain attention in expectancy of a stimulus. The subtest "Covert Attention" measures the ability to direct visual attention toward a stimulus without change of gaze direction (Posner, 1980) and is a sensitive measure of visual neglect. A central cue (arrow) indicates the side on which a target stimulus (cross) may appear (presentation time of 2 s). The arrow either points in the direction of where the stimulus appears (valid trials) or in the opposite direction (invalid trials). As in invalid trials attentional focus is initially shifted in the opposite direction, re-orientation is needed. Visuospatial neglect is indicated by prolonged reaction times (RTs) in invalid trials toward the contralesional hemi-field. RT to invalid left-sided stimuli was therefore the main outcome measure. Visual field deficits were assessed with the subtest "Visual Field." In this test peripheral flicker stimuli appear on a black screen (with fixation control) and the subject indicates with a keystroke whether it was perceived.

Line bisection, cancelation, and copying figures were assessed with subtests of the Neglect-Test (NET, Fels and Geissner, 1996), which is a German adaptation of the "Behavioral Inattention Test" (BIT, Wilson et al., 1987). In order to control for transfer effects on ADL, a questionnaire to measure visuospatial disorders (Beobachtungsbogen für räumliche Störungen, BRS, Neumann and Kerkhoff, 2007) was filled out by the occupational therapist and a family member. It measures impairments in ADL such as eating, self-care, dressing, and communication. Furthermore, side effects of tDCS were assessed with a questionnaire.

TREATMENT

Computerized training batteries (OK-Neglect: Psycware, Sulzbach-Rosenberg, Germany; RehaCom: Schuhfried GmbH, Moedling, Austria) were presented on a large screen (ca. 1.5 × 2 m) with the patient seated on the right side of the screen. Training was started 5 min after the onset of stimulation and continued for 30 min. Therapies were adapted to the patient's individual needs according to best clinical practice. The main focus was on amelioration of smooth pursuit eye movements (SPEM) and training of saccades toward the neglected hemifield, as well as visual exploration and reading combined with optokinetic stimulation.

Direct current of 1 mA was delivered for 20 min via two saline-soaked sponge electrodes (7 × 5 cm), which were fixed on the head with a rubber bandage (NeuroConn DC-stimulator, Eldith, Electro-Diagnostic and Therapeutic Systems GmbH, Ilmenau, Germany). The anode was placed over P4 and the cathode was placed over P3 (international 10–20 EEG system). The current intensity used in this study has been used in several publications with stroke patients (Fregni et al., 2005; Hummel et al., 2005, 2006; Hummel and Cohen, 2005; Boggio et al., 2007). In order to achieve comparable sensations for sham stimulation, all sessions started with a slow up-ramping of current over 30 s. At the end of the stimulation current was turned off slowly in order not to elicit perceptions (Gandiga et al., 2006).

ANALYSIS

The TAP provides norms for adults (TAP 2.2, Zimmermann and Fimm, 2002). Significance levels of intraindividual single-subject differences of T-values for the used subtests (intrinsic and phasic alertness, covert attention) were calculated with the software

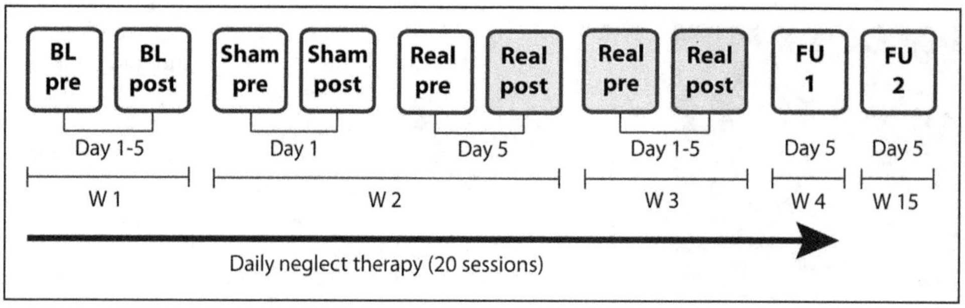

FIGURE 2 | Study design. N.H. received daily standard cognitive neglect therapy for 4 weeks (20 sessions). During W1 the patient received standard therapy only (5 sessions). During W2 the patient additionally received sham tDCS on the first day and real biparietal tDCS on the fifth day. During W3 the patient additionally received real biparietal tDCS (5 sessions) and covert attention was assessed after each session. Post-stimulation measures of day 5 (Real post) served as pre-measures for FU1 and FU2. During W4 he received standard therapy only (5 sessions, FU1). Long-term outcome was assessed 3 months after the end of the stimulation (FU2). BL, baseline assessment; FU, follow-up; W, week. Shaded cells depict real stimulation.

CASE123 (Willmes, 1985, 1990; Guillot and Willmes, 1993) using T-values (percent ranks transformed into standard values), test–retest reliability, and subtest correlations. CASE123 is used to perform psychometric single-case analyses according to Huber (1973), which are based on the classical test theory model and are used for tests with standard norms from large standardization samples with satisfactory reliability estimates such as the used TAP. We compared performance pre- vs. post each single session (Sham 1, Real 1, Real 1/5), pre vs. post repeated sessions (Real 5/5), pre vs. post the 1-week control period (FU1), as well as pre vs. post the 3-month control period (FU2). Post-stimulation measures (Real 5/5) served as pre-measures for FU1 and FU2. Paper-pencil test results (line bisection, cancelation, figure copying) are described qualitatively.

In order to evaluate whether coupling stimulation with cognitive training was more effective than cognitive training alone, a 2 × 4 × 3 ANOVA was performed with the within-subjects factors of Time (Pre and Post), Condition (Single Sham, Single Active, Repeated Active, Repeated Training Only), and Test (Invalid Left, Invalid Right, Phasic Alertness).

RESULTS

COMPUTERIZED MEASURES

At admission a complete hemianopia of the left visual field was diagnosed, which persisted until long-term follow up 3 months after the end of stimulation.

Intrinsic and phasic alertness were impaired at admission (intrinsic: $T = 40$; phasic: $T = 38$) with phasic alertness improving significantly after 1 week of standard therapy ($T = 45$, $p = 0.002$). After the single sham session combined with neglect therapy alertness worsened significantly (intrinsic: $T = 39$, $p < 0.001$; phasic: $T = 38$, $p < 0.001$), whereas after the single real session, alertness improved significantly (intrinsic: $T = 45$, $p = 0.008$; phasic: $T = 49$, $p < 0.001$). Both alertness parameters remained within normal levels after the first combined real tDCS treatment (**Tables 1, 2, Figures 3E,F**).

Covert attention to *valid right-sided stimuli* was within normal performance levels throughout the study. *Covert attention to valid left-sided stimuli* was strongly impaired at admission, showed significant improvements during standard therapy also reaching a stable and normal level after the first combined real tDCS treatment, and was maintained until long-term follow-up (**Tables 1, 2**).

Covert attention to invalid right-sided stimuli fluctuated at training onset, but stayed below average levels before stimulation onset. After the first single real stimulation it also reached normal levels ($T = 50$). After the weekend on the first day of repeated stimulations RTs had declined again ($T = 34$), but again showed a significant improvement immediately after the first of the repeated stimulation sessions ($T = 50$, $p < 0.001$), remained within normal levels during repeated stimulation sessions ($T = 44$, $p < 0.001$), further improved after the end of stimulation until follow-up 1 ($T = 53$, $p < 0.001$), and returned to post-stimulation levels until the long-term follow-up ($T = 42$, $p = 0.232$) (**Tables 1, 2, Figure 3**).

Invalid left-sided stimuli were not perceived at baseline. By the beginning of week 2 the patient was able to perceive them, however, he showed no improvement after single sham stimulation ($T < 20$, no p-value), while significant improvements were observed after a single real stimulation ($T = 28$, $p = 0.025$). Similar as for invalid right-sided stimuli this improvement was not maintained, however, performance improved again even further after the first stimulation session of repeated stimulations ($T = 43$, $p < 0.001$) and remained significantly improved after repeated stimulations ($T = 31$, $p = 0.002$). During the 1-week follow-up with standard therapy performance remained within post-stimulation levels ($T = 29$, $p = 0.576$) and was maintained until long-term follow-up ($T = 31$, $p = 1.000$) (**Tables 1, 2, Figure 3**).

The main interaction of Time, Condition, and Test was highly significant [$F_{(12, 456)} = 19.51$, $p < 0.001$, $\eta_p^2 = 0.34$]. This interaction was due to a significant interaction for Time and Condition for RTs for left invalid stimuli [$F_{(1, 80)} = 7.42$, $p < 0.001$, $\eta_p^2 = 0.22$], but not for right invalid stimuli [$F_{(3, 64)} = 0.50$, $p = 0.687$, $\eta_p^2 = 0.23$], or phasic alertness [$F_{(3, 312)} = 2.00$, $p = 0.113$, $\eta_p^2 = 0.02$]. The significant interaction for left invalid stimuli was partly explained by a strong trend of the single active condition leading to a larger improvement than the single sham condition [$F_{(1, 40)} = 4.00$, $p = 0.052$, $\eta_p^2 = 0.09$], but was mainly explained by a significantly larger improvement after repeated combined

Table 1 | Raw data alertness and covert attention.

Test	Pre (5) BL	Post (5) BL	Pre (1) sham	Post (1) sham	Pre (1) real	Post (1) real	Pre (5) real	Post (5) real	FU 11 week	FU 23 mo
Intrinsic alertness	309 ± 64	317 ± 89	276 ± 45	316 ± 51	311 ± 86	287 ± 64	249 ± 54	289 ± 80	299 ± 71	267 ± 46
Phasic alertness	301 ± 43	268 ± 64	262 ± 42	302 ± 72	301 ± 55	247 ± 44	232 ± 44	217 ± 47	214 ± 35	258 ± 38
Covert attention valid left	1859 ± 606	1083 ± 493	682 ± 239	413 ± 192	444 ± 213	347 ± 162	378 ± 221	343 ± 150	350 ± 158	350 ± 145
Covert attention valid right	403 ± 135	351 ± 71	316 ± 166	282 ± 66	321 ± 109	304 ± 90	299 ± 98	329 ± 81	298 ± 93	372 ± 71
Covert attention invalid left	–	–	1184 ± 652	874 ± 735	1310 ± 292	686 ± 365	1346 ± 364	650 ± 329	675 ± 368	569 ± 138
Covert attention invalid right	500 ± 174	764 ± 148	495 ± 149	495 ± 83	484 ± 98	446 ± 69	553 ± 70	472 ± 74	425 ± 40	488 ± 39

Abbreviations: BL, baseline standard therapy; (1): 1 therapy session; (5): 5 therapy sessions; FU 1: Follow-up 1 week after the end of stimulation (5 days of standard therapy); FU 2, Follow-up 3 months after the end of stimulation; Mo, months. –: Patient was not able to perceive stimuli. Shading indicates time-periods of combined real tDCS and standard therapy (light gray: single real stimulation; dark gray: repeated real stimulation). Values are presented as median reaction time ± standard deviation.

Table 2 | *T*- and *p*-values alertness and covert attention.

Test	Pre (5) BL	Post (5) BL	*p*-value	Pre (1) sham	Post (1) sham	*p*-value	Pre (1) real	Post (1) real	*p*-value	Pre (5) real	Post (5) real	*p*-value	FU 1 1 week	*p*-value	FU 2 3 mo	*p*-value
Intrinsic alertness	40 (42)	39 (36)	0.598	**48 (50)**	39 **(49)**	<0.001	40 (36)	**45** (42)	**0.008**	**51 (47)**	**45** (38)	0.002	**43** (40)	0.292	**51 (51)**	**0.002**
Phasic alertness	38 (51)	**45 (44)**	**0.002**	**46 (52)**	38 (42)	<0.001	38 **(48)**	**49 (51)**	**<0.001**	**50 (51)**	**56 (49)**	**0.009**	**57 (57)**	0.661	**46 (54)**	<0.001
Posner valid left	<20 (<20)	<20 (<20)	–	<20 (21)	**46** (25)	**<0.001***	40 (23)	**54** (26)	**<0.001**	**52** (23)	**54** (32)	0.264	**50** (27)	0.025	**50** (26)	0.025
Posner valid right	**45** (35)	**51 (51)**	0.099	**56** (32)	**66 (51)**	**0.006**	**55** (39)	**59** (42)	0.271	**61** (40)	**54 (46)**	0.054	**61** (41)	0.054	**51 (45)**	0.409
Posner invalid left	–	–	–	<20 (24)	<20 (24)	–	<20 (26)	28 (26)	**0.025***	<20 (26)	31 (26)	**0.002***	29 (26)	0.576	31 (33)	1.000
Posner invalid right	40 (28)	24 (30)	<0.001	40 (30)	40 (40)	1.000	42 (37)	**50 (45)**	**<0.001**	34 **(45)**	**44** (43)	**<0.001**	**53 (58)**	**0.000**	42 **(59)**	0.232

Abbreviations: BL, baseline standard therapy; (1): 1 therapy session; (5): 5 daily therapy sessions; FU 1, Follow-up 1 week after the end of stimulation (5 days of standard therapy); FU 2, Follow-up 3 months after the end of stimulation; Mo, months. –: Patient was not able to perceive stimuli and/or p-values could not be calculated ($T < 20$). Shading indicates time-periods of combined real tDCS and standard therapy (light gray: single real stimulation; dark gray: repeated real stimulation). T-values of median reaction time and of standard deviations are presented. P-values are two-sided. Bold font indicates performance levels within normal range of the norm population (T-values) or significant improvements (p-values).

**For $T < 20$ p-values were calculated using $T = 20$, significance of p-values for these time-points are therefore underestimated.*

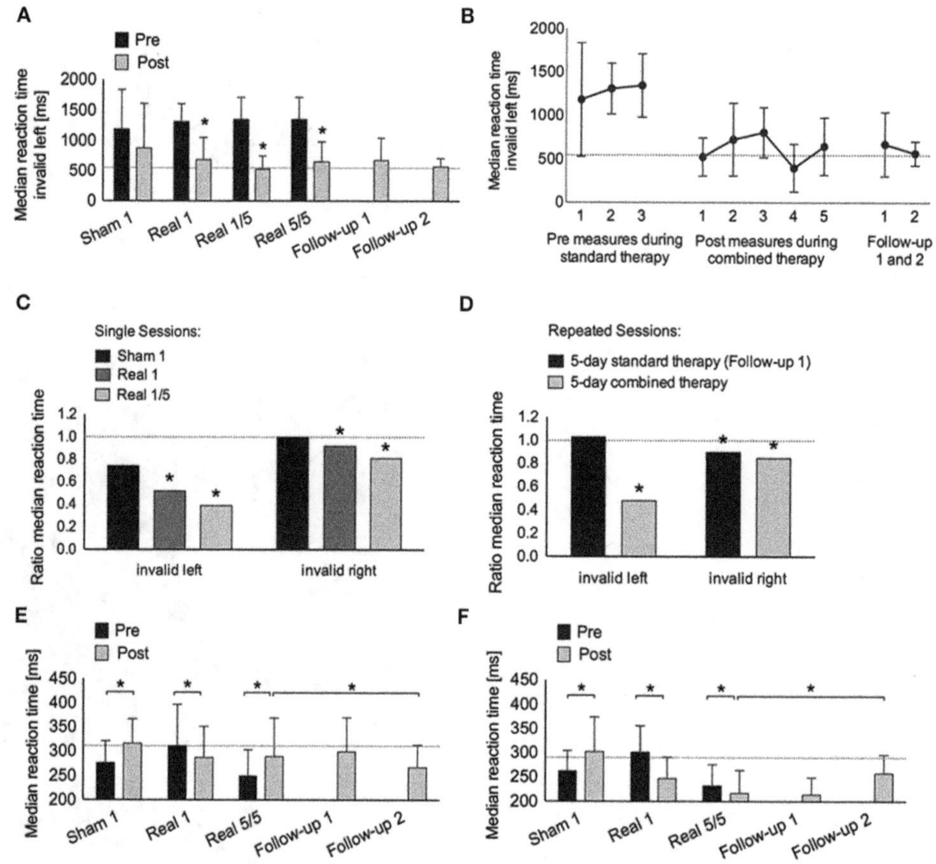

FIGURE 3 | Covert attention task (Posner paradigm, A–D) and alertness (E,F). (A) Median reaction time (±*SD*) to invalid left-sided stimuli pre (dark gray bars) and post (light gray bars) treatment: single-sham (Sham 1), single-real (Real 1), single-real on the first day of repetitive stimulation (Real 1/5), repeated-real during 5 days (Real 5/5), standard therapy during 1 week after the end of stimulation (Follow-up 1), and 3 months after the end of stimulation (Follow-up 2). **(B)** Median reaction time (±*SD*) to invalid left-sided stimuli on three different days before real stimulation (pre-measures), after five consecutive sessions with real stimulation (post-measures), and at Follow-up 1 and 2. **(C)** Ratio of median reaction time post-pre to invalid left- and right-sided stimuli after single-sham (Sham 1), single-real (Real 1), single-real on the first day of repetitive stimulation (Real 1/5), and **(D)** after repeated-real during 5 days, and standard therapy during 1 week after the end of stimulation (Follow-up 1). **(E,F)** Median reaction time (±*SD*) in intrinsic **(E)** and phasic **(F)** alertness. *at least $p < 0.05$.

treatment as compared to cognitive training alone [$F_{(1, 40)} = 21.12, p < 0.001, \eta_p^2 = 0.35$].

PAPER-PENCIL MEASURES

Star cancelation performance fluctuated over the course of rehabilitation and did not vary with stimulation. However, both line bisection and figure copying improved after real stimulation sessions.

Line bisection was deviated toward the right after the single real stimulation session (5.3 ± 1.5 cm) and before beginning repeated stimulation (4.7 ± 1.4 cm). By the end of the stimulation-week the bisection had deviated toward the left side (−2.5 ± 1.7 cm) and was maintained over 3 days without stimulation (−1.8 ± 1.6 cm). However, by the end of the 1-week follow-up it returned to a rightward deviation (3.9 ± 0.7 cm), but reimproved until the long-term follow-up (0.9 ± 2.3 cm) (**Figure 4**).

Figure copying was clearly impaired at baseline (5/9 points). After the single real stimulation it improved by 1 point (6/9 points) and improved another 2 points (8/9 points) after repeated stimulation sessions. However, performance declined again after the end of real stimulation (6/9 points both at the 1-week as well as the 3-month follow-up) (**Figure 5**).

ACTIVITIES OF DAILY LIVING

During his stay at the rehabilitation center, N.H. did not show an improvement in ADL as measured with the BRS (Baseline: 0.9 points; after repeated stimulations: 1.22 points). Only at the 3-month follow-up all parameters showed an improvement (0.16 points).

SIDE-EFFECTS

The patient reported tingling sensations after the single sham as well as after each of the real stimulation sessions.

DISCUSSION

This single-case study investigated the long-term impact of repetitive, biparietal tDCS on neglect symptoms in subacute stroke. We found a significantly larger improvement in therapy outcome after combined biparietal tDCS and cognitive training, while cognitive training on its own after single treatment sessions as well as repeated sessions over a time-period of 5 days did not lead to significant changes. Improvements in covert attention as well as alertness were maintained over a follow-up period of 1 week as well as a follow-up period of 3 months after the end of stimulation, whereas performance improvements in paper-pencil tasks were transient, returning to pre-stimulation levels at follow-up.

The main outcome measure (covert attention to left-sided stimuli according to the Posner paradigm) showed the strongest improvement, which was maintained until long-term follow-up, however, without reaching normal levels. Though RTs to invalid stimuli presented in the right hemi-field were also significantly modulated by stimulation, the effects were not as strong as for RTs to left-sided invalid stimuli. When comparing stimulation effects on RTs toward left and right invalid stimuli as well as alertness over the different stimulation conditions (single/repeated, with/without tDCS), only RTs toward left invalid stimuli were significantly modulated by stimulation. This finding supports the assumption of an asymmetrical distribution of brain activity in spatial attention, where the right hemisphere is dominant for orientation of covert attention to either hemi-field (Heilman and Van Den Abell, 1980; Corbetta et al., 1993). On the other hand it corroborates the hypothesis that reducing over-excitability in the undamaged hemisphere can have a beneficial impact.

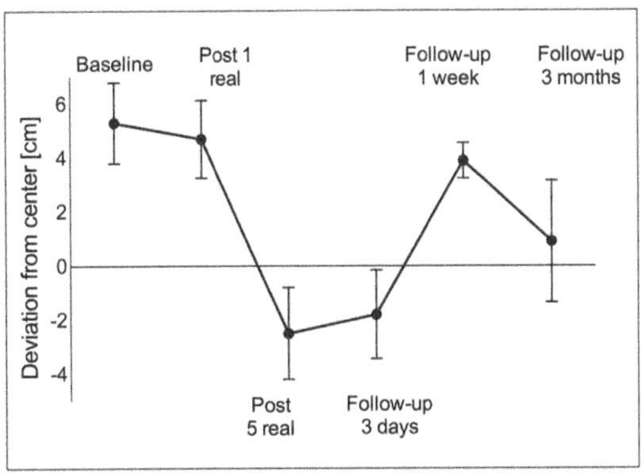

FIGURE 4 | Line bisection. A right-sided deviation was observed at baseline and remained right-sided after one real stimulation session. However, after five daily stimulation sessions the deviation turned to the left (over-compensation) and remained left-sided for another 3 days of standard therapy. At the 1-week follow-up as well as at the 3-month follow-up the deviation returned to the right again. Values are presented as mean ± standard deviation (SD).

Alertness measures were used as control measures. After one session of sham tDCS combined with neglect therapy intrinsic and phasic alertness were reduced, which could be due to fatigue. However, after one session of real tDCS, alertness improved significantly. Right frontoparietal areas are specifically important for alertness functions, which might explain why the placement of the anode over the right parietal cortex showed a beneficial impact. Nevertheless, alertness was not the driving factor for the improvement in the RTs toward left-invalid stimuli as we could show that after this initial improvement alertness measures remained within an age-matched norm level and did not show the same pattern of change as RTs toward left-invalid stimuli.

Interestingly, an improvement in most cognitive measures was observed after only one real stimulation session. However, further improvement and stabilization might arise only during repeated and specific combined treatment, which might trigger physiological processes that promote ongoing spontaneous recovery processes. Previous studies found significant long-term changes after only one tDCS session (e.g., Flöel et al., 2012). Effects of tDCS have been associated with NMDA-receptor dependent changes that reflect processes of long-term potentiation (LTP) and depression (LTD) that can become apparent even during or immediately after non-invasive brain stimulation (Liebetanz et al., 2002; Nitsche et al., 2003).

Qualitative performance in the cancelation task was not modulated by stimulation, while performance in figure copying as well as line bisection showed a maximal increase after 5 days of repeated stimulation. In the line bisection task an initially strong ipsilesional deviation, which can be typically observed in neglect patients, turned into a contralesional deviation after repeated tDCS sessions. Such a pattern can be interpreted as over-compensation and occurs usually in patients with hemianopia. Interestingly, over-compensation could still be observed 3 days

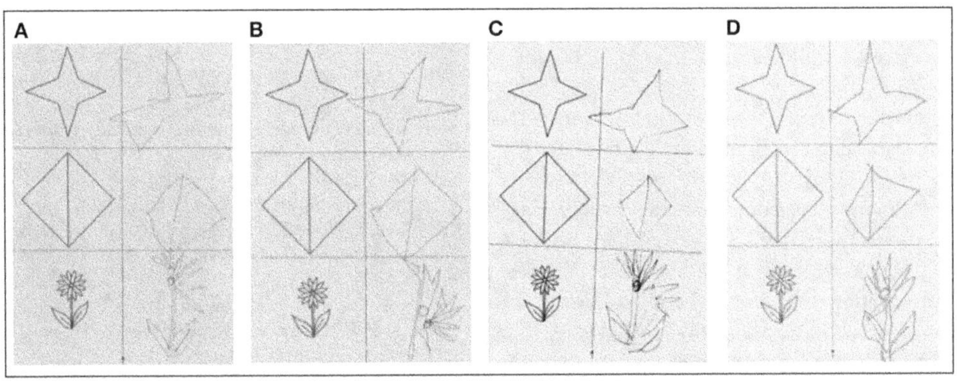

FIGURE 5 | Figure copying. (A) Before single real stimulation (5/9 points); **(B)** after single real stimulation (6/9 points); **(C)** before 5 daily real stimulations (6/9 points); **(D)** after 5 daily real stimulations (8/9 points).

after the end of stimulation but returned to an ipsilesional deviation at the 1-week follow-up, and finally approached normal levels at the 3-month follow-up. Sparing et al. (2009) also observed a reduction of deviation in a line bisection task but no over-compensation. This effect may be related to the bilateral approach used in the present study. In sum, improvements in paper-pencil tasks were not maintained until the 1-week and 3-month follow-up.

During the rehabilitation period, no measurable transfer of positive effects on ADL was observed. Improvements were only noticeable at the 3-month follow-up. Therefore, it is not possible to determine the association of changes in ADL with stimulation effects. However, in a study by Shindo et al. (2006) most improvement occurred 2–4 weeks after repeated rTMS sessions, which supports the assumption of a kick-off effect of stimulation, which may only later translate into ADL improvements.

It remains to be confirmed in future studies in larger patient samples and including a longer follow-up period that repeated sessions may not only result in a long-term improvement but also have a positive transfer effect on ADL functions. Additional assessments of physiological correlates could furthermore help to elucidate possible delayed stimulation effects.

Several drawbacks of this study need to be mentioned, which are mostly due to the fact that the investigation took place during the subacute stage. First, spontaneous recovery processes need to be taken into account (Cramer, 2008). Furthermore, we cannot rule out the possibility that effects are due to cognitive training alone. Second, the patient participated in other neurorehabilitative programs and practiced by himself. Both of these factors could explain the observed improvements. However, specific effects during the active and sham single sessions contradict these explanations. Furthermore, we would expect continuous improvement over time. Third, some of the paper-pencil tasks could not be assessed at all test-times due to fatigue and time restrictions. Fourth, one could argue that positive effects were caused by a mere improvement of alertness. Though alertness functions might modulate neglect symptoms (Sturm et al., 2006), they do not alone account for this improvement (e.g., after sham stimulation we observe opposite effects on alertness and covert attention). Furthermore, while alertness remained variable within normal levels during repeated stimulation, RTs to invalid stimuli in the covert attention measure improved further. Nyffeler et al. (2009) also suggested that effects were not due to an unspecific increase of alertness, as RTs to right-sided stimuli did not change significantly in their study. We found neither a significant modulating effect of stimulation for alertness nor for invalid right-sided stimuli. Finally, it is in the nature of single-case studies that it is not possible to generalize results to a greater population. Nevertheless, they are helpful in guiding future studies with larger patient populations and can give us valuable insight into specific diseases, providing unique information that might be useful for individualized treatment approaches. Specifically in the subacute stage after a stroke many factors contribute to a large variability, which is a reason why few studies investigate the impact of brain stimulation in subacute patients, although this might be the most fruitful period to stimulate the brain. We may be able to support and guide ongoing compensatory and restitution processes not only through behavioral therapies, but combine them with non-invasive brain stimulation in order to increase beneficial effects.

In sum, during combined therapy functional improvement was significantly higher than during standard therapy alone and was maintained over a follow-up period of 1 week and 3 months. A transfer effect to ADL was only observed at the long-term follow up. Future studies should investigate larger patient populations and longer treatments periods.

AUTHOR CONTRIBUTIONS

Anna-Katharine Brem and Lutz Jäncke designed the study. Anna-Katharine Brem, Evelyn Unterburger, and Irving Speight contributed to data collection and analysis. Anna-Katharine Brem prepared the draft report, which was critically reviewed by all authors.

ACKNOWLEDGMENTS

We would like to express our gratitude to N.H. for his participation. Furthermore, we would like to thank the neuropsychological team for support with the therapy sessions, and the occupational therapy team as well as N.H.'s partner for assessments of ADL functions. We would like to thank Prof. Peter Brugger for providing additional data and Giulia Maistrello for helping with data entry. Work on this study was supported by the Zürcher Höhenklinik Wald ZHW, Switzerland, and the University of Zurich.

REFERENCES

Boggio, P. S., Nunes, A., Rigonatti, S. P., Nitsche, M. A., Pascual-Leone, A., and Fregni, F. (2007). Repeated sessions of noninvasive brain DC stimulation is associated with motor function improvement in stroke patients. *Restor. Neurol. Neurosci.* 25, 123–129.

Bowen, A., Hazelton, C., Pollock, A., and Lincoln, N. B. (2013). Cognitive rehabilitation for spatial neglect following stroke. *Cochrane Database Syst. Rev.* 7:CD003586. doi: 10.1002/14651858.CD003586

Brighina, F., Bisiach, E., Oliveri, M., Piazza, A., La Bua, V., Daniele, O., et al. (2003). 1 Hz repetitive transcranial magnetic stimulation of the unaffected hemisphere ameliorates contralesional visuospatial neglect in humans. *Neurosci. Lett.* 336, 131–133. doi: 10.1016/S0304-3940(02)01283-1

Carod-Artal, J., Egido, J. A., González, J. L., and Varela de Seijas, E. (2000). Quality of life among stroke survivors evaluated 1 year after stroke: experience of a stroke unit. *Stroke* 31, 2995–3000. doi: 10.1161/01.STR.31.12.2995

Clarke, P., Marshall, V., Black, S. E., and Colantonio, A. (2002). Well-being after stroke in Canadian seniors: findings from the Canadian Study of Health and Aging. *Stroke* 33, 1016–1021. doi: 10.1161/01.STR.0000013066.24300.F9

Corbetta, M., Miezin, F. M., Shulman, G. L., and Petersen, S. E. (1993). A PET study of visuospatial attention. *J. Neurosci.* 13, 1202–1226.

Cramer, S. C. (2008). Repairing the human brain after stroke: I. Mechanisms of spontaneous recovery. *Ann. Neurol.* 63, 272–287. doi: 10.1002/ana.21393

Declaration of Helsinki. (1964). Available online at: http://www.wma.net/en/20activities/10ethics/10helsinki/

Doricchi, F., Thiebaut de Schotten, M., Tomaiuolo, F., and Bartolomeo, P. (2008). White matter (dis)connections and gray matter (dys)functions in visual neglect: gaining insights into the brain networks of spatial awareness. *Cortex* 44, 983–995. doi: 10.1016/j.cortex.2008.03.006

Duncan, P. W., Zorowitz, R., Bates, B., Choi, J. Y., Glasberg, J. J., Graham, G. D., et al. (2005). Management of Adult Stroke Rehabilitation Care: a clinical practice guideline. *Stroke* 36, e100–e143. doi: 10.1161/01.STR.0000180861.54180.FF

Fels, M., and Geissner, E. (1996). *Neglect-Test (NET)*. Goettingen: Hogrefe.

Flöel, A., Suttorp, W., Kohl, O., Kürten, J., Lohmann, H., Breitenstein, C., et al. (2012). Non-invasive brain stimulation improves object-location learning in the elderly. *Neurobiol. Aging* 33, 1682–1689. doi: 10.1016/j.neurobiolaging.2011.05.007

Fregni, F., Boggio, P. S., Mansur, C. G., Wagner, T., Ferreira, M. J. L., Lima, M. C., et al. (2005). Transcranial direct current stimulation of the unaffected hemisphere in stroke patients. *Neuroreport* 16, 1551–1555. doi: 10.1097/01.wnr.0000177010.44602.5e

Gandiga, P. C., Hummel, F. C., and Cohen, L. G. (2006). Transcranial DC stimulation (tDCS): a tool for double-blind sham-controlled clinical studies in brain stimulation. *Clin. Neurophysiol.* 117, 845–850. doi: 10.1016/j.clinph.2005.12.003

Guillot, G., and Willmes, K. (1993). *CASE123: Ein Programmpaket zur Analyse von Testdaten mit Methoden der Psychometrischen Einzelfalldiagnostik.* Aachen: Neurologische Klinik, RWTH Aachen.

Heilman, K. M., and Van Den Abell, T. (1980). Right hemisphere dominance for attention: the mechanism underlying hemispheric asymmetries of inattention (neglect). *Neurology* 30, 327–330. doi: 10.1212/WNL.30.3.327

Huber, H. P. (1973). *Psychometrische Einzelfalldiagnostik.* Weinheim: Beltz.

Hummel, F., Celnik, P., Giraux, P., Floel, A., Wu, W.-H., Gerloff, C., et al. (2005). Effects of non-invasive cortical stimulation on skilled motor function in chronic stroke. *Brain* 128, 490–499. doi: 10.1093/brain/awh369

Hummel, F., and Cohen, L. G. (2005). Improvement of motor function with noninvasive cortical stimulation in a patient with chronic stroke. *Neurorehabil. Neural Repair* 19, 14–19. doi: 10.1177/1545968304272698

Hummel, F. C., Voller, B., Celnik, P., Floel, A., Giraux, P., Gerloff, C., et al. (2006). Effects of brain polarization on reaction times and pinch force in chronic stroke. *BMC Neurosci.* 7:73. doi: 10.1186/1471-2202-7-73

Intercollegiate Stroke Working Party. (2008). *National Clinical Guidelines for Stroke, 3rd Edn.* London: Royal College of Physicians.

Jäncke, L., Specht, K., Shah, J. N., and Hugdahl, K. (2003). Focused attention in a simple dichotic listening task: an fMRI experiment. *Brain Res. Cogn. Brain Res.* 16, 257–266. doi: 10.1016/S0926-6410(02)00281-1

Kerkhoff, G. (2001). Spatial hemineglect in humans. *Prog. Neurobiol.* 63, 1–27. doi: 10.1016/S0301-0082(00)00028-9

Kim, B. R., Chun, M. H., Kim, D.-Y., and Lee, S. J. (2013). Effect of high- and low-frequency repetitive transcranial magnetic stimulation on visuospatial neglect in patients with acute stroke: a double-blind, sham-controlled trial. *Arch. Phys. Med. Rehabil.* 94, 803–807. doi: 10.1016/j.apmr.2012.12.016

Kinsbourne, M. (1987). "Mechanisms of unilateral neglect," in *Neurophysiological and Neuropsychological Aspects of Unilateral Neglect*, ed M. Jeannerod (Amsterdam: Elsevier), 69–86.

Kinsbourne, M. (1993). "Orientation bias model of unilateral neglect: evidence from attentional gradients within hemispace," in *Unilateral Neglect: Clinical and Experimental Studies*, eds I. Robertson and J. Marshall (New York, NY: L. Erlbaum Associates), 63–86.

Ko, M.-H., Han, S.-H., Park, S.-H., Seo, J.-H., and Kim, Y.-H. (2008). Improvement of visual scanning after DC brain polarization of parietal cortex in stroke patients with spatial neglect. *Neurosci. Lett.* 448, 171–174. doi: 10.1016/j.neulet.2008.10.050

Koch, G., Oliveri, M., Cheeran, B., Ruge, D., Lo Gerfo, E., Salerno, S., et al. (2008). Hyperexcitability of parietal-motor functional connections in the intact left-hemisphere of patients with neglect. *Brain* 131, 3147–3155. doi: 10.1093/brain/awn273

Liebetanz, D., Nitsche, M. A., Tergau, F., and Paulus, W. (2002). Pharmacological approach to the mechanisms of transcranial DC-stimulation-induced after-effects of human motor cortex excitability. *Brain* 125, 2238–2247. doi: 10.1093/brain/awf238

Lim, J. Y., Kang, E. K., and Paik, N.-J. (2010). Repetitive transcranial magnetic stimulation to hemispatial neglect in patients after stroke: an open-label pilot study. *J. Rehabil. Med.* 42, 447–452. doi: 10.2340/16501977-0553

Neumann, G., and Kerkhoff, G. (2007). *Beobachtungsbogen für Räumliche Störungen (BRS). Manual.* Göttingen: Hogrefe.

Nitsche, M. A., Fricke, K., Henschke, U., Schlitterlau, A., Liebetanz, D., Lang, N., et al. (2003). Pharmacological modulation of cortical excitability shifts induced by transcranial direct current stimulation in humans. *J. Physiol. (Lond.)* 553, 293–301. doi: 10.1113/jphysiol.2003.049916

Nyffeler, T., Cazzoli, D., Hess, C. W., and Muri, R. M. (2009). One session of repeated parietal theta burst stimulation trains induces long-lasting improvement of visual neglect. *Stroke* 40, 2791–2796. doi: 10.1161/STROKEAHA.109.552323

Oliveri, M., Bisiach, E., Brighina, F., Piazza, A., La Bua, V., Buffa, D., et al. (2001). rTMS of the unaffected hemisphere transiently reduces contralesional visuospatial hemineglect. *Neurology* 57, 1338–1340. doi: 10.1212/WNL.57.7.1338

Posner, M. I. (1980). Orienting of attention. *Q. J. Exp. Psychol.* 32, 3–25. doi: 10.1080/00335558008248231

Posner, M. I., Walker, J. A., Friedrich, F. J., and Rafal, R. D. (1984). Effects of parietal injury on covert orienting of attention. *J. Neurosci.* 4, 1863–1874.

Ringman, J. M., Saver, J. L., Woolson, R. F., Clarke, W. R., and Adams, H. P. (2004). Frequency, risk factors, anatomy, and course of unilateral neglect in an acute stroke cohort. *Neurology* 63, 468–474. doi: 10.1212/01.WNL.0000133011.10689.CE

Shindo, K., Sugiyama, K., Huabao, L., Nishijima, K., Kondo, T., and Izumi, S.-I. (2006). Long-term effect of low-frequency repetitive transcranial magnetic stimulation over the unaffected posterior parietal cortex in patients with unilateral spatial neglect. *J. Rehabil. Med.* 38, 65–67. doi: 10.1080/16501970500441807

Song, W., Du, B., Xu, Q., Hu, J., Wang, M., and Luo, Y. (2009). Low-frequency transcranial magnetic stimulation for visual spatial neglect: a pilot study. *J. Rehabil. Med.* 41, 162–165. doi: 10.2340/16501977-0302

Sparing, R., Thimm, M., Hesse, M. D., Küst, J., Karbe, H., and Fink, G. R. (2009). Bidirectional alterations of interhemispheric parietal balance by non-invasive cortical stimulation. *Brain* 132, 3011–3020. doi: 10.1093/brain/awp154

Sturm, W., Thimm, M., Küst, J., Karbe, H., and Fink, G. R. (2006). Alertness-training in neglect: behavioral and imaging results. *Restor. Neurol. Neurosci.* 24, 371–384.

Sturm, W., and Willmes, K. (2001). On the functional neuroanatomy of intrinsic and phasic alertness. *Neuroimage* 14, S76–S84. doi: 10.1006/nimg.2001.0839

Vuilleumier, P., Hester, D., Assal, G., and Regli, F. (1996). Unilateral spatial neglect recovery after sequential strokes. *Neurology* 46, 184–189. doi: 10.1212/WNL.46.1.184

Willmes, K. (1985). An approach to analyzing a single subject's scores obtained in a standardized test with application to the Aachen Aphasia Test (AAT). *J. Clin. Exp. Neuropsychol.* 7, 331–352. doi: 10.1080/01688638508401268

Willmes, K. (1990). Statistical methods for a single-case study approach to aphasia therapy research. *Aphasiology* 4, 415. doi: 10.1080/02687039008249092

Wilson, B. A., Cockburn, J., and Halligan, P. (1987). *Behavioural Inattention Test.* Titchfield: Thames Valley Test Company.

Zimmermann, P., and Fimm, B. (2002). "A test battery for attentional performance," in *Applied Neuropsychology of Attention. Theory, Diagnosis and Rehabilitation*, eds M. Leclercq and P. Zimmermann (London: Psychology Press), 110–151.

Should I stay or should I go? Conceptual underpinnings of goal-directed actions

Giovanni Mirabella[1,2] *

[1] Istituto Neurologico Mediterraneo, IRCCS Neuromed, Pozzilli, Italy
[2] Department of Physiology and Pharmacology 'V. Erspamer,' La Sapienza University, Rome, Italy

Edited by:
Manuel Casanova, University of Louisville, USA

Reviewed by:
Satoshi Tsujimoto, Kobe University, Japan
Mikhail Lebedev, Duke University, USA

***Correspondence:**
Giovanni Mirabella, Istituto Neurologico Mediterraneo, IRCCS Neuromed, via Atinense 18, 86077 Pozzilli, Italy
e-mail: giovanni.mirabella@uniroma1.it

All actions, even the simplest like moving an arm to grasp a pen, are associated with energy costs. Thus all mobile organisms possess the ability to evaluate resources and select those behaviors that are most likely to lead to the greatest accrual of valuable items (reward) in the near or, especially in the case of humans, distant future. The evaluation process is performed at all possible stages of the series of decisions that lead to the building of a goal-directed action or to its suppression. This is because all animals have a limited amount of energy and resources; to survive and be able to reproduce they have to minimize the costs and maximize the outcomes of their actions. These computations are at the root of behavioral flexibility. Two executive functions play a major role in generating flexible behaviors: (i) the ability to predict future outcomes of goal-directed actions; and (ii) the ability to cancel them when they are unlikely to accomplish valuable results. These two processes operate continuously during the entire course of a movement: during its genesis, its planning and even its execution, so that the motor output can be modulated or suppressed at any time before its execution. In this review, functional interactions of the extended neural network subserving generation and inhibition of goal-directed movements will be outlined, leading to the intriguing hypothesis that the performance of actions and their suppression are not specified by independent sets of brain regions. Rather, it will be proposed that acting and stopping are functions emerging from specific interactions between largely overlapping brain regions, whose activity is intimately linked (directly or indirectly) to the evaluations of pros and cons of an action. Such mechanism would allow the brain to perform as a highly efficient and flexible system, as different functions could be computed exploiting the same components operating in different configurations.

Keywords: decision-making, reward, voluntary motor control, behavioral flexibility, countermanding task, reaching arm movements

INTRODUCTION

Our survival depends on the ability to gather, parse and evaluate the stream of constantly changing environmental stimuli and to flexibly adapt our behavioral responses according to the context in which we are embedded. This is because all animals operate with limited resources, and thus the way they value their internal states, sensory experience, and behavioral output influences directly how they will invest their time and energy (Rangel et al., 2008). The bottom line is that the opportunity of executing any action needs to be continuously evaluated in order to minimize its costs and to maximize its payoffs. In fact, the value associated with a certain stimulus is not an intrinsic property of the stimulus, but can change as a function of the internal states of the agent at the time the stimulus is encountered and as a function of agent's previous experience with that stimulus. For instance, for a thirsty gazelle the water of a pond might represent a highly valuable stimulus, unless it perceives the presence of hungry lions.

Central to this process are two executive functions: (i) the ability to predict the future outcomes of a given action; and (ii) the ability to suppress inappropriate, i.e., not sufficiently valuable, actions. Importantly, these two executive functions operate not only during the genesis of an action, but also during the planning of an already selected action. In fact, during the temporal gap between the time when an action has been chosen and the moment when the motor output is going to be generated, the context might have changed, altering the computed value of the action and thus requiring a radical change of the planned motor strategy. For instance, the sight of a tasty cake is likely to drive a child to plunge his fingers into the cream, but if, when he is about to act, he suddenly feels he is observed by his parents, he will refrain from executing the planned movement. In this instance, the fear of being punished has overcome the potential reward of a sweet food, causing the suppression of the pending action.

Conceptually, a goal-directed action can be modeled as multi-step decision process to which several brain regions contribute (see **Figure 1**; **Table 1**). The different stages leading up to the execution or the inhibition of an action are described in the next sections. The model I propose has been inspired by that suggested by Haggard (2008). However, there are two key differences between the former and the latter. First of all, the new model does not necessarily subserve human volition (see paragraph 'Concluding Thoughts'). Secondly, in this new

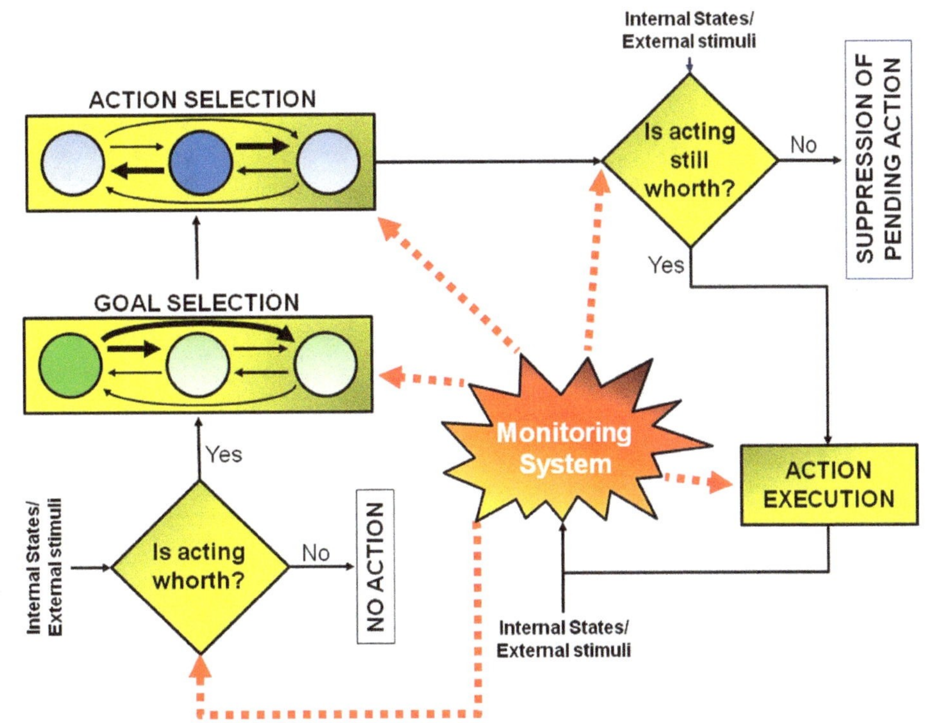

FIGURE 1 | Model of goal-directed actions. The model consists of a set of a multi-step decision processes leading either to the execution or to the inhibition of an action, according to the evaluation of its pros and cons. This model does not have a strictly serial or parallel architecture. Some processes must occur before others (e.g., the early "should-I-stay-or-should-I-go" decision aimed at evaluating whether acting is worthwhile must occur before goal or action selection), but other processes occur in parallel (e.g., the monitoring system, whose role is to compute predictions about future reward and to measure discrepancies between expected and actual outcomes, is active during all the steps). See text for further details.

model, each stage of the process can be influenced by a component named monitoring system, according to the results of the outcomes of previous decisions (see paragraph 'The Monitoring System'). As a consequence the model I propose does not work strictly in a serial fashion, but both serially and in parallel.

Before proceeding, I want to remark that I will mostly deal with upper limb action control, leaving aside saccadic eye movement control. This is because the saccadic system has a different functional organization from that controlling arm and hand movements (e.g., see Churchland and Shenoy, 2007; Schall and Godlove, 2012). For instance, a number of studies have provided evidence that the inhibitory controls of eye and hand movements are independent (e.g., Logan and Irwin, 2000; Boucher et al., 2007; Sumner et al., 2007; Mirabella et al., 2011). Interestingly, Mirabella et al. (2009) and Stevenson et al. (2009) studied the effect of introducing a temporal gap between the end of the fixation and target presentation on the reaction times (RTs) and on the speed of inhibition of reaching movements and saccades, respectively. They found contrasting results: in the former study the gap produced a decrease in the inhibitory speed and in the latter an increase. This is not odd, as saccades have a different ecological relevance from hand and arm movements in primates. In fact, outside neurophysiology laboratories, they allow physical interactions with the environment, thus leading to material outcomes such as acquisition of food or tools. Nevertheless, it is likely that the very general principles, not the fine details, of the genesis of eye and limb movements are rather similar.

THE MOTIVATION TO ACT (EARLY "SHOULD-I-STAY-OR-SHOULD-I-GO" DECISION)

The first step is represented by the motivation to act (early "should-I-stay-or-should-I-go" decision). This is determined by an evaluation process which is aimed at determining whether or not the individual's current needs are satisfied. The evaluative process can be primed because of a change in either the external environment (e.g., the sight of a cake) or the internal states (e.g., a sudden hungry feeling), or both (e.g., the sight of a cake prompts a hungry feeling). Thus, these first computations would evaluate whether or not the current state has to be changed to pursue a desire (e.g., eating) against several possible constraints (e.g., eating too much might cause weight gain). If the motivation is considered worthwhile then movement preparation will jump to the next stage, otherwise it will be canceled.

This is an essential process and one which is continuously performed by our motor system. In fact, in most places where we live, if not all, we are surrounded by tools whose sight automatically activates motor schemas that would normally be employed to interact with those objects. These actions are prompted by the features of the objects, the so-called affordances (Gibson,

Table 1 | Summary of the main brain regions involved in each stage of the model describing the genesis of an arm goal oriented action, together with the most relevant references.

Early "should-I-stay-or-should-I-go" decision	SMA/pre-SMA	Boccardi et al. (2002), Grezes and Decety (2002), Biran and Chatterjee (2004), Sumner et al. (2007), Forstmann et al. (2008), Ridderinkhof et al. (2011), van Gaal et al. (2011)
	Sector F5 (subregion of PMv)/PPC	Murata et al. (1997), Rizzolatti and Luppino (2001)
	Basal ganglia (dopaminergic neurons; putamen and pallidum)	Mazzoni et al. (2007), Schmidt et al. (2008), Bonanni et al. (2010), for a review see Turner and Desmurget (2010)
Goal selection	OFC	Damasio (1994), Padoa-Schioppa and Assad (2006), Fellows and Farah (2007), Padoa-Schioppa and Assad (2008), for a review see Wallis (2007)
	LPFC	Hoshi et al. (2000), Barraclough et al. (2004), Genovesio et al. (2005, 2012), for a review see Wise (2008)
Action selection	PMd	Cisek and Kalaska (2005), Klaes et al. (2011), for a review see Cisek and Kalaska (2010)
	PRR	Calton et al. (2002), Cui and Andersen (2007), Scherberger and Andersen (2007)
Late "should-I-stay-or-should-I-go" decision	IFG/DLPFC (subregions of LPFC)	Aron et al. (2003), Aron and Poldrack (2006), Chambers et al. (2006), Aron et al. (2007), Zheng et al. (2008), Zandbelt and Vink (2010), Jahfari et al. (2012), Zandbelt et al. (2013), for a review see Aron et al. (2014)
	Pre-SMA	Aron et al. (2007), Li et al. (2008), Chen et al. (2010), Zandbelt and Vink (2010), Jahfari et al. (2012), Zandbelt et al. (2013)
	Basal ganglia (striatum, STN)	Aron and Poldrack (2006), Van den Wildenberg et al. (2006), Aron et al. (2007), Li et al. (2008), Zandbelt and Vink (2010), Swann et al. (2011), Mirabella et al. (2012)
	PMd and M1	Coxon et al. (2006), Swann et al. (2009), Mirabella et al. (2011), Mattia et al. (2012), Mattia et al. (2013)
	PPC	Chikazoe et al. (2009), Jahfari et al. (2010), Zandbelt et al. (2013)
Action execution	PMd and M1	Tanji and Evarts (1976), Georgopoulos et al. (1982), Weinrich et al. (1984), Riehle and Requin (1989), Hoshi and Tanji (2000), Hoshi and Tanji (2002), Churchland et al. (2006), for a review see Shenoy et al. (2013)
	Spinal cord	Prut and Fetz (1999)
	Basal ganglia (STN)	Paradiso et al. (2003), Loukas and Brown (2004), Mirabella et al. (2013)
Monitoring system	ACC	Bernstein et al. (1995), Brown and Braver (2005), Kennerley et al. (2006), Sheth et al. (2012)
	Basal ganglia (dopaminergic neurons; ventral striatum)	Schultz et al. (1997), O'Doherty et al. (2003), Montague et al. (2004), Bayer and Glimcher (2005), Chikazoe et al. (2009), Zandbelt and Vink (2010), Jahfari et al. (2012), Zandbelt et al. (2013)
	Frontal pole cortex (subregion of PFC)	Tsujimoto et al. (2010), for a review see Tsujimoto et al. (2011)
	SMA/pre-SMA	Chikazoe et al. (2009), Chen et al. (2010), Scangos and Stuphorn (2010), Zandbelt and Vink (2010), Jahfari et al. (2012), Zandbelt et al. (2013), Bonini et al. (2014)

SMA, supplementary motor area; pre-SMA, pre-supplementary motor area; PMv, ventral premotor cortex; PPC, posterior parietal cortex; LPFC, lateral prefrontal cortex; DLPFC, dorsolateral prefrontal cortex; PMd, dorsal premotor cortex; PRR, parietal reach region; IFG, inferior frontal gyrus; STN, subthalamic nucleus; M1, primary motor cortex; ACC, anterior cingulate cortex; FPC, frontal pole cortex.

1979). It has been shown that even the simple observation of pictures depicting affordable objects (such as graspable objects) activates a sub-region of the medial frontal cortex, the supplementary motor area (SMA; see **Figure 2**), even when there is no requirement to actually act on those stimuli (Grezes and Decety, 2002). These stimulus-driven activations are rapid, involuntary, and unconscious.

Sumner et al. (2007), using subliminal stimuli to prime movements in a direction opposite to the requested one, showed that while control subjects were able to withhold unwanted actions, patients with microlesions of the SMA or the supplementary eye fields (SEFs) were impaired during the execution of hand or eye movements, respectively. They concluded that the SMA and SEF mediate automatic effector-specific suppression of motor plans.

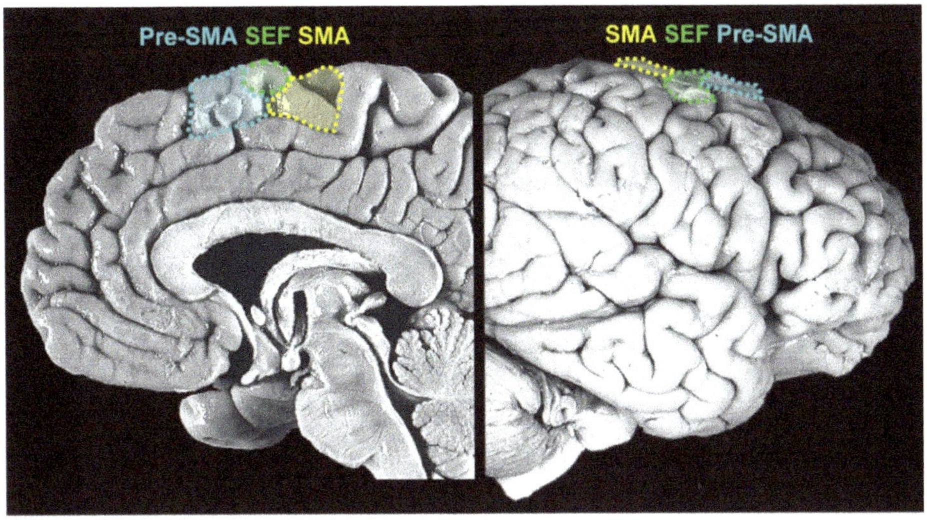

FIGURE 2 | Medial frontal cortex (details of the medial portion of Brodmann areas 6 and 8). Midsagittal view of the medial wall **(left)** and lateral prefrontal cortex (LPFC) surface **(right)**, delineating the supplementary motor area (SMA), supplementary eye field (SEF) and pre-supplementary motor area (pre-SMA). Reproduced with permission from Ridderinkhof et al. (2011).

However, there is another way to look at those automatic activations: they might represent the activity of the network subserving the evaluative process which is at the base of the early "should-I-stay-or-should-I-go" decision. In other words, affordances might increase the motivation to act, but to execute an action they have to be coupled with an internal state congruent with the primed action (e.g., the sight of a glass of water will prime the action if and only if an individual is thirsty; see **Figure 1**).

From this perspective the suppression of a triggered action might be seen not as an active process, but rather as an automatic consequence of the evaluative procedure. Using this framework, is possible to put forward a functional hypothesis underling two rare neuropsychological disorders, the alien limb syndrome and the utilization behavior. Both diseases are characterized by the fact that patients cannot resist objects' affordance, and they are automatically forced to perform stimulus-driven motor responses even when they do not need those objects (Humphreys and Riddoch, 2000). Patients with the alien hand syndrome perform involuntary actions with the limb contralateral to a focal brain lesion most frequently located in the medial frontal cortex, usually involving the SMA (Della Sala et al., 1991; Biran and Chatterjee, 2004). Patients suffering from utilization behavior compulsively grasp and use objects placed within their reach. This syndrome has been linked to bilateral damage to the medial frontal region involving the SMA, pre-SMA, and cingulate motor areas (Boccardi et al., 2002). Therefore, at least to some extent, the sites of the lesions causing those syndromes are largely overlapping, with the difference that in the former case it is located just in one hemisphere whereas in the latter case it affects both hemispheres. Possibly what is affected in both syndromes is the circuitry underlying the early "should-I-stay-or-should-I-go" evaluation, so that most stimulus-driven activations are no longer matched with our internal needs and thus they cannot be filtered out.

The discovery of the so-called canonical neurons in monkeys' lateral premotor area F5 may represent the neural mechanisms underlying responsiveness to object affordances (Murata et al., 1997). These neurons become active both when grasping an object and when seeing the same object without moving (Murata et al., 1997), and they are likely to feed the neural network of the medial frontal region which presides over the evaluation of whether to act. In fact, the lateral premotor area F5 receives projections from several regions of the posterior parietal cortex (PPC; Rizzolatti and Luppino, 2001), which is the end point of a crucial pathway for the visual guidance of actions toward objects, named the dorsal stream (Milner and Goodale, 1995). As such, PPC and F5 are likely to play a key role in visuomotor transformations, providing a neurophysiological correlate of stimulus-driven action affordance.

Several lines of evidence indicate that the fate of these activations might be decided in pre-SMA, which would act as a gate through which the available action affordances might be translated into actual actions (Ridderinkhof et al., 2011). First of all, a functional magnetic imaging (fMRI) study has shown that the strength of activation in pre-SMA covaries with the extent of inappropriate responses driven by stimulus-action association, i.e., the selection of appropriate action engages stronger activation of the pre-SMA in the face of many competing alternatives (Forstmann et al., 2008). Second, a strong negative correlation has been demonstrated between pre-SMA gray-matter volume and the inability to efficiently deal with competing response tendencies (van Gaal et al., 2011).

It would be very reductive to limit this first stage to the filtering of stimulus-driven action affordances and to the medial frontal regions. In fact, a role is surely also played by those brain regions that underlie arousal regulation (in particular the dopaminergic system), increasing or decreasing the readiness of animals to react. There are a wide variety of stimuli that can trigger arousal, from relatively simple sensory stimuli (e.g., the smell of blood or the sound of a mating call) to much more complex situations (e.g., the feeling of social exclusion or the feeling of being idolized). These signals prompt some basic instincts or learned memories which, according to the current contextual situation, might change the internal state of the animals, triggering an alert state. In these instances, animals do not yet have a goal, but they are more ready to act. The dopaminergic system is likely to play an important role in this stage of action genesis as witnessed by one of the symptoms of the most severe form Parkinson's disease (PD), the akinesia, i.e., the inability to initiate any goal-directed movement. Akinesia is not a pure motor disturbance, because it has been shown that in situations of great emergency (e.g., a missile attack, an earthquake) otherwise akinetic PD patients can show a sudden transient ability to move (paradoxical kinesia; Glickstein and Stein, 1991; Schlesinger et al., 2007; Bonanni et al., 2010). Evidently, when dopamine neurons are remarkably reduced in number, all behavioral options or internal mental states would appear to have the same value as the current state. In the face of this flat value function, the best choice for PD patients is to freeze. In extreme situations, salient stimuli may elicit stronger discharge of dopaminergic cells than normal, driving the patient to act. Recently, Mazzoni et al. (2007) suggested that even in less dramatic situations the slowness of movements (bradikinesia) in PD patients may be attributable to an improper evaluation of movement energy costs. In these experiments, PD patients and healthy controls were asked to move their arm to a previously specified target at different speeds a given number of times. Both were able to make required movements with the same accuracy, but PD patients needed significantly more trials before reaching the required number of repetitions. As the accuracy of patients was the same as that of controls, authors concluded that the loss of dopamine did not cause bradykinesia through a speed-accuracy trade-off. Rather, it affected decision-making through a faulty evaluation of the costs of movements, i.e., allocation of the correct amount of energy to meet the demands of the task. In other words, PD weakened the key link between motivation and movement gain. In fact, the dopaminergic system has been shown to play a major role in reward-dependent learning (e.g., Schultz et al., 1997; Montague et al., 2004).

Other evidence indicates that the regulation of action motivation based on previous experiences is one of the main functions of the basal ganglia, not just of the dopaminergic system (Turner and Desmurget, 2010). This hypothesis is supported by one symptom which often accompanies focal damage of the basal ganglia, the so-called auto-activation deficit or abulia (Habib, 2004), in which patients suffer from a marked deficit in motivation to perform spontaneous acts despite an absence of overt motor impairment. In particular, Schmidt et al. (2008) asked patients suffering from auto-activation deficit, due to bilateral lesions of the putamen or pallidum, to control grip forces in response either to explicit sensory instructions or to monetary incentives. Although they fully understood the instructions, patients were capable of modulating their movement only in the former, not in the latter, condition.

All in all, it is clear that there are several brain regions that regulate the willingness to act. This early "should-I-stay-or-should-I-go" decision should play a key role because it would activate (or stop) the chain of other decisions that will potentially lead to action execution. While many other subsequent stages might be performed in parallel, this first one is likely to be a stand-alone process during which no actions are planned and thus there is no need for any neural signal to inhibit them.

GOAL SELECTION

Once performance of an action is considered worthwhile, because a need has to be satisfied, the next set of decisions will be devoted to the selection of the most opportune goal among the several different alternatives usually available (e.g., to satisfy the feeling of hunger we might decide to eat the cake in front of us or to leave the room and go to a restaurant). This process possibly entails two stages: first, values are assigned to each available option and subsequently a decision is taken weighting these values according to the behavioral context (e.g., Glimcher et al., 2005). Even though this schema is conceptually logical, it is very unlikely that neural processing would be strictly organized in distinct serial stages. As depicted in **Figure 1**, it is very likely that multiple potential goals are simultaneously represented. To each goal a given value would be assigned and weighted according to the situation. As multiple goals cannot be pursued at the same time, these representations probably start to compete with each other, perhaps through mutual inhibition (**Figure 1**). This competition can be biased by several factors which ultimately influence the expected outcome of the action[1]. In this review I will argue that these biasing signals might come from the brain regions of the "monitoring system," i.e., the system that evaluates and stores the outcome of past actions (see **Figure 1** and see The Monitoring System). Value assignment and the competition might occur at the same time, probably in different sectors of the prefrontal cortex (PFC). PFC is not a homogeneous structure but is composed of multiple areas that differ in terms of cytoarchitecture and anatomical connections with other areas (Petrides and Pandya, 1999, 2002; **Figure 3**). Thus, it is likely that each area might perform its own function; however, their exact roles are not yet clear. Part of the reason is that the PFC contributes to a bewildering array of functions (Wise, 2008).

Nevertheless, converging evidence argues that orbitofrontal cortex (OFC) plays a key role in linking stimuli to their values (for a review see Wallis, 2007). Indeed, lesions to the OFC impair choice behavior, leading to unreliable choices (e.g., Damasio, 1994; Fellows and Farah, 2007) or abnormal gambling (e.g., Camille et al., 2004; Koenigs and Tranel, 2007). Padoa-Schioppa and Assad (2006), recording single-units in monkeys, demonstrated that a particular class of neurons of the OFC ("chosen neurons") encode the subjective value of two different drinks (juice and water) irrespective of their taste, volume or the action that needs to be taken to obtain them. Thus these cells encoded value *per se*, allowing a comparison for qualitatively different goods. Later on, Padoa-Schioppa and Assad (2008) also showed that the discharge of these neurons was independent of the presence of other goods. These findings indicate that the OFC produces stable value representations, i.e., a key trait of choices, because it allows abstract comparisons such as

[1]An exception to this model might occur when the number of potential goals exceeds the capacity of working memory. In these instances goals might be processed differently.

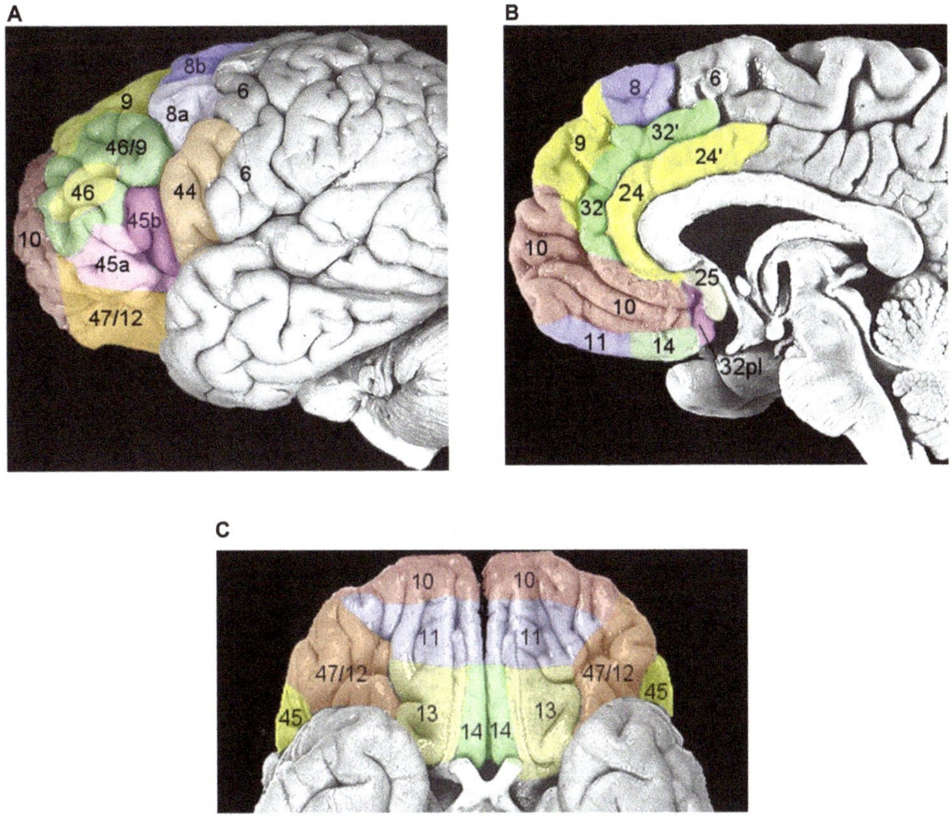

FIGURE 3 | Areas composing the prefrontal cortex (PFC) according to the parcellation of Petrides and Pandya (1999, 2002). (A) Areas of the lateral PFC. The inferior frontal gyrus (IFG) corresponds to Brodmann area (BA) 44, or pars opercolaris, to BA45, or pars triangularis, and to BA47/12, or pars orbitalis. The dorsolateral prefrontal cortex (DLPFC) corresponds to BA9/46 and BA46. **(B)** Areas of the medial wall of the PFC. The anterior cingulate cortex (ACC) corresponds to BA32, BA24, and BA25 (dorsocaudal portions are indicated with a hyphen). BA10 corresponds to the frontopolar cortex. The orbitofrontal cortex (OFC) corresponds to BA11 and BA14. **(C)** Areas of ventral orbital surface of the PFC. BA10 corresponds to the frontopolar cortex. Area BA47/12 corresponds to the pars orbitalis of the IFG. The OFC corresponds to BA11, BA13, and BA14. Reproduced with permission from Ridderinkhof et al. (2004).

transitivity between different goods which are not available at the same time.

On the other hand, to select properly the more appropriate goal, the values of the options must be evaluated in light of the situation which an animal has to face (e.g., if an animal is starving even a non-preferred food represents a good choice). Therefore, to represent value efficiently in different situations, a neuronal representation should flexibly adapt to the current context. These computations are probably carried on in lateral prefrontal cortex (LPFC). Several studies have shown that neural activities of those areas specify the so-called task sets. A task set is a configuration of perceptual, attentional, mnemonic, and motor processes that is actively maintained to perform a given task. It specifies the rules needed to solve the specific task, but it is independent of the stimuli as long as they have to be processed in the same way. Therefore it is not surprising that the PFC contributes to an enormous array of functions ranging from selective attention (Lebedev et al., 2004) to working memory (Funahashi et al., 1989), problem-solving strategies (Genovesio et al., 2005) and categorization of sensory stimuli (Freedman et al., 2002). This list is by no means exhaustive, but it is intended to give an idea of the several kinds of knowledge that are processed in the LPFC. Recently, a series of studies has provided evidence about the way in which this array of cognitive processes can be combined to produce sophisticated behavior (Genovesio et al., 2005, 2006, 2012). The logic underlying all these experiments was that of setting tasks which require several kinds of long-term and short-term knowledge, while recording single-unit activity in the LPFC. For instance, Genovesio et al. (2005) trained monkeys to make a saccade to the left, right, or upward direction in response to a visual object, depending on the cue and on the goal that had occurred on the previous trial (**Figure 4**). This way the monkeys could not learn a fixed stimulus-response association. Instead, they had to adopt repeat-stay and change-shift strategies, i.e., if the cue was the same as in the previous successful trial the monkeys repeated the response, while if the cue was different they had to change their response. Genovesio et al. (2005) found that the activity of some single-neurons in the dorsolateral prefrontal cortex (DLPFC) represent different strategies, that is, special kinds of abstract rules acquired on the basis of task performance history. Similarly, Barraclough et al. (2004) found that DLPFC neurons encoded monkeys' past decisions and payoffs, providing crucial

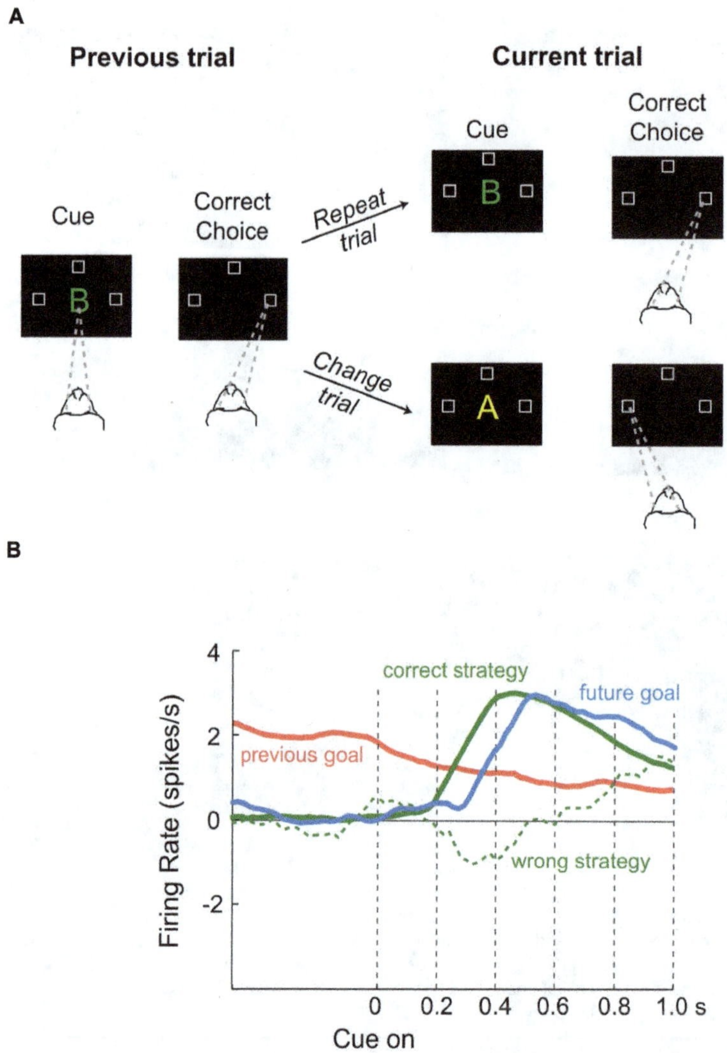

FIGURE 4 | Role of dorsolateral prefrontal cortex during a "strategy task." (A) Temporal sequence of the visual displays during the task and behavioral responses required of the monkeys. Each trial began when monkeys fixated on a spot at the center of the display (gaze direction is indicated by the dashed lines). After a delay, a cue appeared. When it disappeared, the monkeys had to make a saccadic eye movement to one of three positions (unfilled squares). Monkeys were required to remember both the cue and the goal of the trial just performed because the response on the next trial (current trial) depended on the previous choice, i.e., if the cue was the same as in the previous successful trial, the monkeys repeated the response (repeat trial), while if the cue was different they had to change their response (change trial). Thus, monkeys were forced to change strategy according to the past trial history, adopting either a repeat-stay strategy or a change-shift strategy **(B)** Neural activity reflecting the previous goal (red), the future goal (blue), the correct strategy (solid green line), and the wrong strategy (dashed green line). Previous-goal signal decreased after cue onset as the signals for the correct strategy and future goal increased. In contrast, when monkeys chose the wrong strategy, a weak or absent strategy signal occurred during the time of goal selection. Reproduced with permission from Wise (2008).

signals to update estimates of expected reward. Thus, according to the authors the activity of these cells subserves the optimization of decision-making strategies. Other neurons in the same area represented fixed stimulus–response mappings learned previously (Hoshi et al., 2000).

All in all it seems that the different subregions of the LPFC process several types of knowledge and, taking into account the context in which the animals operate and the outcome of the action performed, allow the performance of non-routine, i.e., flexible, behaviors (Wise, 2008). Clearly such complex elaborations cannot be done in isolation. In fact, it has been recently proposed that information about several different metrics of available resources in the surrounding environment (e.g., numerosity, duration, distance) are provided to the LPFC by the PPC (Genovesio et al., 2014). Certainly, along the fronto-parietal network attentive signals flow bidirectionally, allowing the selection of salient stimuli during visually guided movements (e.g., Lebedev and Wise, 2001; for reviews see Corbetta and Shulman, 2002; Reynolds and Chelazzi, 2004). Two other relevant sources of information are the OFC, which, as described at the beginning of this paragraph, delivers knowledge about the value of the stimuli, and the anterior cingulate cortex (ACC) and/or the pre-SMA, which deliver signals dealing with prediction of expected outcome (see The Monitoring System). In addition, sensory areas could also contribute to this process. For instance, it has been found that activity of neurons in macaque area V4 can underlie the selection of elemental object features and their translation into a response-related format that can directly contribute to the control of the animal's actions (Mirabella et al., 2007).

These are just a few examples; many cortical and subcortical structures are connected with the PFC, which is optimally situated to gather and synthesize information to select the more appropriate goal, and the best task set to achieve it in a given context.

ACTION SELECTION

Even though goal and strategies are selected in the PFC, there are several lines of evidence indicating that choosing between alternative actions to achieve an identified goal and the generation of specific motor commands (i.e., motor plans) are accomplished by neural populations in the dorsal premotor cortex (PMd; Cisek and Kalaska, 2005; Klaes et al., 2011), in the primary motor cortex (Tanji and Evarts, 1976) and in the so-called parietal reach region (PRR), a subregion of the PPC (Cui and Andersen, 2007; Scherberger and Andersen, 2007). Therefore goal selection and the selection of movements to reach them are two separate processes that, to some extent, are likely to occur one after the other.

As most goals can be achieved in any of several ways, multiple potential actions are possibly represented at the same time and start to compete for implementation[2]. That this was the case was demonstrated by Cisek and Kalaska (2005) in a seminal experiment. While recording from PMd, they set a task in which two spatial cues indicated two opposite potential reaching actions. After a delay, a non-spatial cue specified the correct choice (**Figure 5**). Soon after the presentation of the two cues, the neural activity of PMd specified both directions of potential reach targets simultaneously. When information for selecting the correct action became available, its neural representation was strengthened while the other was suppressed.

On these grounds, the authors hypothesized that PMd prepares multiple actions in parallel and selects between them through a process of biased competition taking place within the same neural substrate that guides the execution of those actions (Cisek, 2006; Cisek and Kalaska, 2010). Thus, the mechanism of action selection is likely to occur in a similar way to that underlying goal selection (**Figure 1**).

Dorsal premotor cortex is not the only site where multiple potential actions can be represented. In fact, it has been shown that if a monkey is presented with a spatial target, but not instructed about whether an arm or a saccadic eye movement is required, neurons begin to discharge simultaneously in different regions of the PPC, the lateral and the medial intraparietal sulcus (LIP and MIP, respectively; Calton et al., 2002; Cui and Andersen, 2007). These discharges represent the simultaneous coding of saccade

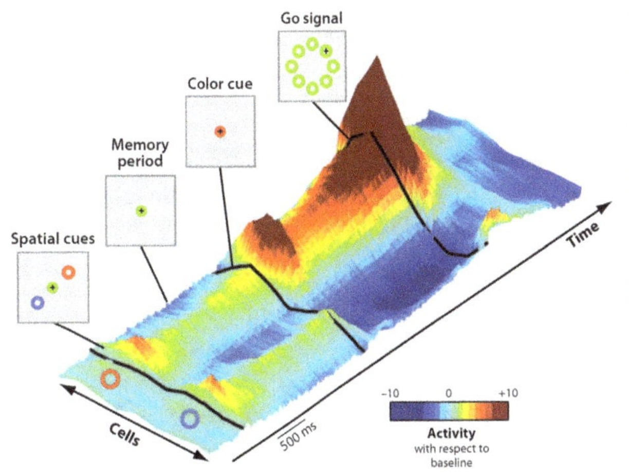

FIGURE 5 | Time course of population activity in the dorsal premotor cortex during a reach-selection task. The diagrams on the left replicate the temporal sequence of the visual displays during the task. Each trial began with the monkeys moving the cursor (+) into a central green circle. Next, a red and a blue cue circle appeared at two of eight possible target positions, in opposite directions from the center for about a second (first display, "Spatial cues"). Then the cues disappeared (second display, "Memory period") and after a variable period the central circle changed color to red or blue (third display, "Color cue"). Finally, the go signal was delivered (fourth display). The central circle disappeared and green circles appeared at all eight positions. To perform correctly the monkeys had to move the cursor from the central circle to the target indicated by the color cue. The 3-D colored surface on the right depicts changes of neural activity along time with respect to baseline, with cells sorted by their preferred direction along the bottom edge. Note that during the entire period of ambiguity until the presentation of the color cue, the population encoded both potential directions. When the color cue provided the information for selecting the correct action, its neural representation was strengthened while the other was suppressed. Reproduced with permission from Cisek and Kalaska (2010).

and reach plans. Later, if an arm movement is cued (Calton et al., 2002) or freely chosen (Cui and Andersen, 2007), the activity of MIP becomes stronger than that of LIP, and vice versa if a saccade is instructed or chosen.

Recently, Klaes et al. (2011) confirm and extended these findings by demonstrating that in situations of uncertain choice, the frontoparietal reach areas (PRR and PMd) construct all potential motor alternatives. However, Klaes et al. (2011) made a further step showing that that potential actions were also biased by the monkeys' subjective desirability, confirming the model proposed by Cisek (2006).

All in all, these findings seem to indicate that in the frontoparietal reach areas there is a continuous and simultaneous processing of multiple movement options. Possibly, as some computational models predict (e.g., Smith and Ratcliff, 2004), neural activity related to response choices, i.e., the motor plans, builds up in separate accumulators as a function of the evidence for or against them until one reaches a threshold, winning the competition.

What a motor plan is or what it represents is a very debated issue. It is generally accepted that the motor plan is formed in the premotor cortex and in M1 (Tanji and Evarts, 1976; Weinrich et al., 1984), but what is encoded by the neural activity of the motor cortices and how it relates to movement activity are matters of some

[2]As previously stated for the representation of multiple goals, even in this instance the representation of multiple potential movements may be limited by the capacity of working memory.

controversy. It has been proposed that the discharge of single-unit might represent a subthreshold version of movement (Tanji and Evarts, 1976) or that population activity represents some movement parameters (e.g., reach direction and distance Georgopoulos et al., 1982; Riehle and Requin, 1989) or even the combination between information about the target and about the effector used (Hoshi and Tanji, 2000, 2002). However, all these approaches have been proven to be inconsistent or equivocal in fully explaining the activity in the motor system (for a review see Shenoy et al., 2013).

An alternative proposal is that this activity reflects a mix of signals: "*some will be outputs to drive the spinal cord and muscles, but many will be internal processes that help to compose the outputs, but are themselves only poorly described in terms of the movement*" (Shenoy et al., 2013, p. 339). In other words, the activity that precedes a movement would represent the initial state of a dynamic system which will determine the temporal patterns needed to drive actions. Under this hypothesis the motor plan does not explicitly represent movement parameters; it is still closely related to movement activity, but the reciprocal relationship is not transparent at the level of the individual cells. This framework seems to reconcile several past, apparently contradictory, findings and to provide a wider comprehension of the functioning of the cortical motor system (Shenoy et al., 2013). One possible limit of the dynamic system hypothesis, that future studies will have to overcome, is that most of the data come from experiments in which there is a delay between the appearance of the target and the go signal (delayed-reach task, e.g., Churchland et al., 2006). Clearly, to be fully validated the hypothesis should be tested in tasks featuring performance or inhibition of reaching movements in different contexts (but see Mattia et al., 2013).

In conclusion, the same substrates where the action selections occur are also those that are used to prepare and guide the execution of the movement that is ultimately selected.

THE FINAL EVALUATION (LATE "SHOULD-I-STAY-OR-SHOULD-I-GO" DECISION)

By the end of the previous stages, what had been evaluated as the best action to achieve the desired goal is planned, but before the corresponding motor plan can be executed it has to pass a further final check (late "should-I-stay-or-should-I-go" decision). This is a fundamental step, because from the moment at which the decision to act has been taken to the time when the motor output is about to be generated, the continuous flow of information might signal that something has changed in the external environment, in the internal states or in both. These changes might impact on the previous evaluations as the selected action might turn out to be no longer appropriate (Haggard, 2008). A common experience might be that of a person about to cross a road but, just before stepping onto the road, he hears the sound of an ambulance siren clearly approaching. In the most common instance, the person would halt his step to avoid being hit. However, the evaluation might be radically different if his/her child is already in the middle of the road. In the former case suppressing the action is clearly the most valuable decision but, in the latter, the risk of losing the parental investment might trigger the person to act even faster in order to secure the child. The evaluation could be also influenced by endogenous signals, for instance the same person in the above example could take the risk of crossing the road because he suddenly remembers that his plane is leaving.

Computationally this last check could be realized by comparing the output of a predictive forward model with a goal description (e.g., see Wolpert and Miall, 1996). When the mismatch between the predicted result and the goal becomes too large, i.e., the action is unlikely to allow the achievement of the desired result, the pending action is canceled. There are several tasks that are currently exploited to study the inhibitory function and each has some advantages over the others (for a review see Ridderinkhof et al., 2011); however, in order to design a potential neural network capable of augmenting inhibition of pending actions, I will focus on the stop-signal paradigm (Logan and Cowan, 1984). There are two reasons to choose this as a paradigmatic task. Firstly it is the only one which allows study of the suppression of ongoing movements, and secondly it has been widely used exploiting several effectors (the eyes, e.g., see Hanes and Schall, 1996; the finger, e.g., see Logan and Cowan, 1984; the arm, e.g., see Mirabella et al., 2006); thus a wealth of data are available. The stop-signal (or countermanding) paradigm probes a subject's ability to withhold a planned movement triggered by a go signal when an infrequent stop-signal is presented after a variable delay (see **Figure 6A**).

Starting from the behavioral performance during the countermanding task it is possible to yield an estimate of the duration of the suppression process [stop-signal reaction time (SSRT); Logan and Cowan, 1984; Band et al., 2003; Boucher et al., 2007]. The SSRT is a key behavioral parameter for uncovering the neural substrates of inhibition. In fact, those brain regions showing a change in activity when a movement is produced with respect to when it is suppressed, and where the onset of this shift precedes the end of the SSRT, can be assumed to be causally related to the suppression process.

Thus the stop-signal task allows to study of the way subjects react to an unexpected imperative stop instruction. This is referred to as "reactive inhibition." At the same time, this approach also allows assessment of changes in the response strategies of individuals embedded in such an experimental context. In fact, the rules of the countermanding task create a conflict on all no-stop trials because subjects are instructed to move as fast as possible, but, at the same time, they tend to delay movement initiation to wait for the occurrence of a possible stop-signal. As a consequence, healthy subjects had longer RTs when executing go-trials intermixed with stop-trials than when executing go-trials alone (e.g., Mirabella et al., 2006; Verbruggen and Logan, 2009). In addition, the occurrence of stop trials induces a lengthening of the RTs of responses produced in the immediately subsequent no-stop trials (Mirabella et al., 2006, 2012; Verbruggen and Logan, 2009; Zandbelt and Vink, 2010). This form of control over response execution in anticipation of known task demands, driven by endogenous signals, i.e., the awareness of the possible presentation of stop-signals, has been called "proactive control/inhibition." In the following, I will describe results mainly related to reactive inhibition, while I will mainly focus on proactive inhibition in the next paragraph where

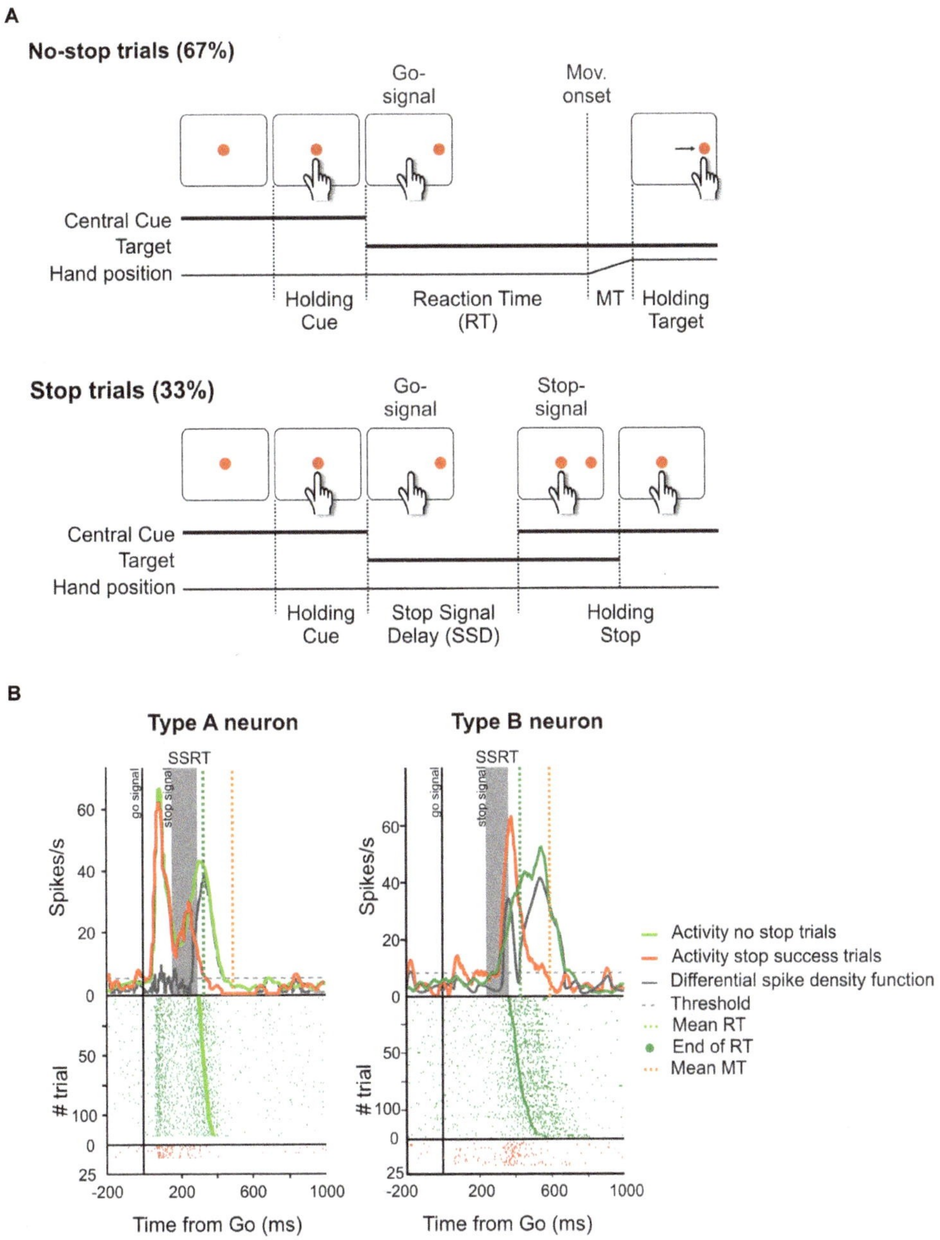

FIGURE 6 | Causal role of neurons of the dorsal premotor cortex (PMd) in reactive inhibition. (A) Temporal sequence of the visual displays for no-stop and stop trials in the reaching version of the countermanding task. All trials began with the presentation of a central stimulus. After a variable holding delay (500–800 ms) it disappeared and simultaneously a target appeared to the right, acting as a go-signal. In the no-stop trials subjects had to start a speeded reaching movement toward the peripheral target. Randomly, on a fraction of interleaved trials (33%), the central stimulus reappeared after variable delays (SSDs), instructing subjects to inhibit movement initiation. In these stop trials, if subjects countermanded the planned movement keeping the arm on the central stimulus the trial was scored as a stop-success trial. Otherwise, if subjects executed the reaching movement the trial was scored as a stop-failure trial (not shown). Reproduced with permission from Mattia et al. (2012). **(B)** Changes of activity driven by the stop-signal onset in PMd neurons modulated during the preparation of the movement. In each panel the upper graph represents the average spike density function while the lower graph shows the raster plots of neural activity in no-stop trials (green tick-marks) and stop-success trials (red tick-marks). Neural activity was always aligned to the go-signal onset (first vertical line). The gray band represents the estimated duration of the stop-signal reaction time (SSRT) in that session. The gray line represents the differential spike density function, while the dashed gray line represents the threshold value for significant divergence. The green and the orange vertical dotted lines in the top panels indicate the average RT and the average end of MT, respectively. The green dots in the rasters represent the end of the RTs. On the right, the activity of a representative "type A" countermanding neuron is shown. In this cell, neural activity during stop-success trials (red line) initially resembles that of no-stop trials (green line) but, with a delay after the stop-signal presentation, it suddenly starts to decrease and the differential spike density function crosses the threshold 34.4 ms before the end of the SSRT. On the left, the activity of a representative "type B" countermanding neuron is shown. In this instance, the activity in stop-success trials increases after stop-signal presentation with respect to that recorded during no-stop trials 39.9 ms before the end of the SSRT. Therefore both these two types of neurons exhibit a modulation of activity sufficient to control the suppression of an ongoing arm movement.

I will deal with the monitoring system (but see also Action Execution). Clearly, all proactive strategies necessarily derive from these computations. This does not mean the neural substrates of reactive and proactive inhibition have to be different. In fact, it has been shown that there is an overlap between them (e.g., Jahfari et al., 2012; Zandbelt et al., 2013; for a review see Aron, 2011); however, reactive and proactive inhibition might derive from two conceptually different modules (the late "should-I-stay-or-should-I-go" decision module and the monitoring system; see **Figure 1**).

Variants of the stop-signal task have been used several times in association with different techniques [e.g., single-unit recordings, fMRI, electroencephalographic scalp recordings (EEG), intracranial electroencephalographic recordings (iEEF), lesions, transcranial magnetic stimulation (TMS), deep brain stimulation (DBS)], different effectors (the eyes, the arm, and the fingers), and different pathologies (e.g., PD, attention deficit and hyperactivity disorder, Tourette syndrome, obsessive–compulsive disorder). From this large number of studies, a network of brain regions that seem to be involved in implementing inhibition has been identified. To this network belong both cortical and subcortical structures, that largely overlap with those involved in movement generation, planning, and even movement execution.

One of the prefrontal regions that more frequently has been reported to have an inhibitory role is the inferior frontal gyrus (IFG), especially in the right hemisphere (see Aron et al., 2014 for a recent review). For instance, Aron et al. (2003) have shown that humans with a lesion to the right, but not to the left IFG exhibit longer SSRTs than healthy subjects. Furthermore they showed that the lengthening of the SSRT was proportional to the extent of damage in the right IFG. Less frequently, the DLPFC has also been claimed to participate in this executive function (e.g., Zheng et al., 2008). However, its role is controversial. In fact, while Zheng et al. (2008) showed that individuals who were more proficient at inhibition had a greater activation in DLPF, Chambers et al. (2006) found that temporary deactivation of the same region, with repetitive TMS, did not significantly alter the speed of inhibition.

Imagining studies revealed the involvement in this form of inhibition of the pre-SMA (e.g., Aron et al., 2007; Li et al., 2008; Zandbelt and Vink, 2010; Jahfari et al., 2012) as well as of the striatum (Li et al., 2008; Zandbelt and Vink, 2010). Even in this instance the exact role of these structures is unclear and debated. Li et al. (2008) compared the fMRI brain activation of individuals with short versus long SSRTs who were identical in all other aspects of stop-signal performance. Their aim was to isolate the neural correlates of response inhibition from those of response monitoring and/or attentional control. Under these experimental conditions, Li et al. (2008) found that the caudate head had greater activation in individuals with short than with long SSRT, and the extent of its activation was positively correlated with activity in the pre-SMA. In contrast, Scangos and Stuphorn (2010), by recording single-neuron activity of SMA and pre-SMA of monkeys during an arm countermanding task, found that these cells could not contribute directly to response inhibition as most of them modulate after the SSRT. Instead, the majority of neurons signaled expectation of reward, as they were modulated by the amount of expected reward.

Another basal ganglion implicated in stopping ongoing actions is the subthalamic nucleus (STN; see Aron and Poldrack, 2006). Mirabella et al. (2012) demonstrated that bilateral STN DBS selectively improves inhibitory functions as its electrical stimulation significantly shortened the SSRT, but did not influence the RTs of no-stop trials. These results agree with those of Van den Wildenberg et al. (2006) and Swann et al. (2011), but not with those of Li et al. (2008). In the above-described study, they found that neither the STN nor the IFG were active during reactive stop and thus concluded that both structures had a role in attentional monitoring of the stop-signal. Similarly, Zandbelt and Vink (2010) did not find evidence of STN activation during movement cancelation.

Finally, two other areas have been found to be involved in inhibitory function, i.e., the PMd (Mirabella et al., 2011; Mattia et al., 2012, 2013) and the primary motor cortex (M1; Coxon et al., 2006; Swann et al., 2009; Mattia et al., 2012). Mirabella et al. (2011) showed that about 30% of PMd cells changed their discharge before the end of the SSRT when the monkey had to stop a reaching movement. Thus these neurons seem to be causally involved in reactive inhibition (see **Figure 6B**). These findings were confirmed and extended by a subsequent study (Mattia et al., 2012), in which epicortical event-related potentials (ERPs) were recorded from the lateral surface of the fronto-temporal lobes of epileptic patients performing the countermanding task. It was found that an ERP complex was selectively expressed before the end of the SSRT in M1, and in the premotor cortex (**Figure 7**). Thus, Mattia et al. (2012) deduced that motor cortices are causally involved in inhibitory control. In conclusion, even though the exact role of each of the brain regions involved in the stop task remains controversial, it clearly emerges a considerable overlap between brain region subserving the preparation of an action and its suppression (see **Table 1**).

To summarize, the late "should-I-stay-or-should-I-go" decision represents a hinge of our goal-directed behavior because it allows crucial, last-minute changes of strategies when the cost of an action overcomes the benefits. Unlike the early "should-I-stay-or-should-I-go" decision, which does not require active suppression, in this instance some neural signals aiming to halt the activity linked to the ongoing action have to be produced by the nervous system (**Figure 1**). Given this, it should not come as a surprise that such a large network of brain regions has to be involved.

ACTION EXECUTION

Once the last check is passed, the motor commands are sent to the spinal cord, activate the muscles, and produce the movement. It must be remarked that it is very unlikely that even the spinal cord would be a passive relay of "higher directives." In fact, Prut and Fetz (1999) have shown that spinal interneurons show pre-movement activity during a delayed task, similarly to PMd (Wise et al., 1983). This indicates that, at least under some experimental conditions, movement preparation may occur simultaneously over widely distributed regions, including spinal levels.

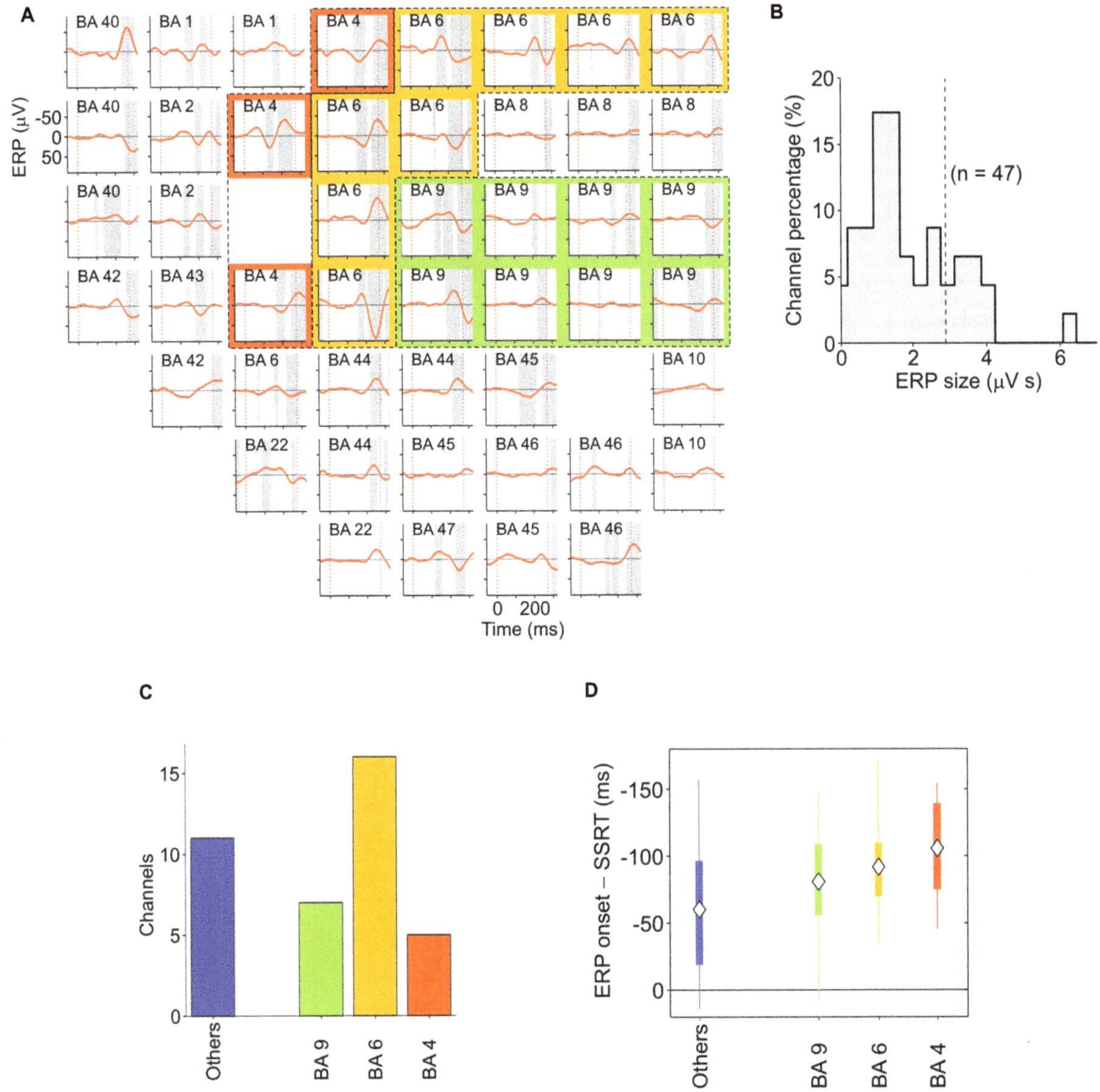

FIGURE 7 | Spatiotemporal distribution of stop-event related potentials (ERPs) in successful-stop (SS) trials. (A) Average stop-ERPs (solid red curves) of SS trials centered on stop-signal appearance corresponding to the selected channels for one pharmacoresistant epileptic patient. Gray areas, time intervals at which the stop-ERP was significantly different from 0 (Wilcoxon signed-rank test, $P < 0.01$). Subplot labels: Brodmann areas (BAs) over which electrodes were positioned. Colored areas: electrodes placed over the primary motor cortex (red, BA4), the premotor cortex (yellow, BA6) and the DLPFC (green, BA9). **(B)** Histogram of the stop-ERP sizes of panel **(A)**. Stop-ERP sizes were computed as the integral of absolute values of stop-ERP voltage deflections in the interval periods marked by gray areas within SSRT. Dashed line: threshold value for selecting the subset of channels with large enough stop-ERPs used for population analyses (see Mattia et al., 2012 for details). **(C)** Number of channels showing large enough average stop-ERPs across five patients ($n = 39$) grouped by BA. Blue bar (others) represents those areas where channels were not selected more than twice across all patients. **(D)** Box plot of stop-ERP onsets measured with respect to the end of SSRT across all selected channels in all patients. Stop-ERP onset was defined as the first time that an electrode voltage was significantly different from 0. Diamonds indicate average onset times. Tick bars indicate the first and the third quartile. Vertical lines indicate the extreme time lags in the channel group. Freely adapted from Mattia et al. (2012), with permission.

Additionally, it must be taken into account that arm movements, unlike saccades, are not ballistic movements as they can be stopped at any point along their path (De Jong et al., 1990; Scangos and Stuphorn, 2010). As a consequence, their planning can be modified even during the execution phase. This is in line with the findings of Mirabella et al. (2008), who compared RTs and movement times (MTs) of reaching movements toward visual targets executed either during an RT task (go-only task) or during a countermanding task. In both tasks subjects executed the same movements, but in the countermanding task subjects were aware that a stop-signal could randomly appear during movement preparation, indicating that the pending action should be suppressed. The awareness of the possible appearance of the stop-signal creates a conflict on all no-stop trials because, despite the instructions to always move as fast as possible, subjects spontaneously tend to delay movement initiation to wait for the possible occurrence of a stop-signal (e.g., Mirabella et al., 2006, 2012). This is a common proactive strategy that subjects implicitly adopt to have a greater chance of stopping their movements. However, the proactive strategy was also found to affect the MTs, which were shorter during the no-stop trials and longer during the go-only trials. Probably the increased length of RTs during the no-stop trials allowed subjects to fully process movement parameters and thus to move faster. In contrast, in go-only trials the absence of a proactive brake allows a shortening of RTs, at the cost of leaving some details of the motor program uncompleted, so that the planning must be completed during the movement. This strategy represents an optimization of costs versus benefits because shorter RTs are compensated by longer MTs and vice versa.

Interestingly, Mirabella et al. (2013) demonstrated that STN takes part in this process. In fact PD patients in which both DBS were turned on behaved similarly to healthy subjects, whereas when both DBS were off the same patients had both RTs and MTs longer in no-stop trials than in go-only trials (**Figure 8**). Therefore this study demonstrated the existence of a causal link between the DBS of STN and the motor strategy exploited. Once again this evidence favors the hypothesis that STN is not involved in a single function (e.g., reactive inhibition); instead, more generally, it can compute the payoff of an ongoing action.

THE MONITORING SYSTEM

In order to learn how to make good decisions, the brain needs to compute, learn, and store the results of the outcomes that were generated by its previous decisions. To this end the ability of computing predictions about future reward and the ability of measuring discrepancies between attended and actual outcomes are fundamental. These functions are performed by a set of brain regions that collectively I will call the "monitoring system" (**Figure 1**). This system is composed of a set of cortical and subcortical structures that allow coding of reward expectations, detection of errors and implementation of behavioral adjustments, aiming to cope with more or less demanding context in order to optimize future choices. Therefore signals produced by the monitoring system can influence any stage of action implementation.

A key role in this set of processes is played by the ACC, located in the frontal medial wall (**Figure 3**). It has been known for

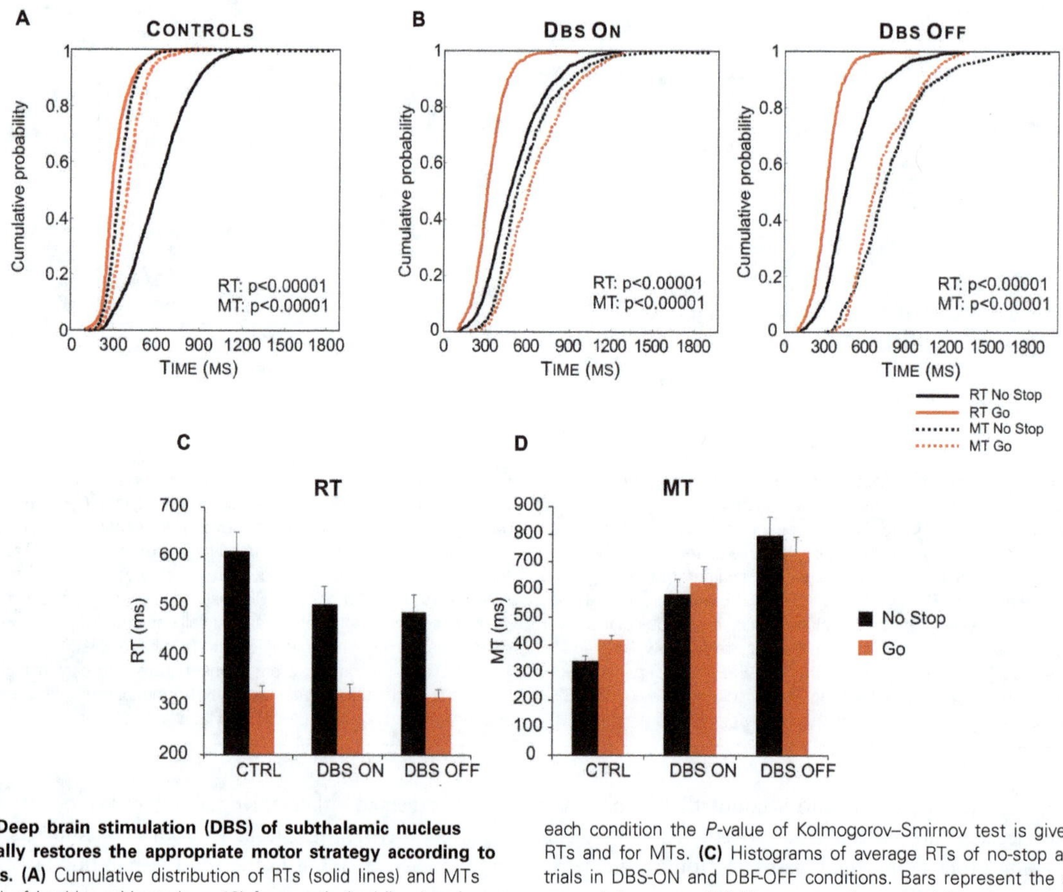

FIGURE 8 | Deep brain stimulation (DBS) of subthalamic nucleus (STN) partially restores the appropriate motor strategy according to the contexts. (A) Cumulative distribution of RTs (solid lines) and MTs (dotted lines) of healthy subjects ($n = 13$) for go-only (red lines) and no-stop (black lines) trials. **(B)** Cumulative distributions of RTs (solid lines) and MTs (dotted lines) of DBS patients ($n = 12$) in DBS-ON and DBF-OFF conditions for both go-only (red lines) and no-stop (black lines) trials. For each condition the *P*-value of Kolmogorov–Smirnov test is given, both for RTs and for MTs. **(C)** Histograms of average RTs of no-stop and go-only trials in DBS-ON and DBF-OFF conditions. Bars represent the standard error of the mean. **(D)** Histograms of average MTs of no-stop and go-only trials in each DBS-ON and DBF-OFF condition. Bars represent the standard error of the mean. Reproduced from Mirabella et al. (2013), with permission from PLOS.

a long time that this area is involved in cognitive control over behavior (e.g., Bernstein et al., 1995; Botvinick et al., 1999); however, its precise role remains considerably debated. One influential hypothesis is that the activity of ACC might represent the likelihood of obtaining or losing reward in response to particular actions. Evidence in support of this idea comes from the results of Brown and Braver (2005). They administered to human volunteers a stop-change task while recording the fMRI BOLD signal. The task, (**Figure 9**), required participants to make rapid left- or right-hand button-press responses according to the direction of an arrow. In 33% of cases, during the RTs, a second arrow pointing in the opposite direction was presented and the responses had to be reversed. Using a staircase algorithm, authors adjusted the time of presentation of the second arrow, hence controlling the likelihood of making mistakes (either 10 or 50%). At the beginning of each trial, participants were informed of the error likelihood by a color cue: a blue bar indicated 50% error probability, while a white bar indicated 10% error probability. The activity of ACC was greater during the high error than during the low error conditions. This held true not only during change trials, but also during trials in which participants did not have to change the responses (**Figure 9**). Therefore ACC does not simply indicate response conflict (occurring when the two arrows are presented) or error occurrence; instead more generally it signals the perceived likelihood of potential errors. Crucially, Brown and Braver (2005) exploiting a neural-network model, showed that this pattern of response gradually emerged over the course of the experimental session, i.e., after individuals learned the associations between color cue and error likelihood.

Other studies point to a slightly different role for the ACC. According to these accounts, ACC would provide a continuously updated prediction of expected cognitive demand which will be used to optimize future behavior. For instance, Sheth et al. (2012) showed that ACC activity speeds up behavioral responses when cognitive demand remain stable, but, in more challenging situations, it slows down responses to allow a greater accuracy. Kennerley et al. (2006), studying the behavioral responses of monkeys before and after ACC lesions, confirmed that this region adaptively guides future behaviors, but exploiting a different mechanism. In a key experiment, monkeys were rewarded when performing a certain action (e.g., lifting a lever) until the rewarded action was changed (e.g., to get the reward it had to turn the lever). Non-lesioned monkeys had no difficult in this task, while ACC-lesioned monkeys following an unrewarded lift response switched to turning, but could not sustain this response on subsequent trials. Thus, the lesion compromised the ability to associate pay-offs with the outcome of past actions to adaptively guide future behavior.

Whatever the exact role of ACC in monitoring behavioral performance, it appears that this capability develops through experience. It is very probable that the knowledge of past experiences is built through reinforcement-learning processes, mediated by the discharge of midbrain dopamine neurons. The discharge of these neurons measures deviations from individuals' previous reward expectations, i.e., they compute the so-called prediction errors (Schultz et al., 1997; O'Doherty et al., 2003; Bayer and Glimcher, 2005). Every time an event is better than expected, dopaminergic neurons phasically increase their discharge. In contrast, they do not change firing rate when an event occurs as predicted, while they decrease their discharge if something worse than expected takes place. Prediction errors are thought to play a key role in guiding decision-making by signaling the need to adjust future behavior, i.e., they are fundamental to learning processes (Schultz et al., 1997; Montague et al., 2004).

Dopaminergic neurons project widely to the striatum and to several regions of PFC including the ACC (Freund et al., 1984; Smith et al., 1994). The activity of ventral striatum seems to correlate with prediction error computation (Bray and O'Doherty, 2007; Hare et al., 2008) and thus it is likely to contribute to some further elaboration of action-outcome predictions. However, ACC plays a different role from ventral striatum, exploiting prediction errors as training signals to build extended action-outcome histories, that later could be exploited to adapt goal-directed behaviors (Holroyd and Coles, 2002; Brown and Braver, 2005; Kennerley et al., 2006). Given such a complex function, it is unlikely that ACC would rely solely on signals coming from dopaminergic neurons. In fact, other brain regions have been shown to produce signals promoting learning. For instance, it has been shown that neurons of the frontal pole cortex code the outcome of actions (Tsujimoto et al., 2010; for a review see Tsujimoto et al., 2011). Also, neurons in SMA and pre-SMA of monkeys have been shown to be modulated by the amount of expected reward and thus these regions might, among other things, be signaling expectation of reward too (Scangos and Stuphorn, 2010). Not all studies point to this conclusion, e.g., recently Bonini et al. (2014), by recording evoked field potentials in pharmacoresistant epileptic patients, claimed that SMA continuously assesses ongoing actions and, when an error occurs, it signals to ACC.

Whatever the exact role of each of these components, they form a system that is capable of monitoring actions, evaluating their behavioral outcomes, and learning the association between a certain environmental context and the likelihood that a certain action or strategy will lead to the desired goal. Thus, the monitoring system is the ideal candidate for implementing proactive preparation of action plans in anticipation of known task demands. Such advance preparation has been studied in the context of response inhibition, in particular when the countermanding task is employed. This is because the rules of this paradigm produce a conflict every time subjects have to execute no-stop trials (see **Figure 6A**). As described above, this context induces a lengthening of the RTs and at the same time a shortening of MTs with respect to situations in which the same movements have to be performed, but stop-signals are never presented (e.g., Mirabella et al., 2008, 2013).

The study of the neural underpinnings of proactive control revealed that the network of brain regions that subserve this function largely overlaps with those subserving reactive inhibition. This conclusion stems from several fMRI studies which employed a probabilistic stop task with cues indicating the likelihood of stop trial occurrence (e.g., Chikazoe et al., 2009; Zandbelt and Vink, 2010; Jahfari et al., 2012; Zandbelt et al., 2013). Some cues indicate that go-signals are never followed by a stop-signal (certain go-signals), whereas others indicate that go-signals have a

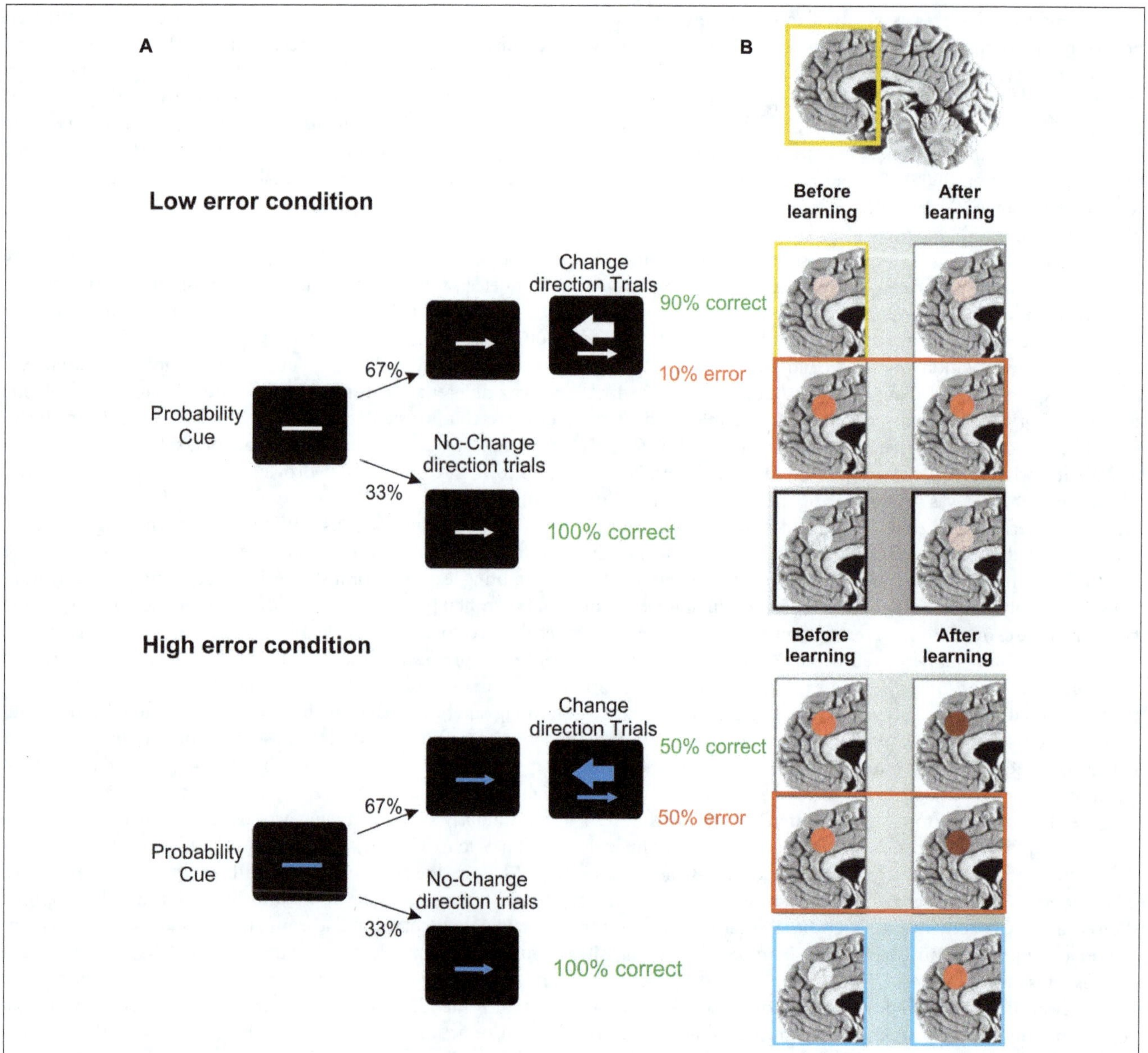

FIGURE 9 | Role of ACC in predicting error likelihood. (A) Temporal sequence of the visual displays for the change-signal task. Initially a probability cue (plain line) was displayed. The cue could be either white or blue, predicting low or high error likelihood respectively. After a delay, a go signal was presented (left or right pointing arrow) indicating the required button-press response (left or right index press for left or right pointing arrow, respectively). Randomly on 33% of the trials a change signal was displayed (a larger arrow pointing in the opposite direction with respect to that presented as go signal). To this signal, subjects had to reverse the response from that indicated by the go signal. Error rates were controlled by a staircase procedure so that in the low error condition the delay between the go signal and the change signal was kept shorter and subjects made around 90% of correct responses. In the high error condition the delay was kept longer and subjects made around 50% correct responses. **(B)** Brain regions highlighted indicate the activation of ACC during the stop-change before and after learning (the greater the activation, the deeper the red color) for correct, wrong change-direction trials and for no-change trials (for the top to the bottom row) in the low and high error conditions. Interestingly, during no-change trials ACC activity increased with practice, especially in response to blue color cues, reflecting an improved ability to predict the likelihood of making an error. Freely adapted from Ridderinkhof and van den Wildenberg (2005), with permission.

certain likelihood of being followed by a stop-signal (uncertain go-signals). By comparing brain activity between these conditions, it has been possible to uncover the neural substrate of advanced action preparation. Overall it emerged that when subjects expect the occurrence of a stop-signal, they proactively engage the network subserving reactive inhibition in a progressively increasing fashion according to the likelihood of stop presentation. A lower stop probability would correspond to a weaker activation of the network and to less marked slowing of responses, while when the stop is presented the activation is much stronger and the motor output is completely blocked (Aron, 2011).

These studies did not show clear activations of either of ACC or midbrain dopaminergic neurons in the ventral tegmental area and in the substantia near pars compacta (but see Zandbelt et al., 2013). However, these might be due either to the fact that commonly a region-of-interest approach had been chosen or because of limitations of the fMRI technique. Nevertheless, the activation of other components of the monitoring system, i.e., striatum, SMA and pre-SMA, has been shown several times (Chikazoe et al., 2009; Zandbelt and Vink, 2010; Jahfari et al., 2012; Zandbelt et al., 2013). This activity might reflect the computations which underlie learning of the association between the experimental context and the likelihood of performing (or stopping) an action. Thus, these signals should drive the proactive network so as to maximize the probability of moving without missing stop trials. Further studies are needed to test this hypothesis.

CONCLUDING THOUGHTS

On the whole, it seems clear that the neural network subserving goal-directed actions is very extensive, encompassing both frontal and parietal area as well as subcortical brain structures. This does not come as a surprise, as we live in a complex and ever-changing environment, which continuously offers an enormous variety of opportunities for potential actions. Thus, our motor system is called on to perform a continuous evaluation of alternative actions that may become available, in order to decide whether to persist in a given activity or to stop it and switch to a different one. This is the hinge of our behavioral flexibility. Central to this feature are the abilities of predicting the likelihood of achieving the desired goal with a certain action or strategy, and of canceling pending actions when they are no longer valuable. These two processes operate continuously during the entire course of a movement, during its genesis, its planning, and even its execution, so that the motor output can be modulated or suppressed at any time before its execution.

These considerations are clearly at odds with the old-fashioned serial framework according to which "*we sense the world, think about it, and then act upon it*" (Cisek and Kalaska, 2010, p. 271). Instead, they are compatible with the idea of parallel processing. Thus, one or more goals or actions can be coded at the same time, so that alternatives can be ready for release at short notice. Importantly, the evaluation of an action can also lead to its suppression when it has already been selected. Very probably the neural machinery underling action preparation and the neural substrates underling action inhibition are simultaneously active. From what is stated above, it is not too surprising that many of the regions mediating the decisions to act appear to be involved also in decisions to refrain from acting (Coxon et al., 2006; Mirabella et al., 2011; Mattia et al., 2012; see **Table 1**). This leads to the main point of the present review. Many, if not all, brain regions belonging to the network which controls goal-oriented movements are involved in more stages of this process. For instance, the SMA and the pre-SMA are involved in the early "should-I-stay-or-should-I-go" decision as they are involved in gating action affordances (e.g., Sumner et al., 2007; Ridderinkhof et al., 2011). However, they are also part of the monitoring system (see The Monitoring System) and they contribute to the late "should-I-stay-or-should-I-go" decision (Aron and Poldrack, 2006; Aron et al., 2007). In addition it has been shown that stimulation of SMA generates a feeling of an urge to move a particular body part, without necessarily causing any actual movement (Fried et al., 1991). The involvement of SMA in the feeling of volition has recently been confirmed by Fried et al. (2011) who recorded single-neuron activity in epileptic pharmacoresistant patients. Both PMd and M1 are involved both in the genesis of motor plans (Tanji and Evarts, 1976; Weinrich et al., 1984; Hoshi and Tanji, 2000, 2002; Churchland et al., 2006; Mattia et al., 2013; Shenoy et al., 2013) and also in their inhibition (Coxon et al., 2006; Mirabella et al., 2011; Mattia et al., 2012). Most of the network subserving reactive inhibition is also involved in proactive inhibition (see Action Execution).

Some other brain regions are involved not solely in motor controls, but also in very different tasks. The ACC has been shown to be involved in monitoring behavioral performance (see The Monitoring System), but also in pain processing (Singer et al., 2004). The role of the IFG is even more controversial as it seems to perform several different functions, some of which are lateralized (see Liakakis et al., 2011 for a review). The left IFG is implicated in both perceptive and productive aspects of language (see Uddén and Bahlmann, 2012 for a review). Some studies indicate that the right IFG plays a key role in redirecting selective attention toward unexpected stimuli (Corbetta and Shulman, 2002); others suggest that it has a specific role in motor inhibition (Aron et al., 2014) or in suppression of unwanted memories (Benoit and Anderson, 2012). In addition, the IFG of both hemispheres are involved in processing of symbolic gestures used for social non-verbal communication (Lindenberg et al., 2012), and they are regions belonging to the core of the human mirror-neuron system, i.e., of the system that is thought to allow the ability of understanding the intentions of others (for a review see Rizzolatti and Craighero, 2004). Finally, the PFC contribute to an enormous array of functions (for a review see Wise, 2008).

Given this picture, I believe that is rather hard to assign a very specific role to most of those regions when performing complex cognitive functions, such as the augmentation of adaptive behaviors. Possibly, complex cognitive functions are not performed by a unique structure. Rather, they might emerge from the coordinated activity of large-scale neuronal networks that are dynamically configured on fixed anatomical connections (von der Malsburg et al., 2010). The mechanisms underlying the dynamic coordination of neural populations are poorly understood. Nevertheless, it has been suggested that the formation of functional networks is achieved by modulating the degree of coherence among temporally structured responses of widely distributed neurons. In its turn, coherence might be modulated by rhythmic modulation of activity and synchronization among these populations (see Fries, 2005 for a review). According to this framework a given brain region can perform specific operations, e.g., the right IFG might subserve the reorienting of selective attention (Corbetta and Shulman, 2002) or the ACC might compute the likelihood of a successful action, but its functional features can be exploited in a variety of tasks. Thus the outcome of complex processes would depend not upon the activation of one or a few brain regions, but on the specific interactions of the network activated during the ongoing task. This hypothesis would explain why the same regions are active under many different contexts, and it might also help to understand the limited success achieved by brain–machine interfaces (BMIs; for reviews see Baranauskas, 2014; Bensmaia and Miller, 2014).

The large majority of BMI interfaces are aimed at restoring body mobility in patients suffering from motor deficits caused by brain injury, neurologic diseases and limb loss (Bensmaia and Miller, 2014). BMIs record brain signals, decode movement-related information and use these to control external devices (e.g., prosthetic limbs, wheelchairs). Although at present the BMI approach had been fruitful (e.g., Hatsopoulos and Donoghue, 2009) it has also shown several limitations. Patients have to undergo a long period of training before learning how to use the BMIs, and signals extracted from the brain are noisy and difficult to interpret so the error rate is rather high and the response speed is slow. All in all, the guidance of external devices is still far from approximating natural behaviors. This applies to both non-invasive and invasive BMIs. Non-invasive BMIs are mainly based on EEG signals recorded from the scalp. Activity recorded at the scalp level lacks selectivity; it is made up of a mix of signals coming from different cortical regions and thus the amount of useable information conveyed is likely to be too low (Baranauskas, 2014). On the other hand, invasive BMIs employ multiple electrodes surgically inserted into the brain (usually in M1 and/or the somatosensory cortex). Even though the quality of the recorded signals is definitely better, information transfer rate is still not dramatically improved (Baranauskas, 2014). The BMI approach has been shown to reproduce relatively simple behaviors such as two-dimensional center-out reaching tasks (e.g., Wolpaw and McFarland, 2004). Other much more complex tasks, e.g., those entailing suppression of pending actions (Mirabella, 2012), have almost never been tested (but see Ifft et al., 2012). The relatively low degree of success of invasive BMI might be due to the fact that, due to ethical reasons, it has been possible to capture only a very limited amount of the activity of the neural network underling goal-directed actions. However, as stated above, flexible control of behavior can be achieved only through the functional interactions of several brain regions, so it is possible that signals recorded from a limited cortical area fail to provide enough information to reproduce natural movements. To overcome these limitations, it would be necessary to find a way to record simultaneously from several key regions underlying goal-directed actions. Clearly, this is currently not feasible on humans beings, though it could be tested on non-human primates.

Before concluding, I would like to make an important remark: all processes described in the present review, i.e., genesis and suppression of goal-directed actions, do not require either intention, volition, or awareness. These computations can be performed by most animals, and surely by all primates. Not by chance, many of the data described here come from studies on non-human primates. What exactly volition or free will is and how and when it is generated from brain activity is, at best, unclear. There is a consensus around the idea originally proposed by Libet et al. (1983) that the awareness of intention precedes movements by some 100s of milliseconds. Thus, it is possible that the brain generates a action and, only subsequently, some pre-motor processes produce the subjective experience of willing to execute that action, which is perceived as being freely chosen (Hallett, 2007). To overcome the impasse of these findings, Libet (1985) proposed that because awareness of intention precedes movements, our free will should rely on the ability to withhold upcoming actions (see Mirabella, 2007; Haggard, 2008 for reviews). However, it has been shown that action suppression can be implemented unintentionally and unconsciously (see van Gaal et al., 2008). Furthermore, both monkeys (e.g., Mirabella et al., 2011) and rats (e.g., Eagle et al., 2008) can cancel pending movements. It has to be recognized that most studies on action inhibition in humans rely on externally and not on internally triggered stops (see Brass and Haggard, 2007 for an original approach), so further evidence has to be collected before venturing conclusions around the relationship between the veto power and willingness. As Roskies (2010) stated: "*For now, [. . .], the most significant contribution neuroscience has made has been in allowing us to formulate novel questions about the nature of voluntary behavior, and in providing new ways of addressing them.*" I hope that the present review will also help to circumscribe what free will is not.

ACKNOWLEDGMENTS

I thank Maurizio Mattia, Leonardo Chelazzi, and Richard Ridderinkhof for valuable comments and helpful discussions.

REFERENCES

Aron, A. R. (2011). From reactive to proactive and selective control: developing a richer model for stopping inappropriate responses. *Biol. Psychiatry* 69, e55–e68. doi: 10.1016/j.biopsych.2010.07.024

Aron, A. R., Behrens, T. E., Smith, S., Frank, M. J., and Poldrack, R. A. (2007). Triangulating a cognitive control network using diffusion-weighted magnetic resonance imaging (MRI) and functional MRI. *J. Neurosci.* 27, 3743–3752. doi: 10.1523/JNEUROSCI.0519-07.2007

Aron, A. R., Fletcher, P. C., Bullmore, E. T., Sahakian, B. J., and Robbins, T. W. (2003). Stop-signal inhibition disrupted by damage to right inferior frontal gyrus in humans. *Nat. Neurosci.* 6, 115–116. doi: 10.1038/nn1003

Aron, A. R., and Poldrack, R. A. (2006). Cortical and subcortical contributions to stop signal response inhibition: role of the subthalamic nucleus. *J. Neurosci.* 26, 2424–2433. doi: 10.1523/JNEUROSCI.4682-05.2006

Aron, A. R., Robbins, T. W., and Poldrack, R. A. (2014). Inhibition and the right inferior frontal cortex: one decade on. *Trends Cogn. Sci.* 18, 177–185. doi: 10.1016/j.tics.2013.12.003

Band, G. P., van der Molen, M. W., and Logan, G. D. (2003). Horse-race model simulations of the stop-signal procedure. *Acta Psychol. (Amst.)* 112, 105—142. doi: 10.1016/S0001-6918(02)00079-3

Baranauskas, G. (2014). What limits the performance of current invasive brain machine interfaces? *Front. Syst. Neurosci.* 8:68. doi: 10.3389/fnsys.2014.00068

Barraclough, D. J., Conroy, M. L., and Lee, D. (2004). Prefrontal cortex and decision making in a mixed-strategy game. *Nat. Neurosci.* 7, 404–410. doi: 10.1038/nn1209

Bayer, H. M., and Glimcher, P. W. (2005). Midbrain dopamine neurons encode a quantitative reward prediction error signal. *Neuron* 47, 129–141. doi: 10.1016/j.neuron.2005.05.020

Benoit, R. G., and Anderson, M. C. (2012). Opposing mechanisms support the voluntary forgetting of unwanted memories. *Neuron* 76, 450–460. doi: 10.1016/j.neuron.2012.07.025

Bensmaia, S. J., and Miller, L. E. (2014). Restoring sensorimotor function through intracortical interfaces: progress and looming challenges. *Nat. Rev. Neurosci.* 15, 313–325. doi: 10.1038/nrn3724

Bernstein, P. S., Scheffers, M. K., and Coles, M. G. (1995). "Where did I go wrong?" A psychophysiological analysis of error detection. *J. Exp. Psychol. Hum. Percept. Perform.* 21, 1312–1322. doi: 10.1037/0096-1523.21.6.1312

Biran, I., and Chatterjee, A. (2004). Alien hand syndrome. *Arch. Neurol.* 61, 292–294. doi: 10.1001/archneur.61.2.292

Boccardi, E., Della Sala, S., Motto, C., and Spinnler, H. (2002). Utilisation behaviour consequent to bilateral SMA softening. *Cortex* 38, 289–308. doi: 10.1016/S0010-9452(08)70661-0

Bonanni, L., Thomas, A., and Onofrj, M. (2010). Paradoxical kinesia in parkinsonian patients surviving earthquake. *Mov. Disord.* 25, 1302–1304. doi: 10.1002/mds.23075

Bonini, F., Burle, B., Liégeois-Chauvel, C., Régis, J., Chauvel, P., and Vidal, F. (2014). Action monitoring and medial frontal cortex: leading role of supplementary motor area. *Science* 343, 888–891. doi: 10.1126/science.1247412

Botvinick, M., Nystrom, L. E., Fissell, K., Carter, C. S., and Cohen, J. D. (1999). Conflict monitoring versus selection-for-action in anterior cingulate cortex. *Nature* 402, 179–181. doi: 10.1038/46035

Boucher, L., Palmeri, T. J., Logan, G. D., and Schall, J. D. (2007). Inhibitory control in mind and brain: an interactive race model of countermanding saccades. *Psychol. Rev.* 114, 376–397. doi: 10.1037/0033-295X.114.2.376

Brass, M., and Haggard, P. (2007). To do or not to do: the neural signature of self-control. *J. Neurosci.* 27, 9141–9145. doi: 10.1523/JNEUROSCI.0924-07.2007

Bray, S., and O'Doherty, J. (2007). Neural coding of reward-prediction error signals during classical conditioning with attractive faces. *J. Neurophysiol.* 97, 3036–3045. doi: 10.1152/jn.01211.2006

Brown, J. W., and Braver, T. S. (2005). Learned predictions of error likelihood in the anterior cingulate cortex. *Science* 307, 1118–1121. doi: 10.1126/science.1105783

Calton, J. L., Dickinson, A. R., and Snyder, L. H. (2002). Non-spatial, motor-specific activation in posterior parietal cortex. *Nat. Neurosci.* 5, 580–588. doi: 10.1038/nn0602-862

Camille, N., Coricelli, G., Sallet, J., Pradat-Diehl, P., Duhamel, J. R., and Sirigu, A. (2004). The involvement of the orbitofrontal cortex in the experience of regret. *Science* 304, 1167–1170. doi: 10.1126/science.1094550

Chambers, C. D., Bellgrove, M. A., Stokes, M. G., Henderson, T. R., Garavan, H., Robertson, I. H., et al. (2006). Executive "brake failure" following deactivation of human frontal lobe. *J. Cogn. Neurosci.* 18, 444–455. doi: 10.1162/089892906775990606

Chen, X., Scangos, K. W., and Stuphorn, V. (2010). Supplementary motor area exerts proactive and reactive control of arm movements. *J. Neurosci.* 30, 14657–14675. doi: 10.1523/JNEUROSCI.2669-10.2010

Chikazoe, J., Jimura, K., Hirose, S., Yamashita, K., Miyashita, Y., and Konishi, S. (2009). Preparation to inhibit a response complements response inhibition during performance of a stop-signal task. *J. Neurosci.* 29, 15870–15877. doi: 10.1523/JNEUROSCI.3645-09.2009

Churchland, M. M., and Shenoy, K. V. (2007). Delay of movement caused by disruption of cortical preparatory activity. *J. Neurophysiol.* 97, 348–359. doi: 10.1152/jn.00808.2006

Churchland, M. M., Yu, B. M., Ryu, S. I., Santhanam, G., and Shenoy, K. V. (2006). Neural variability in premotor cortex provides a signature of motor preparation. *J. Neurosci.* 26, 3697–3712. doi: 10.1523/JNEUROSCI.3762-05.2006

Cisek, P. (2006). Integrated neural processes for defining potential actions and deciding between them: a computational model. *J. Neurosci.* 26, 9761–9770. doi: 10.1523/JNEUROSCI.5605-05.2006

Cisek, P., and Kalaska, J. F. (2005). Neural correlates of reaching decisions in dorsal premotor cortex: specification of multiple direction choices and final selection of action. *Neuron* 45, 801–814. doi: 10.1016/j.neuron.2005.01.027

Cisek, P., and Kalaska, J. F. (2010). Neural mechanisms for interacting with a world full of action choices. *Annu. Rev. Neurosci.* 33, 269–298. doi: 10.1146/annurev.neuro.051508.135409

Corbetta, M., and Shulman, G. L. (2002). Control of goal-directed and stimulus-driven attention in the brain. *Nat. Rev. Neurosci.* 3, 201–215. doi: 10.1038/nrn755

Coxon, J. P., Stinear, C. M., and Byblow, W. D. (2006). Intracortical inhibition during volitional inhibition of prepared action. *J. Neurophysiol.* 95, 3371–3383. doi: 10.1152/jn.01334.2005

Cui, H., and Andersen, R. A. (2007). Posterior parietal cortex encodes autonomously selected motor plans. *Neuron* 56, 552–559. doi: 10.1016/j.neuron.2007.09.031

Damasio, A. R. (1994). *Descartes' Error: Emotion, Reason, and the Human Brain.* New York: Putman.

De Jong, R., Coles, M. G., Logan, G. D., and Gratton, G. (1990). In search of the point of no return: the control of response processes. *J. Exp. Psychol. Hum. Percept. Perform.* 16, 164–182. doi: 10.1037/0096-1523.16.1.164

Della Sala, S., Marchetti, C., and Spinnler, H. (1991). Right-sided anarchic (alien) hand: a longitudinal study. *Neuropsychologia* 29, 1113–1127. doi: 10.1016/0028-3932(91)90081-I

Eagle, D. M., Baunez, C., Hutcheson, D. M., Lehmann, O., Shah, A. P., and Robbins, T. W. (2008). Stop-signal reaction-time task performance: role of prefrontal cortex and subthalamic nucleus. *Cereb. Cortex* 18, 178–188. doi: 10.1093/cercor/bhm044

Fellows, L. K., and Farah, M. J. (2007). The role of ventromedial prefrontal cortex in decision making: judgment under uncertainty or judgment per se? *Cereb. Cortex* 17, 2669–2674. doi: 10.1093/cercor/bhl176

Forstmann, B. U., van den Wildenberg, W. P. M., and Ridderinkhof, K. R. (2008). Neural mechanisms, temporal dynamics, and individual differences in interference control. *J. Cogn. Neurosci.* 20, 1854–1865. doi: 10.1162/jocn.2008.20122

Freedman, D. J., Riesenhuber, M., Poggio, T., and Miller, E. K. (2002). Visual categorization and the primate prefrontal cortex: neurophysiology and behavior. *J. Neurophysiol.* 88, 929–941.

Freund, T. F., Powell, J. F., and Smith, A. D. (1984). Tyrosine hydroxylase-immunoreactive boutons in synaptic contact with identified striatonigral neurons, with particular reference to dendritic spines. *Neuroscience* 13, 1189–1215. doi: 10.1016/0306-4522(84)90294-X

Fried, I., Katz, A., McCarthy, G., Sass, K. J., Williamson, P., Spencer, S. S., et al. (1991). Functional organization of human supplementary motor cortex studied by electrical stimulation. *J. Neurosci.* 11, 3656–3666.

Fried, I., Mukamel, R., and Kreiman, G. (2011). Internally generated preactivation of single neurons in human medial frontal cortex predicts volition *Neuron* 69, 548–562. doi: 10.1016/j.neuron.2010.11.045

Fries, P. (2005). A mechanism for cognitive dynamics: neuronal communication through neuronal coherence. *Trends Cogn. Sci.* 9, 474–480. doi: 10.1016/j.tics.2005.08.011

Funahashi, S., Bruce, C. J., and Goldman-Rakic, P. S. (1989). Mnemonic coding of visual space in the monkey's dorsolateral prefrontal cortex. *J. Neurophysiol.* 61, 331–349.

Genovesio, A., Brasted, P. J., Mitz, A. R., and Wise, S. P. (2005). Prefrontal cortex activity related to abstract response strategies. *Neuron* 47, 307–320. doi: 10.1016/j.neuron.2005.06.006

Genovesio, A., Brasted, P. J., and Wise, S. P. (2006). Representation of future and previous spatial goals by separate neural populations in prefrontal cortex. *J. Neurosci.* 26, 7305–7316. doi: 10.1523/JNEUROSCI.0699-06.2006

Genovesio, A., Tsujimoto, S., and Wise, S. P. (2012). Encoding goals but not abstract magnitude in the primate prefrontal cortex. *Neuron* 74, 656–662. doi: 10.1016/j.neuron.2012.02.023

Genovesio, A., Wise, S. P., and Passingham, R. E. (2014). Prefrontal-parietal function: from foraging to foresight. *Trends Cogn. Sci.* 18, 72–81. doi: 10.1016/j.tics.2013.11.007

Georgopoulos, A. P., Kalaska, J. F., Caminiti, R., and Massey, J. T. (1982). On the relations between the direction of two-dimensional arm movements and cell discharge in primate motor cortex. *J. Neurosci.* 2, 1527–1537.

Gibson, J. J. (1979). *The Ecological Approach to Visual Perception.* Boston, MA: Houghton-Mifflin.

Glickstein, M., and Stein, J. (1991). Paradoxical movement in Parkinson's disease. *Trends Neurosci.* 14, 480–482. doi: 10.1016/0166-2236(91)90055-Y

Glimcher, P. W., Dorris, M. C., and Bayer, H. M. (2005). Physiological utility theory and the neuroeconomics of choice. *Games Econ. Behav.* 52, 213–256. doi: 10.1016/j.geb.2004.06.011

Grezes, J., and Decety, J. (2002). Does visual perception of object afford action? Evidence from a neuroimaging study. *Neuropsychologia* 40, 212–222. doi: 10.1016/S0028-3932(01)00089-6

Habib, M. (2004). Athymhormia and disorders of motivation in basal ganglia disease. *J. Neuropsychiatry Clin. Neurosci.* 16, 509–524. doi: 10.1176/appi.neuropsych.16.4.509

Haggard, P. (2008). Human volition: towards a neuroscience of will. *Nat. Rev. Neurosci.* 9, 934–946. doi: 10.1038/nrn2497

Hallett, M. (2007). Volitional control of movement: the physiology of free will. *Clin. Neurophysiol.* 118, 1179–1192. doi: 10.1016/j.clinph.2007.03.019

Hanes, D. P., and Schall, J. D. (1996). Neural control of voluntary movement initiation. *Science* 274, 427–430. doi: 10.1126/science.274.5286.427

Hare, T. A., O'Doherty, J., Camerer, C. F., Schultz, W., and Rangel, A. (2008). Dissociating the role of the orbitofrontal cortex and the striatum in the computation of goal values and prediction errors. *J. Neurosci.* 28, 5623–5630. doi: 10.1523/JNEUROSCI.1309-08.2008

Hatsopoulos, N. G., and Donoghue, J. P. (2009). The science of neural interface systems. *Annu. Rev. Neurosci.* 32, 249–266. doi: 10.1146/annurev.neuro.051508.135241

Holroyd, C. B., and Coles, M. G. (2002). The neural basis of human error processing: reinforcement learning, dopamine, and the error-related negativity. *Psychol. Rev.* 109, 679–709. doi: 10.1037/0033-295X.109.4.679

Hoshi, E., Shima, K., and Tanji, J. (2000). Neuronal activity in the primate prefrontal cortex in the process of motor selection based on two behavioral rules. *J. Neurophysiol.* 83, 2355–2373.

Hoshi, E., and Tanji, J. (2000). Integration of target and body-part information in the premotor cortex when planning action. *Nature* 408, 466–470. doi: 10.1038/35044075

Hoshi, E., and Tanji, J. (2002). Contrasting neuronal activity in the dorsal and ventral premotor areas during preparation to reach. *J. Neurophysiol.* 87, 1123–1128.

Humphreys, G. W., and Riddoch, M. J. (2000). One more cup of coffee for the road: object-action assemblies, response blocking and response capture after frontal lobe damage. *Exp. Brain Res.* 133, 81–93. doi: 10.1007/s002210000403

Ifft, P. J., Lebedev, M. A., and Nicolelis, M. A. (2012). Reprogramming movements: extraction of motor intentions from cortical ensemble activity when movement goals change. *Front. Neuroeng.* 5:16. doi: 10.3389/fneng.2012.00016

Jahfari, S., Stinear, C. M., Claffey, M., Verbruggen, F., and Aron, A. R. (2010). Responding with restraint: what are the neurocognitive mechanisms? *J. Cogn. Neurosci.* 22, 1479–1492. doi: 10.1162/jocn.2009.21307

Jahfari, S., Verbruggen, F., Frank, M. J., Waldorp, L. J., Colzato, L., Ridderinkhof, K. R., et al. (2012). How preparation changes the need for top-down control of the basal ganglia when inhibiting premature actions. *J. Neurosci.* 32, 10870–10878. doi: 10.1523/JNEUROSCI.0902-12.2012

Kennerley, S. W., Walton, M. E., Behrens, T. E. J., Buckley, M. J., and Rushworth, M. F. S. (2006). Optimal decision making and the anterior cingulate cortex. *Nat. Neurosci.* 9, 940–947. doi: 10.1038/nn1724

Klaes, C., Westendorff, S., Chakrabarti, S., and Gail, A. (2011). Choosing goals, not rules: deciding among rule-based action plans. *Neuron* 70, 536–548. doi: 10.1016/j.neuron.2011.02.053

Koenigs, M., and Tranel, D. (2007). Irrational economic decision-making after ventromedial prefrontal damage: evidence from the Ultimatum Game. *J. Neurosci.* 27, 951–956. doi: 10.1523/JNEUROSCI.4606-06.2007

Lebedev, M. A., Messinger, A., Kralik, J. D., and Wise, S. P. (2004). Representation of attended versus remembered locations in prefrontal cortex. *PLoS Biol.* 2:e365. doi: 10.1371/journal.pbio.0020365

Lebedev, M. A., and Wise, S. P. (2001). Tuning for the orientation of spatial attention in dorsal premotor cortex. *Eur. J. Neurosci.* 13, 1002–1008. doi: 10.1046/j.0953-816x.2001.01457.x

Li, C. S., Yan, P., Sinha, R., and Lee, T. W. (2008). Subcortical processes of motor response inhibition during a stop signal task. *Neuroimage* 41, 1352–1363. doi: 10.1016/j.neuroimage.2008.04.023

Liakakis, G., Nickel, J., and Seitz, R. J. (2011). Diversity of the inferior frontal gyrus – a meta-analysis of neuroimaging studies. *Behav. Brain Res.* 225, 341–347. doi: 10.1016/j.bbr.2011.06.022

Libet, B. (1985). Unconscious cerebral initiative and the role of conscious will in voluntary action. *Behav. Brain Sci.* 8, 529–566. doi: 10.1017/S0140525X00044903

Libet, B., Gleason, C. A., Wright, E. W., and Pearl, D. K. (1983). Time of conscious intention to act in relation to onset of cerebral activity (readiness-potential). The unconscious initiation of a freely voluntary act. *Brain* 106, 623–642. doi: 10.1093/brain/106.3.623

Lindenberg, R., Uhlig, M., Scherfeld, D., Schlaug, G., and Seitz, R. J. (2012). Communication with emblematic gestures: shared and distinct neural correlates of expression and reception. *Hum. Brain Mapp.* 33, 812–823. doi: 10.1002/hbm.21258

Logan, G. D., and Cowan, W. B. (1984). On the ability to inhibit thought and action: a theory of an act of control. *Psychol. Rev.* 91, 295–327. doi: 10.1037/0033-295X.91.3.295

Logan, G. D., and Irwin, D. E. (2000). Don't look! Don't touch! Inhibitory control of eye and hand movements. *Psychon. Bull. Rev.* 7, 107–112. doi: 10.3758/BF03210728

Loukas, C., and Brown, P. (2004). Online prediction of self-paced hand-movements from subthalamic activity using neural networks in Parkinson's disease. *J. Neurosci. Methods* 137, 193–205. doi: 10.1016/j.jneumeth.2004.02.017

Mattia, M., Pani, P., Mirabella, G., Costa, S., Del Giudice, P., and Ferraina, S. (2013). Heterogeneous attractor cell assemblies for motor planning in premotor cortex. *J. Neurosci.* 33, 11155–11168. doi: 10.1523/JNEUROSCI.4664-12.2013

Mattia, M., Spadacenta, S., Pavone, L., Quarato, P., Esposito, V., Sparano, A., et al. (2012). Stop-event-related potentials from intracranial electrodes reveal a key role of premotor and motor cortices in stopping ongoing movements. *Front. Neuroeng.* 5:12. doi: 10.3389/fneng.2012.00012

Mazzoni, P., Hristova, A., and Krakauer, J. W. (2007). Why don't we move faster? Parkinson's disease, movement vigor, and implicit motivation. *J. Neurosci.* 27, 7105–7116. doi: 10.1523/JNEUROSCI.0264-07.2007

Milner, D., and Goodale, M. (1995). *The Visual Brain in Action.* Oxford: Oxford University press.

Mirabella, G. (2007). Endogenous Inhibition and the neural basis of "free won't." *J. Neurosci.* 27, 13919–13920. doi: 10.1523/JNEUROSCI.4943-07.2007

Mirabella, G. (2012). Volitional inhibition and brain-machine interfaces: a mandatory wedding. *Front. Neuroeng.* 5:20. doi: 10.3389/fneng.2012.00020

Mirabella, G., Bertini, G., Samengo, I., Kilavik, B. E., Frilli, D., Della Libera, C., et al. (2007). Neurons in area V4 of the macaque translate attended features into behaviorally relevant categories. *Neuron* 54, 303–318. doi: 10.1016/j.neuron.2007.04.007

Mirabella, G., Iaconelli, S., Modugno, N., Giannini, G., Lena, F., and Cantore, G. (2013). Stimulation of subthalamic nuclei restores a near normal planning strategy in Parkinson's patients. *PLoS ONE* 8:e62793. doi: 10.1371/journal.pone.0062793

Mirabella, G., Iaconelli, S., Romanelli, P., Modugno, N., Lena, F., Manfredi, M., et al. (2012). Deep brain stimulation of subthalamic nuclei affects arm response inhibition in Parkinson's patients. *Cereb. Cortex* 22, 1124–1132. doi: 10.1093/cercor/bhr187

Mirabella, G., Pani, P., and Ferraina, S. (2008). Context influences on the preparation and execution of reaching movements. *Cogn. Neuropsychol.* 25, 996–1010. doi: 10.1080/02643290802003216

Mirabella, G., Pani, P., and Ferraina, S. (2009). The presence of visual gap affects the duration of stopping process. *Exp. Brain Res.* 192, 199–209. doi: 10.1007/s00221-008-1570-y

Mirabella, G., Pani, P., and Ferraina, S. (2011). Neural correlates of cognitive control of reaching movements in the dorsal premotor cortex of rhesus monkeys. *J. Neurophysiol.* 106, 1454–1466. doi: 10.1152/jn.00995.2010

Mirabella, G., Pani, P., Paré, M., and Ferraina, S. (2006). Inhibitory control of reaching movements in humans. *Exp. Brain Res.* 174, 240–255. doi: 10.1007/s00221-006-0456-0

Montague, P. R., Hyman, S. E., and Cohen, J. D. (2004). Computational roles for dopamine in behavioural control. *Nature* 431, 760–767. doi: 10.1038/nature03015

Murata, A., Fadiga, L., Fogassi, L., Gallese, V., Raos, V., and Rizzolatti, G. (1997). Object representation in the ventral premotor cortex (area F5) of the monkey. *J. Neurophysiol.* 78, 2226–2230.

O'Doherty, J. P., Dayan, P., Friston, K., Critchley, H., and Dolan, R. J. (2003). Temporal difference models and reward-related learning in the human brain. *Neuron* 38, 329–337. doi: 10.1016/S0896-6273(03)00169-7

Padoa-Schioppa, C., and Assad, J. A. (2006). Neurons in the orbitofrontal cortex encode economic value. *Nature* 441, 223–226. doi: 10.1038/nature04676

Padoa-Schioppa, C., and Assad, J. A. (2008). The representation of economic value in the orbitofrontal cortex is invariant for changes of menu. *Nat. Neurosci.* 11, 95–102. doi: 10.1038/nn2020

Paradiso, G., Saint-Cyr, J. A., Lozano, A. M., Lang, A. E., and Chen, R. (2003). Involvement of the human subthalamic nucleus in movement preparation. *Neurology* 61, 1538–1545. doi: 10.1212/01.WNL.0000096021.28967.57

Petrides, M., and Pandya, D. N. (1999). Dorsolateral prefrontal cortex: comparative cytoarchitectonic analysis in the human and the macaque brain and corticocortical connection patterns. *Eur. J. Neurosci.* 11, 1011–1136. doi: 10.1046/j.1460-9568.1999.00518.x

Petrides, M., and Pandya, D. N. (2002). Comparative cytoarchitectonic analysis of the human and the macaque ventrolateral prefrontal cortex and corticocortical connection patterns in the monkey. *Eur. J. Neurosci.* 16, 291–310. doi: 10.1046/j.1460-9568.2001.02090.x

Prut, Y., and Fetz, E. E. (1999). Primate spinal interneurons show pre-movement instructed delay activity. *Nature* 401, 590–594. doi: 10.1038/44145

Rangel, A., Camerer, C., and Montague, P. R. (2008). A framework for studying the neurobiology of value-based decision making. *Nat. Rev. Neurosci.* 9, 545–556. doi: 10.1038/nrn2357

Reynolds, J. H., and Chelazzi, L. (2004). Attentional modulation of visual processing. *Annu. Rev. Neurosci.* 27, 611–647. doi: 10.1146/annurev.neuro.26.041002.131039

Ridderinkhof, K. R., Forstmann, B. U., Wylie, S. A., Burle, B., and van den Wildenberg, W. P. M. (2011). Neurocognitive mechanisms of action control: resisting the call of the sirens. *Cogn. Sci.* 2, 174–192. doi: 10.1002/wcs.99

Ridderinkhof, K. R., and van den Wildenberg, W. P. (2005). Adaptive coding. *Science* 307, 1059–1060. doi: 10.1126/science.1109837

Ridderinkhof, K. R., van den Wildenberg, W. P., Segalowitz, S. J., and Carter, C. S. (2004). Neurocognitive mechanisms of cognitive control: the role of prefrontal cortex in action selection, response inhibition, performance monitoring, and reward-based learning. *Brain Cogn.* 56, 129–140. doi: 10.1016/j.bandc.2004.09.016

Riehle, A., and Requin, J. (1989). Monkey primary motor and premotor cortex: single-cell activity related to prior information about direction and extent of an intended movement. *J. Neurophysiol.* 61, 534–549.

Rizzolatti, G., and Craighero, L. (2004). The mirror-neuron system. *Annu. Rev. Neurosci.* 27, 169–192. doi: 10.1146/annurev.neuro.27.070203.144230

Rizzolatti, G., and Luppino, G. (2001). The cortical motor system. *Neuron* 31, 889–901. doi: 10.1016/S0896-6273(01)00423-8

Roskies, A. L. (2010). How does neuroscience affect our conception of volition? *Annu. Rev. Neurosci.* 33, 109–130. doi: 10.1146/annurev-neuro-060909-153151

Scangos, K. W., and Stuphorn, V. (2010). Medial frontal cortex motivates but does not control movement initiation in the countermanding task. *J. Neurosci.* 30, 1968–1982. doi: 10.1523/JNEUROSCI.4509-09.2010

Schall, J. D., and Godlove, D. C. (2012). Current advances and pressing problems in studies of stopping. *Curr. Opin. Neurobiol.* 22, 1012–1021. doi: 10.1016/j.conb.2012.06.002

Scherberger, H., and Andersen, R. A. (2007). Target selection signals for arm reaching in the posterior parietal cortex. *J. Neurosci.* 27, 2001–2012. doi: 10.1523/JNEUROSCI.4274-06.2007

Schlesinger, I., Erikh, I., and Yarnitsky, D. (2007). Paradoxical kinesia at war. *Mov. Disord.* 22, 2394–2397. doi: 10.1002/mds.21739

Schmidt, L., d'Arc, B. F., Lafargue, G., Galanaud, D., Czernecki, V., Grabli, D., et al. (2008). Disconnecting force from money: effects of basal ganglia damage on incentive motivation. *Brain* 131, 1303–1310. doi: 10.1093/brain/awn045

Schultz, W., Dayan, P., and Montague, P. R. (1997). A neural substrate of prediction and reward. *Science* 275, 1593–1599. doi: 10.1126/science.275.5306.1593

Shenoy, K. V., Sahani, M., and Churchland, M. M. (2013). Cortical control of arm movements: a dynamical systems perspective. *Annu. Rev. Neurosci.* 36, 337–359. doi: 10.1146/annurev-neuro-062111-150509

Sheth, S. A., Mian, M. K., Patel, S. R., Asaad, W. F., Williams, Z. M., Dougherty, D. D., et al. (2012). Human dorsal anterior cingulate cortex neurons mediate ongoing behavioural adaptation. *Nature* 488, 218–221. doi: 10.1038/nature11239

Singer, T., Seymour, B., O'Doherty, J., Kaube, H., Dolan, R. J., and Frith, C. D. (2004). Empathy for pain involves the affective but not sensory components of pain. *Science* 303, 1157–1162. doi: 10.1126/science.1093535

Smith, P. L., and Ratcliff, R. (2004). Psychology and neurobiology of simple decisions. *Trends Neurosci.* 27, 161–168. doi: 10.1016/j.tins.2004.01.006

Smith, Y., Bennett, B. D., Bolam, J. P., Parent, A., and Sadikot, A. F. (1994). Synaptic relationships between dopaminergic afferents and cortical or thalamic input in the sensorimotor territory of the striatum in monkey. *J. Comp. Neurol.* 344, 1–19. doi: 10.1002/cne.903440102

Stevenson, S. A., Elsley, J. K., and Corneil, B. D. (2009). A "gap effect" on stop signal reaction times in a human saccadic countermanding task. *J. Neurophysiol.* 101, 580–590. doi: 10.1152/jn.90891.2008

Sumner, P., Nachev, P., Morris, P., Jackson, S. R., Kennard, C., and Husain, M. (2007). Human medial frontal cortex mediates unconscious inhibition of voluntary action. *Neuron* 54, 697–711. doi: 10.1016/j.neuron.2007.05.016

Swann, N., Poizner, H., Houser, M., Gould, S., Greenhouse, I., Cai, W., et al. (2011). Deep brain stimulation of the subthalamic nucleus alters the cortical profile of response inhibition in the beta frequency band: a scalp EEG study in Parkinson's disease. *J. Neurosci.* 31, 5721–5729. doi: 10.1523/JNEUROSCI.6135-10.2011

Swann, N., Tandon, N., Canolty, R., Ellmore, T. M., McEvoy, L. K., Dreyer, S., et al. (2009). Intracranial EEG reveals a time-and frequency-specific role for the right inferior frontal gyrus and primary motor cortex in stopping initiated responses. *J. Neurosci.* 29, 12675–12685. doi: 10.1523/JNEUROSCI.3359-09.2009

Tanji, J., and Evarts, E. V. (1976). Anticipatory activity of motor cortex neurons in relation to direction of an intended movement. *J. Neurophysiol.* 39, 1062–1068.

Tsujimoto, S., Genovesio, A., and Wise, S. P. (2010). Evaluating self-generated decisions in frontal pole cortex of monkeys. *Nat. Neurosci.* 13, 120–126. doi: 10.1038/nn.2453

Tsujimoto, S., Genovesio, A., and Wise, S. P. (2011). Frontal pole cortex: encoding ends at the end of the endbrain. *Trends Cogn. Sci.* 15, 169–176. doi: 10.1016/j.tics.2011.02.001

Turner, R. S., and Desmurget, M. (2010). Basal ganglia contributions to motor control: a vigorous tutor. *Curr. Opin. Neurobiol.* 20, 704–716. doi: 10.1016/j.conb.2010.08.022

Uddén, J., and Bahlmann, J. (2012). A rostro-caudal gradient of structured sequence processing in the left inferior frontal gyrus. *Philos. Trans. R. Soc. Lond. B Biol. Sci.* 367, 2023–2032. doi: 10.1098/rstb.2012.0009

Van den Wildenberg, W. P., van Boxtel, G. J., van der Molen, M. W., Bosch, D. A., Speelman, J. D., and Brunia, C. H. (2006). Stimulation of the subthalamic region facilitates the selection and inhibition of motor responses in Parkinson's disease. *J. Cogn. Neurosci.* 18, 626–636. doi: 10.1162/jocn.2006.18.4.626

van Gaal, S., Ridderinkhof, K. R., Fahrenfort, J. J., Scholte, H. S., and Lamme, V. A. (2008). Frontal cortex mediates unconsciously triggered inhibitory control. *J. Neurosci.* 28, 8053–8062. doi: 10.1523/JNEUROSCI.1278-08.2008

van Gaal, S., Scholte, H. S., Lamme, V. A., Fahrenfort, J. J., and Ridderinkhof, K. R. (2011). Pre-SMA graymatter density predicts individual differences in action selection in the face of conscious and unconscious response conflict *J. Cogn. Neurosci.* 23, 382–390. doi: 10.1162/jocn.2010.21444

Verbruggen, F., and Logan, G. D. (2009). Proactive adjustments of response strategies in the stop-signal paradigm. *J. Exp. Psychol. Hum. Percept. Perform.* 35, 835–854. doi: 10.1037/a0012726

von der Malsburg, C., Phillips, W. A., and Singer, W. (2010). *Dynamic Coordination in the Brain: From Neurons to Mind.* Cambridge, MA: The MIT Press. doi: 10.7551/mitpress/9780262014717.001.0001

Wallis, J. D. (2007). Orbitofrontal cortex and its contribution to decision-making. *Annu. Rev. Neurosci.* 30, 31–56. doi: 10.1146/annurev.neuro.30.051606.094334

Weinrich, M., Wise, S. P., and Mauritz, K. H. (1984). A neurophysiological study of the premotor cortex in the rhesus monkey. *Brain* 107, 385–414. doi: 10.1093/brain/107.2.385

Wise, S. P. (2008). Forward frontal fields: phylogeny and fundamental function. *Trends Neurosci.* 31, 599–608. doi: 10.1016/j.tins.2008.08.008

Wise, S. P., Weinrich, M., and Mauritz, K. H. (1983). Motor aspects of cue-related neuronal activity in premotor cortex of the rhesus monkey. *Brain Res.* 260, 301–305. doi: 10.1016/0006-8993(83)90685-6

Wolpaw, J. R., and McFarland, D. J. (2004). Control of a two-dimensional movement signal by a noninvasive brain-computer interface in humans. *Proc. Natl. Acad. Sci. U.S.A.* 101, 17849–17854. doi: 10.1073/pnas.0403504101

Wolpert, D. M., and Miall, R. C. (1996). Forward models for physiological motor control. *Neural Netw.* 9, 1265–1279. doi: 10.1016/S0893-6080(96)00035-4

Zandbelt, B. B., Bloemendaal, M., Neggers, S. F., Kahn, R. S., and Vink, M. (2013). Expectations and violations: delineating the neural network of proactive inhibitory control. *Hum. Brain Mapp.* 34, 2015–2024. doi: 10.1002/hbm.22047

Zandbelt, B. B., and Vink, M. (2010). On the role of the striatum in response inhibition. *PLoS ONE* 5:e13848. doi: 10.1371/journal.pone.0013848

Zheng, D., Oka, T., Bokura, H., and Yamaguchi, S. (2008). The key locus of common response inhibition network for nogo and stop signals. *J. Cogn. Neurosci.* 20, 1–9. doi: 10.1162/jocn.2008.20100

21

When "altering brain function" becomes "mind control"

Andrew Koivuniemi[1]* and Kevin Otto[2,3]

[1] *Indiana University School of Medicine, Indianapolis, IN, USA*
[2] *Weldon School of Biomedical Engineering, Purdue University, West Lafayette, IN, USA*
[3] *J. Crayton Pruitt Family Department of Biomedical Engineering, University of Florida, Gainesville, FL, USA*

Edited by:
Mikhail Lebedev, Duke University, USA

Reviewed by:
Mikhail Lebedev, Duke University, USA
Brian D. Earp, University of Oxford, UK
Jan-Hendrik Heinrichs, Forschungszentrum Jülich, Germany

****Correspondence:***
Andrew Koivuniemi, Indiana University School of Medicine, 340 W 10th Street, Indianapolis, IN 46202, USA
e-mail: akoivuni@iupui.edu

Functional neurosurgery has seen a resurgence of interest in surgical treatments for psychiatric illness. Deep brain stimulation (DBS) technology is the preferred tool in the current wave of clinical experiments because it allows clinicians to directly alter the functions of targeted brain regions, in a reversible manner, with the intent of correcting diseases of the mind, such as depression, addiction, anorexia nervosa, dementia, and obsessive compulsive disorder. These promising treatments raise a critical philosophical and humanitarian question. "Under what conditions does 'altering brain function' qualify as 'mind control'?" In order to answer this question one needs a definition of mind control. To this end, we reviewed the relevant philosophical, ethical, and neurosurgical literature in order to create a set of criteria for what constitutes mind control in the context of DBS. We also outline clinical implications of these criteria. Finally, we demonstrate the relevance of the proposed criteria by focusing especially on serendipitous treatments involving DBS, i.e., cases in which an unintended therapeutic benefit occurred. These cases highlight the importance of gaining the consent of the subject for the new therapy in order to avoid committing an act of mind control.

Keywords: philosophy of mind, ethics, neurosurgery, deep brain stimulation, psychiatry

INTRODUCTION

The use of deep brain stimulation (DBS) technology for the treatment of psychiatric disorders is one of the most promising and rapidly evolving areas of neurosurgical research (Abelson et al., 2005; Mayberg et al., 2005; Lozano and Lipsman, 2013). Nonetheless, in treating diseases of the mind by directly altering the brain's functioning, neurosurgeons, neurologists, psychiatrists, and neuro-engineers run the risk of having this effort interpreted as "mind control". The purpose of this paper is to address that specific concern in the context of DBS as it is currently practiced and studied by providing a definition of "mind control" that applies to DBS. That is, it is not intended to account for the neurosurgeons staffing the wards of philosophical thought experiments, whose powers to monitor and manipulate the brain and their patients' actions know no limits (Frankfurt, 1969). Therefore, this paper seeks to cover adult patients who have given informed consent for the treatment of their psychiatric or neurologic illness.

By narrowing the scope of the article, we hope to maximize its relevance while minimizing distracting (though philosophically interesting) cases. It is important to point out that the conditions under discussion (adults, undergoing treatment, who are capable of informed consent—including patients in states such as locked-in syndrome) describe nearly all individuals currently receiving DBS with the exception of those treated for persistent vegetative state who lack the capacity to do anything, including the ability to provide consent (Yamamoto et al., 2010).

While the phrase "mind control" appears in the contemporary literature discussing advances in DBS, it is often brought up dismissively (Fins et al., 2009) or to catch the reader's attention (Horgan, 2004) but never with an accompanying formal definition. This is surprising, especially given a sophisticated and robust ethics literature on DBS and psychiatry that deals with related topics such as autonomy and informed consent (Bell et al., 2009; Clausen, 2010), authenticity (Kraemer, 2013), enhancement (Earp et al., 2014), and paternalism (Sjöstrand and Juth, 2014) as well as unintended side effects of stimulation which alter personality (Synofzik and Schlaepfer, 2008) and the way in which DBS can influence patients' perceptions of their identity (Lipsman et al., 2009). Common features in this literature are an agreement that autonomy is one of the key features that must be preserved in the ethical practice of DBS and that this can been accomplished in psychiatric patients through the practice of informed consent (Dunn et al., 2011).

Beyond the contemporary neuro-ethics literature, mind control has been the subject of numerous books and articles. One of the most thorough accounts of mind control in the context of electrical stimulation of the human mind appears in Elliot Valenstein's aptly titled *Brain Control* (Valenstein, 1973). While Valenstein never supplies a formal definition of mind control, his primary argument focuses on discrediting the notion that a subject's thoughts, choices or actions could be manipulated through electrical stimulation of the brain by giving a detailed account of its known capabilities and limitations. Other discussions of mind control tend to have focused on psychopharmacologic methods or behavioral methods of altering brain function, such as those employed in the Central Intelligence Agency's MKULTRA program (Senate, 1977).

Possibly the richest source of accounts of mind control is not in the formal academic literature but in the online accounts of individuals who claim to have witnessed acts of mind control or who claim to be the target of mind control. In 2006 Bell et al. provided a formal textual analysis of 10 characteristic examples. Though the authors make it clear that they take these narratives as signs of a delusional disorder and their analysis focused primarily on the social network of the reports, they managed to highlight several themes which the accounts shared. These shared features help to establish an intuitive basis for what people believe qualifies as mind control. The accounts often focused on: (1) an authoritarian organization, such as "the police," "the Dutch government," or "freemasonic intelligence agencies;" (2) employing some tool to augment brain function, such as a "frequency weapon," "brain implant" or "network of transmitters," in order to; (3) alter the subject's thoughts or actions; (4) without the subjects consent.

In proposing our criteria for mind control we retained and formalized all of the common themes of the internet accounts with the exception of the authoritarian organization. The authoritarian element was dropped because the authors saw no reason to exclude individuals acting alone from being capable of committing an act of mind control. This is especially true in the context of DBS where typically only one person or a few people are responsible for the management of the treatment. Therefore, we are proposing the phrase "mind control" be used to describe instances when researchers or clinicians using DBS intentionally alter patients' behavior without consent and define those instances using the criteria below.

After stating our formal criteria, we explain why the criteria are limited to the subject's behavior and neutral with regards to the subject's mental events during the act of mind control. Then we provide test cases, which we argue intuitively do and do not qualify as mind control and are correctly included and excluded by the proposed criteria respectively. Next, we apply the criteria to a non-obvious case of mind control. Finally, we conclude with a discussion of mind control in the context of serendipitous therapy, i.e., cases where an individual sees a therapeutic effect for a psychiatric illness for which he or she did not give consent to have treated, such as in a patient treated with DBS for anxiety who saw a remission of his alcoholism. We argue that in such cases one should gain the individual's explicit consent for the treatment of the serendipitously improved comorbid illness or else one would qualify as committing an act of mind control.

CRITERIA OF MIND CONTROL

Alteration of the brain's functioning through direct stimulation (either activation or suppression of action potentials) within the subject's brain qualifies as mind control when it meets all of the following three criteria:

Result Criterion: Direct alteration of the brain's function must result in a behavioral change in the subject.

Consent Criterion: The behavioral change does not need to be against the expressed will of the patient. The change must simply have taken place without the subject's consent.

Intent Criterion: The behavioral change must have been the goal or the purpose of the person or the group controlling the DBS. It cannot be an accident or an unintended consequence, including side effects, of the stimulation.

In summary, mind control must alter the patient's behavior in an observable way without the subject's consent and must be enacted for that purpose.

LIMITING MIND TO BEHAVIOR

The above criteria rest on an assumption that the ultimate purpose of "mind control" is to modify the behavior of an individual, and the word "mind" is used in a folk psychology manner to describe the intuitive mechanism of the control (Dennett, 1982). It is important to spell out the definition of "mind control" in the context of behavior because that is the relevant way DBS is currently employed. This is because neurosurgeons and neurologists cannot make perfectly reliable *a priori* guesses about what effect a given instance of DBS will have on a given patient. They must therefore rely entirely on their observations of the patients' behaviors, which include their patients' reports.

To understand this point, consider that neurosurgeons have a great deal of information about what parts of the brain are associated with certain faculties, such as the formation and comprehension of speech, sensation of touch over the body, execution of intended movement, and sight. Further, they know that the destruction of these regions will leave the patient with a deficit so protecting them during surgery is one of the surgeon's highest priorities. However, the surgeons cannot predict exactly where these regions are located in specific patients based on previous studies alone (Penfield and Perot, 1963; Kim et al., 2009). Therefore, some neurosurgical cases are performed with the patient awake so that he or she can report the sensations he or she experiences when the neurosurgeon applies electric current to the brain region of interest. Based on the patient's reports, the surgeon will individualize his approach in order to resect the pathological tissue while sparing the functionally important, so called eloquent, cortex. If the procedure were performed without the patient's behavioral feedback there would be a very high probability that an important cortical region would be damaged leaving the patient with a neurological deficit (Penfield and Boldrey, 1937).

The same type of procedure is also essential to the practice of DBS. For example patients must be closely observed intraoperatively for behavioral signs, such as a reflexive smile, in order for the surgical team to determine the effect of stimulation (Okun et al., 2004; Haq et al., 2011). Once the electrode and stimulator are implanted, specially trained neurologists adjust the stimulation parameters and closely observe the effect on the patient's symptoms (Volkmann et al., 2006). Finally, patients must be closely followed during treatment for signs of cognitive decline (Parsons et al., 2006), mood disorders (Bejjani et al., 1999; Kulisevsky et al., 2002), or other, sometimes serendipitous, behavioral changes (Kuhn et al., 2007). In summary, the use of DBS relies entirely on the patient's behavior as the sole feedback mechanism for targeting the electrode as well for modifying the stimulation parameters in order to achieve the desired effect. Because the person or persons controlling the DBS rely on observation of behavior, any instance of mind control using DBS would necessarily rely entirely on the subject's behavior. Therefore, a practical definition of mind control can be limited solely to behavior without directly addressing metaphysical questions related to the mind itself.

OBVIOUS TEST CASES

Having proposed the criteria for mind control, it is important to test them. This is best done by asking whether the criteria account for cases of obvious mind control while excluding cases that are obviously not mind control.

For a clear example of mind control, we must (fortunately) look beyond the current practice of DBS into its murkier past. One such case was published in 1963 in the journal *Science* by a psychosurgery group working under Dr. Robert Heath at Tulane University (Bishop et al., 1963). This article detailed a "self-stimulation" experiment in which a 35 year old man was implanted with electrodes in eight different brain structures, including in the head of the caudate, the septal area, and the amygdala. These electrodes were labeled by researchers as either "rewarding" or "aversive" and the subject was given a lever and a button which, when operated, would activate one of the electrodes. As the experiment proceeded, the researchers varied the electrodes which the lever and button activated and also varied the stimulation parameters delivered through the electrodes.

This experiment was based on studies previously done in rats, cats, dogs, goats, monkeys, and bottle nosed dolphins (Olds, 1962) which had shown that the animals' behavior could be predictably controlled by placing stimulating electrodes into "rewarding" and "aversive" regions of the brain and then correlating stimulation through the electrodes to elements of the animals' environment. Therefore, the researchers had good reason to anticipate specific behavioral responses in the human subject. Further, at no point do the authors say that the subject, who was referred to as "clearly nonnormal," gave consent for the experiment or understood why the experiment was conducted.

Looking back to the proposed criteria for mind control, we see that this case satisfies all three. First, electrical stimulation of the brain was employed in a manner that clearly influenced the subject's behavior, satisfying the *Result Criterion*. Second, at no point did the authors state that the patient gave consent to have his behavior manipulated in this manner, satisfying the *Consent Criterion*. Finally, the behavior change was anticipated by the researchers controlling the stimulation of the subject's brain, satisfying the *Intent Criterion*.

Next, we must ask is there an example of altering brain function which obviously is not mind control and, also, is correctly excluded by the *Result, Consent*, and *Intent Criteria*? Consider the treatment of essential tremor with DBS. It is safe, effective, and has been approved by the FDA (Koller et al., 2001). It is believed to work through altering the function of the brain (more specifically by causing a reversible, functional lesion (Grill et al., 2004) in a malfunctioning part of the brain), ultimately permitting the patient to accomplish routine daily activities free from the violent hand tremors that are the hallmark of the disease. This relief of symptoms is the direct result of the electrical pulses in the brain, which alter its standard pattern of firing; however, it is not an instance of mind control.

Why is DBS for the treatment of essential tremor not an example of mind control? After all, it could be argued that one is altering the behavior of the patient's hands, from a tremulous grasp to a stable grip, and that this was explicitly the purpose of the individual programing the DBS device. However, while this example meets the requirements of the *Result Criterion* as well as the *Intent Criterion*, it fails to meet the *Consent Criterion* because in all cases of DBS for essential tremor, all patients give consent for stimulation with the explicit desire to see this behavioral change. Interestingly, DBS for essential tremor could be thought of as "mind freedom," as opposed to "mind control" because, instead of preventing the patient from carrying out a desired behavior or forcing an undesired behavior, it allows the patient to act on his choices with less difficulty.

The same argument also holds for DBS treatments of psychiatric diseases like depression (Lozano et al., 2008). One might make the argument that being a psychiatric disease, depression is classically described as a disease of the mind. Therefore, if one can control the patient's disease one must be controlling the patient's mind, i.e., committing an act of mind control. The proposed criteria would exclude this case of mind control because, as in the case of DBS for the treatment of essential tremor, the effect on the patient was with the patient's consent, and, thus, it fails the *Consent Criterion*.

NON-OBVIOUS TEST CASE

While it is important that the criteria capture one's intuition, they should also go beyond and clarify murkier territory. The criteria should be able to help one examine non-obvious cases and arrive at a reasoned judgment about their status as mind control or as non-mind control. Thus, the criteria above are especially useful when attempting to identify borderline instances of mind control.

Turning again to the past, consider the following case of an experiment conducted by Jose Delgado and his collaborators Drs. Obrador and Martin-Rodriguez into the stimulation of the caudate nucleus of an epileptic patient:

> As shown by direct observation and by analysis of the record, within 30 s after application of caudate stimulation there was a significant change in the patient's mood. During controls, he was reserved, his conversation was limited and he was concerned about his illness. After caudate stimulation, his spontaneous verbalization increased more than twofold and contained expressions of friendliness and euphoric behavior which culminated in jokes and loud singing in a gay *cante jondo* style, accompanied by tapping with his right hand, which lasted for about 2 min. The euphoria continued for about 10 min and then the patient gradually reverted to his usual, more reserved attitude. This increase in friendliness was observed following three different stimulation sessions of the caudate, and did not appear when other areas were tested (Valenstein, 1973).

In the above description, the researchers are attempting to correct the patient's epilepsy with the use of electrical current. In testing one of their hypothesized targets, they managed to elicit a strong behavioral effect. The patient's attitude changed from quiet reserve to expressive joviality, i.e., the researchers significantly altered the patient's behavior and in doing so satisfied the *Result Criterion*, as well as the *Consent Criterion* because they did not have the patient's consent to alter his behavior in this manner. At this point one could argue, correctly, that this was an accident. The experimenters had no *a priori* knowledge that the patient would respond to stimulation in this fashion so it could not have been their intention to do so; thus, they failed to satisfy the *Intent Criterion*.

The essential issue arose when the stimulation was repeated, three different times, without any documentation that the patient wanted to have his personality manipulated in this manner. While this might, at first, seem like nit picking, it is important to appreciate that the experimenters now had reason to believe that the behavior of the individual would be affected in a specific way. When they activated the stimulation and produced the anticipated effect, it was purposeful. In this way, the experimenters fulfilled the *Intent Criterion*. As in the case of a schizophrenic patient subjected to the self-stimulation experiment above, it seems clear that the researchers' motivation was intellectual curiosity and not malice. Nevertheless, both of these cases demonstrate that malice is not necessary for mind control.

SERENDIPITY AND MIND CONTROL

The above case raises a critical question with regard to several recently published studies in which subjects received DBS in an effort to treat one illness, but instead saw serendipitous improvement in a comorbid psychiatric illness. One serendipitous discovery was reported by Kuhn et al. (2007) who attempted to treat a man with anxiety disorder by placing DBS electrodes into his nucleus accumbens, a major component in the reward circuit of the mammalian brain. While the patient's anxiety did not improve, he did see significant remission in his alcohol dependency, leading the group to propose the target as a potential treatment for alcoholism and addiction.

A second example comes from Hamani et al. (2008) who used DBS of the hypothalamus in an effort to help control a patient with morbid obesity. Although the patient continued to gain weight (a fact left out of the primary article and only included in the online supplemental materials) he did experience a flashback while receiving intra-operative test stimulation. This led the researchers to do a battery of studies to determine if stimulation to the same area at a lower level, which did not cause a flashback, could improve memory. To the surprise of the researchers, they found a significant increase in the subject's verbal memory. Based on this finding the authors proposed the anterior fornix (a structure adjacent to the hypothalamus) as a target for the treatment of dementia and began enrolling patients to study it further.

Finally, Israël et al. (2010) describes a case in which a woman was receiving DBS of the subgenual cingulate gyrus (Cg25) for treatment of depression. The authors noted that, although the patient continued to have relapses of major depression, she stopped experiencing symptoms related to a significant comorbid anorexia nervosa. Based on the remarkable improvement the patient experienced, despite her less remarkable improvement for her depression, the authors proposed Cg25 as a target for the treatment of anorexia nervosa.

There are several curious similarities among the cases above. First, the intended effect of DBS was either not seen or was not particularly robust. Second, the serendipitous effect on the comorbid illness (or enhancement of normal faculties in the case of anterior fornix stimulation for memory) was remarkable. Third, based on these cases all authors proposed that the stimulated sites be tested as targets for monotherapy for the responding illness. A final common feature was that at no point did the authors describe the patient receiving informed consent for the managing of the comorbid illness or for enhancing the patient's faculties (Earp et al., 2014), with DBS. The only paper that commented on informed consent was Hamani et al. which stated:

> The procedure was approved by the University Health Network Research Ethics Board, and written informed consent was obtained under the guidance of a hospital ethicist, who served as a consent monitor. The basis of the approval for this man was the refractory nature of the obesity, the exhaustion of reasonable therapeutic alternatives, and the possibility of reducing the health risks of chronic obesity should the intervention prove successful (Hamani et al., 2008).

In the passage above, the authors clearly stated a reasonable approach for obtaining informed consent for the treatment of the patient's obesity. However, they did not describe receiving the patient's consent for the use of DBS in order to enhance his verbal memory. Despite not reporting the patient's informed consent to have his memory augmented, they proceeded to run a battery of tests on the patient's memory function and, furthermore, did not mention discontinuing the treatment once it became apparent that DBS was not effective for the treatment of obesity.

The above cases raises a critical question: were these examples of "mind control"? The patients had unexpected alterations in their behavior and it appears, based on the descriptions of the cases, that the DBS was continued primarily because of these unexpected results. Further, the authors did not report that they repeated the informed consent process for the serendipitous alteration in the patient's behavior. The authors of this paper could conjecture that, once the researchers realized the unexpected effect DBS was having on their patient they consulted with him or her and received his or her blessing to continue therapy. Nonetheless, if they (or others) had not secured the consent of their patients for these new treatment indications, then they would be satisfying the *Result* (behavior change) *Consent* (happening without patient's consent) and *Intent* (behavioral change was the goal of DBS) criteria of mind control. Therefore, it is critical for clinicians and researchers to secure additional consent in the case of serendipitous therapeutic benefit in order to avoid the charge that they are committing an act of mind control.

CONCLUSION

We have argued that DBS is not synonymous with mind control; however, if not appropriately safeguarded, patients can be vic-tims of mind control even without malice on the part of those controlling the stimulation, especially in the case of serendipi-tous treatment of co-morbid psychiatric illnesses. While many instances of mind control are easily identified, there are certain instances where the distinction is more ambiguous. This paper outlines a clear set of criteria to help more effectively and reliably clarify those ambiguous cases. For an act to be considered mind control it must alter the individual's behavior (*Result Criterion*) without his consent (*Consent Criterion*) and this alteration to the behavior of the individual must be the goal of the person or group controlling the alteration (*Intent Criterion*). Relying on the researchers' or clinicians' intuitions alone is not sufficient because those intuitions might easily become clouded such as in the serendipitous discovery of an effect of DBS. It is, therefore, important to note that in cases of serendipitous treatments of psychiatric illness patients also require the explicit consent for the treatment of the co-morbid illness, or else the case would qualify as mind control. It is the intention of the authors to minimize the risk of such accidents by clarifying the underlying concepts.

REFERENCES

Abelson, J. L., Curtis, G. C., Sagher, O., Albucher, R. C., Harrigan, M., Taylor, S. F., et al. (2005). Deep brain stimulation for refractory obsessive-compulsive disorder. *Biol. Psychiatry* 57, 510–516. doi: 10.1016/j.biopsych.2004.11.042

Bejjani, B.-P., Damier, P., Arnulf, I., Thivard, L., Bonnet, A.-M., Dormont, D., et al. (1999). Transient acute depression induced by high-frequency deep-brain stimulation. *N. Engl. J. Med.* 340, 1476–1480. doi: 10.1056/NEJM199905133401905

Bell, E., Mathieu, G., and Racine, E. (2009). Preparing the ethical future of deep brain stimulation. *Surg. Neurol.* 72, 577–586. doi: 10.1016/j.surneu.2009.03.029

Bishop, M. P., Elder, S. T., and Heath, R. G. (1963). Intracranial self-stimulation in man. *Science* 140, 394–396. doi: 10.1126/science.140.3565.394

Clausen, J. (2010). Ethical brain stimulation—neuroethics of deep brain stimulation in research and clinical practice. *Eur. J. Neurosci.* 32, 1152–1162. doi: 10.1111/j.1460-9568.2010.07421.x

Dennett, D. C. (1982). How to study human consciousness empirically or nothing comes to mind. *Synthese* 53, 159–180. doi: 10.1007/bf00484895

Dunn, L. B., Holtzheimer, P. E., Hoop, J. G., Mayberg, H. S., Roberts, L. W., and Appelbaum, P. S. (2011). Ethical issues in deep brain stimulation research for treatment-resistant depression: focus on risk and consent. *AJOB Neurosci.* 2, 29–36. doi: 10.1080/21507740.2010.533638

Earp, B. D., Sandberg, A., Kahane, G., and Savulescu, J. (2014). When is diminishment a form of enhancement? Rethinking the enhancement debate in biomedical ethics. *Front. Syst. Neurosci.* 8:12. doi: 10.3389/fnsys.2014.00012

Fins, J. J., Krames, E., Peckham, P., and Rezai, A. (2009). "Deep brain stimulation: ethical issues in clinical practice and neurosurgical research," in *Neuromodulation*, eds Elliot S. Krames, P. Hunter Peckham and Ali R. Rezai (London: Elsevier), 81–91.

Frankfurt, H. G. (1969). Alternate possibilities and moral responsibility. *J. Philos.* 66, 829–839. doi: 10.2307/2023833

Grill, W. M., Snyder, A. N., and Miocinovic, S. (2004). Deep brain stimulation creates an informational lesion of the stimulated nucleus. *Neuroreport* 15, 1137–1140. doi: 10.1097/00001756-200405190-00011

Hamani, C., McAndrews, M. P., Cohn, M., Oh, M., Zumsteg, D., Shapiro, C. M., et al. (2008). Memory enhancement induced by hypothalamic/fornix deep brain stimulation. *Ann. Neurol.* 63, 119–123. doi: 10.1002/ana.21295

Haq, I. U., Foote, K. D., Goodman, W. G., Wu, S. S., Sudhyadhom, A., Ricciuti, N., et al. (2011). Smile and laughter induction and intraoperative predictors of response to deep brain stimulation for obsessive-compulsive disorder. *Neuroimage* 54, S247–S255. doi: 10.1016/j.neuroimage.2010.03.009

Horgan, J. (2004). The myth of mind control. *Discover* 25, 40–47.

Israël, M., Steiger, H., Kolivakis, T., McGregor, L., and Sadikot, A. F. (2010). Deep brain stimulation in the subgenual cingulate cortex for an intractable eating disorder. *Biol. Psychiatry* 67, e53–e54. doi: 10.1016/j.biopsych.2009.11.016

Kim, S. S., McCutcheon, I. E., Suki, D., Weinberg, J. S., Sawaya, R., Lang, F. F., et al. (2009). Awake craniotomy for brain tumors near eloquent cortex: correlation of intraoperative cortical mapping with neurological outcomes in 309 consecutive patients. *Neurosurgery* 64, 836–846. doi: 10.1227/01.NEU.0000342405.80881.81

Koller, W. C., Lyons, K. E., Wilkinson, S. B., Troster, A. I., and Pahwa, R. (2001). Long-term safety and efficacy of unilateral deep brain stimulation of the thalamus in essential tremor. *Mov. Disord.* 16, 464–468. doi: 10.1002/mds.1089

Kraemer, F. (2013). Me, myself and my brain implant: deep brain stimulation raises questions of personal authenticity and alienation. *Neuroethics* 6, 483–497. doi: 10.1007/s12152-011-9115-7

Kuhn, J., Lenartz, D., Huff, W., Lee, S., Koulousakis, A., Klosterkoetter, J., et al. (2007). Remission of alcohol dependency following deep brain stimulation of the nucleus accumbens: valuable therapeutic implications? *J. Neurol. Neurosurg. Psychiatry* 78, 1152–1153. doi: 10.1136/jnnp.2006.113092

Kulisevsky, J., Berthier, M., Gironell, A., Pascual-Sedano, B., Molet, J., and Parés, P. (2002). Mania following deep brain stimulation for Parkinson's disease. *Neurology* 59, 1421–1424. doi: 10.1212/wnl.59.9.1421

Lipsman, N., Zener, R., and Bernstein, M. (2009). Personal identity, enhancement and neurosurgery: a qualitative study in applied neuroethics. *Bioethics* 23, 375–383. doi: 10.1111/j.1467-8519.2009.01729.x

Lozano, A., and Lipsman, N. (2013). Probing and regulating dysfunctional circuits using deep brain stimulation. *Neuron* 77, 406–424. doi: 10.1016/j.neuron.2013.01.020

Lozano, A. M., Mayberg, H. S., Giacobbe, P., Hamani, C., Craddock, R. C., and Kennedy, S. H. (2008). Subcallosal cingulate gyrus deep brain stimulation for treatment-resistant depression. *Biol. Psychiatry* 64, 461–467. doi: 10.1016/j.biopsych.2008.05.034

Mayberg, H. S., Lozano, A. M., Voon, V., Mcneely, H. E., Seminowicz, D., Hamani, C., et al. (2005). Deep brain stimulation for treatment-resistant depression. *Neuron* 45, 651–660. doi: 10.1016/j.neuron.2005.02.014

Okun, M. S., Bowers, D., Springer, U., Shapira, N. A., Malone, D., Rezai, A. R., et al. (2004). What's in a "smile?" Intra-operative observations of contralateral smiles induced by deep brain stimulation. *Neurocase* 10, 271–279. doi: 10.1080/13554790490507632

Olds, J. (1962). Hypothalamic substrates of reward. *Physiol. Rev.* 42, 554–604.

Parsons, T. D., Rogers, S. A., Braaten, A. J., Woods, S. P., and TrÖster, A. I. (2006). Cognitive sequelae of subthalamic nucleus deep brain stimulation in Parkinson's disease: a meta-analysis. *Lancet Neurol.* 5, 578–588. doi: 10.1016/s1474-4422(06)70475-6

Penfield, W., and Boldrey, E. (1937). Somatic motor and sensory representation in the cerebral cortex of man as studied by electrical stimulation. *Brain* 60, 389–443. doi: 10.1093/brain/60.4.389

Penfield, W., and Perot, P. (1963). The brain's record of auditory and visual experience. A final summary and discussion. *Brain* 86, 595–696. doi: 10.1093/brain/86.4.595

Senate, U. (1977). Select committee on intelligence and subcommittee on health and scientific research of the committee on human resources. Project MKULTRA: the CIA's program of research in behavioral modification. US Government Printing Office, Washington, DC.

Sjöstrand, M., and Juth, N. (2014). Authenticity and psychiatric disorder: does autonomy of personal preferences matter? *Med. Health Care Philos.* 17, 115–122. doi: 10.1007/s11019-013-9509-x

Synofzik, M., and Schlaepfer, T. E. (2008). Stimulating personality: ethical criteria for deep brain stimulation in psychiatric patients and for enhancement purposes. *Biotechnol. J.* 3, 1511–1520. doi: 10.1002/biot.200800187

Valenstein, E. S. (1973). *Brain Control.* New York: John Wiley and Sons.

Volkmann, J., Moro, E., and Pahwa, R. (2006). Basic algorithms for the programming of deep brain stimulation in Parkinson's disease. *Mov. Disord.* 21, S284–S289. doi: 10.1002/mds.20961

Yamamoto, T., Katayama, Y., Kobayashi, K., Oshima, H., Fukaya, C., and Tsubokawa, T. (2010). Deep brain stimulation for the treatment of vegetative state. *Eur. J. Neurosci.* 32, 1145–1151. doi: 10.1111/j.1460-9568.2010.07412.x

22

Using virtual reality to augment perception, enhance sensorimotor adaptation, and change our minds

W. Geoffrey Wright*

Physical Therapy and Bioengineering, Motion Analysis and Perception Laboratory, Temple University, Philadelphia, PA, USA

Edited by:
Mikhail Lebedev, Duke University, USA

Reviewed by:
Christopher K. Rhea, University of North Carolina – Greensboro, USA
Mohammad Al-Amri, Cardiff University, UK

***Correspondence:**
W. Geoffrey Wright, Physical Therapy and Bioengineering, Motion Analysis and Perception Laboratory, 1301 Cecil B. Moore Ave., Ritter Annex, Room 992, Temple University, Philadelphia, PA 19122, USA
e-mail: wrightw@temple.edu

Technological advances that involve human sensorimotor processes can have both intended and unintended effects on the central nervous system (CNS). This mini review focuses on the use of virtual environments (VE) to augment brain functions by enhancing perception, eliciting automatic motor behavior, and inducing sensorimotor adaptation. VE technology is becoming increasingly prevalent in medical rehabilitation, training simulators, gaming, and entertainment. Although these VE applications have often been shown to optimize outcomes, whether it be to speed recovery, reduce training time, or enhance immersion and enjoyment, there are inherent drawbacks to environments that can potentially change sensorimotor calibration. Across numerous VE studies over the years, we have investigated the effects of combining visual and physical motion on perception, motor control, and adaptation. Recent results from our research involving exposure to dynamic passive motion within a visually-depicted VE reveal that short-term exposure to augmented sensorimotor discordance can result in systematic aftereffects that last beyond the exposure period. Whether these adaptations are advantageous or not, remains to be seen. Benefits as well as risks of using VE-driven sensorimotor stimulation to enhance brain processes will be discussed.

Keywords: virtual reality environment, vection, sensorimotor integration, motor adaptation, prism adaptation cross-modal processing, posture control, brain augmentation

INTRODUCTION

The use of technology to augment brain function has a nebulous history, in part, because the term *brain augmentation* can be defined in so many ways. It implies an enhancement of brain function, but how it is measured introduces some uncertainty. To clarify this further, it should be recognized that the function of the brain is nothing short of control of the entire body and all one's experiences, both internal processes and externally-directed actions. Therefore augmenting brain function could include a wide range of easy or difficult to identify enhancements, such as boosting immune system response, improving mood, memory, or perception, optimizing motor control, or increasing sub-optimal function after injury. To make brain augmentation even harder to define, sometimes the only measure we have of its effective implementation is through observation of external behavior.

A simple definition of brain augmentation could be enhancement of sensation, such as the use of spectacles to improve myopia. Most glasses wearers will be familiar with the initial adaptation to a slight magnification and/or shift in close-up visual space that occurs with new glasses. This type of adaptation is even more evident when using light-refracting prism glasses to intentionally shift the visually perceived world. Facilitation of adaptive processes could be considered another form of brain augmentation. For example, prism adaptation has been used to correct strabismus by helping the eyes accomplish perceptual convergence and reducing the angle of squint (Pigassou, 1972). In hemispatial neglect wearing prism glasses can augment the brain's ability to adapt its sensorimotor representation of the external world and reduce the perceptual deficit (Rossetti et al., 1998).

Augmenting brain function by enhancing perception or compensating for a deficit is an area in which virtual reality (VR) technology is also being applied. Similar to prism adaptation, VR technology can be used to alter the egocentric and allocentric representations of the world (Castiello et al., 2004). In this paper, the issue of identifying enhancement in the realm of sensory perception, motor control, and sensorimotor adaptation by using virtual environments (VE) will be reviewed. The sensorimotor and perceptual processes that may cause these changes will be examined while also highlighting the difficulty that goes along with defining, measuring, and quantifying enhancement. Not all changes are enhancement, since some are not adaptive or are accompanied by unwanted degradation of other functions or cause unintended responses.

AUGMENTING PERCEPTION

A fundamental aspect of creating an immersive experience within a VE is in creating a sense of three-dimensionality so that one believes one can move about within the virtual world. A common barrier to this is that one may wish to travel further in the VE than is possible in a limited space (e.g., a flight simulation).

Although the perception of self-motion typically occurs as a result of combined visual and physical motion stimuli, its long been known that visually-induced self-motion perception (i.e., vection) can occur in the absence of actual motion (Mach, 1875; Young et al., 1973; Pavard and Berthoz, 1977; Howard, 1986; Frigon and Delorme, 1992; Harris et al., 2000; Palmisano, 2002; Wright, 2002). However, optic flow when walking about the real world is different than when rotating the eyes or head while the body remains stationary (Gibson, 1954). That our central nervous system (CNS) can accurately detect this difference likely evolved as an essential part of navigating through the world searching for food or mates and avoiding danger. The exact selective pressures that shaped these neural processes can only be inferred, however, its very likely that in the pre-modern world earth-bound species (flightless and terrestrial) were less frequently exposed to the visual-vestibular discordance that occurs during passive motion to which we are often exposed in the modern world (e.g., during any vehicle transport). Although the multiple sensory inputs that occur during self-motion do not always have a prescribed relation, they co-occur with greater probability in certain relations to one another than others. For example, terrestrial animals experience sustained vection (very low frequency) in a direction orthogonal to vertical more frequently than parallel to it. Furthermore, the sensory organs are oriented upright relative to gravity more frequently than inverted. Despite this, it seems there was a strong selective advantage for omnidirectional sensory organs that could be mapped to each other rather flexibly. One need only don a pair of prism glasses to experience visuomotor remapping that makes even a completely inverted world eventually feel "normal" (Stratton, 1896). This sensorimotor lability can be used to induce a compelling sense of immersion in a VE even when sensory inputs are incongruent, sub-threshold, or absent.

The flexible, adaptable sensorimotor integration described above is how the brain's perceptual abilities can be augmented in a VE. For example, self-motion perception can be induced even when sensory input is below threshold. In a VE, the inertial stimulus is often sub-threshold or even absent, yet perception of self-motion is still experienced. In our VE studies, we have tested how this perception is affected by manipulating the concordance of visual and inertial sensory inputs (see **Table 1**; Wright, 2002, 2009; Wright and Glasauer, 2003, 2006; Wright and Schneider, 2009). To enhance the level of immersion, subjects viewed a high-fidelity, realistic visual scene from a first person perspective while wearing a head-mounted display (HMD; Wright et al., 2005, 2006, 2009). To further enhance the perceptual experience, we drew on previously established knowledge about motion perception. The visual system primarily transduces velocity information from the visual stimulus, and is less sensitive to acceleration (Berthoz et al., 1975; Telford et al., 1992; Warren and Kurtz, 1992). Acceleration information is primarily derived from the inertial stimulus, which even in the absence of vision plays an important part of the experience of motion (Wright et al., 2005). Gravitoinertial input resulting from physical motion and background gravity stimulate the vestibular and somatosensory systems (i.e., the graviceptors) which provide linear acceleration

Table 1 | Perceptual and/or motor behavior in immersive VE.

Study	Visual stimulus	Physical stimulus	Instructed response (DV)	Unintended response
Wright and Glasauer (2003)	Static or Roll tilting VE scene	Roll tilt of whole body while sitting	Subjective vertical (joystick/glass orientation)	Motor response depends on type of object wielded even if similar size and weight
Wright et al. (2005)	Up-down translation of VE scene depicting various amplitudes of motion	Up-down whole body translation either matching or mismatching visual amplitude	Subjective estimate of self-motion amplitude	Visual-vestibular weighting not always linear summation
Wright et al. (2009)	Left-right translation of VE scene	Roll tilt of whole body while sitting	Subjective vertical (joystick orientation)	Joystick Translations
Wright and Schneider (2009)	Left-right or up-down translation of VE scene	None	Subjective vertical (joystick orientation)	Joystick Translations
Wright (2009)	Left-right translation of VE scene	Up-down whole body translation of various amplitudes	Subjective estimate of self-motion amplitude	Left-right self-motion perception increased as physical up-down motion increased
Wright et al. (2013)	Left-right translation of VE scene	Fore-aft whole body translation while sitting	Stabilize head (yaw, pitch, roll angular velocity)	Yaw head movement
Wright (2013)	Fore-aft translation of VE scene in 3-walled, earth-fixed cave	Left-right whole-body translation while standing	Maintain balance (center of pressure)	Postural response to visual+physical stimulus. Postural aftereffects during post-adaptation visual stimulation

and rotation information (Guedry, 1974). But like the visual system, there is an overlap in what qualifies as an adequate stimulus, as suggested by the fact that graviceptors may also be sensitive to velocity cues (Jones and Young, 1978). Our investigations suggest that combinations of physical and visual stimulation can result in sensory summation. This can increase how compelling perceived self-motion is when stimuli are matched directionally and temporally (Wright et al., 2005). However, we have also found that perceived self-motion can be enhanced by adding together discordant stimuli, such as by combining physical tilt with visually-depicted translation (Wright et al., 2009). In fact, the "compellingness" of visually-induced self-motion can be enhanced in the direction of the visual stimulus by increasing the amplitude of a discordant inertial input. This is true even if the visual and inertial vectors are 90–180° out of alignment with each other (Wright et al., 2005; Wright, 2009; Ash et al., 2011).

Another contributing factor that augments the VE-user's immersion by enhancing the self-motion experience is predicated on the idea of tilt-translation ambiguity (Young et al., 1984; Parker et al., 1985; Merfeld et al., 2005; Holly et al., 2006). Accurate perception of tilt versus translation is obfuscated in part because gravitational and inertial accelerations are physically indistinguishable, and in part because the adequate stimulus for the visual system is velocity-dependent while the adequate stimulus for graviceptors is acceleration-dependent. Thus, tilt in a gravitational field could conceivably be perceived as translation. However, when multiple sensory inputs are combined, a unified sense of self-motion can be derived. Whether this perception is rotation or translation or some combination of both is, in part, determined by spatial, temporal, and cognitive factors (Wertheim et al., 2001; Wright et al., 2006; Holly and McCollum, 2008; Riecke, 2009). The perception also depends on the independence of the velocity and acceleration vectors. In nature, a positive velocity could be experienced with an infinite number of positive or negative acceleration vectors. This is important because the visual system's velocity-sensitive and the vestibular system's acceleration-sensitive. All these factors contribute to how VE can be used to induce unusual self-motion perceptions, despite the fact that the sensory pattern has never been experienced (Wright, 2009). This fact has been capitalized on by IMAX®-based rides for decades, where an individual can experience compelling self-motion while completely stationary; moreover, the perception can be further enhanced when subtle movements of the theater seat are added.

The phenomenological evidence above suggests that veridical self-motion perception is dependent on the integration of multiple sensory inputs that do not have a prescribed relation to one another. Moreover, perception can be extended beyond the normal limits of the senses by combining sensory inputs in VE to induce non-veridical self-motion perception. A sense of immersion in a VE can be enhanced by the belief that movement within the VE is actually happening. But if the VE is augmenting perception of a "false" reality, does this also alter one's actions? And more importantly, is there a real-world benefit? The first question has been brought up before (Stanney et al., 1998; Cohn et al., 2000) but lately the focus of attention has shifted to the latter question. Many researchers and clinicians have embarked upon systematic investigation of how VR can augment the brain's ability to recover from disease and injury (e.g., Liebermann et al., 2012). In the next sections we delve into these questions, first by determining whether motor behaviors are altered by VE immersion then by looking at sensorimotor adaptation within a VE.

THE PERCEPTION-ACTION LINK IN VE

Perception can be defined as the organization of sensory stimuli (both externally received or internally generated) resulting in a conscious awareness of a phenomenon. Perception and action are tightly linked processes, with the interaction of sensory input and motor output being fundamental to the calibration of fine and gross motor skills. Accurate perception of the body's movements is critical to fine-tuning motor skills. However, there are many examples of dissociations between perception and action (e.g., Goodale and Milner, 1992; Merfeld et al., 2005). Thus, even though perception of self-motion and orientation can be altered in a VE, how it affects motor output has required investigation. In a series of studies, we looked at manual motor control, head stabilization, and postural control while immersed in a VE to evaluate whether the perception-action link reliably occurs in VE.

Much like in the perceptual studies, we tested conditions that combined visually-depicted motion both with and without actual physical motion. Subjects performed a manual motor control task while sitting in a tiltable motion device and viewing a visual depiction of linear translation in an HMD (Wright and Glasauer, 2003, 2006; Wright et al., 2009; Wright and Schneider, 2009). During this VE immersion, subjects were instructed to align a handheld object to the perceived vertical. Perceptual reports confirmed self-translation to be more compelling when physical tilt of the subject was added to the linear visual motion (Wright et al., 2009; Wright and Schneider, 2009). But interestingly, despite being asked only to align the handheld object to vertical, subjects also showed automatic, unconscious translation of the unconstrained arm. These unintended motor actions were entrained with the visually-depicted motion, as if experiencing accelerations due to actual translation (see **Table 1**). Although its been shown that constant velocity visual rotation in a VE can affect the direction of reaching (Cohn et al., 2000; Dvorkin et al., 2009), our findings also revealed that vision could induce vection with both velocity and acceleration components. Automatic motor responses occurred as if a compensatory force was required to counter the illusory acceleration. Moreover, the more compelling the perceived self-motion, the larger the motor response.

We were also interested in determining how VE immersion might affect other motor control processes such as head stabilization (Wright et al., 2013) and whole-body postural control (Wright, 2013). In one study, subjects were exposed to physical accelerations while viewing a directionally discordant visual scene. Significant head stabilization responses were dependent on the direction of visual flow even though visual input was discordant with the physical stimulus (Wright et al., 2013). In another study applying a similar experimental test protocol to investigate posture control, we paired visually-depicted translation in one direction with an orthogonally directed translation of the support surface. This cross-axis stimulation resulted in a postural response in standing humans that showed entrainment with both the visual and the support surface stimuli (Wright, 2013). These findings may not be unexpected, since studies predating VR technology have shown that postural control can be entrained to a visual stimulus by simulating movement of the entire room, when the floor is kept stationary (Lishman and Lee, 1973). Furthermore, the postural response can be influenced by the characteristics of the discordant visual input (Lestienne et al., 1977). If an immersive VE is used the postural response to a visual input can be potentiated even if the input is temporally discordant with surface movement (Keshner et al., 2004). Together these results suggest that VE can be used to induce a motor response to a non-veridical virtual input, even in the presence of a strong destabilizing physical stimulus that requires an appropriate postural response to keep from falling. Thus, VE can cause an unintended postural response leading to instability.

INDUCING SENSORIMOTOR ADAPTATION AND MALADAPTIVE AFTEREFFECTS

To study postural adaptation in VE, we exposed subjects to cross-axis postural stimulation for an extended period of time. By looking for aftereffects, as is often done in prism-adaptation research, we wished to see if the postural response seen during discordant stimulation involved adaption or was simply a transient response that would disappear as soon as one of the stimuli was removed (Wright, 2013). The plasticity of the CNS, which allows discordance to be reduced by sensorimotor re-mapping, is present at birth and plays an essential role in shaping motor development through interaction with the environment (Held and Freedman, 1963). Seminal work on visuospatial adaptation using light-refracting prism glasses dating back a century and a half (von Helmholtz, 1867; Stratton, 1896) has shown us that although neural plasticity may diminish with age, this form of plasticity does not have a critical period; rather to some extent it lasts well into adulthood (Hardt et al., 1971). Therefore, determining whether VE exposure will automatically cause sensorimotor adaptation is important. If one considers VE usage in everyday life, for training purposes, or for rehabilitation, one might expect very large exposure times, which could have long lasting aftereffects.

We exposed standing subjects for an extended period of time (5 min) to the cross-axis stimulation. After the adaptation period, we stopped the dynamic support stimulation while subjects continued to view the same visual translation stimulus as before. What was found in the post-adaptation phase is that subjects indeed showed an aftereffect in the COP, which was rotated as much as 45° from the direction of the visual stimulation. This finding is complementary to the finding which showed sensorimotor adaptation of the vestibulo-ocular reflex (VOR) in monkeys after prolonged pairing of physical rotation with an orthogonally directed optic flow (Wei and Angelaki, 2001). The evidence from our study on humans show that long lasting (>2 min) whole-body sensorimotor adaption can also be induced after prolonged exposure (<5 min) to discordant combinations of inertial and visual stimulation in a VE (Wright, 2013). Preliminary evidence suggests that these adaptations may even last for a few days. Specifically, after a few exposures staggered over multiple days, aftereffects appear immediately upon re-immersion into the VE without requiring a fresh dose of cross-axis adaptation.

This raises the question whether these residual aftereffects seen in healthy individuals who spend extended time in a VE are adaptive in the real world or unwanted aftereffects. Inaccurate automatic motor responses due to recalibration of visual, vestibular, and somatosensory coordination certainly involves a risk. However, for those with a perceptual or motor deficit, VE immersion may move them from a maladaptive state towards an adaptive one. Although this requires further investigation, what is apparent is that VE can be used to facilitate the brain's natural ability to adapt to changes in the sensory environment. In fact, VE-based brain augmentation applications have already begun to appear in clinical applications. They have been used to ameliorate hemi-neglect symptoms by remapping the neglected space (Castiello et al., 2004), thus reducing a perceptual deficit, and improving function.

CONCLUSIONS

The fidelity of immersive VE has increased with amazing speed over the last two decades. One need only play the latest release of any popular first person shooter or sports-themed video game to be astounded by its verisimilitude. Because of the level of immersion one can experience, the question arises as to how quickly our CNS adapts to such simulated reality. More importantly, how robust are these adaptations, not only to the accurate attributes of the manufactured environments, but also to their inaccuracies. Even if visual fidelity such as spatial resolution, update rates, perspective geometry, monocular and binocular cues, et cetera are all perfectly programmed to match reality in a VE, the absence of inertial cues to accompany simulated translation through such environments will affect how the CNS calibrates the perceptuomotor system to these non-veridicalities. In other words, exposure to a VE will automatically cause sensorimotor adaptation, whether desired or not. But hopefully, VE's ability to augment brain functions by enhancing perception, eliciting automatic motor behavior, and inducing sensorimotor adaptation can be applied in useful ways.

Trusting what we can measure as evidence of brain enhancement may not solve the problem of defining brain augmentation, when short-term benefits may accompany long-term deficits. Conversely, long-term enhancements may be overlooked because of a more immediate decrement in brain function that can happen as the brain adapts to or learns a new technology. What can be certain is that benefits from brain augmentation, if understood and applied, can be far-reaching. If used to recover loss of function following neurological damage, brain augmentation can potentially bring function back to healthy levels. The ways in which scientist, technologist, and clinicians are applying VR technology to rehabilitation is already happening and the hopes are that the individuals involved in this collective creative process will have the foresight to exploit the potential of neural plasticity, while recognizing that not all change is good.

ACKNOWLEDGMENTS

This work is supported, in part, by the US Army Medical Research and Materiel Command under Contract No. W81XWH-13-C-0189 (W. Geoffrey Wright).

REFERENCES

Ash, A., Palmisano, S., and Kim, J. (2011). Vection in depth during consistent and inconsistent multisensory stimulation. *Perception* 40, 155–174. doi: 10.1068/p6837

Berthoz, A., Pavard, B., and Young, L. R. (1975). Perception of linear horizontal self-motion induced by peripheral vision (linearvection): basic characteristics and visual-vestibular inter-actions. *Exp. Brain Res.* 23, 471–489. doi: 10.1007/bf00234916

Castiello, U., Lusher, D., Burton, C., Glover, S., and Disler, P. (2004). Improving left hemispatial neglect using virtual reality. *Neurology* 62, 1958–1962. doi: 10.1212/01.wnl.0000128183.63917.02

Cohn, J. V., DiZio, P., and Lackner, J. R. (2000). Reaching during virtual rotation: context specific compensations for expected coriolis forces. *J. Neurophysiol.* 83, 3230–3240.

Dvorkin, A. Y., Kenyon, R. V., and Keshner, E. A. (2009). Effects of roll visual motion on online control of arm movement: reaching within a dynamic virtual environment. *Exp. Brain Res.* 193, 95–107. doi: 10.1007/s00221-008-1598-z

Frigon, J.-Y., and Delorme, A. (1992). Roll, pitch, longitudinal and yaw vection visually induced by optical flow in flight simulation conditions. *Perceptual and Motor Skills* 74, 935–955.

Gibson, J. (1954). The visual perception of objective motion and subjective movement. *Psychol. Rev.* 61, 304–314. doi: 10.1037/h0061885

Goodale, M. A., and Milner, A. D. (1992). Separate visual pathways for perception and action. *Trends Neurosci.* 15, 20–25. doi: 10.1016/0166-2236(92)90344-8

Guedry, F. E. (1974). "Psychophysics of vestibular sensation," *Handbook of Sensory Physiology* (Vol. 6), ed H. H. Kornhuber (New York: Springer-Verlag), 1–154.

Hardt, M. E., Held, R., and Steinbach, M. J. (1971). Adaptation to displaced vision: a change in the central control of sensorimotor coordination. *J. Exp. Psychol.* 89, 229–239. doi: 10.1037/h0031159

Harris, L. R., Jenkin, M., and Zikovitz, D. C. (2000). Visual and non- visual cues in the perception of linear self motion. *Exp. Brain Res.* 135, 12–21. doi: 10.1007/s002210000504

Held, R., and Freedman, S. J. (1963). Plasticity in the human sensorimotor control. *Science* 142, 455–462. doi: 10.1126/science.142.3591.455

Holly, J. E., and McCollum, G. (2008). Constructive perception of self-motion. *J. Vestib. Res.* 18, 249–266.

Holly, J. E., Pierce, S. E., and McCollum, G. (2006). Head tilt-translation combinations distinguished at the level of neurons. *Biol. Cybern.* 95, 311–326.

Howard, I. P. (1986). "The perception of posture, self motion and the visual vertical," in *Sensory Processes and Perception, Handbook of Human Perception and Performance* (Vol. 1), eds K. R. Boff, L. Kaufman and J. P. Thomas (New York: Wiley), 18.1–18.62.

Jones, G. M., and Young, L. R. (1978). Subjective detection of vertical acceleration: a velocity-dependent response? *Acta Otolaryngol.* 85, 45–53. doi: 10.3109/00016487809121422

Keshner, E. A., Kenyon, R. V., and Langston, J. (2004). Postural responses exhibit multisensory dependencies with discordant visual and support surface motion. *J. Vestib. Res.* 14, 307–319.

Lestienne, F., Soechting, J., and Berthoz, A. (1977). Postural readjustments induced by linear motion of visual scenes. *Exp. Brain Res.* 28, 363–384. doi: 10.1007/bf00235717

Liebermann, D. G., Berman, S., Weiss, P. L., and Levin, M. F. (2012). Kinematics of reaching movements in a 2-D virtual environment in adults with and without stroke. *IEEE Trans. Neural Syst. Rehabil. Eng.* 20, 778–787. doi: 10.1109/tnsre.2012.2206117

Lishman, J. R., and Lee, D. N. (1973). The autonomy of visual kinaesthesis. *Perception* 2, 287–294. doi: 10.1068/p020287

Mach, E. (1875). *Grundlinien der Lehre von den Bewegungsempfindungen.* Leipzig: Engelmann.

Merfeld, D. M., Sukyung, P., Gianna-Poulin, C., Black, F. O., and Wood, S. (2005). Vestibular perception and action employ qualitatively different mechanisms. II. VOR and perceptual responses during combined Tilt and Translation. *J. Neurophysiol.* 94, 199–205. doi: 10.1152/jn.00905.2004

Palmisano, S. (2002). Consistent stereoscopic information increases the perceived speed of vection in depth. *Perception* 31, 463–480. doi: 10.1068/p3321

Parker, D. E., Reschke, M. F., Arrott, A. P., Homick, J. L., and Lichtenberg, B. K. (1985). Otolith tilt-translation reinterpretation following prolonged weightlessness: implications for preflight training. *Aviat. Space Environ. Med.* 56, 601–606.

Pavard, B., and Berthoz, A. (1977). Linear acceleration modifies the perceived velocity of a moving visual scene. *Perception* 6, 529–540. doi: 10.1068/p060529

Pigassou, R. (1972). The functional treatment of strabismus. *Can. J. Ophthalmol.* 7, 331–335.

Riecke, B. E. (2009). Cognitive and higher-level contributions to illusory self-motion perception ("vection"): does the possibility of actual motion affect vection? *Jpn. J. Psychon. Sci.* 28, 135–139.

Rossetti, Y., Rode, G., Pisella, L., Farne, A., Li, L., Boisson, D., et al. (1998). Prism adaptation to a rightward optical deviation rehabilitates left hemispatial neglect. *Nature* 395, 166–169. doi: 10.1038/25988

Stanney, K., Salvendy, G., Deisinger, J., DiZio, P., Ellis, S., Ellison, J., et al. (1998). Aftereffects and sense of presence in virtual environments: formulation of a research and development agenda. *Int. J. Hum. Comput. Interact.* 10, 135–187. doi: 10.1207/s15327590ijhc1002_3

Stratton, G. (1896). Some preliminary experiments on vision without inversion of the retinal image. *Psychol. Rev.* 3, 611–617. doi: 10.1037/h0072918

Telford, L., Spratley, J., and Frost, B. J. (1992). Linear vection in the central visual field facilitated by kinetic depth cues. *Perception* 21, 337–349. doi: 10.1068/p210337

von Helmholtz, H. (1867). *Handbuch der physiologischen Optik.* Leipzig: Voss.

Warren, W. H., and Kurtz, K. J. (1992). The role of central and peripheral vision in perceiving the direction of self-motion. *Percept. Psychophys.* 51, 443–454. doi: 10.3758/bf03211640

Wei, M., and Angelaki, D. E. (2001). Cross-axis adaptation of the translational vestibulo-ocular reflex. *Exp. Brain Res.* 138, 304–312. doi: 10.1007/s002210100695

Wertheim, A. H., Mesland, B. S., and Bles, W. (2001). Cognitive suppression of tilt sensations during linear horizontal self-motion in the dark. *Perception* 30, 733–741. doi: 10.1068/p3092

Wright, W. G. (2002). *Human Self-motion Perception During Vertical Linear Oscillation and Virtual Environment Exposure.* PhD Dissertation Waltham, MA: Brandeis University.

Wright, W. G. (2009). Linear vection in virtual environments can be strengthened by discordant inertial input. *Conf. Proc. IEEE Eng. Med. Biol. Soc.* 1157–1160. doi: 10.1109/iembs.2009.5333425

Wright, W. G. (2013). Using virtual reality to induce cross-axis adaptation of postural control: implications for rehabilitation. *IEEE Proc. ICVR2013* 289–294. doi: 10.1109/icvr.2013.6662095

Wright, W. G., Agah, M., Darvish, K., and Keshner, E. A. (2013). Head stabilization shows multisensory dependence on spatiotemporal characteristics of visual and inertial passive stimulation. *IEEE Trans. Neural Syst. Rehabil. Eng.* 21, 191–197. doi: 10.1109/icvr.2011.5971869

Wright, W. G., DiZio, P., and Lackner, J. R. (2005). Vertical linear self-motion perception during virtual visual and inertial stimulation: more than weighted summation of sensory inputs. *J. Vest. Res.* 15, 185–195.

Wright, W. G., DiZio, P., and Lackner, J. R. (2006). Apparent self-motion in two visual contexts: dissociable mechanisms underlie perception. *J. Vest. Res.* 16, 23–28.

Wright, W. G., and Glasauer, S. (2003). Haptic subjective vertical shows context dependence: task and vision play a role during dynamic tilt stimulation. *Ann. N Y Acad. Sci.* 1004, 531–535. doi: 10.1196/annals.1303.069

Wright, W. G., and Glasauer, S. (2006). Subjective somatosensory vertical during dynamic tilt is dependent on task, inertial condition and multisensory concordance. *Exp. Brain Res.* 172, 310–321. doi: 10.1007/s00221-006-0347-4

Wright, W. G., and Schneider, E. (2009). Manual motor control during "virtual" self-motion: implications for VR rehabilitation. *IEEE Proc. ICVR2009* 166–172. doi: 10.1109/icvr.2009.5174226

Wright, W. G., Schneider, E., and Glasauer, S. (2009). Compensatory motor responses of object-wielding during combined linear visual and physical roll tilt stimulation. *Exp. Brain Res.* 192, 683–694. doi: 10.1007/s00221-008- 1581-8

Young, L. R., Dichgans, J., Murphy, R., and Brandt, T. (1973). Interaction of optokinetic and vestibular stimuli in motion perception. *Acta Otolaryngol.* 76, 24–31. doi: 10.3109/00016487309121479

Young, L. R., Oman, C. M., Watt, D. G. D., Money, K. E., and Lichtenberg, B. K. (1984). Spatial orientation in weightlessness and readaptation to earth's gravity. *Science* 225, 205–208. doi: 10.1126/science.6610215

23

Cognitive biases can affect moral intuitions about cognitive enhancement

Lucius Caviola[1]*, Adriano Mannino[2], Julian Savulescu[3,4] and Nadira Faulmüller[1,4,5]*

[1] Department of Experimental Psychology, University of Oxford, Oxford, UK
[2] Department of Philosophy, University of Bern, Bern, Switzerland
[3] Oxford Uehiro Centre for Practical Ethics, University of Oxford, Oxford, UK
[4] Oxford Centre for Neuroethics, University of Oxford, Oxford, UK
[5] Department Values, Technology and Innovation, Delft University of Technology, Delft, Netherlands

Edited by:
Mikhail Lebedev, Duke University, USA

Reviewed by:
Peter B. Reiner, University of British Columbia, Canada
Ioan Opris, Wake Forest University, USA
Nick J. Davis, Swansea University, UK

***Correspondence:**
Lucius Caviola and Nadira Faulmüller, Department of Experimental Psychology, University of Oxford, 9 South Parks Road, Oxford, OX1 3UD, UK
e-mail: lucius.caviola@psy.ox.ac.uk; nadira.faulmueller@psy.ox.ac.uk

Research into cognitive biases that impair human judgment has mostly been applied to the area of economic decision-making. Ethical decision-making has been comparatively neglected. Since ethical decisions often involve very high individual as well as collective stakes, analyzing how cognitive biases affect them can be expected to yield important results. In this theoretical article, we consider the ethical debate about cognitive enhancement (CE) and suggest a number of cognitive biases that are likely to affect moral intuitions and judgments about CE: status quo bias, loss aversion, risk aversion, omission bias, scope insensitivity, nature bias, and optimistic bias. We find that there are more well-documented biases that are likely to cause irrational aversion to CE than biases in the opposite direction. This suggests that common attitudes about CE are predominantly negatively biased. Within this new perspective, we hope that subsequent research will be able to elaborate this hypothesis and develop effective de-biasing techniques that can help increase the rationality of the public CE debate and thus improve our ethical decision-making.

Keywords: cognitive enhancement, rationality, cognitive bias, attitudes, de-biasing, moral intuitions, brain function augmentation

COGNITIVE ENHANCEMENT AND BIASED REASONING

The enhancement of cognitive brain functions by means of technology has become a reality. Recent research has demonstrated that various pharmaceuticals can have—at least modest—performance-enhancing effects in healthy individuals (for reviews, see Repantis et al., 2010; Husain and Mehta, 2011). In line with these findings, the off-label use of pharmacological substances like methylphenidate (e.g., Ritalin-®) or modafinil (e.g., Provigil-®) seems to be prevalent, in particular among students (Herman-Stahl et al., 2007; Smith and Farah, 2011; Dietz et al., 2013), and professionals in very responsible jobs like physicians (Franke et al., 2013). It has even been argued that the use of such substances might become an implicit requirement for individuals in certain professions (e.g., Maslen et al., in press). Non-pharmacological methods of cognitive enhancement (CE), such as gene therapy or neural implants, could become more widely used in the future (Bostrom and Sandberg, 2009). Even though there is considerable use of CE, recent research shows that the general public has strongly negative attitudes regarding the introduction and use of CE (for a review, see Schelle et al., 2014).

In this article, we argue that these concerns are partly driven by pervasive cognitive biases. A bias is a systematic deviation from a standard of rationality (Baron, 2005), an error frequently committed by the human mind. We use the definition of "rationality" common in cognitive science, referring to normative models of accurate belief formation (Foley, 1987; Audi, 2001) and optimal decision-making in order to achieve one's goal (Dawes, 1998). (Ir)rationality is therefore relative to the goal of having accurate beliefs or to goals in general. Thus, while some cognitive patterns may be suboptimal with regard to a particular goal, they may be perfectly optimal with regard to another. For illustration, consider "status quo bias", which we will address in the following section. If, upon reflection, an agent consciously and stably places some intrinsic value on the status quo, then in no sense can the agent be said to irrationally prefer the status quo (i.e., to make a cognitive mistake in doing so). However, the available evidence suggests that human agents do not, upon reflection, intrinsically care about the status quo, or at least to a significantly lesser degree than their immediate intuitions would have it: the experiments documenting our intuitive status quo preference (e.g., Samuelson and Zeckhauser, 1988) are interesting because they reveal a fact about our intuitive decision-making which our reflection disapproves of and is thus irrational. Also, nearly all action-guiding moral theories have an account of when the status quo should be modified, which is why the general bias towards it will tend to bring about suboptimal moral outcomes (c.f. Bostrom and Ord, 2006). Furthermore, if by "moral" decision-making we mean decision-making that is optimal from an "altruist" or "impartial" perspective, then non-related goals such as status quo preservation will lead to irrationality, too. Hence, it is justifiable to classify the status quo bias and the other biases we are discussing below as, indeed, biases.

The aim of this paper is to offer a new perspective on the debate about CE by identifying cognitive biases that affect our common intuitions and moral reactions. We will first give a rough overview of the academic debate and the public's view of CE and then discuss a number of potential biases that are likely to influence widespread judgments about CE.

In the academic debate about CE, opinions of critics (often bioconservatives) and supporters (often transhumanists) are quite sharply divided. Critics often question its medical safety, considering the potential side effects and unknown long-term health risks (Healey and Rayner, 2008). Critics also see CE as a threat to human autonomy (Habermas, 2003), authenticity (Elliott, 2004) humility and solidarity (Sandel, 2004) and equality and fairness (Fukuyama, 2004). Proponents, on the other hand, focus on the potential positive aspects and potentials of CE. For instance, Savulescu (2006) points out that the introduction of CE could help decrease unfair natural differences in abilities. Bostrom (2008) emphasizes the enormous positive leverage effect that CE could generate in the future. He speculates that a 1% increase in all scientists' cognitive performance "would amount to an indirect contribution equal to 100,000 times what the average scientist contributes" (p. 2). Others note that CE is not relevantly different from traditional forms of enhancement, such as information technology (Harris, 2010).

Recent research reviewing the general public's attitudes towards CE has shown that lay people share many of the critics' concerns about CE (Schelle et al., 2014). Participants from samples of students or parents, for example, fear that safety is not ensured (Forlini and Racine, 2012; Partridge et al., 2013). They think that CE could lead to peer pressure and thus undermine our autonomous decisions (Forlini and Racine, 2009). Also, they worry that unequal distribution of CE would result in an unfair advantage of a privileged few (Fitz et al., 2013). These views are often reflected in exaggerated reports by the media and might even lead to severe aversive social consequences for users (Faulmüller et al., 2013). The Guardian, for example, has described CE substances as "capitalism's wonder-pills", which "turn you into the closest human approximation there is to a machine" (Mahdawi, 2012).

We believe that the common concerns about CE are justified at least to some extent, and a greater scientific understanding of CE is required in order to draw confident conclusions (Maslen et al., 2014). Most importantly, long-term safety of CE is not currently ensured (c.f. Husain and Mehta, 2011) and is being called into question (e.g., Urban and Gao, 2014). Nevertheless, we speculate that the public's views on CE are negatively biased. While the involved biases do not necessarily undermine any specific argument for or against CE—these would need to be evaluated on their philosophical and scientific merits—they might partially explain the general opposition to CE as well as the selective focus on certain arguments and exaggeration of their relative weight. It is not unusual for human cognition to selectively search for certain classes of arguments and systematically neglect or undervalue certain others (c.f. Kunda, 1990 on "motivated reasoning")—a bias that might affect the judgments of both opponents and proponents of CE. Biases may lead people to come up with a set of arguments that expresses sound considerations but is significantly incomplete or weighted wrongly. We thus propose that in order to fully explain prevalent opposition to CE, it is necessary to look into the role biases play in the CE context. Awareness of these biases is a precondition of rational public debate about CE, which in turn is needed for developing and establishing optimal social and legal regulations.

Empirical research into biases over the last four decades has shown that human reasoning is very prone to systematic irrational patterns, i.e., cognitive biases (e.g., Tversky and Kahneman, 1974), especially when the subject matter is as complex, novel, abstract and ideologically loaded as is the use and regulation of CE (Cosmides and Tooby, 1992; Kahan et al., 2013). We argue that a number of cognitive biases well-documented in psychology and behavioral economics partly explain prevalent negative attitudes towards CE. While we believe that attitudes towards CE are predominantly negatively biased, there may also be biases leading us to irrationally favor CE. We will indicate some biases likely to affect judgments about CE and illustrate why and how they may be impairing our judgments in this context. Thus, our aim is to suggest several hypotheses about potential irrational sources of the prevalent (negative or positive) attitudes towards CE. Some of the biases on our below list have been studied in behavioral economics, such as status quo bias, loss aversion, risk aversion, scope insensitivity. The others—omission bias, nature bias, and optimistic bias—have been addressed more in psychology and philosophy. Our application of the knowledge about biases to the CE debate is comparatively novel, as is the application to ethical issues in general. We hope to offer a valuable perspective as a contribution to more rational public debate on controversial ethical issues involving new practices or technologies. Since ethical questions often involve high stakes, this endeavor can be expected to yield important results for public ethical debate.

POTENTIAL COGNITIVE BIASES

STATUS QUO BIAS

Status quo bias describes the tendency to prefer the current state of affairs over a change even if a change would result in better expected outcomes. For instance, Samuelson and Zeckhauser (1988) presented participants with hypothetical choice tasks about financial investment, which either were defined with a clear status quo or not. Participants were significantly more likely to choose the option designated as the status quo compared to the same option that was not labeled the status quo. Numerous further experiments reliably demonstrate this effect (e.g., Kahneman et al., 1991). It seems plausible that popular aversion to CE is partly due to status quo bias: it may partly result from the pure fact that CE constitutes a novelty. Historically, new ideas and technologies have often encountered strong aversion and opposition at first (Jay, 1981; Weil and Rosen, 1995), but became accepted at a later point in time. Coffee—a traditional form of CE—provides an instructive example: it was first considered an unacceptable drug and even forbidden in some countries (Weinberg and Bealer, 2001; Cowan, 2005). Bostrom and Ord (2006) have already drawn attention to the role status quo bias likely plays in the debate about CE. They also suggest a de-biasing tool—the *Reversal Test*—designed to expose and overcome status quo bias. If we believe that the enhancement of certain cognitive abilities will have negative consequences, we should consider the reverse: if an increase in intelligence is judged as negative, would a decrease in intelligence be judged favorable? If not, we are committed to claiming that our current level of intelligence is at an at least local optimum. This is, of course, possible but would require further justification. Obviously, it is an empirical question whether the introduction of CE actually results in net positive consequences or not. In case it would, however, status quo bias still exerts a psychological force against its endorsement. Empirical research can potentially expose the prevalence of status quo bias by, for example, observing whether people come to a different conclusion after reflecting on the rationale of the Reversal Test and applying it to the context of CE.

LOSS AVERSION

Loss aversion describes the tendency to weigh losses more than gains (Kahneman and Tversky, 1984). In monetary contexts, for example, loss aversion results in a stronger dissatisfaction after losing $1 than satisfaction after gaining $1 (Kahneman and Tversky, 1984). Whether something is perceived as a loss or as a gain depends on how the decisional situation is framed: one can either "get a $1 discount" or "avoid a $1 surcharge". Loss aversion can act on its own, but may also be a source of status quo bias (Bostrom and Ord, 2006). Maybe we recognize positive as well as negative consequences that the introduction of CE likely entails, such as the potential benefits due to enhanced intelligence on the one hand and the fear of increased unfairness in society due to unequal access to CE on the other hand (Fitz et al., 2013). But due to loss aversion, we likely tend to exaggerate the weight of the negative consequences relative to the positive ones.

RISK AVERSION

Risk aversion describes the tendency to undervalue an option that is less certain compared to a more certain option with equal expected outcome value (Kahneman and Tversky, 1984). Since preserving the status quo usually involves less uncertainty than a change does, risk aversion may be a further source of status quo bias, and it can act on its own as well. Consider a gamble where you have the option A of winning $1000 with a chance of 85% or the option B of winning $800 for sure. Most people prefer option B to A. However, option A has a higher expected value of 0.85 * $1000 = $850 and is therefore the rational decision if one values money linearly. As we are constantly faced with uncertainty, we are in fact dealing with such gambles all the time. We may be reluctant to introduce CE simply because its expected consequences involve probabilities that deviate more strongly from 100% and 0% than do the ones of the status quo. For example, methylphenidate almost certainly improves memory (for a meta-analysis, see Repantis et al., 2010), but there is a chance of long-term adverse effects (King et al., 2006). Though the expected utility calculation may favor the use of methylphenidate in certain cases, people are likely to retain a preference against it due to risk aversion and a resulting "precautionary principle" heuristic.

OMISSION BIAS

Omission bias describes the tendency to judge decisions differently depending on whether the same outcome is brought about through an act or an omission (Spranca et al., 1991). More specifically, people consider harms that have been caused by action worse than equal harms caused by omission. Ritov and Baron (1990) observed that parents often show reluctance to vaccinate their children. The expected harm of non-prevented disease is much greater than the expected harm of vaccination (Gangarosa et al., 1998), but parents seem to overvalue the expected harm caused by the vaccination because it is the result of their action. Similarly, we may fear that the introduction of CE is likely to or may cause harm. However, CE may also prevent harms from occurring and thus refraining from introducing may be a harmful omission, i.e., a missed opportunity for reducing harm. Due to our general omission bias, we are likely to systematically overvalue the harm of introducing CE compared to the harm resulting from not introducing it. For example, people might believe that the use of CE substances by medical doctors potentially causes active harm by inducing sleep disorders (Partridge et al., 2013)—but they might neglect or underestimate the potential positive consequences of doctors' increased ability to focus, i.e., the potential negative consequences of inaction. Rejecting CE may lead to greater harms suffered by more people overall. This question cannot be settled by unreflective intuition but requires open—un-biased—scientific investigation.

SCOPE INSENSITIVITY

Scope insensitivity occurs when people don't assign appropriate weight to the quantity of a decisional option (Kahneman, 2000; Desvousges et al., 2010). For example, a study has demonstrated that people are willing to pay the same amount of money to either help 9,000 people or 90,000 people who are at risk (Kahneman and Knetsch, 1992; Baron and Greene, 1996). This is irrational if one's goal is to help people and have everyone count the same, for the money one is willing to pay should then scale linearly with the number of people affected. It seems that our ability to intuitively represent such large numbers and their relations correctly is quite limited. In the context of CE, a probable implication is that we are not giving appropriate weight to the enormously high number of individual decisions, people (and generations) potentially affected by the consequences of introducing CE and thus to the importance and priority of the CE issue.

NATURE BIAS

Several studies on peoples' attitudes towards CE have revealed that natural CE substances are seen as less harmful and less ethically problematic than artificial ones (e.g., Bergström and Lynöe, 2008). For example, in a study with university students, participants were more likely to consider the use of artificial CE substances morally wrong than herbal ones (Scheske and Schnall, 2012). These judgments seem to be impaired by a form of nature bias (c.f. the fallacy of *appealing to nature*), i.e., a tendency to view the "natural" as good and the "unnatural" as bad. Given that many examples of "natural and bad" (e.g., diseases) as well as "unnatural and good" (e.g., medicine) things exist, it is highly questionable whether tracking the "natural" tracks what people (would) actually assign value to, and it is clear that it is not intrinsically morally relevant according to the "altruistically/impartially optimal decision-making" criterion.

OPTIMISTIC BIAS

Some biases may also be pushing people towards an overly optimistic evaluation of the consequences of introducing CE. An example is the optimistic bias described by Chapin and Coleman (2009), which causes people to underestimate the possibility of negative outcomes. Examples include people underestimating the risk of becoming a victim of crime, of losing money in the markets, or of getting lung cancer after smoking (Weinstein and Klein, 1996). In the context of CE, people might underestimate the dangers, such as negative side effects, that CE could entail.

An additional source of optimistically skewed views of CE might result from biased reduction of cognitive dissonance by people who are already using forms of CE. When confronted with falsificatory information about CE, such as documented health concerns, users might experience discomfort—cognitive dissonance—and be likely to selectively adopt beliefs that justify their behavior (Festinger, 1957).

Thus, there are potential biases leading to an overly positive attitude towards CE. Overall, however, it seems there are more well-documented highly prevalent biases likely to cause irrational aversion to CE than biases in the opposite direction.

CONCLUSION

We have aimed to offer and motivate the perspective that biases are likely to impair judgments about CE, mostly in the negative direction. We are aware that the above list of biases is incomplete and speculative and hope that empirical research will further elaborate on our suggestions. It must be emphasized that "biases" often do provide sensible decisional rules of thumb—after all, many of them seem to have proven to be successful heuristics for our evolutionary ancestors. However, the practical scope of this argument is very limited first because our current environment is different from our evolutionary environment, and second because the metaphorical goals of our genes that have been served by some "bias-heuristics" need not coincide with our goals (Stanovich, 2004). Nevertheless, the existence of such biases cannot alone undermine the soundness of any objection to CE. But they can explain why people, including policy makers, may take an unreflective or one-sided position on such debates. More generally, many of our moral intuitions about controversial practices are likely to be influenced by such cognitive biases. Not only do we require psychological interventions such as remedial heuristics, we require good ethical argument and relevant scientific evidence to identify which of our moral intuitions are justified, and which are not.

We believe the CE debate would benefit from research investigating the role cognitive biases play in judgments about CE and from the subsequent development of techniques that help people judge the relevant issues in a less biased way. These techniques should be simple heuristics (Larrick, 2004) that are easily applicable in the context of CE. Bostrom and Ord (2006) *Reversal Test* or Savulescu (2007) *Loss/Gain Heuristic* are examples of such heuristics. Psychological research could test whether people's attitudes towards CE change after applying de-biasing techniques, i.e., by being made aware of the biases potentially impairing their judgments. If they do change, we have reason to assume that cognitive biases play a role in the current attitudes towards CE.

ACKNOWLEDGMENTS

This work was supported by the Wellcome Trust (grant code 086041/Z/08/Z) and the Oxford Martin School (Oxford Martin Programme on Resource Stewardship), supporting Julian Savulescu and Nadira Faulmüller. This work was supervised by Nadira Faulmüller.

REFERENCES

Audi, R. (2001). *The Architecture of Reason: The Structure and Substance of Rationality.* New York, NY: Oxford University Press.

Baron, J. (2005). *Thinking and Deciding.* Cambridge, MA: Cambridge University Press.

Baron, J., and Greene, J. (1996). Determinants of insensitivity to quantity in valuation of public goods: contribution, warm glow, budget constraints, availability and prominence. *J. Exp. Psychol. Appl.* 2, 107–125. doi: 10.1037/1076-898x.2.2.107

Bergström, L. S., and Lynöe, N. (2008). Enhancing concentration, mood and memory in healthy individuals: an empirical study of attitudes among general practitioners and the general population. *Scand. J. Public Health* 36, 532–537. doi: 10.1177/1403494807087558

Bostrom, N. (2008). "Three ways to advance science," in *Nature Podcast.* Available online at: http://www.nickbostrom.com/views/science.pdf. Accessed on January 31, 2008.

Bostrom, N., and Ord, T. (2006). The reversal test: eliminating status quo bias in applied ethics. *Ethics* 116, 656–679. doi: 10.1086/505233

Bostrom, N., and Sandberg, A. (2009). Cognitive enhancement: methods, ethics, regulatory challenges. *Sci. Eng. Ethics* 15, 311–341. doi: 10.1007/s11948-009-9142-5

Chapin, J., and Coleman, G. (2009). Optimistic bias: what you think, what you know, or whom you know?. *N. Am. J. Psychol.* 11, 121–132. Available online at: http://www.questia.com/library/journal/1G1-195427665/optimistic-bias-what-you-think-what-you-know-or

Cosmides, L., and Tooby, J. (1992). "Cognitive adaptations for social exchange," in *The Adapted Mind: Evolutionary Psychology and the Generation of Culture*, eds J. Barkow, L. Cosmides and J. Tooby (New York, NY: Oxford University Press), 163–228.

Cowan, B. W. (2005). *The Social Life of Coffee: The Emergence of the British Coffee House.* New Haven, CT: Yale University Press.

Dawes, R. M. (1998). "Behavioral decision making and judgment," in *The Handbook of Social Psychology* (Vol. 1), eds D. T. Gilbert, S. T. Fiske and G. Lindzey 4th Edn. (Boston, MA: McGraw-Hill), 497–548.

Desvousges, W. H., Johnson, F. R., Dunford, R. W., Boyle, K. J., Hudson, S. P., Wilson, K. N., et al. (2010). *Measuring Nonuse Damages Using Contingent Valuation: An Experimental Evaluation of Accuracy.* 2nd Edn. Research Triangle Park, NC: RTI Press.

Dietz, P., Striegel, H., Franke, A. G., Lieb, K., Simon, P., and Ulrich, R. (2013). Randomized response estimates for the 12-month prevalence of cognitive-enhancing drug use in university students. *Pharmacotherapy* 33, 44–50. doi: 10.1002/phar.1166

Elliott, C. (2004). *Better Than Well: American Medicine Meets the American Dream.* New York: W. W. Norton and Company.

Faulmüller, N., Maslen, H., and Santoni de Sio, F. (2013). The indirect psychological costs of cognitive enhancement. *Am. J. Bioeth.* 13, 45–47. doi: 10.1080/15265161.2013.794880

Festinger, L. (1957). *A Theory of Cognitive Dissonance.* Stanford, CA: Stanford University Press.

Fitz, N. S., Nadler, R., Manogaran, P., Chong, E. W. J., and Reiner, P. B. (2013). Public attitudes toward cognitive enhancement. *Neuroethics* 7, 173–188. doi: 10.1007/s12152-013-9190-z

Foley, R. (1987). *The Theory of Epistemic Rationality.* Cambridge, MA: Harvard University Press.

Forlini, C., and Racine, E. (2009). Autonomy and coercion in academic "Cognitive Enhancement" using methylphenidate: perspectives of key stakeholders. *Neuroethics* 2, 163–177. doi: 10.1007/s12152-009-9043-y

Forlini, C., and Racine, E. (2012). Stakeholder perspectives and reactions to "academic" cognitive enhancement: unsuspected meaning of ambivalence and analogies. *Public Underst. Sci.* 21, 606–625. doi: 10.1177/0963662510385062

Franke, A. G., Bagusat, C., Dietz, P., Hoffmann, I., Simon, P., Ulrich, R., et al. (2013). Use of illicit and prescription drugs for cognitive or mood enhancement among surgeons. *BMC Med.* 11:102. doi: 10.1186/1741-7015-11-102

Fukuyama, F. (2004). Transhumanism. *Foreign Policy* 144, 42–43. doi: 10.2307/4152980

Gangarosa, E. J., Galazka, A. M., Wolfe, C. R., Phillips, L. M., Gangarosa, R. E., Miller, E., et al. (1998). Impact of anti-vaccine movements on pertussis control: the untold story. *Lancet* 351, 356–361. doi: 10.1016/s0140-6736(97)04334-1

Habermas, J. (2003). *The Future of Human Nature.* Cambridge, UK: Polity Press.

Harris, J. (2010). *Enhancing Evolution: The Ethical Case for Making Better People.* Princeton: Princeton University Press.

Healey, P., and Rayner, S. (2008). *Unnatural Selection: The Challenges of Engineering Tomorrow's People.* London: Earthscan.

Herman-Stahl, M. A., Krebs, C. P., Kroutil, L. A., and Heller, D. C. (2007). Risk and protective factors for methamphetamine use and nonmedical use of prescription stimulants among young adults aged 18 to 25. *Addict. Behav.* 32, 1003–1015. doi: 10.1016/j.addbeh.2006.07.010

Husain, M., and Mehta, M. A. (2011). Cognitive enhancement by drugs in health and disease. *Trends Cogn. Sci.* 15, 28–36. doi: 10.1016/j.tics.2010.11.002

Jay, T. B. (1981). Computerphobia: what to do about it. *Educ. Technol.* 21, 47–48.

Kahan, D. M., Peters, E., Dawson, E. C., and Slovic, P. (2013). "Motivated numeracy and enlightened self-government," in *Yale Law School Public Law Working Paper 307* (New Haven, CT).

Kahneman, D. (2000). "Evaluation by moments: past and future," in *Choices, Values and Frames*, eds D. Kahneman and A. Tversky (New York, NY: Cambridge University Press and Russell Sage Foundation), 693–708.

Kahneman, D., and Knetsch, J. L. (1992). Valuing public goods: the purchase of moral satisfaction. *J. Environ. Econ. Manage.* 22, 57–70. doi: 10.1016/0095-0696(92)90019-s

Kahneman, D., Knetsch, J. L., and Thaler, R. H. (1991). Anomalies: the endowment effect, loss aversion and status-quo bias. *J. Econ. Perspect.* 5, 193–206. doi: 10.1257/jep.5.1.193

Kahneman, D., and Tversky, A. (1984). Choices, values and frames. *Am. Psychol.* 39, 341–350. doi: 10.1037//0003-066x.39.4.341

King, S., Griffin, S., Hodges, Z., Weatherly, H., Asseburg, C., Richardson, G., et al. (2006). A systematic review and economic model of the effectiveness and cost-effectiveness of methylphenidate, dexamfetamine and atomoxetine for the treatment of attention deficit hyperactivity disorder in children and adolescents. *Health Technol. Assess.* 10, iii–iv, xiii–146. doi: 10.3310/hta10230

Kunda, Z. (1990). The case for motivated reasoning. *Psychol. Bull.* 108, 480–498. doi: 10.1037//0033-2909.108.3.480

Larrick, R. P. (2004). "Debiasing," in *Blackwell Handbook of Judgment and Decision Making*, eds J. Koehler and N. Harvey (Malden, MA: Blackwell), 316–337.

Mahdawi, A. (2012). "Speed and the city: meet the Adderall-addled adults of New York," in *The Guardian.* Available online at: http://www.theguardian.com/commentisfree/2012/oct/12/adderall-new-york-capitalism. Accessed on October 12, 2012.

Maslen, H., Faulmüller, N., and Savulescu, J. (2014). Pharmacological cognitive enhancement—how future neuroscientific research could advance ethical debate. *Front. Syst. Neurosci.* 8:107. doi: 10.3389/fnsys.2014.00107

Maslen, H., Santoni de Sio, F., and Faulmüller, N. (in press). "With cognitive enhancement comes great responsibility?," in *Responsible Innovation* (Vol. 2), eds B. J. Koops (Dordrecht: Springer).

Partridge, B., Bell, S., Lucke, J., and Hall, W. (2013). Australian university students' attitudes towards the use of prescription stimulants as cognitive enhancers: perceived patterns of use, efficacy and safety. *Drug Alcohol Rev.* 32, 295–302. doi: 10.1111/dar.12005

Repantis, D., Schlattmann, P., Laisney, O., and Heuser, I. (2010). Modafinil and methylphenidate for neuroenhancement in healthy individuals: a systematic review. *Pharmacol. Res.* 62, 187–206. doi: 10.1016/j.phrs.2010.04.002

Ritov, I., and Baron, J. (1990). Reluctance to vaccinate: omission bias and ambiguity. *J. Behav. Decis. Mak.* 3, 263–277. doi: 10.1002/bdm.3960030404

Samuelson, W., and Zeckhauser, R. (1988). Status quo bias in decision making. *J. Risk Uncertain.* 1, 7–59. doi: 10.1007/bf00055564

Sandel, M. J. (2004). The case against perfection: what's wrong with designer children, bionic athletes and genetic engineering. *Atl. Mon.* 292, 50–54, 56–60, 62.

Savulescu, J. (2006). "Justice, fairness and enhancement," in *Progress in Convergence: Technologies for Human Wellbeing*, eds W. S. Bainbridge and M. C. Roco (Danvers, MA: Wiley-Blackwell), 321–338.

Savulescu, J. (2007). "Genetic interventions and the ethics of enhancement of human beings," in *The Oxford Handbook of Bioethics*, ed B. Steinbock (Oxford: Oxford University Press), 516–535. doi: 10.1093/oxfordhb/9780199562411.003.0023

Schelle, K. J., Faulmüller, N., Caviola, L., and Hewstone, M. (2014). Attitudes toward pharmacological cognitive enhancement—a review. *Front. Syst. Neurosci.* 8:53. doi: 10.3389/fnsys.2014.00053

Scheske, C., and Schnall, S. (2012). The ethics of 'Smart Drugs': moral judgments about healthy people's use of cognitive-enhancing drugs. *Basic Appl. Soc. Psychol.* 34, 508–515. doi: 10.1080/01973533.2012.711692

Smith, M. E., and Farah, M. J. (2011). Are prescription stimulants "smart pills"? The epidemiology and cognitive neuroscience of prescription stimulant use by normal healthy individuals. *Psychol. Bull.* 137, 717–741. doi: 10.1037/a0023825

Spranca, M., Minsk, E., and Baron, J. (1991). Omission and commission in judgment and choice. *J. Exp. Soc. Psychol.* 27, 76–105. doi: 10.1016/0022-1031(91)90011-t

Stanovich, K. E. (2004). *The Robot's Rebellion. Finding Meaning in the Age of Darwin.* Chicago: Chicago University Press.

Tversky, A., and Kahneman, D. (1974). Judgment under uncertainty—heuristics and biases. *Science* 185, 1124–1131. doi: 10.1126/science.185.4157.1124

Urban, K. R., and Gao, W.-J. (2014). Performance enhancement at the cost of potential brain plasticity: neural ramifications of nootropic drugs in the healthy developing brain. *Front. Syst. Neurosci.* 8:38. doi: 10.3389/fnsys.2014.00038

Weil, M. M., and Rosen, L. D. (1995). The psychological impact of technology from a global perspective: a study of technological sophistication and technophobia in university students from twenty-three countries. *Comput. Hum. Behav.* 11, 95–133. doi: 10.1016/0747-5632(94)00026-e

Weinberg, B. A., and Bealer, B. K. (2001). *The World of Caffeine: The Science and Culture of the World's Most Popular Drug.* New York, NY: Routledge.

Weinstein, N. D., and Klein, W. M. (1996). Unrealistic optimism: present and future. *J. Soc. Clin. Psychol.* 15, 1–8. doi: 10.1521/jscp.1996.15.1.1

Permissions

All chapters in this book were first published in ABFFFC, by Frontiers; hereby published with permission under the Creative Commons Attribution License or equivalent. Every chapter published in this book has been scrutinized by our experts. Their significance has been extensively debated. The topics covered herein carry significant findings which will fuel the growth of the discipline. They may even be implemented as practical applications or may be referred to as a beginning point for another development.

The contributors of this book come from diverse backgrounds, making this book a truly international effort. This book will bring forth new frontiers with its revolutionizing research information and detailed analysis of the nascent developments around the world.

We would like to thank all the contributing authors for lending their expertise to make the book truly unique.

They have played a crucial role in the development of this book. Without their invaluable contributions this book wouldn't have been possible. They have made vital efforts to compile up to date information on the varied aspects of this subject to make this book a valuable addition to the collection of many professionals and students.

This book was conceptualized with the vision of imparting up-to-date information and advanced data in this field. To ensure the same, a matchless editorial board was set up. Every individual on the board went through rigorous rounds of assessment to prove their worth. After which they invested a large part of their time researching and compiling the most relevant data for our readers.

The editorial board has been involved in producing this book since its inception. They have spent rigorous hours researching and exploring the diverse topics which have resulted in the successful publishing of this book. They have passed on their knowledge of decades through this book. To expedite this challenging task, the publisher supported the team at every step. A small team of assistant editors was also appointed to further simplify the editing procedure and attain best results for the readers.

Apart from the editorial board, the designing team has also invested a significant amount of their time in understanding the subject and creating the most relevant covers. They scrutinized every image to scout for the most suitable representation of the subject and create an appropriate cover for the book.

The publishing team has been an ardent support to the editorial, designing and production team. Their endless efforts to recruit the best for this project, has resulted in the accomplishment of this book. They are a veteran in the field of academics and their pool of knowledge is as vast as their experience in printing. Their expertise and guidance has proved useful at every step. Their uncompromising quality standards have made this book an exceptional effort. Their encouragement from time to time has been an inspiration for everyone.

The publisher and the editorial board hope that this book will prove to be a valuable piece of knowledge for researchers, students, practitioners and scholars across the globe.

List of Contributors

Puiu F. Balan and Annelies Gerits
Laboratory for Neuro-and Psychophysiology, Katholieke Universiteit Leuven Medical School, Leuven, Belgium

Wim Vanduffel
Laboratory for Neuro-and Psychophysiology, Katholieke Universiteit Leuven Medical School, Leuven, Belgium
Athinoula A. Martinos Center for Biomedical Imaging, Massachusetts General Hospital, Charlestown, MA, USA
Department of Radiology, Harvard Medical School, Charlestown, MA, USA

David Zarka, Carlos Cevallos, Mathieu Petieau and Thomas Hoellinger
Laboratory of Neurophysiology and Movement Biomechanics, Université Libre de Bruxelles, Brussels, Belgium

Bernard Dan
Laboratory of Neurophysiology and Movement Biomechanics, Université Libre de Bruxelles, Brussels, Belgium
Department of Neurology, Hopital Universitaire des Enfants reine Fabiola, Université Libre de Bruxelles, Bruxelles, Belgium

Guy Cheron
Laboratory of Neurophysiology and Movement Biomechanics, Université Libre de Bruxelles, Brussels, Belgium
Laboratory of Electrophysiology, Université de Mons-Hainaut, Bruxelles, Belgium

Caroline Di Bernardi Luft, Michael J. Banissy and Joydeep Bhattacharya
Department of Psychology, Goldsmiths, University of London, London, UK

Ernesto Pereda
Lab. of Electrical Engineering and Bioengineering, Department of Industrial Engineering, Institute of Biomedical Technology, University of La Laguna, Tenerife, Spain
Elaine Astrand, Claire Wardak and Suliann Ben Hamed
CNRS, Cognitive Neuroscience Center, UMR 5229, University of Lyon 1, Bron Cedex, France

Felix Duecker, Tom A. de Graaf and Alexander T. Sack
Department of Cognitive Neuroscience, Faculty of Psychology and Neuroscience, Maastricht University, Maastricht, Netherlands
Maastricht Brain Imaging Center, Maastricht University, Maastricht, Netherlands

Irina A. Solopova and Victor A. Selionov
Laboratory of Neurobiology of Motor Control, Institute for Information Transmission Problems, Russian Academy of Science, Moscow, Russia

Francesca Sylos-Labini
Laboratory of Neuromotor Physiology, IRCCS Fondazione Santa Lucia, Rome, Italy
Centre of Space Bio-medicine, University of Rome Tor Vergata, Rome, Italy

Victor S. Gurfinkel
Biomedical Engineering Department, Oregon Health and Science University, Portland, OR, USA

Francesco Lacquaniti
Laboratory of Neuromotor Physiology, IRCCS Fondazione Santa Lucia, Rome, Italy
Centre of Space Bio-medicine, University of Rome Tor Vergata, Rome, Italy
Department of Systems Medicine, University of Rome Tor Vergata, Rome, Italy

Yuri P. Ivanenko
Laboratory of Neuromotor Physiology, IRCCS Fondazione Santa Lucia, Rome, Italy

Jenni Deveau and Aaron R. Seitz
Department of Psychology, University of California, Riverside, Riverside, CA, USA

Susanne M. Jaeggi
School of Education, University of California, Irvine, Irvine, CA, USA
Department of Cognitive Sciences, University of California, Irvine, Irvine, CA, USA

Victor Zordan and Calvin Phung
Department of Computer Science, University of California, Riverside, Riverside, CA, USA

Giovanni Di Pino
Institute of Neurology and Fondazione Alberto Sordi - Research Institute for Ageing, Campus Bio Medico University of Rome, Rome, Italy
Laboratory of Biomedical Robotics and Biomicrosystems CIR - Centre for Integrated Research, Campus Bio Medico University of Rome, Rome, Italy

Angelo Maravita
Department of Psycology, Università di Milano-Bicocca, Milano, Italy

Loredana Zollo and Eugenio Guglielmelli
Laboratory of Biomedical Robotics and Biomicrosystems CIR - Centre for Integrated Research, Campus Bio Medico University of Rome, Rome, Italy

Vincenzo Di Lazzaro
Institute of Neurology and Fondazione Alberto Sordi - Research Institute for Ageing, Campus Bio Medico University of Rome, Rome, Italy

Sandra B. Chapman
Center for BrainHealth®, The University of Texas at Dallas, Dallas, TX, USA

Raksha A. Mudar
Department of Speech and Hearing Science, University of Illinois at Urbana-Champaign, Champaign, IL, USA

Arthur Saniotis and Maciej Henneberg
Biological Anthropology and Comparative Anatomy Unit, School of Medical Sciences, The University of Adelaide, Adelaide, SA, Australia
Centre for Evolutionary Medicine, University of Zürich, Zürich, Switzerland

Jaliya Kumaratilake and James P. Grantham
Biological Anthropology and Comparative Anatomy Unit, School of Medical Sciences, The University of Adelaide, Adelaide, SA, Australia

Kimberly J. Schelle
Radboud Honours Academy, Radboud University, Nijmegen, Netherlands
Department of Industrial Design, Eindhoven University of Technology, Eindhoven, Netherlands

Bas M. J. Olthof
Radboud Honours Academy, Radboud University, Nijmegen, Netherlands
Faculty of Medical Sciences, Institute of Neuroscience, Newcastle University, Newcastle upon Tyne, UK

Wesley Reintjes
Radboud Honours Academy, Radboud University, Nijmegen, Netherlands
Department of Neurology, Isala Clinics, Zwolle, Netherlands

Carsten Bundt
Radboud Honours Academy, Radboud University, Nijmegen, Netherlands
Department of Experimental Psychology, Ghent University, Ghent, Belgium

Joyce Gusman-Vermeer
Radboud Honours Academy, Radboud University, Nijmegen, Netherlands

Anke C. C. M. vanMil
Radboud Honours Academy, Radboud University, Nijmegen, Netherlands
Department of Physiology, Radboud Institute for Health Sciences, Radboud University Medical Center, Nijmegen, Netherlands

Hui-Xin Qi*, Jon H. Kaas and Jamie L. Reed
Department of Psychology, Vanderbilt University, Nashville, TN, USA

Valentina Pieramico, Stefano Cesinaro and Valerio Frazzini
Molecular Neurology Unit, Center of Excellence on Aging, University "G. d'Annunzio", Chieti-Pescara, Chieti, Italy

Roberto Esposito
Department of Neuroscience, Imaging and Clinical Sciences, University "G. d'Annunzio", Chieti-Pescara, Chieti, Italy

Stefano L. Sensi
Molecular Neurology Unit, Center of Excellence on Aging, University "G. d'Annunzio", Chieti-Pescara, Chieti, Italy
Department of Neuroscience, Imaging and Clinical Sciences, University "G. d'Annunzio", Chieti-Pescara, Chieti, Italy
Departments of Neurology and Pharmacology, Institute for Memory Impairments and Neurological Disorders, University of California-Irvine, Irvine, CA, USA

Alexander V. Lebedev and Françoise J. Siepel
Department of Psychiatry, Centre for Age-Related Medicine, Stavanger University Hospital, Stavanger, Norway

Eric Westman, Aleksandra Lebedeva and Joana B. Pereira
Department of Neurobiology, Care Sciences and Society, Karolinska Institutet, Stockholm, Sweden

Andrew Simmons
Department of Neuroimaging, Institute of Psychiatry, King's College London, London, UK
NIHR Biomedical Research Centre for Mental Health and Biomedical Research Unit for Dementia, London, UK

Dag Aarsland
Department of Psychiatry, Centre for Age-Related Medicine, Stavanger University Hospital, Stavanger, Norway
Department of Neurobiology, Care Sciences and Society, Karolinska Institutet, Stockholm, Sweden

Christoph Kapeller and Robert Prueckl
Guger Technologies OG, Graz, Austria g.tec medical engineering GmbH, Schiedlberg, Austria
Department of Computational Perception, Johannes Kepler University, Linz, Austria

Kyousuke Kamada and Hiroshi Ogawa
Department of Neurosurgery, Asahikawa Medical University, Asahikawa, Japan

Josef Scharinger
Department of Computational Perception, Johannes Kepler University, Linz, Austria

Christoph Guger
Guger Technologies OG, Graz, Austria
g.tec medical engineering GmbH, Schiedlberg, Austria

Naoki Tajiri, Kelsey Duncan, Alesia Antoine, Mibel Pabon, Sandra A. Acosta, Ike de la Pena, Diana G. Hernadez-Ontiveros, Kazutaka Shinozuka, Hiroto Ishikawa, Yuji Kaneko and Cesar V. Borlongan
Center of Excellence for Aging and Brain Repair, Department of Neurosurgery and Brain Repair, Morsani College of Medicine, University of South Florida, Tampa, FL, USA

Ernest Yankee, Michael McGrogan and Casey Case
Sanbio Inc., Mountain View, CA, USA

Eric J. Blumberg, Matthew S. Peterson and Raja Parasuraman
Arch Lab, Department of Psychology, George Mason University, Fairfax, VA, USA

Marieke E. Thurlings
Information and Computing Sciences, Utrecht University, Utrecht, Netherlands
Perceptual and Cognitive Systems, TNO, Soesterberg, Netherlands

Anne-Marie Brouwer and Jan B. F. Van Erp
Perceptual and Cognitive Systems, TNO, Soesterberg, Netherlands

Peter Werkhoven
Information and Computing Sciences, Utrecht University, Utrecht, Netherlands

Anna-Katharine Brem
Berenson-Allen Center for Noninvasive Brain Stimulation, Division of Cognitive Neurology, Department of Neurology, Beth Israel Deaconess Medical Center, Harvard Medical School, Boston, MA, USA

Evelyn Unterburger
Department of Neuropsychology, University Hospital Zurich, Zurich, Switzerland

Irving Speight
Department of Neuropsychology, Zürcher Höhenklinik Wald ZHW, Rehabilitation Center, Faltigberg-Wald, Switzerland

Lutz Jäncke
Division Neuropsychology, Institute of Psychology, University of Zurich, Zurich, Switzerland
Center for Integrative Human Physiology, University of Zurich, Zurich, Switzerland
International Normal Aging and Plasticity Imaging Center, University of Zurich, Zurich, Switzerland
University Research Priority Program "Dynamic of Healthy Aging," University of Zurich, Zurich, Switzerland
Department of Special Education, King Abdulaziz University, Jeddah, Saudi Arabia

Giovanni Mirabella
Istituto Neurologico Mediterraneo, IRCCS Neuromed, Pozzilli, Italy
Department of Physiology and Pharmacology 'V. Erspamer,' La Sapienza University, Rome, Italy

Andrew Koivuniemi
Indiana University School of Medicine, Indianapolis, IN, USA

Kevin Otto
eldon School of Biomedical Engineering, Purdue University, West Lafayette, IN, USA
J. Crayton Pruitt Family Department of Biomedical Engineering, University of Florida, Gainesville, FL, USA

W. Geoffrey Wright
Physical Therapy and Bioengineering, Motion Analysis and Perception Laboratory, Temple University, Philadelphia, PA, USA

Lucius Caviola
Department of Experimental Psychology, University of Oxford, Oxford, UK

Adriano Mannino
Department of Philosophy, University of Bern, Bern, Switzerland

Julian Savulescu
Oxford Uehiro Centre for Practical Ethics, University of Oxford, Oxford, UK
Oxford Centre for Neuroethics, University of Oxford, Oxford, UK

Nadira Faulmüller
Department of Experimental Psychology, University of Oxford, Oxford, UK
Oxford Centre for Neuroethics, University of Oxford, Oxford, UK
Department Values, Technology and Innovation, Delft University of Technology, Delft, Netherlands

Index

www.ingramcontent.com/pod-product-compliance
Lightning Source LLC
LaVergne TN
LVHW080927210926
848485LV00004B/745